Improving Human Health through the Healing Power of Medicinal Mushrooms

Scott A. Johnson

Improving human health through the healing power of medicinal mushrooms / Scott A. Johnson

Cover design: Scott A. Johnson
Cover Copyright: © 2023, by Scott A. Johnson

ISBN-13: 979-8988720621

Discover more books by Scott A. Johnson at authorscott.com
Published by Scott A. Johnson Professional Writing Services, LLC: Orem, UT

Dedication

To my family for their continued support and love; and to The Creator for providing an array of natural solutions to improve human health. Thank you to you, the reader, for supporting me in my efforts to help others feel better with the simple, yet powerful, natural solutions offered in my books.

Contents

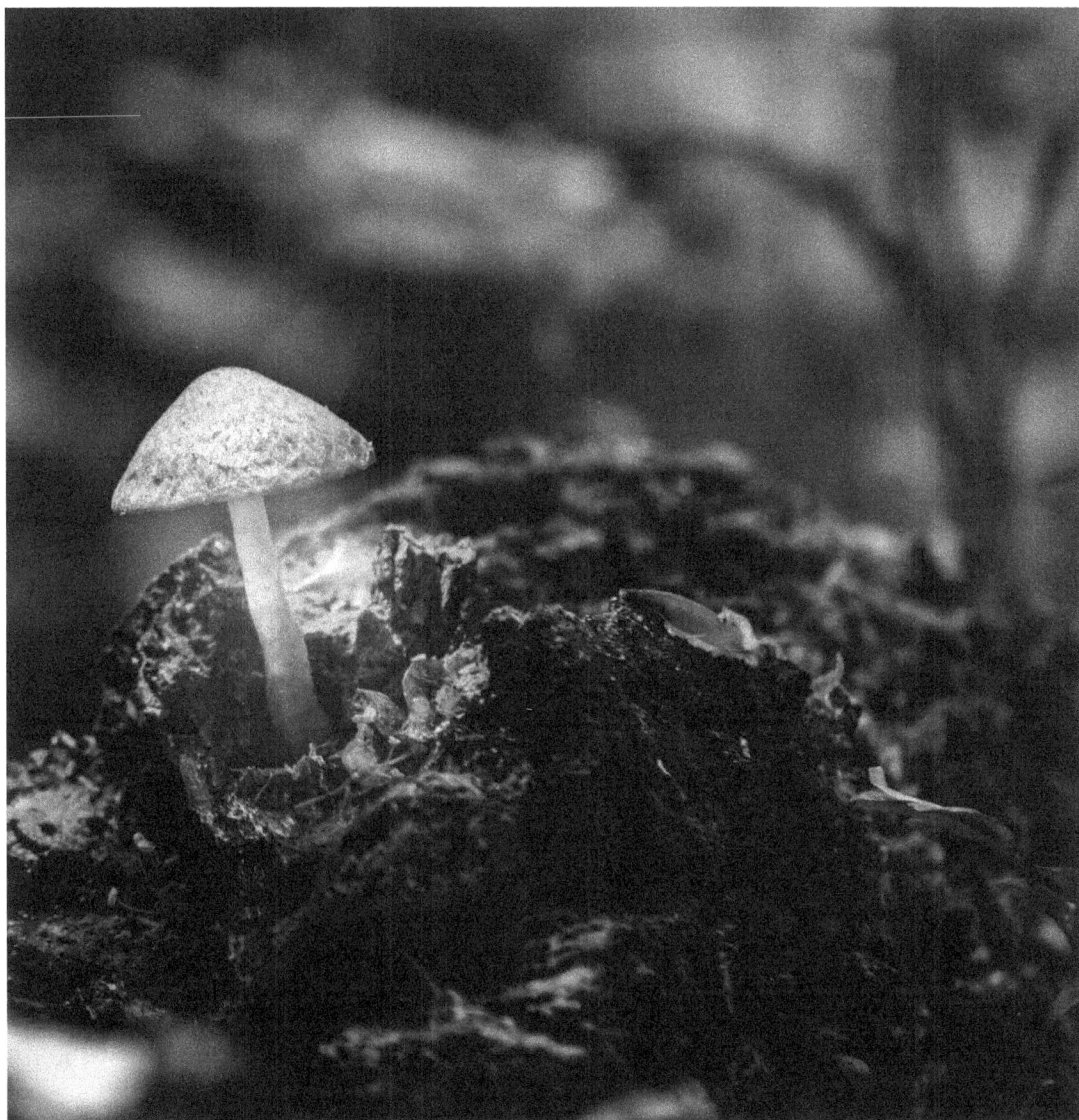

In the vast tapestry of nature's pharmacy, there exists a group of remarkable organisms that have quietly played a pivotal role in human health and wellness for millennia— medicinal mushrooms. Science has taken us to the point that we fully understand that human health is remarkably tied to and affected by microbial exposure. Both beneficial and harmful microbes come in contact with us every single day, which can shift our health in a positive or negative direction. The key for health and homeostasis is to increase your exposure to healthy microbes, including medicinal mushrooms, and keep your immune system functioning in an optimum way to handle the harmful microbes you are exposed to.

Relied upon for their health-giving benefits for centuries, medicinal mushrooms are powerful fungi loaded with antioxidants, phytonutrients, and novel compounds that provide myriad benefits. While over two thousand species of edible mushrooms are currently known, medicinal mushrooms are those that uniquely contain phytocompounds that promote human health. Many of these mushrooms were identified by ancient cultures through trial and error before science could reveal the phytocompounds that provide mushrooms with their therapeutic properties. Fortunately, this ancient art of using mushrooms to maintain and restore human health is merging with science to help us better use these fungi to achieve maximum results. Medicinal mushrooms have recently experienced a renaissance in the health-and-wellness scene, with researchers, clinicians, and the general public seeking to reveal the wisdom of how the ancients used them to treat and prevent diseases and enhance overall well-being.

Mushrooms, a diverse group of organisms belonging to the fungal kingdom, come in a multitude of shapes, sizes, and colors. While many are known for their culinary uses, such as the beloved button mushroom (*Agaricus bisporus*), others, like reishi and cordyceps, have garnered attention for their remarkable medicinal properties. These fungi are collectively referred to as medicinal mushrooms, functional mushrooms, or adaptogenic—improve your ability to respond to stress, anxiety, and fatigue, and improve overall well-being—mushrooms, and they have a long history of traditional use for health and wellness.

Mycology is the study of fungi, which includes mushrooms. These often overlooked and underappreciated functional organisms play crucial roles in ecosystems, agriculture, medicine, and industry. The history of mycology is intertwined with the broader history of biology and natural sciences. Fungi have been part of human existence since ancient times, but systematic study and classification only began to take shape in the seventeenth and eighteenth centuries when scientific instruments capable of looking into their composition became available.

Early humans had practical knowledge of fungi, using some for food and others as medicine. They discovered the medicinal value of mushrooms through painstaking trial and error, relying wholly on experience and intuition to guide their selection and use. Cave paintings dating back thousands of years depict mushrooms, suggesting their cultural significance throughout the centuries. The Greek physician Hippocrates used amadou mushroom (*Fomes fomentarius*) as a potent anti-inflammatory agent. Tao Hongjing, an alchemist from the fifth century, described the use of several mushrooms for medicine. Even the famous Ice Man, who lived nearly 5,300 years ago, was found carrying amadou and a birch polypore mushroom in his pouch, suggesting the importance of these remedies for his survival in the Alps of northern Italy. The lag for modern medicine to catch up to these ancient healers in their use of medicinal mushrooms is now rapidly changing as mushrooms are being embraced as part of contemporary medical systems.

The seventeenth-century Flemish botanist Carolus Clusius is often credited with initiating the systematic study of fungi. However, it was not until the eighteenth century that the Swedish mycologist Elias Magnus Fries laid the foundation for modern mycology by introducing a standardized system of fungal taxonomy. Pioneers like Pier Antonio Micheli, Carl Linnaeus, and Lewis David von Schweinitz made significant contributions to the understanding and classification of fungi in the eighteenth and nineteenth centuries. The development of microscopy, molecular biology, and DNA sequencing in the twentieth century revolutionized mycology, allowing for a deeper understanding of fungal diversity and relationships.

Fungi play diverse and vital roles in nature, agriculture, medicine, industry, and more. Their significance extends far beyond the commonly known roles of mushrooms as food. Fungi are integral to the functioning of ecosystems, influencing nutrient cycling, decomposition, and the health of plants and animals. Fungi are essential decomposers, breaking down dead organic matter and recycling nutrients, which releases them back into ecosystems. Without them, the planet would be buried in organic waste. Mycorrhizal fungi form mutualistic relationships with the roots of most plants, aiding in nutrient absorption, particularly phosphorus and nitrogen. Saprophytic fungi feed on dead or decaying organic matter, helping to recycle nutrients and contributing to the decomposition of leaf litter and wood. Lichens are complex organisms consisting of fungi and photosynthetic partners (algae or cyanobacteria). They are important pioneers in colonizing harsh environments. In this way, fungi have symbiotic relationships with plants, and this symbiosis extends to humans.

Fungi have yielded invaluable medicines, including antibiotics like penicillin (*Penicillium*), immunosuppressants, and cholesterol-lowering drugs. Moreover, fungi have become sources of potential treatments for various diseases, including diseases that plague modern humans like cancer. We are just beginning to unravel and understand the potential of these unassuming organisms to improve human health, but their growing acceptance is exciting.

The classification of fungi is a complex endeavor, given their incredible diversity. In the case of mushrooms, mycologists are constantly changing things, making classification an ever-evolving science. Fungi are not plants but belong to their own kingdom, distinct from animals and plants. They can be classified into several major groups:

Zygomycota: These fungi are characterized by their ability to produce zygospores resistant to some antifungals during sexual reproduction. They include bread molds and some plant pathogens.

Ascomycota: Also known as sac fungi, this group includes many edible fungi (like morel and truffle) and plant pathogens. Ascomycota produce sexual spores in saclike structures called asci.

Basidiomycota: Basidiomycetes are famous for their club-shaped reproductive structures called basidia. This group includes mushrooms, toadstools, and shelf fungi.

Glomeromycota: These fungi form mycorrhizal associations with plants and are essential for nutrient exchange in ecosystems.

Chytridiomycota: Chytrids are unique among fungi as they have flagellated spores and are often found in aquatic environments. Some chytrids are responsible for amphibian declines.

Microsporidia: These are intracellular parasites, mostly affecting insects but also capable of infecting humans and other animals.

Cryptomycota: Recently discovered, these fungi are relatively unknown but could play significant roles in aquatic ecosystems.

Fungi also have profound effects on human life, both directly and indirectly, in various aspects. First, they are an important food source used in dishes around the world. Edible mushrooms like the common button mushroom (*Agaricus bisporus*) and oyster mushroom (*Pleurotus ostreatus*) are widely consumed. Fungi also play an important role in brewing, winemaking, baking, and the production of fermented foods and beverages. As mentioned previously, important medicines have been derived from fungi, including penicillin. Certain fungi break down and detoxify pollutants and harmful chemicals, making them useful in bioremediation efforts, and affording humans protection from their harmful effects. Fungi are used in biotechnological processes to produce enzymes, biofuels, and other valuable products. Some fungi, like *Psilocybe* mushrooms, contain psychoactive compounds and have cultural and spiritual significance. These fungi are also being studied for potential therapeutic use, particularly among those conditions that are very difficult to treat with chemical medicines (e.g., PTSD and other mental health conditions).

Despite the wealth of knowledge about fungi, many aspects of mycology remain unexplored. Fungal taxonomy is continually evolving because of advances in genetic techniques. The classification of fungi is complex, and many fungal species are yet to be discovered and described. Some fungi are threatened by habitat loss and overharvesting. Conservation efforts are needed to protect rare and ecologically important species, and hopefully, their cultivation will increase as demand from consumers grows. The exploration of the bioactive compounds found in mushrooms is rapidly advancing, but we still have much to learn about how to use them for specific health conditions and to discover which constituents are most important for specific conditions.

Mushrooms are part of the fungal kingdom, with most belonging to the phylum Basidiomycota. Another significant phylum is Ascomycota, which includes important fungi like yeast and truffles. These two phyla constitute the subkingdom Dikarya, which is often referred to as the higher fungi within the fungal kingdom.

The phylum Basidiomycota is home to a wide range of mushrooms, and it is characterized by the presence of basidia—club-shaped structures that produce sexual spores. This phylum is divided into numerous classes, orders, families, and genera based on various features, including the structure of the basidiomata (the fruiting body, which is the part of the mushroom we commonly recognize), the arrangement of spores, and the presence of specific microscopic structures.

Agaricomycetes is the largest class within the Basidiomycota phylum, encompassing most of the familiar mushroom-forming fungi. It includes a diverse range of mushroom species, from the common button mushroom to the iconic shiitake mushroom (*Lentinula edodes*). This class is further divided into orders, families, and genera based on shared characteristics and evolutionary relationships.

Within the class Agaricomycetes, there are various orders and families that further narrow down the classification of mushrooms. For example:

Order Agaricales: This order includes many familiar gilled mushrooms, such as the genus Agaricus. It also encompasses the Amanita genus, which includes both edible and toxic species.

Family Tricholomataceae: This family includes mushrooms like the commercially cultivated shiitake mushroom and the inedible but striking fly agaric (*Amanita muscaria*).

These are just a few examples, and there are numerous other orders, families, and genera within the class Agaricomycetes, each representing a diverse range of mushroom species.

The genus and species names are the most specific levels of classification for mushrooms. Each genus groups together species that share significant similarities in terms of morphology, genetics, and other characteristics. The species name is unique to a particular organism and is often associated with a specific ecological niche, geographical location, or distinguishing feature.

For example, the common button mushroom belongs to the genus Agaricus, and its species name is bisporus. Therefore, its scientific name is *Agaricus bisporus*. This naming system, known as binomial nomenclature, allows scientists to precisely identify and communicate information about individual mushroom species, rather than creating confusion by relying upon commonly used local names.

Mycology is a dynamic and interdisciplinary field that continues to unveil the secrets of the fungal kingdom. Fungi, with their diverse roles in ecosystems, their impact on human life, and their potential in medicine and industry, offer a vast and fascinating realm for exploration and discovery. As our understanding of fungi deepens, we can harness their potential for the betterment of both the natural world and human health, unlocking new frontiers in science and medicine.

Mushrooms, with their diverse shapes, sizes, and colors, are the fruiting bodies of fungi. While they may seem simple at first glance, a closer examination reveals a complex anatomy. Understanding the anatomy of mushrooms is not only essential for identifying and appreciating these organisms but also for recognizing their ecological, medicinal, and culinary significance. The key components of mushroom anatomy include:

Cap (Pileus): The cap is the uppermost part of the mushroom and is often the most conspicuous. It varies widely in size, shape, and color among different mushroom species. The cap's surface can be smooth, wrinkled, scaly, or covered in a layer of protective tissue called the cuticle. Beneath the cap, the gills or pores (depending on the type of mushroom) are attached. Together, the cap and stalk are called the fruiting body, and these contain large amounts of polysaccharides, such as beta-glucans. They also contain antioxidants, phenolic compounds, minerals, and vitamins.

Gills and Pores: Gills are thin, blade-like structures found under the cap of many mushroom species. They radiate outward from the stalk and are responsible for producing and holding the mushroom's spores. The arrangement, color, and attachment of gills can vary significantly between mushroom species and are important features for identification. Pores, on the other hand, are found in mushrooms like boletes. Instead of gills, these mushrooms have a sponge-like underside covered in small pores. Spores are produced within these pores and are released when they mature.

Stalk (Stipe): The stalk is the stem or "leg" of the mushroom. It connects the cap to the substrate (the surface on which the mushroom is growing). The stalk provides support and elevates the cap above the ground, allowing for better spore dispersal. The size, shape, color, and texture of the stalk vary among mushroom species.

Ring (Annulus) and Veil: Not all mushrooms have a ring, but it's a distinctive feature when present. The ring is a collar-like or skirtlike structure encircling the upper part of the stalk, just below the cap. It is the remnant of the partial veil, a protective membrane that covers and protects the developing gills or pores. As the mushroom matures, the veil often ruptures or falls away, leaving the ring behind.

Spore Print: The color of a mushroom's spore print is a crucial diagnostic feature. To create a spore print, a mature mushroom is placed, gills or pores down, on a piece of paper or glass. As the mushroom releases its spores, they collect on the surface below, forming a pattern that can vary in color, such as white, brown, pink, or black, depending on the mushroom species. Spores can contain ergosterol, proteins, and enzymes useful for therapeutic use.

Mycelium: The mycelium is the vegetative part of the fungus. It consists of a network of fine, thread-like structures called hyphae. Mycelium is typically hidden underground or within the substrate, where it grows and absorbs nutrients. The mycelium is responsible for the mushroom's growth, and it can persist for years, even decades, depending on the species. The mycelium of mushrooms can contain unique polysaccharides—frequently different from those found in the fruiting bodies—and other bioactive metabolites like organic acids and enzymes.

Rhizomorphs: Some mushrooms, like oak root fungus (*Armillaria mellea*), form specialized structures called rhizomorphs. These are dense, cord-like bundles of mycelium that allow the fungus to spread and explore new areas efficiently. Rhizomorphs play a crucial role in the fungal life cycle, particularly in the case of wood-decaying fungi.

Hyphal Knots: Hyphal knots are clusters of mycelial hyphae that give rise to the primordia (the initial fruiting body, or the first recognizable undifferentiated mass of the hyphae that develops into the mushroom fruit body), which eventually develop into mature mushrooms. They are often the first visible sign of mushroom formation and appear as small, round structures on the substrate surface.

Volva: In some mushroom species, you may find a volva, a cuplike or sack-like structure that surrounds the base of the stalk. It is the remnant of the universal veil, a membrane that initially enveloped the entire mushroom. The presence and characteristics of the volva are important for identification in certain mushroom families.

MUSHROOM ANATOMY

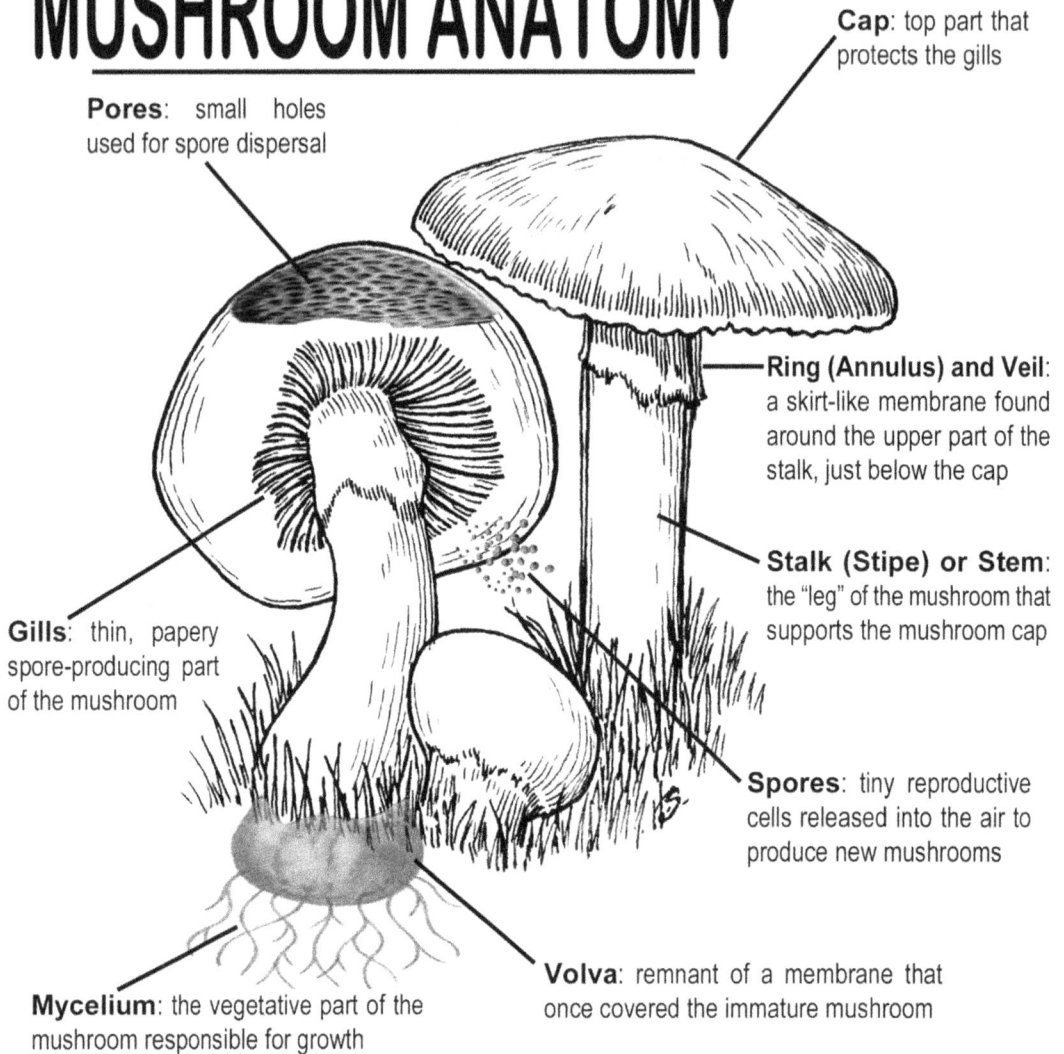

Cap: top part that protects the gills

Pores: small holes used for spore dispersal

Ring (Annulus) and Veil: a skirt-like membrane found around the upper part of the stalk, just below the cap

Stalk (Stipe) or Stem: the "leg" of the mushroom that supports the mushroom cap

Gills: thin, papery spore-producing part of the mushroom

Spores: tiny reproductive cells released into the air to produce new mushrooms

Mycelium: the vegetative part of the mushroom responsible for growth

Volva: remnant of a membrane that once covered the immature mushroom

The concentration of bioactive compounds within a mushroom varies according to its maturity and growth cycle. Some mushrooms, like common button mushrooms, contain higher levels of ergosterol and vitamin D2 when they are immature. The levels of phenolic compounds vary greatly according to maturity as well. This is why it is so important to evaluate the chemistry and presence of bioactive compounds in mushrooms at varying stages to determine the best time to harvest them to maximize their medicinal and therapeutic value.

Understanding mushroom anatomy is crucial for identifying different species, especially for foragers and mycologists who want to distinguish between edible and toxic mushrooms or find those with high medicinal value. Additionally, mushroom anatomy sheds light on the ecological roles and life cycles of these important organisms, highlighting their significance in ecosystems and their contribution to human culture and cuisine.

Mushrooms are unassuming fungi, often overlooked in the grand scheme of botanical diversity, that have garnered the attention of scientists, healers, and health enthusiasts around the world. With a rich history deeply rooted in traditional medicine systems, these mushrooms are now emerging as a promising frontier in modern medicine, offering a vast array of potential therapeutic benefits. As scientific research continues to unveil the myriad of compounds and properties within medicinal mushrooms, we find ourselves on the cusp of a new era in health care—one where fungi take a prominent role.

As this resurgence of interest in medicinal mushrooms grows, science is beginning to reveal what the ancients knew through experience, that mushrooms have many biological properties that can benefit humans. Improved cognition, enhanced immunity, better sleep, reduced inflammation, and even anticancer activity are just a few of the benefits revealed so far. As our understanding of the intricate relationship between medicinal mushrooms and human health deepens, modern scientific research is shedding light on the mechanisms behind their therapeutic effects. Based on their known therapeutic activities, clinicians and researchers are now exploring how fungi may play a role in managing conditions such as cancer, diabetes, cardiovascular disease, mental health disorders, autoimmune conditions, and neurodegenerative disorders.

The use of mushrooms for medicinal purposes traces back thousands of years, with evidence from various cultures highlighting their importance. In ancient China, mushrooms like reishi were considered symbols of longevity and vitality, and they were reserved for emperors and nobility. Similarly, indigenous peoples of North America have a rich tradition of using mushrooms like turkey tail for their healing properties. The diverse array of traditional uses reflects the versatility of medicinal mushrooms in addressing a wide range of health concerns.

This concise introduction to medicinal mushrooms endeavors to unravel the world of mycology, exploring the scientific discoveries and potential therapeutic applications that make these fungi a compelling scientific subject and a beacon of hope for many seeking natural and holistic health solutions. Mycological research has led to the development of well-known drugs such as penicillin, tetracycline, streptomycin, and statins. While these discoveries isolated a single component from a fungus to create a chemical medicine, those seeking natural solutions often prefer to enjoy the whole, natural, complex substance with its built-in polypharmacology of dozens of compounds, or at least a complex extract that concentrates the key bioactive compounds. This plethora of bioactive and useful constituents creates a synergistic (significantly amplifies the activity of compounds), antagonistic (buffers the harmful effects of potent compounds), and additive (enhances the activity of compounds) effects within a single fungus.

The therapeutic potential of medicinal mushrooms can be attributed to the presence of various bioactive compounds. These include polysaccharides, beta-glucans, triterpenoids, and secondary metabolites like ergosterol and hericenones, among others. These compounds interact with the human body in intricate ways, influencing various physiological processes and contributing to the mushrooms' medicinal properties.

Medicinal mushrooms can be taken in their natural state but are more commonly consumed as a powder or extract. Adaptogens, like medicinal mushrooms, initiate measured biological adjustments that can take a few weeks to observe and experience. You shouldn't expect immediate results—with the exception of *Psilocybe* mushroom extracts. Rather, patiently await their powerful and lasting effects. In essence, mushrooms are adjusting the function of key biological systems within the human body to allow it to do what it does when roadblocks are removed—maintain a state of balance and homeostasis. The human body is the real hero and healer, while the mushrooms simply act as the means that permits the body to perform the biological processes necessary for us to be healthy.

Each variety of medicinal mushroom offers a distinctive set of benefits. The benefits of the top twenty types of medicinal mushrooms will be explored in this book. This includes preclinical research (laboratory, animal, or computer-based simulations), clinical research (in humans), their potential adverse effects, cautions and contraindications, and, of course, how to use them and in what dosage. Preclinical research helps us understand their mechanisms of action and how they interact with the human body, and reveals their therapeutic potential. The clinical research confirms the preclinical findings and helps determine how to use them and at what dose you are most likely to realize the desired benefits.

In the amazingly vast world of natural remedies, medicinal mushrooms stand as a testament to the wisdom of ancient traditions and the potential of uniting this wisdom with modern science. Their rich history, diverse array of species, and myriad bioactive compounds make them an exciting discipline within natural medicine. Indeed, there is so much potential among these functional fungi that Paul Stamets, a mycologist and author of multiple books on mushrooms, declared that "mushrooms can help save the world" because of their environmental and medicinal applications.[1] As research continues to unravel the mysteries of mushrooms and their potential applications in modern health care, medicinal mushrooms may soon take their rightful place as valuable contributors to our well-being.

AGARIKON

(Laricifomes officinalis, syn. Fomitopsis officinalis)

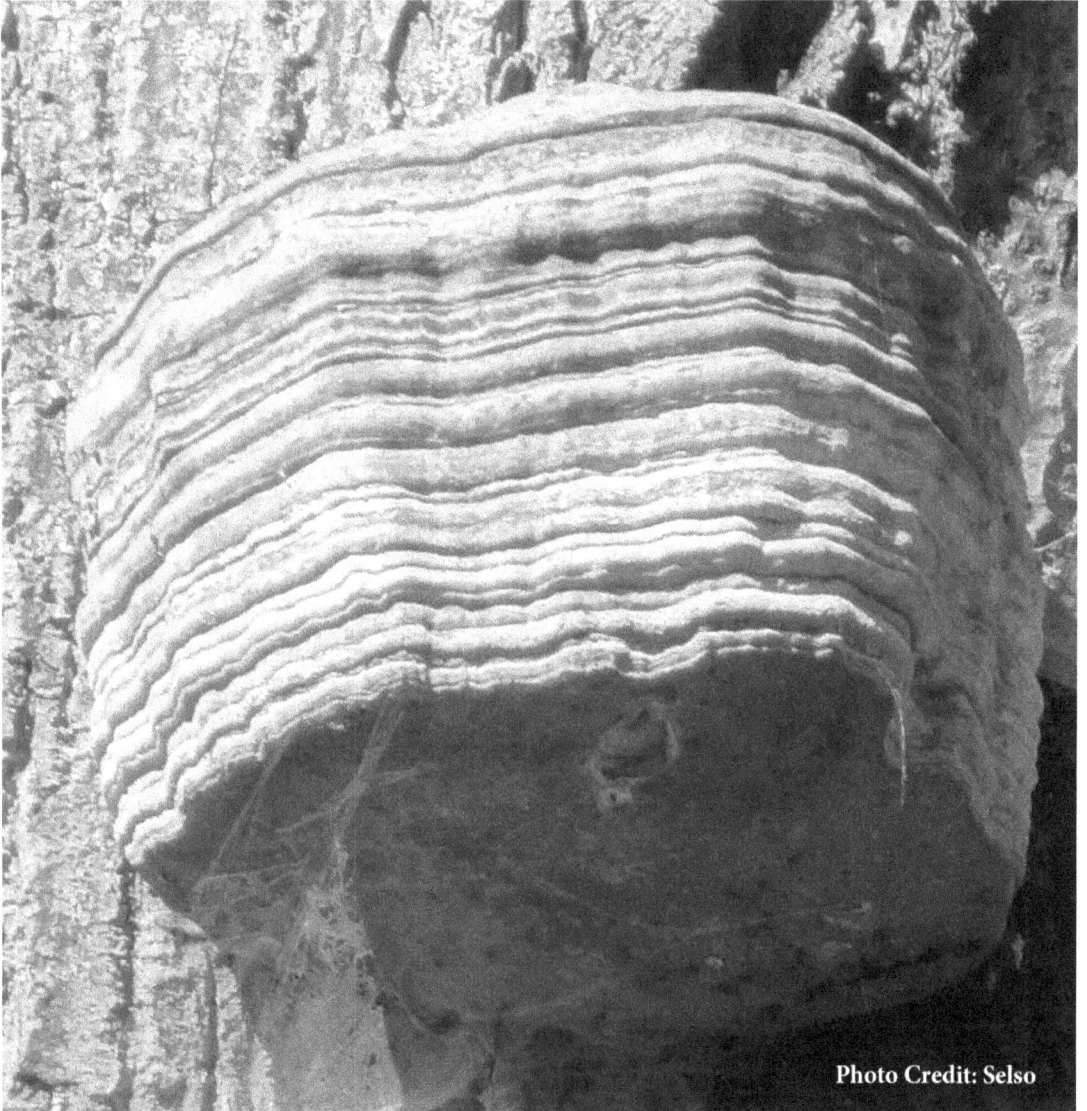

Photo Credit: Selso

Kingdom: Fungi
Phylum: Basidiomycota
Class: Agaricomycetes
Order: Polyporales
Family: Fomitopsidaceae
Genus: Laricifomes | Fomitopsis
Species: officinalis
Native Habitat: Europe, Asia, North America, and Morocco

Laricifomes officinalis (syn. *Fomitopsis officinalis*) is a wood-decay polypore—fungi that forms large fruiting bodies with pores or tubes on the underside—mushroom that goes by the common name agarikon. Although lesser known and used as a medicinal mushroom, they stand out for their historical use in traditional medicine dating back to ancient Greece, where they were used almost as a panacea for various health conditions. These mushrooms were such popular ancient remedies that they were once called the "elixir for long life" in ancient times.

Agarikon is primarily found in old-growth coniferous and deciduous forests in temperate and boreal forests across North America, Europe, and Asia. It is becoming rarer because of this unique growing enviornment. Its appearance is distinctive, featuring a large, elongated, and often gnarled fruiting body with a brown-to-blackish crust-like surface. The agarikon mushroom is known for its slow growth and can reach impressive sizes, with some specimens living for several decades. Sometimes called the tinder or hoof fungus because of its characteristic tough woody appearance with a dark, velvety upper surface and a lighter, porous underside, agarikon somewhat resembles a hoof or bracket. It is frequently found growing on birch and beech trees.

Agarikon mushrooms have a rich history of use in traditional medicine among indigenous cultures in Europe and Asia. They were revered for their healing properties and traditionally used to address various ailments. Some of their most common traditional uses include immune support, respiratory health, inflammatory conditions, wound healing, and digestive support.

In recent years, agarikon mushrooms have attracted greater attention from the scientific community. Modern research has unveiled a wealth of information about their active compounds and potential health benefits. Like many other ancient remedies, the ancient uses of agarikon mushrooms discovered by painstaking trial and error have been validated by modern science. Their antiviral, immune-regulating, anti-inflammatory, respiratory-supporting, and wound-healing effects have each been observed by modern-day researchers. Additionally, antioxidant properties have been noted. With more and more research revealing the properties of this mushroom, its use has increased among natural healers.

Agarikon mushrooms have stood the test of time and continue to have a place in supporting human health. With their origins rooted in traditional medicine and their active compounds increasingly studied by modern science, these fungi offer an intriguing union of the ancient healing arts and modern science.

As research into their properties and applications expands, these mushrooms are likely to find their way into a broader array of natural remedies, herbal medicine, and wellness products. Whether you are seeking immune support, natural wound care, or relief from inflammatory conditions, they are worthy tools for your natural medicine cabinet.

NOTABLE COMPOUNDS: Lanostane triterpenoids, polysaccharides, mannofucogalactan, organic acids, coumarins, phenolic compounds, beta-glucans

BENEFITS ACCORDING TO PRECLINICAL RESEARCH:

- ♈ Anticancer (liver)[2,3,4]
- ♈ Anticancer (lung)[5,6]
- ♈ Anticancer (colorectal)[7,8]
- ♈ Anticancer (breast)[9]
- ♈ Anticancer (cervical)[10]
- ♈ Anticancer (rodent liver)[11]
- ♈ Anticancer (rodent sarcoma)[12]
- ♈ Combats rheumatoid arthritis[13]
- ♈ Anti-inflammatory[14]
- ♈ Stimulates immune function[15]
- ♈ Antiviral (hepatitis C, influenza H5N1, smallpox)[16,17]
- ♈ Antimicrobial[18,19,20]
- ♈ Relieves painful menstruation[21]
- ♈ Alleviates hemorrhoids[22]
- ♈ Antituberculosis[23]
- ♈ Relieves cough[24]
- ♈ Trypanocidal[25]
- ♈ Antioxidant[26,27]

BENEFITS ACCORDING TO CLINICAL RESEARCH:

- ➢ None found

THERAPEUTIC POTENTIAL: Inflammatory conditions, respiratory conditions, viral infections

CLINICAL DOSAGES: Unknown; typical doses are: 500 mg daily; intensive use of 500 mg, two to three times daily

POTENTIAL ADVERSE EFFECTS: Diarrhea, stomachache, nausea

CAUTIONS AND CONTRAINDICATIONS: Pregnancy, lactation, agarikon mushroom allergy

ALMOND MUSHROOM

(Agaricus subrufescens; syn. *Agaricus rufotegulis, Agaricus fiardii; Agaricus brasiliensis* (misidentified), *Agaricus blazei* (misidentified))

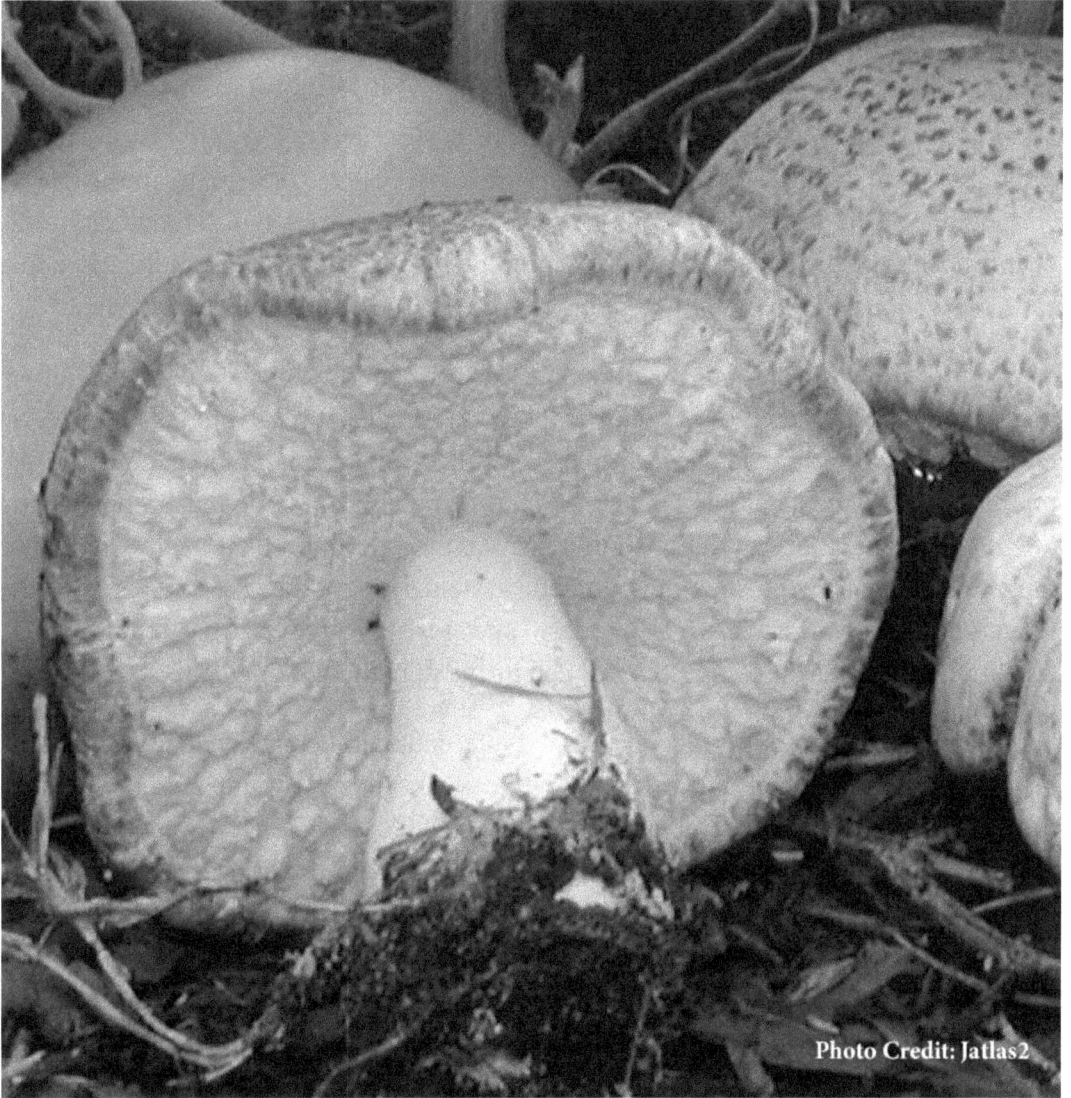

Photo Credit: Jatlas2

Kingdom: Fungi
Phylum: Basidiomycota
Class: Agaricomycetes
Order: Agaricales
Family: Agaricaceae
Genus: Agaricus
Species: subrufescens | rufotegulis | fiardii | brasiliensis | blazei
Native Habitat: Brazil | Europe | Dominican Republic, Mexico | Brazil | United States, Canada

The almond mushroom, also known as the Brazilian mushroom, royal sun mushroom, or mushroom of the sun, is a fascinating and versatile fungus with a rich history of medicinal use. This mushroom, native to the Atlantic rainforest in Brazil, has garnered global attention for its numerous health benefits. It was discovered in Brazil in the 1960s and misidentified as a species found in the United States (*Agaricus blazei*). Further complicating this issue, *Agaricus blazei* was rejected as a proper species name for the almond mushroom in 2002, but the name of another existing species, *Agaricus brasiliensis*, was proposed. Analysis of European *Agaricus rufotegulis* discovered that it is the same species as *Agaricus subrufescens*. Given the great confusion and comingling of the different species, research for each species will be included in this chapter, with the understanding that research for one species may actually apply to all species since they are used as synonyms in the research despite their differences.

A brown, gilled mushroom that belongs to the family Agaricaceae, the almond mushroom is considered a national treasure in Brazil. It was first discovered and documented in the Piedade region of São Paulo, Brazil, but its indigenous use as a traditional medicine dates back much further. In Brazil, the almond mushroom has been utilized for generations by indigenous communities and traditional healers for a wide range of health concerns, including immune system support, digestive issues, and stress reduction. The mushroom's adaptability and resistance to various environmental conditions make it a hardy species that can thrive in both wild and cultivated settings.

The almond mushroom has recently gained international recognition and is now being studied and incorporated into modern healthcare practices. The mushroom contains a diverse array of bioactive compounds that contribute to its therapeutic potential. One of the most well-documented medicinal properties of the almond mushroom is its ability to bolster the immune system. The mushroom is rich in β-glucans, a type of complex sugar that has been linked to immune-modulating effects. β-glucans can stimulate the production of immune cells, such as macrophages and natural killer cells, enhancing the body's defense against pathogens and malignant cells. This makes it an attractive option for individuals looking to fortify their immune response.

Inflammation is a natural and essential response to injury or infection, but chronic inflammation is associated with numerous diseases, including arthritis, heart disease, and cancer. The almond mushroom has shown promise in mitigating chronic inflammation due to its anti-inflammatory properties. Some studies suggest that the mushroom's compounds can inhibit the release of pro-inflammatory molecules, making it a potential tool for managing inflammatory conditions.

The high content of antioxidants in the almond mushroom is another reason it is valued for its medicinal use. Antioxidants help neutralize free radicals in the body, which are unstable molecules that can cause cellular damage. By reducing oxidative stress, this mushroom may help prevent various chronic diseases and contribute to overall well-being.

Research has explored the potential antitumor effects of the almond mushroom, which are largely attributed to its β-glucans and other bioactive compounds. These substances may inhibit the growth of cancer cells and promote apoptosis (programmed cell death) in malignant cells.

With the increasing number of people struggling to manage their blood sugar, many mushrooms have been investigated for their blood sugar-balancing activity, and this includes the almond mushroom. Some research suggests that it can help regulate blood sugar levels by improving insulin sensitivity and enhancing glucose metabolism. These properties make it a candidate for inclusion in diabetes management strategies.

The potential cardiovascular benefits of the almond mushroom are also noteworthy. Its antioxidant and anti-inflammatory properties can help reduce the risk of heart disease. Additionally, some studies have indicated that it may contribute to lower blood pressure, improve lipid profiles, and protect vascular tissues, further promoting cardiovascular health.

The liver plays a crucial role in detoxification and metabolic processes within the body. The almond mushroom has demonstrated liver protective properties, which is especially relevant in the context of liver diseases, including non-alcoholic fatty liver disease (NAFLD).

In a world filled with stress and anxiety, finding natural solutions to promote mental health is vital. The almond mushroom has been studied for its potential to reduce stress and anxiety. It is believed that its bioactive compounds may influence neurotransmitters and neural pathways associated with mood regulation, providing a potential natural remedy for mental well-being.

This mushroom has been used traditionally to address gastrointestinal complaints and some studies suggest that it does indeed have a protective effect on the digestive system by promoting gut health and balancing the gut microbiome. This makes it a candidate for individuals with conditions such as irritable bowel syndrome (IBS) and inflammatory bowel disease (IBD).

The mushroom's antioxidant and anti-inflammatory properties may have benefits for skin health. Almond mushroom extracts have been incorporated into skincare products to combat signs of aging and protect the skin from damage caused by free radicals.

With all the emerging science revealing its therapeutic value, the almond mushroom holds great promise as a medicinal mushroom. Boasting a rich history and diverse array of bioactive compounds, it has a promising future in healthcare and significant therapeutic potential. From immune system support to its potential in cancer treatment, the almond mushroom continues to be a subject of scientific research and a source of healing for health enthusiasts. As our understanding of this remarkable mushroom continues to grow, it may find a more prominent place in modern medicine, offering a natural and holistic approach to health and well-being.

NOTABLE COMPOUNDS: Polysaccharides, beta-glucans, alpha-glucans, phenolics, ergostanes, agaritine, agarol, ergosterol, blazeispirols, blazein, fructogalactans

AGARICUS SUBRUFESCENS, AGARICUS RUFOTEGULIS, AGARICUS FIARDII—BENEFITS ACCORDING TO PRECLINICAL RESEARCH:

- Anticancer (rodent sarcoma)[28]
- Enhances the gut microbiome (promotes balance in microbiome)[29]
- Improves intestinal immunity and immune system development[30]
- Stimulates immune function[31]
- Shields against DNA mutation[32]
- Defends against damage caused by UV rays[33]
- Antiviral (flavivirus)[34]
- Inhibits mycotoxin production[35]

AGARICUS BLAZEI, AGARICUS RUFOTEGULIS, AGARICUS FIARDII—BENEFITS ACCORDING TO CLINICAL RESEARCH:

➢ None found

AGARICUS BLAZEI—BENEFITS ACCORDING TO PRECLINICAL RESEARCH:

- Anticancer (chronic myeloid leukemia, acute lymphoblastic leukemia, acute myeloid leukemia)[36-46]
- Anticancer (myeloma)[47]
- Anticancer (prostate)[48]
- Anticancer (pancreatic)[49]
- Anticancer (liver)[50,51,52,53,54]
- Prevents liver cancer[55,56]
- Anticancer (osteosarcoma)[57]
- Anticancer (ovarian)[58]
- Anticancer (lung)[59,60,61]
- Anticancer, mildly (colorectal)[62]

- ☬ Anticancer (gastric)[63,64]
- ☬ Prevents colon cancer;[65,66] other research suggests it has no effect[67,68]
- ☬ Enhances the activity of doxorubicin against liver cancer[69]
- ☬ Defends against DNA damage caused by cyclophosphamide[70]
- ☬ Anticancer (rodent sarcoma)[71-80]
- ☬ Anticancer (rodent Ehrlich carcinoma)[81,82]
- ☬ Anticancer (rodent fibrosarcoma)[83,84]
- ☬ Anticancer (rodent melanoma)[85]
- ☬ Relieves anxiety[86]
- ☬ Neuroprotective[87]
- ☬ Preserves brain function during aging[88]
- ☬ Ameliorates Parkinson's disease[89,90,91]
- ☬ Stimulates immune function[92-111]
- ☬ Enhances immune system activity against cancer (inhibits myeloid-derived suppressor cells, promotes natural killer cell activity and phagocytosis, activates NLRP3 inflammasome)[112,113,114,115,116,117]
- ☬ Upregulates genes associated with immune function[118]
- ☬ Balances immune function[119,120,121,122]
- ☬ Restores Th1/Th2 balance in TH2-skewed conditions (cancer, asthma)[123]
- ☬ Anti-inflammatory[124,125,126,127,128]
- ☬ Reduces inflammation in a model of osteoporosis[129]
- ☬ Suppresses allergies[130,131,132]
- ☬ Mitigates anaphylaxis-like reactions[133]
- ☬ Improves the gut microbiome (reduces the relative abundance of harmful bacteria and increases the relative abundance of healthy bacteria, improves the Firmicutes/Bacteroidetes ratio)[134]
- ☬ Combats obesity[135]
- ☬ Antidiabetic[136-142]
- ☬ Promotes pancreatic tissue recovery in diabetic subjects[143]
- ☬ Protects pulmonary tissues against damage caused by diabetic-related oxidative stress[144]
- ☬ Shields against liver and brain tissue injury caused by paracetamol (acetaminophen)[145]
- ☬ Liver protective[146-152]
- ☬ Protects against lethal septicemia in a model of fecal peritonitis (inflammation of the thin membrane that lines the inside of the abdomen)[153]
- ☬ Minimizes damage caused by atherosclerosis;[154,155] may also increase immune and inflammatory reaction in an atherosclerotic state[156]
- ☬ Reduces blood pressure and improves circulation[157]

- ♀ Support healthy lipid levels[158,159,160]
- ♀ Protects against gastric ulcers[161]
- ♀ Defends against testicular damage[162]
- ♀ Prevents DNA damage—may be genotoxic in some cases (the majority of the research showed a protective effect)[163-174]
- ♀ Alleviates damage caused by oxidative stress[175,176]
- ♀ Antioxidant[177-183]
- ♀ Stimulates estrogenic activity[184,185]
- ♀ Antiviral (human immunodeficiency virus 1)[186]
- ♀ Mitigates cerebral malaria[187]
- ♀ Antiviral (inhibits structural changes in host cells caused by the western equine encephalitis)[188]
- ♀ Antimicrobial[189,190,191]
- ♀ Leishmanicidal, anti-leishmaniasis[192,193,194,195]
- ♀ Promotes healthy aging[196]
- ♀ Alleviates periodontitis[197]
- ♀ Accelerates wound healing[198,199,200]

AGARICUS BLAZEI—BENEFITS ACCORDING TO CLINICAL RESEARCH:

- ➤ Reduced birch allergies (lowered IgE levels and decreased basophil activation to allergen) in people with birch allergies[201]
  - 60 mL of AndoSan (a Agaricus blazei-based mushroom extract) daily for seven weeks
- ➤ Normalizes liver function in people with hepatitis B (carrier for more than three years)[202]
  - 1,500 mg daily for twelve months
- ➤ Altered the expression of genes involved in the G-protein coupled receptor signaling pathway, in cell cycling, and in transcriptional regulation, and slightly reduced viral load in people with chronic hepatitis C[203]
  - 20 mL AbM extract three times daily
- ➤ Reverses insulin resistance in people with type 2 diabetes when used in combination with metformin and gliclazide[204]
  - 1,500 mg daily for twelve weeks
- ➤ Improves symptoms of ulcerative colitis and reduces fatigue in people with mild–moderate ulcerative colitis[205]
  - 30 mL of AndoSan twice daily for three weeks
- ➤ Decreases levels of pathogenic cytokines in blood and calprotectin in feces in people with inflammatory bowel disease (ulcerative colitis and Chron's disease)[206]
  - 20 mL AndoSan three times daily for twelve days

- Improves symptoms of and fatigue associated with Crohn's diseases but not statistically significant compared to placebo[207]
    - 30 mL of AndoSan twice daily for three weeks
- Reduced IL-2 cytokine release in people with Crohn's disease and IL-5 in people with ulcerative colitis[208]
    - 30 mL of AndoSan twice daily for three weeks
- Reduces cytokine (IL-1beta, TNF-alpha, IL-17, and IL-2) release in healthy individuals with a trend in the reduction of chemokines (IL-8, IFN-gamma, G-CSF)[209]
    - 20 mL AndoSan three times daily for twelve days
- Enhances quality of life—reduces physical symptoms in males and mental symptoms in females (those aged 66 and older tended to experience improved physical components, while those 65 and under noted improved mental components—in people with cancer in remission[210]
    - 1,800 mg of Sen-Sei-Rio (lyophilized, granulated powder) per day
- Reduces chemotherapy-related side effects (appetite loss, hair loss, emotional instability, general weakness) and enhances natural killer cell activity in women with gynecological cancers undergoing chemotherapy[211]
    - 1,800 mg of Sen-Sei-Rio (lyophilized, granulated powder) per day
- 60 mL per day of AndoSan was not able to produce statistically significant improvements in treatment response or survival in people with multiple myeloma undergoing high dose chemotherapy with autologous stem cell support[212]
- 900 mg/day was insufficient to improve inflammatory markers in elderly women[213]

AGARICUS BRASILIENSIS—BENEFITS ACCORDING TO PRECLINICAL RESEARCH:

- Anticancer (oral)[214]
- Anticancer (breast)[215]
- Suppresses the side effects of 5-fluorouracil[216]
- Ameliorates cancer-related cachexia (ongoing muscle loss)[217]
- Anticancer (rodent sarcoma, fibrosarcoma)[218,219,220]
- Antidepressant[221]
- Relieves anxiety[222]
- Stimulates immune function[223,224,225,226,227,228,229,230,231,232]
- Relieves pain[233]
- Anti-inflammatory[234,235]
- Attenuates the systemic effects of rheumatoid arthritis[236]
- Reduces pulmonary inflammation[237]
- Antidiabetic[238]

- 🍄 Guards against diabetic neuropathy and relieves associated pain[239]
- 🍄 Ameliorates gestational diabetes[240]
- 🍄 Reverses neonatal jaundice by lowering bilirubin levels[241]
- 🍄 Heart protective (increases myocardial SOD activity)[242]
- 🍄 Reduces blood pressure and improves circulation[243]
- 🍄 Improves lipid profiles[244]
- 🍄 Inhibits platelet activation (beneficial for vascular diseases)[245]
- 🍄 Preserves liver function or protects liver health[246,247,248]
- 🍄 Prevents nonalcoholic fatty liver disease[249]
- 🍄 Reverses alcohol-related liver injury[250]
- 🍄 Protects against gastric ulcers[251]
- 🍄 Shields against damage and death caused by sepsis[252]
- 🍄 Protects against DNA damage[253,254]
- 🍄 Antioxidant[255,256,257,258]
- 🍄 Promotes healthy aging[259]
- 🍄 Antiviral (poliovirus type 1)[260]
- 🍄 Antiviral (influenza H1N1 PR8)[261]
- 🍄 Antiviral (herpes simplex virus 1 and 2, bovine herpes virus)[262,263,264,265,266]
- 🍄 Antibacterial[267]
- 🍄 Wound healing[268,269]

AGARICUS BRASILIENSIS—BENEFITS ACCORDING TO CLINICAL RESEARCH:

- ➢ Decreased muscle fatigue and improved muscular strength during and after strength training[270]
  - 2,000 mg daily in the morning for 24 days
- ➢ Promotes the formation of antibody-beta-glucan complexes and activates immune cells to potentially prevent fungal infections in healthy individuals[271]
  - 900–1,500 mg daily after breakfast for twelve weeks
- ➢ Reduces body fat, visceral fat, cholesterol, and blood sugar levels, and increases natural killer cell activity in healthy individuals[272]
  - 1,500–4,500 mg twice daily for seven days
- ➢ Promotes subjective improvements in hair loss, gray hair, fatigue, general malaise, eye strain, shoulder stiffness, coldness of extremities, tiredness during the day, and ease of getting out of bed in healthy people[273]
  - 900–1,500 mg daily after breakfast for twelve weeks

THERAPEUTIC POTENTIAL: Allergies, diabetes, Parkinson's disease, antioxidant support, immune support

CLINICAL DOSAGES: 60 mL of liquid extract daily or 1,500–1,800 mg powder daily; 1,500–4,500 mg twice daily for *A. brasiliensis*; 900–1,500 mg daily for *A. brasiliensis*; recommended dose: 500 mg one to three times daily

POTENTIAL ADVERSE EFFECTS: Nausea, diarrhea, abdominal discomfort, rarely liver toxicity and interstitial lung disease

CAUTIONS AND CONTRAINDICATIONS: Pregnancy, lactation, liver disease, prior to surgery, almond mushroom allergy; diabetes drugs

CHAGA
(Inonotus obliquus)

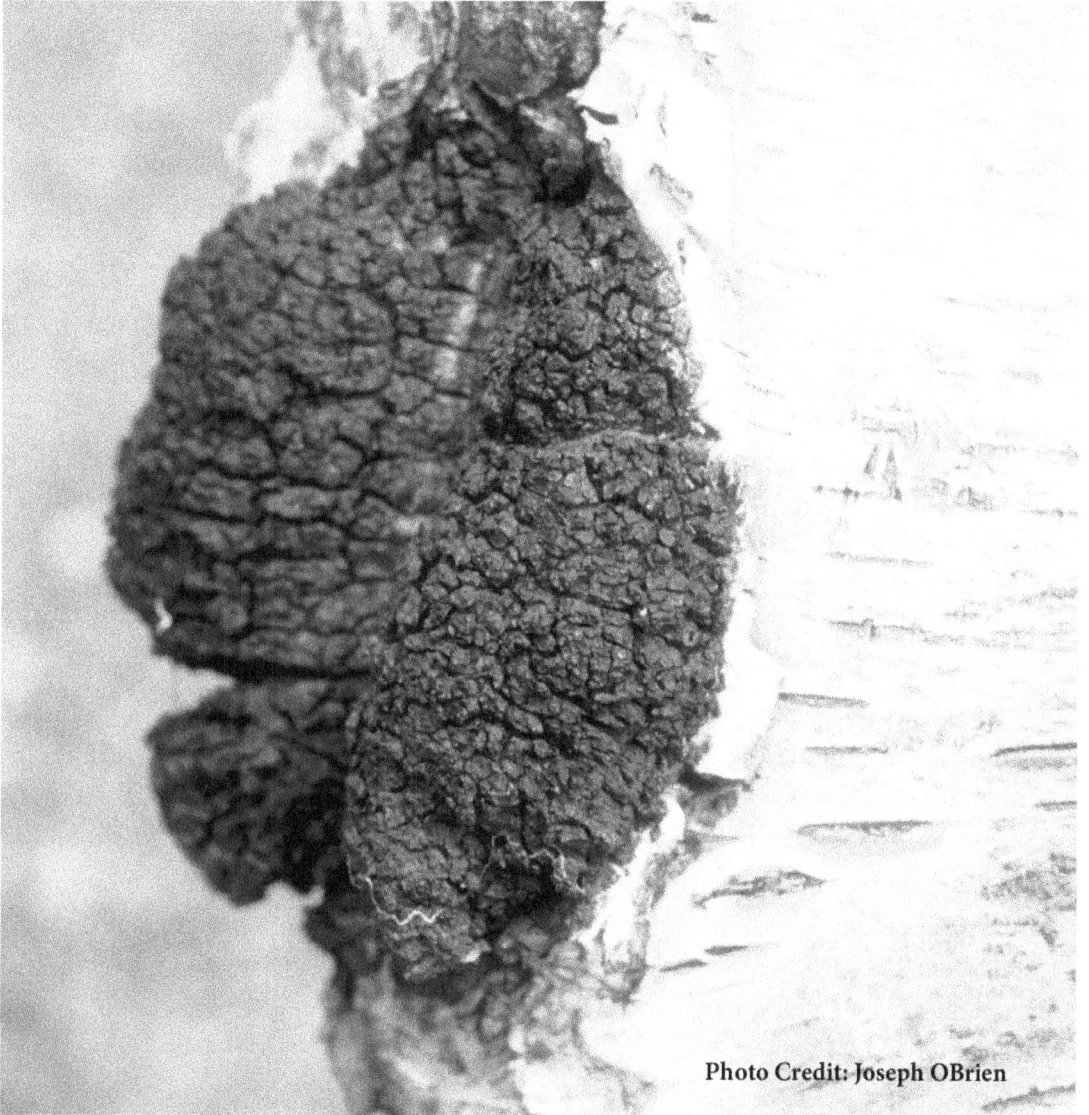

Photo Credit: Joseph OBrien

Kingdom: Fungi
Phylum: Basidiomycota
Class: Agaricomycetes
Order: Hymenochaetales
Family: Hymenochaetaceae
Genus: Inonotus
Species: obliquus
Native Habitat: The Circumboreal Region of North America and Eurasia

Chaga mushrooms (*Inonotus obliquus*) are a parasitic fungus that primarily grows on the bark of birch trees in colder climates, like Siberia, Northern Canada, North America, Russia, and Northern Europe. It is unattractive and looks like a large lump of blackened, crusty, charcoal-like material on the tree. Although it resembles burned charcoal—because of the melanin it contains, it is orange inside. When removed from the tree, it gives off a sweet, woody, and earthy odor. Its taste is woody and sweet, somewhat resembling mocha when brewed in hot water or milk. It was traditionally used for a variety of gastrointestinal conditions, tuberculosis, inflammatory conditions, parasites, heart and liver diseases.[274]

Chaga has captured the attention of both traditional healers and modern scientists. Widely regarded as a medicinal powerhouse, Chaga has a long history of use in traditional medicine, particularly in Siberia, Russia, and other parts of Northern Europe. Chaga use in traditional medicine dates back centuries. Indigenous peoples of Siberia and Northern Europe, such as the Khanty, Mansi, and Chukchi, have long recognized its therapeutic properties. Chaga was traditionally brewed into teas or decoctions and consumed to address various health concerns. Some of its most common uses include to support immune function, reduce inflammation, aid digestion, treat wounds or other skin conditions, and for cancer.

In recent years, Chaga has gained considerable attention from the scientific community, leading to a surge in research aimed at revealing its therapeutic potential. While more studies are needed since the current research is all preclinical, the existing research highlights several promising aspects of Chaga that warrant evaluation in human clinical trials. It has demonstrated antioxidant activity in multiple studies, including combating oxidative stress. Chaga kills various cancers, with much emphasis in the research on its effects against lung cancer. It has also exhibited promising activity against a variety of viruses.

As more research emerges informing the potential therapeutic use of Chaga, it is beginning to transition from traditional folk remedy to a sought-after health-and-wellness product in the modern era. It is available in various forms, including Chaga tea, extracts, capsules, and skin-care products. The Chaga mushroom reminds us of the enduring wisdom of ancient traditional healers and the need for ongoing discoveries of ancient remedies in modern science.

As Chaga continues to gain recognition, more and more consumers are enjoying its benefits. Whether you are looking to boost your immunity, reduce inflammation, or improve your gut microbiome, Chaga offers a wealth of possibilities.

NOTABLE COMPOUNDS: Polysaccharides, polyphenols, antioxidants, triterpenoids, ergosterol, benzoic acid derivatives, ergosterol peroxide, sesquiterpenes, hispidin analogs, melanins, inotodiol, flavan, botulin, betulinic acid, phelligridin D

BENEFITS ACCORDING TO PRECLINICAL RESEARCH:

- 🍄 Protects against stomach ulcer[275]
- 🍄 Relieves colitis[276,277,278,279,280]
- 🍄 Combats colitis-associated cancer (better than *C. militaris*)[281,282]
- 🍄 Prevents tumor formation and metastasis[283]
- 🍄 Anticancer (lung)[284-297]
- 🍄 Reduces lung cancer progression[298]
- 🍄 Anticancer (colorectal)[299-305]
- 🍄 Anticancer (breast)[306,307,308,309,310,311]
- 🍄 Anticancer (prostate)[312,313]
- 🍄 Anticancer (gastric/stomach)[314,315,316]
- 🍄 Anticancer (osteosarcoma)[317]
- 🍄 Anticancer (cervical)[318,319,320,321,322]
- 🍄 Anticancer (ovarian)[323]
- 🍄 Anticancer (uterine)[324]
- 🍄 Anticancer (melanoma)[325]
- 🍄 Anticancer (liver)[326,327,328,329]
- 🍄 Anticancer (fibrosarcoma)[330]
- 🍄 Anticancer (neurogliocytoma)[331]
- 🍄 Anticancer (leukemia, lymphoma)[332,333]
- 🍄 Anticancer (dog bladder)[334]
- 🍄 Anticancer (rodent melanoma)[335,336]
- 🍄 Anticancer (rodent skin)[337,338]
- 🍄 Anticancer (rodent colon)[339]
- 🍄 Anticancer (rodent lymphoma)[340]
- 🍄 Reduces chemotherapy side effects (compromised immunity, gastrointestinal ulcer)[341]
- 🍄 Alleviates histamine-induced microvascular inflammation[342]
- 🍄 Eases uterine inflammation and endometritis[343]
- 🍄 Relieves acute endometriosis[344]
- 🍄 Reduces excess uric acid (hyperuricemia) and related inflammation; helpful for gout[345,346,347]
- 🍄 Anti-inflammatory[348,349,350,351,352]
- 🍄 Blocks pain sensations[353]
- 🍄 Enhances systemic metabolism[354]

- 🍄 Reduces/balances blood glucose[355-371]
- 🍄 Reverses insulin resistance and blood glucose and lowers lipid profiles[372,373,374]
- 🍄 Prevents diabetes[375]
- 🍄 Restores damaged pancreas function (antidiabetic, antioxidative)[376]
- 🍄 Improves type 2 diabetes by modifying the gut microbiome[377]
- 🍄 Reduces blood glucose, body weight, and insulin resistance in model of type 2 diabetes[378]
- 🍄 Reverses dyslipidemia[379,380,381]
- 🍄 Alleviates chronic pancreatitis[382]
- 🍄 Enhances the gut microbiome[383,384,385,386,387,388]
- 🍄 Acts as a prebiotic for *Bifidobacteria*[389]
- 🍄 Increases abundance of antitumor probiotics (*Parabacteroides goldsteinii* and *Bifidobacterium pseudolongum* PV8-2)[390]
- 🍄 Strengthens intestinal barrier function, reduces leaky gut[391]
- 🍄 Regulates immune function[392-401]
- 🍄 Regulates immune responses to and reduces damage caused by *Toxoplasma gondii* infection[402,403,404,405,406]
- 🍄 Weight management, obesity[407,408,409]
- 🍄 Delays cellular aging caused by oxidative stress[410]
- 🍄 Neuroprotective[411-417]
- 🍄 Protect against Alzheimer's disease[418,419]
- 🍄 Inhibits neuroinflammation[420]
- 🍄 Liver protective[421,422,423,424]
- 🍄 Alleviates nonalcoholic fatty liver disease[425]
- 🍄 Heart protective[426]
- 🍄 Kidney protective (diabetic nephropathy)[427,428,429,430,431]
- 🍄 Antiallergic[432,433,434]
- 🍄 Combats asthma[435]
- 🍄 Enhances exercise performance[436]
- 🍄 Postpones physical and mental fatigue[437,438]
- 🍄 Antiviral (SARS-CoV-2)[439,440,441,442,443]
- 🍄 Antiviral (HIV)[444]
- 🍄 Antiviral (influenza virus A/California/07/09—H1N1 pdm09)[445]
- 🍄 Antiviral (hepatitis C—prevents and treats)[446]
- 🍄 Antiviral (prevents HSV-1 infection)[447,448]
- 🍄 Antiviral (feline viruses)[449,450]
- 🍄 Antiviral (murine norovirus)[451]
- 🍄 Anti-infectious[452]
- 🍄 Alleviates erectile dysfunction[453]

- 🍄 Stimulates hair growth[454]
- 🍄 Skin brightening[455]
- 🍄 Protects against UV-B-induced genotoxicity, enhances DNA repair genes[456]
- 🍄 Protects against DNA mutations[457]
- 🍄 Antioxidant[458-486]
- 🍄 Protects against oxidative stress/damage[487,488,489,490,491]

BENEFITS ACCORDING TO CLINICAL RESEARCH:

➢ None found

THERAPEUTIC POTENTIAL: Dysbiosis, leaky gut, colitis, endometriosis, diabetes, metabolic syndrome, gout, cognitive disorders, fatigue, oxidative stress, cancer

CLINICAL DOSAGES: Unknown; typical doses are: Capsules—1,000 mg daily; powder—1,000–2,000 mg daily in a beverage; tea—as instructed on the product label; because no clinical studies have determined an effective clinical dose, follow the supplement manufacturer's instructions

POTENTIAL ADVERSE EFFECTS: The high oxalate content in Chaga mushrooms could lead to kidney failure if excessive Chaga is consumed

CAUTIONS AND CONTRAINDICATIONS: Pregnancy, lactation, kidney disease (oxalate driven), Chaga mushroom allergy, prior to surgery; drugs that thin the blood, antidiabetic drugs, immunosuppressants

(Cordyceps sinensis, syn. Orphiocordyceps sinensis; Cordyceps militaris)

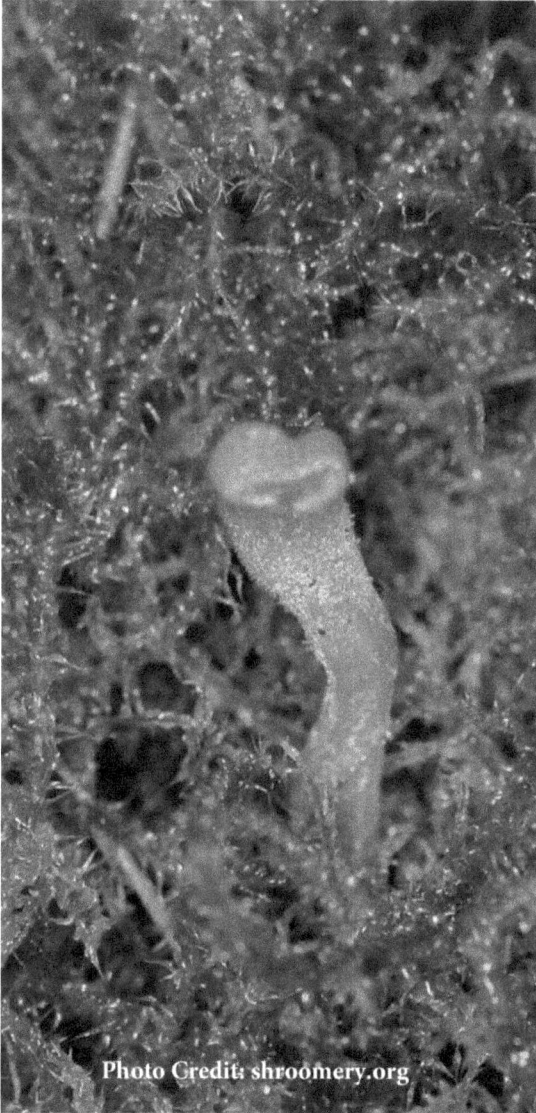

Photo Credit: shroomery.org

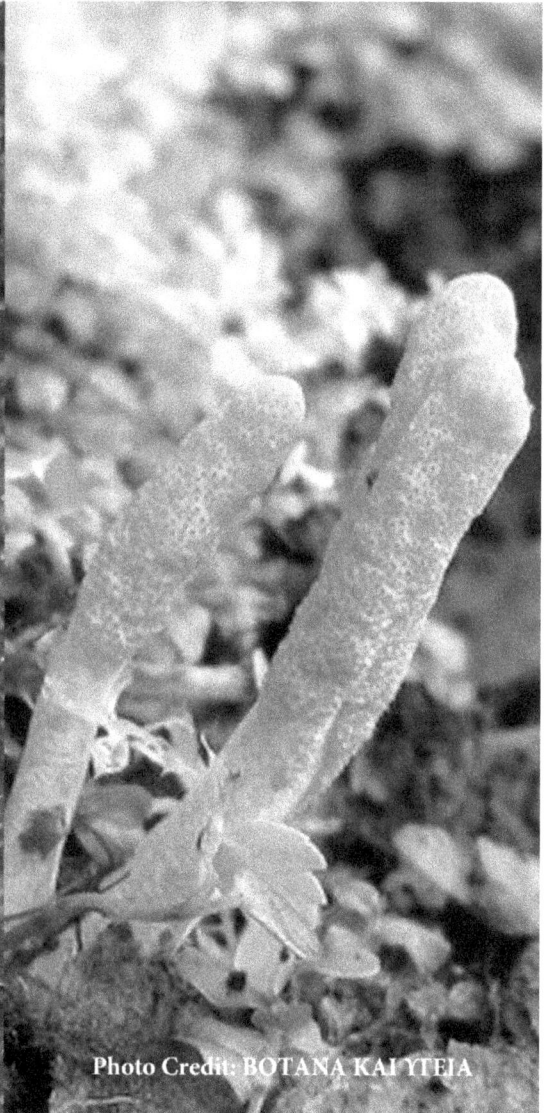

Photo Credit: BOTANA KAI YTEJA

Kingdom: Fungi
Phylum: Ascomycota
Class: Sordariomycetes
Order: Hypocreales
Family: Ophiocordycipitaceae | Cordycipitaceae
Genus: Cordyceps
Species: sinensis | militaris
Native Habitat: High-altitude regions of the Himalayas | North America, Asia, Europe

A remarkable mushroom with a rich tradition in Chinese medicine, cordyceps (most commonly from *Cordyceps sinensis*, but also from *Cordyceps militaris*) mushroom is celebrated for its potential and proven health benefits. This unique fungus is prized for its adaptogenic properties. Cordyceps is a parasitic fungus that primarily targets caterpillars, particularly those found in the Himalayan regions of Tibet, Nepal, Bhutan, and parts of China. This remarkable organism thrives in high-altitude environments, typically above 3,000 meters (9,843 feet). In these harsh, cold, and oxygen-deficient conditions, cordyceps has developed its unique survival strategy.

The life cycle of *Cordyceps sinensis* begins when its spores attach themselves to a caterpillar or other insect larvae. Once attached, the fungus infiltrates the host, slowly consuming it from the inside. As the host insect succumbs to the fungus, a stalklike structure emerges from the caterpillar's head, eventually releasing spores into the air to infect new hosts. This natural process is the source of cordyceps' nickname, the "caterpillar fungus."

Cordyceps usage dates back over two thousand years, where it was frequently used to treat a wide range of ailments, including fatigue, respiratory disorders, and kidney problems. This usage for kidney problems continues today in modern Chinese medicine, and it is commonly employed to improve physical performance and endurance, connecting it to its ancient use for fatigue.

In recent decades, cordyceps has gained significant attention from the scientific community. Researchers have been conducting studies to understand its potential health benefits and therapeutic properties. While more research is needed, some promising findings have emerged, including immune-modulating effects, enhancing of physical performance and endurance, protection of various organs, antioxidant activity, improved energy, and anticancer potential.

The increasing popularity of *Cordyceps sinensis* has led to its incorporation into various wellness products. It is now available in various forms, including capsules, powders, extracts, and even in coffee blends. These products are often marketed as natural remedies to boost energy, improve immunity, and support overall well-being.

One of the key factors driving cordyceps's popularity is its adaptogenic properties. Adaptogens are natural substances that help the body adapt to stress and maintain balance. Cordyceps is believed to help regulate various bodily functions, making it a valuable addition to the toolkit of individuals seeking to optimize their health.

Cordyceps-infused products are commonly used by athletes and fitness enthusiasts to enhance performance, reduce fatigue, and speed recovery. Its potential to improve oxygen utilization is of particular interest to endurance athletes, as it may enhance aerobic capacity.

Cordyceps militaris, often referred to as the "military cordyceps" or "militaris mushroom," is a lesser-known but highly valuable fungus within the Cordyceps genus. While it shares some similarities with the more famous *Cordyceps sinensis*, *Cordyceps militaris* has its unique characteristics and medicinal properties.

Cordyceps militaris is a saprophytic fungus, meaning it grows on dead insects and other organic matter, rather than parasitizing live hosts like *Cordyceps sinensis*. It is commonly found in various regions across the world, including Asia, North America, and Europe. While *Cordyceps militaris* is a more versatile species in terms of habitat and host preferences, it is most notably cultivated on a variety of substrates, making it more accessible and sustainable compared to its caterpillar-fungus counterpart.

The medicinal value of *Cordyceps militaris* is becoming more apparent as research into this strange cordyceps mushroom continues. Like *Cordyceps sinensis*, *Cordyceps militaris* is considered an adaptogen that helps support overall well-being and balance of key body systems' function. It also possesses immune-boosting properties and may be useful to ward off infections and illnesses. Traditionally, this mushroom was used to combat fatigue and increase stamina. It also has antioxidant and anti-inflammatory properties, and has been used to support respiratory health, making it a potential natural remedy for conditions like asthma and bronchitis.

One of the most significant advantages of *Cordyceps militaris* is its cultivation feasibility. Cultivating *Cordyceps militaris* involves growing the fungus on a variety of substrates, such as rice, soybeans, or even synthetic mediums. This cultivation process is less dependent on specific host insects or high-altitude environments, making it more sustainable and cost-effective. Whether you are seeking to boost your immune system, increase your energy levels, or explore new culinary experiences, *Cordyceps militaris* offers a promising avenue for exploration in the realm of natural health.

Both cordyceps species have been well-studied, revealing myriad therapeutic properties and hinting at nearly infinite potential to use these mushrooms for human health. Hundreds of studies show they share similar properties, with the clinical research for *Cordyceps militaris* slowly catching up to its cousin *Cordyceps sinensis*. Remarkably, both species have exhibited anticancer activity against multiple cancer types, significant immunomodulatory activity, and the ability to protect or preserve the function of key organs in the body. With interest in these two related mushrooms growing, the future is bright for cordyceps and human health alike.

NOTABLE COMPOUNDS: Nucleosides, polysaccharides, sterols, protein, amino acids, and polypeptides, dipeptides, cordycepin, CPS-1, CPS-2, ergosterol, H1-A, cordymin, cordysinan, beta-glucans, cordycedipeptide A, cordyceamides A and B, tryptophan, D-mannitol, glucosamine, massoia lactone, chlorogenic acid, and p-coumaric acid

Note: Fermented extracts tend to have higher polyphenol and glucosamine content.[492]

CORDYCEPS SINENSIS—BENEFITS ACCORDING TO PRECLINICAL RESEARCH:

- ♣ Anticancer (breast) [493-499]
- ♣ Anticancer (colorectal)[500,501,502]
- ♣ Anticancer (liver) [503-510]
- ♣ Anticancer (lung)[511,512,513,514,515,516]
- ♣ Anticancer (lung, enhances cisplatin activity)[517]
- ♣ Anticancer (lung, inhibits drug-resistant progression)[518]
- ♣ Anticancer (cervical)[519]
- ♣ Anticancer (endometrial)[520]
- ♣ Anticancer (testicular)[521]
- ♣ Anticancer (testicular, enhances sensitivity to radiation treatment)[522]
- ♣ Anticancer (pancreatic)[523,524]
- ♣ Anticancer (neuroblastoma)[525]
- ♣ Anticancer (glioma)[526]
- ♣ Anticancer (acute promyelocytic leukemia)[527,528,529,530,531,532]
- ♣ Anticancer (prevents leukemia)[533]
- ♣ Anticancer (myeloid leukemia)[534,535,536,537]
- ♣ Anticancer (leukemia, enhances triptolide activity)[538]
- ♣ Anticancer (lymphoma)[539,540,541]
- ♣ Anticancer (melanoma)[542]
- ♣ Anticancer (thyroid)[543]
- ♣ Anticancer (adenocarcinoma)[544]
- ♣ Anticancer (gestational choriocarcinoma)[545]
- ♣ Anticancer (esophageal)[546]
- ♣ Anticancer (oral)[547]
- ♣ Anticancer (oral, enhances response to radiation treatment)[548]
- ♣ Anticancer (head and neck, enhances cisplatin)[549]
- ♣ Enhances immune surveillance against tumor cells[550]
- ♣ Prevents/reduces cancer metastasis[551,552,553,554,555,556]
- ♣ Anticancer (rodent sarcoma/fibrosarcoma)[557,558]
- ♣ Anticancer (rodent liver)[559,560]
- ♣ Anticancer (rodent melanoma) [561-567]

- 🍄 Anticancer (rodent melanoma, amplified by 2'-deoxycoformycin)[568]
- 🍄 Anticancer (rodent breast)[569]
- 🍄 Ameliorates chemotherapy-induced leukopenia[570]
- 🍄 Improves the gut microbiome (*Lactobacillus*, *Bifidobacterium*, *enterococcus cecorum*, Bacteroides, Firmicutes, short-chain fatty acids, reduces Proteobacteria)[571,572,573,574]
- 🍄 Protects Bifidobacteria against antibiotics[575]
- 🍄 Restores intestinal mucosal immunity[576,577]
- 🍄 Strengthens intestinal barrier function[578]
- 🍄 Antidepressant[579]
- 🍄 Alleviates Hashimoto's[580]
- 🍄 Diminishes Parkinson's disease[581]
- 🍄 Lowers high blood pressure, opens blood vessels[582,583,584,585]
- 🍄 Alleviates chronic obstructive pulmonary disease (COPD)[586,587]
- 🍄 Relieves allergic rhinitis and asthma[588,589]
- 🍄 Protects against lung injury or fibrosis[590,591,592]
- 🍄 Decreases allergy-associated airway inflammation[593]
- 🍄 Enhances mucous clearance in pulmonary diseases[594]
- 🍄 Improves immune function in bronchial airway[595]
- 🍄 Counteracts cellular senescence caused by airway cell exposure to cigarette smoke[596]
- 🍄 Ameliorates silicotic pulmonary fibrosis[597]
- 🍄 Ameliorates chemotherapy-induced pulmonary fibrosis (with steroids)[598]
- 🍄 Increases tolerance to inadequate oxygen supply[599,600,601]
- 🍄 Antituberculosis (as an adjunct treatment)[602]
- 🍄 Antidiabetic[603-611]
- 🍄 Reduces insulin resistance, improves glucose metabolism and insulin sensitivity in nondiabetic subjects[612,613,614]
- 🍄 Prevents or delays diabetes[615,616]
- 🍄 Antidepressant[617,618]
- 🍄 Alleviates colitis[619]
- 🍄 Gastrointestinal protective and restorative[620,621]
- 🍄 Anti-inflammatory[622,623,624,625,626]
- 🍄 Relieves pain[627]
- 🍄 Prevents osteoporosis[628,629,630]
- 🍄 Prevents osteoporosis (with strontium)[631,632]
- 🍄 Protects against osteopenia caused by diabetes[633]
- 🍄 Diminishes lupus disease severity[634,635,636]

- ﾃ Reduces autoimmunity/transplant rejection, immunomodulatory (suppresses or balances immune function)[637-650]
- ﾃ Protects against immunosuppression of various causes[651,652,653,654]
- ﾃ Stimulates immune function (likely contingent on which polysaccharides are present and their amounts)[655-675]
- ﾃ Regulates immune function during chronic kidney failure[676]
- ﾃ Alleviates autoimmune encephalomyelitis[677]
- ﾃ Anti-infectious (Group A streptococcus)[678]
- ﾃ Antiviral (HIV-1)[679]
- ﾃ Enhances phagocytosis during group A streptococcal infection[680]
- ﾃ Alleviates polycystic kidney disease[681]
- ﾃ Renal protection after hepatitis B infection[682]
- ﾃ Protects against diabetic kidney damage (nephropathy)[683-691]
- ﾃ Kidney protective[692-712]
- ﾃ Promotes regrowth of injured renal tubular cells[713]
- ﾃ Liver protective[714-726]
- ﾃ Liver protective, except when combined with exercise[727]
- ﾃ Preserves pancreatic beta-cell production despite liver fibrosis[728]
- ﾃ Protects against bone marrow damage caused by radiation[729]
- ﾃ Improves creation of bone marrow[730]
- ﾃ Cardioprotective[731,732,733,734]
- ﾃ Cardio protective (chemotherapy-induced damage)[735]
- ﾃ May help prevent or manage cardiovascular diseases (antiplatelet activity)[736,737,738,739]
- ﾃ Balances heart rate (antiarrhythmic)[740]
- ﾃ Inhibits abdominal aortic thrombosis (blood clot blockage of a main artery)[741]
- ﾃ Alleviates viral myocarditis[742]
- ﾃ Neuroprotective[743-750]
- ﾃ Neurovascular protection[751]
- ﾃ Fights dementia[752]
- ﾃ Improves learning and memory[753]
- ﾃ Protects against arteriosclerosis after aortic transplant[754]
- ﾃ Antiaging (brain, sexual function)[755]
- ﾃ Prolongs lifespan[756]
- ﾃ Triggers autophagy[757]
- ﾃ Improves lipid profiles[758,759,760,761]
- ﾃ Combats obesity (inhibits lipase)[762]
- ﾃ Combats obesity (improves microbiome and bile acid metabolism)[763]
- ﾃ Improves sleep regulation and quality[764]

- 🍄 Increases testosterone[765,766,767,768]
- 🍄 Increases progesterone[769]
- 🍄 Increases estrogen and quality of maturing oocytes (enhances female fertility)[770]
- 🍄 Enhances male reproductive function[771-779]
- 🍄 Stimulates corticosterone production[780,781]
- 🍄 Improves physical performance and endurance, relieves fatigue[782,783,784,785,786]
- 🍄 Increases energy production in the liver, including during iron-deficiency anemia[787,788]
- 🍄 Relieves oral lichen planus[789]
- 🍄 Improves the appearance of the skin[790]
- 🍄 Protects skin against UV-B damage[791]
- 🍄 Antiviral (hepatitis B virus)[792]
- 🍄 Antiviral (feline immunodeficiency virus)[793]
- 🍄 Antibacterial[794,795]
- 🍄 Provides both "Yang" (invigorating) and "Yin" (nourishing) activities (adaptogenic)[796]
- 🍄 Antioxidant[797-810]
- 🍄 Stimulates antioxidant systems[811]
- 🍄 Protects against oxidative stress/damage[812-820]

CORDYCEPS SINENSIS—BENEFITS ACCORDING TO CLINICAL RESEARCH:

- ➤ Supportive after a kidney transplant (primarily to reduce rejection)[821-828]
  - 1,000–6,000 mg daily, in three divided doses
- ➤ Restores immune balance in people with either Graves' disease or Hashimoto's[829]
  - 2,000 mg of fermented powders, three times daily (Corbrin)
- ➤ Chronic obstructive pulmonary disease (COPD)[830]
  - Usually as part of a multi-ingredient product
- ➤ Moderate-to-severe asthma[831]
  - 1,200 mg of fermented cordyceps (Corbin), three times daily
- ➤ Chronic kidney disease[832]
  - 600–2,000 mg, three times daily
- ➤ Protects against aminoglycoside kidney toxicity[833]
  - Article in Chinese, unknown dosage
- ➤ Support during hemodialysis[834]
  - 600–2,500 mg, three times daily
- ➤ Alleviates symptoms of diabetic kidney disease (inflammation, dyslipidemia, excess protein in the urine)[835]
  - 1,000–2,000 mg, three times daily (with angiotensin-converting enzyme inhibitors/angiotensin receptor blockers)

- Prevents renal damage caused by contrast in people with acute coronary syndrome during elective percutaneous coronary intervention[836]
  - Corbrin capsule containing 2,000 mg cordyceps, three times daily, for three days prior to procedure
- Alleviates liver fibrosis/damage in people with chronic hepatitis B[837,838]
  - Articles in Chinese, unknown dosage
- Recovers balance of Th1/Th2 cytokines and enhances Th1 immune response in people with anogenital warts caused by HPV[839]
  - Article in Chinese, unknown dosage
- Improves exercise performance in older adults[840]
  - 1,000 mg, three times daily, for twelve weeks
- Does not improve endurance exercise performance in trained athletes[841]
  - 1,050 mg, three times daily, for five weeks

CORDYCEPS MILITARIS—BENEFITS ACCORDING TO PRECLINICAL RESEARCH:

- Anticancer (lung)[842-857]
- Anticancer (ovarian)[858,859,860]
- Anticancer (cervical)[861,862]
- Anticancer (colorectal)[863-873]
- Anticancer (liver)[874,875,876,877,878]
- Anticancer (kidney)[879,880]
- Anticancer (breast)[881-893]
- Anticancer (prostate)[894,895,896]
- Anticancer (bladder)[897,898,899,900]
- Anticancer (pancreatic)[901]
- Anticancer (gastric)[902]
- Anticancer (glioblastoma)[903,904]
- Anticancer (neuroblastoma)[905]
- Anticancer (melanoma)[906]
- Anticancer (malignant melanoma)[907,908]
- Anticancer (inhibits melanoma metastasis)[909]
- Anticancer (skin; squamous cell carcinoma)[910]
- Anticancer (liver)[911,912,913]
- Anticancer (acute promyelocytic leukemia)[914-922]
- Anticancer (chronic myeloid leukemia)[923,924]
- Anticancer (eosinophilic leukemia)[925]
- Anticancer (histiocytic lymphoma)[926]
- Anticancer (lymphoma)[927]
- Anticancer (oral)[928,929]

- ♈ Anticancer (esophageal)[930]
- ♈ Reverses immunosuppressive tumor microenvironment[931]
- ♈ Inhibits the proliferation of malignant peripheral nerve sheath tumors[932]
- ♈ Reduces the formation of blood vessels (antiangiogenic)[933]
- ♈ Anticancer (rodent lymphoma)[934]
- ♈ Anticancer (rodent liver)[935,936]
- ♈ Anticancer (rodent breast)[937]
- ♈ Anticancer (rodent melanoma)[938,939]
- ♈ Anticancer (rodent oral)[940]
- ♈ Anticancer (rodent sarcoma)[941]
- ♈ Reduces toxicity of chemotherapy to healthy cells[942]
- ♈ Mitigates cognitive impairment caused by chemotherapy[943]
- ♈ Protects DNA against damage caused by radiation therapy[944]
- ♈ Decreases cancer-related fatigue[945]
- ♈ Improves gut microbiome composition (increases short-chain fatty acids, acts as a prebiotic for *Lactobacilli*, increases *Allobaculum, Alistipes, Lachnospiraceae,* and *Muribaculaceae*, decreases *Enterococcus* and *Ruminococcus*, reduces obesity-related microbes)[946-953]
- ♈ Reduces leaky gut[954,955]
- ♈ Alleviates colitis[956,957,958]
- ♈ Antidiabetic[959-975]
- ♈ Alleviates damage caused by diabetes[976]
- ♈ Preserves vascular function during diabetes[977]
- ♈ Protects against kidney damage caused by diabetes (diabetic nephropathy)[978,979,980]
- ♈ Improves glucose and lipid metabolism, reduces insulin resistance (improves insulin sensitivity)[981-989]
- ♈ Maintains sexual function in male diabetics[990]
- ♈ Enhances lipid creation in a hypolipidemic model[991]
- ♈ Reverses metabolic disorders[992]
- ♈ Decreases high cholesterol and triglycerides[993,994,995,996]
- ♈ Improves or prevents atherosclerosis[997,998,999,1000,1001]
- ♈ Inhibits angiotensin-I-converting enzyme (ACE; lowers blood pressure and treats heart failure)[1002,1003,1004]
- ♈ Mitigates blood clots, lowers blood pressure (antiplatelet, antithrombotic)[1005-1011]
- ♈ Increases survival after hypertension[1012]
- ♈ Mitigates thoracic aortic aneurysm[1013]
- ♈ Cardioprotective[1014,1015]
- ♈ Protects against obesity[1016-1025]

- ♈ Supports healthy cognition (inhibits acetylcholinesterase; promotes neurite outgrowth)[1026,1027]
- ♈ Maintains learning function in healthy subjects[1028]
- ♈ Reverses memory and learning impairment[1029,1030,1031,1032]
- ♈ Regulates neuronal transmission[1033]
- ♈ Protects against Alzheimer's disease initiation and progression[1034,1035,1036]
- ♈ Neuroprotective[1037-1047]
- ♈ Reduces neuroinflammation[1048,1049,1050,1051,1052]
- ♈ Improves functional recovery after spinal cord injury[1053]
- ♈ Antidepressant[1054,1055]
- ♈ Improves oxygenation (antihypoxic)[1056]
- ♈ Reduces physical fatigue[1057,1058,1059,1060]
- ♈ Enhances physical performance, endurance, and strength, promotes cellular energy production[1061,1062]
- ♈ Kidney protective[1063,1064,1065]
- ♈ Improves chronic kidney disease[1066]
- ♈ Liver protective[1067,1068,1069]
- ♈ Combats liver fibrosis[1070,1071,1072]
- ♈ Protects against liver damage caused by alcohol[1073]
- ♈ Protects against acute pancreatitis[1074]
- ♈ Protects the reproductive system[1075]
- ♈ Improves bone strength[1076,1077,1078]
- ♈ Suppresses bone loss caused by inflammation[1079]
- ♈ Prevents poor development of bones caused by oxidative stress[1080]
- ♈ Alleviates osteoarthritis[1081]
- ♈ Relieves rheumatoid arthritis[1082]
- ♈ Combats nonalcoholic fatty liver disease[1083-1089]
- ♈ Reduces insomnia[1090]
- ♈ Lung protective[1091,1092]
- ♈ Enhances mucous clearance in pulmonary diseases[1093,1094]
- ♈ Decreases excess mucus production in airways[1095]
- ♈ Alleviates asthma[1096,1097,1098,1099,1100]
- ♈ Relieves bronchitis[1101]
- ♈ Relieves allergies[1102-1109]
- ♈ Stimulates immune function[1110-1136]
- ♈ Suppresses or balances immune function[1137,1138,1139,1140,1141]
- ♈ Preserves mitochondria function (antiaging)[1142,1143]
- ♈ Increases SIRT1 expression (antiaging)[1144]
- ♈ Activates AMPK (antiaging)[1145]

- Preserves vision/eyesight[1146,1147]
- Stimulates myogenesis, which may help treat and prevent degenerative muscle diseases caused by the depletion of muscle stem cells[1148]
- Anti-inflammatory[1149-1166]
- Reduces excess uric acid (hyperuricemia); helpful for gout[1167,1168,1169,1170,1171]
- Prevents or slows cartilage damage in osteoarthritic model[1172]
- Inhibits degeneration and inflammation in an intervertebral disc degeneration model[1173]
- Alleviates *Candida*-induced vaginitis[1174]
- Promotes male reproductive development and sexual function[1175-1183]
- Diminishes benign prostatic hyperplasia (enlarge prostate)[1184]
- Improves male hormones[1185]
- Antiviral (COVID-19)[1186]
- Combats COVID-19-related cytokine storm[1187]
- Antiviral (hepatitis C)[1188,1189]
- Antiviral (influenza H1N1, influenza A)[1190,1191]
- Antiviral (HIV-1)[1192]
- Relieves eczema (atopic dermatitis)[1193,1194,1195,1196]
- Skin antiaging (improves collagen synthesis and skin cell regeneration)[1197]
- Skin brightening[1198]
- Antimicrobial[1199-1207]
- Antioxidant[1208-1230]
- Protects against oxidative stress/damage[1231-1236]
- Larvicidal (diamondback moth—*Plutella xylostella*)[1237]
- Insecticidal (Colorado potato beetle—*Leptinotarsa decelineata*)[1238]
- Herbicidal[1239]

CORDYCEPS MILITARIS—BENEFITS ACCORDING TO CLINICAL RESEARCH:

- Improves tolerance to high-intensity exercise[1240]
  - 1,300 mg, three times daily for one week
- Speeds recovery of mild-moderate COVID-19[1241]
  - 500 mg, three times daily
- Enhances cell-mediated immunity (NKC activity and lymphocyte proliferation, partly increased Th1 cytokine secretion) in healthy men[1242]
  - 1,500 mg daily for four weeks

THERAPEUTIC POTENTIAL: Kidney transplant support, kidney disorders, COPD, asthma, allergies, traumatic brain injury, Hashimoto's, Graves' disease, lupus, dysbiosis, diabetes, fatigue, physical performance and endurance, weight management, gout, eczema, nonalcoholic fatty liver disease

CLINICAL DOSAGES: 600–6,000 mg daily

POTENTIAL ADVERSE EFFECTS: Abdominal discomfort, constipation or diarrhea, nonalcoholic fatty liver in obese individuals (based on a case study)

CAUTIONS AND CONTRAINDICATIONS: Pregnancy, lactation, autoimmune conditions, prior to surgery, cordyceps mushroom allergy; drugs that thin the blood, immunosuppressants

ENOKI

(Flammulina velutipes)

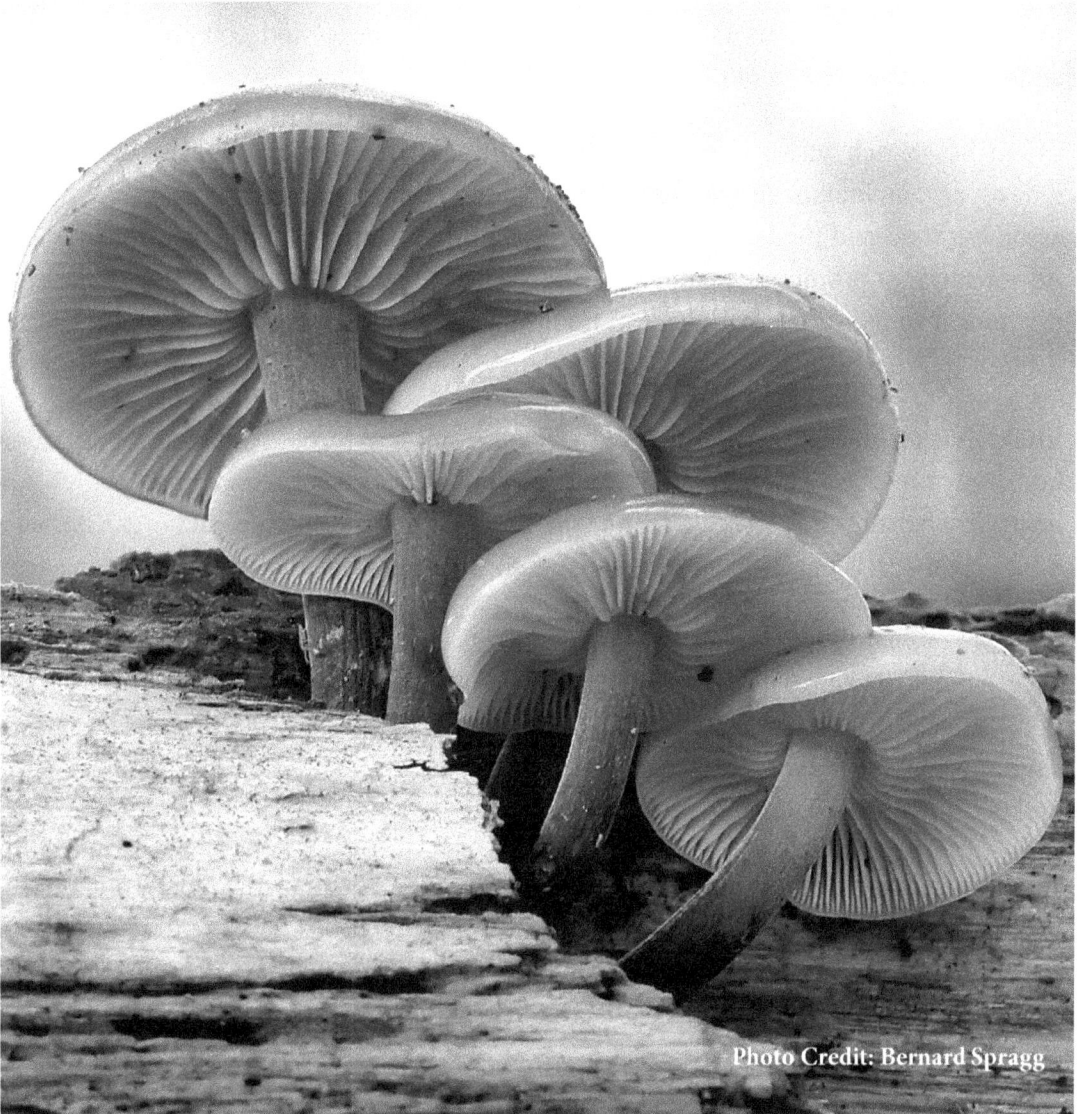

Photo Credit: Bernard Spragg

Kingdom: Fungi
Phylum: Basidiomycota
Class: Agaricomycetes
Order: Agaricales
Family: Physalacriaceae
Genus: Flammulina
Species: velutipes
Native Habitat: East Asia

Concealed in the vast number of mushrooms species, *Flammulina velutipes*, commonly known as the enoki mushroom, velvet shank mushroom, or golden needle mushroom, is a lesser-known fungal species with extraordinary medicinal properties. Native to East Asia but now cultivated and appreciated worldwide, this mushroom offers more than just culinary delights. Its medicinal value, historical uses, and composition make it another valuable mushroom for human health and well-being.

Enoki has a rich history, especially in traditional Chinese and Japanese medicine. Known as "enokitake" in Japanese, this mushroom has been a part of Japanese culture as both a food and medicine for centuries. Both the Chinese and Japanese recognized its potential for promoting health and vitality. Over time, its popularity has spread, and it is now a sought-after ingredient in traditional and modern wellness practices around the world.

Enoki is rich in polysaccharides, which are complex carbohydrates with immune-boosting properties. The mushroom contains antioxidants, such as selenium, which help neutralize harmful free radicals in the body, minimizing cell, tissue, and organ damage. Some compounds in enoki have demonstrated anti-inflammatory activity, which can be beneficial for conditions associated with chronic inflammation, such as arthritis.

As a culinary mushroom, enoki provides vitamins, minerals, protein, and fiber. It is a good source of vitamin D, B-vitamins, potassium, phosphorus, and iron. It has a mild savory or umami flavor and a crunchy texture. Enoki mushrooms lose their crispness and become chewier the longer they are cooked.

Enoki mushrooms have garnered increasing attention for their medicinal potential in natural health. Research is continually uncovering its benefits, leading to its utilization in various applications, including for immune support, inflammatory conditions, respiratory disorders, digestive health, cardiovascular function, and even cancer.

Although a mushroom some are unaware of, hundreds of studies have shed light on the medicinal properties it possesses, making it show up in mushroom complexes available commercially more frequently. Research shows that it has significant antioxidant potential and the ability to reduce inflammation. Its polysaccharides stimulate immune system function improving cancer surveillance and vigilance against infectious pathogens. Enoki can also protect the heart by reducing atherosclerosis and is a focus of research surrounding neurodegenerative conditions like Alzheimer's disease.

There are several ways to incorporate enoki into your wellness routine to harness its medicinal value. The first is to add it to dishes. It is a popular ingredient in Asian cuisine and frequently used in soups, stir-fries, and hot pots. For greater therapeutic value, dietary supplements in the forms of capsules, powders, and tinctures are used. In traditional Chinese and Japanese medicine, health-care practitioners may prescribe enoki as part of herbal formulas tailored to individual health needs. It also has value in personal care and cosmetic products because of its antioxidant and anti-inflammatory properties, which can help reduce the signs of aging.

The Enoki mushroom is not only a delectable ingredient in various culinary dishes but also a remarkable medicinal mushroom with a rich history and promising health benefits. Whether you seek to support your immune system, manage inflammation, reduce the risk of chronic diseases, or explore its potential in cancer prevention and treatment, enoki offers a wide array of health advantages. As scientific research continues to unravel the medicinal value of this mushroom, it remains a promising natural solution to promote a healthier, more vibrant life.

NOTABLE COMPOUNDS: Polysaccharides, phenols, polyphenols, terpenoids, beta-glucans, sterols, ergosterol, 22,23-dihydroergosterol, enokipodins A-D, flammupin A and B, flavonoids, arbutin, epicatechin, phillyrin, apigenin, kaempferol, formononetin, ergothioneine, FIP-fve protein, flammin, velin, chitoglucan, adenosine

BENEFITS ACCORDING TO PRECLINICAL RESEARCH:

- 🍄 Anticancer (liver)[1243,1244]
- 🍄 Anticancer (prostate)[1245]
- 🍄 Anticancer (glioma)[1246]
- 🍄 Anticancer (gastric)[1247]
- 🍄 Anticancer (lung)[1248]
- 🍄 Anticancer (breast)[1249]
- 🍄 Anticancer (myelogenous leukemia)[1250]
- 🍄 Alleviates cisplatin-induced kidney damage[1251]
- 🍄 Anticancer (rodent melanoma)[1252]
- 🍄 Anticancer (rodent lymphocytic leukemia)[1253,1254,1255]
- 🍄 Anticancer (rodent sarcoma)[1256]
- 🍄 Anticancer (rodent liver)[1257]
- 🍄 Neuroprotective[1258]
- 🍄 Suppresses neuroinflammation[1259]
- 🍄 Promotes nerve regeneration[1260]
- 🍄 Reverse memory and learning impairment[1261]
- 🍄 Enhances cognition in Alzheimer's disease[1262]
- 🍄 Reduces motor impairment and demyelination in a multiple sclerosis model[1263]
- 🍄 Improves the gut microbiome (improves flora balance and structure, increases the relative abundance of *Bacteroidaceae, Bifidobacteriaceae,*

Lachnospiraceae, Lactobacillaceae, Saccharomyces, Mycosphaerella, and *Alloprevotella*, remarkably reduces the relative abundance of *Lachnospiraceae, Muribaculaceae, Pleosporaceae,* and *Enterococcaceae*, balances the Firmicutes/Bacteroidetes ratio, enhances production of short-chain fatty acids)[1264-1276]

- Enhances gut health and protects against intestinal inflammation[1277,1278]
- Strengthens gut barrier integrity (reduces leaky gut), although some research suggests that some of its proteins may increase intestinal permeability instead[1279,1280]
- Alleviates ulcerative colitis[1281]
- Stimulates immune function[1282-1302]
- Balances immune function[1303]
- Anti-inflammatory[1304,1305,1306,1307]
- Reduces pulmonary inflammation and respiratory pathogenesis, making it useful for allergic airway diseases[1308-1313]
- Mitigates food allergies[1314]
- Promotes healthy aging[1315,1316]
- Reduces fatigue and slows aging by increasing testosterone production in males[1317]
- Liver protective[1318,1319,1320,1321]
- Improves lipid metabolism and lipid profiles[1322,1323,1324,1325,1326]
- Attenuates metabolic syndrome[1327]
- Aids cardiovascular function[1328]
- Inhibits angiotensin-converting enzyme (ACE), which may lower blood pressure[1329]
- Kidney protective[1330]
- Protects against damage caused by oxidative stress[1331]
- Ameliorates lead poisoning[1332]
- Increases total antioxidant capacity[1333,1334,1335]
- Antioxidant[1336-1351]
- Combats obesity[1352,1353]
- Treats full-thickness skin defects and noncompressible hemorrhages (bleeding in inaccessible sites in the body where compression cannot be applied)[1354]
- Accelerates wound healing[1355,1356,1357]
- Brightens the skin[1358]
- Antiviral (hepatitis B)[1359]
- Antiviral (respiratory syncytial virus replication and inflammation)[1360,1361]
- Antiviral (influenza type A, H1N1)[1362]
- Antimicrobial[1363,1364,1365,1366,1367]

- 🍄 Nematocidal[1368]
- 🍄 Degrades mycotoxins[1369]
- 🍄 Biodegrades or removes chemicals in the environment[1370]

BENEFITS ACCORDING TO CLINICAL RESEARCH:

➢ None found

THERAPEUTIC POTENTIAL: Dysbiosis or improving the gut microbiome, wound healing, allergic asthma

CLINICAL DOSAGES: Unknown; usually as part of a mushroom complex

POTENTIAL ADVERSE EFFECTS: Stomach upset, diarrhea or constipation, vomiting, bloating

CAUTIONS AND CONTRAINDICATIONS: Pregnancy, lactation, enoki mushroom allergy

HONEY

(Armillaria mellea)

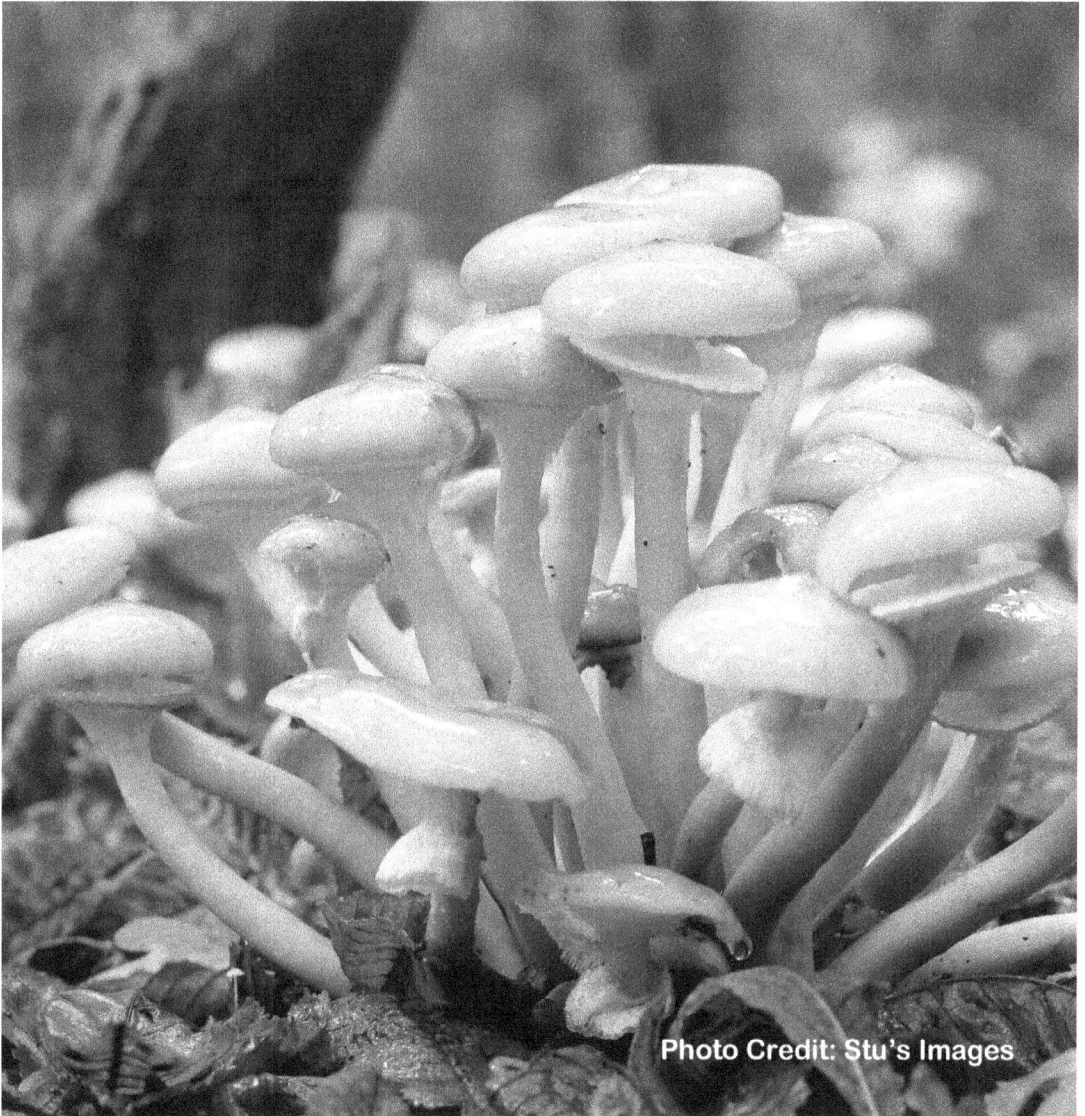

Photo Credit: Stu's Images

Kingdom: Fungi
Phylum: Basidiomycota
Class: Agaricomycetes
Order: Agaricales
Family: Physalacriaceae
Genus: Armillaria
Species: mellea
Native Habitat: North America, Europe, northern Asia

Commonly known as the honey mushroom or honey fungus, *Armillaria mellea* is a fascinating fungus that has drawn the attention of both mycologists and traditional healers alike. Beyond its culinary uses, this mushroom boasts a rich history of medicinal applications, making it a subject of growing interest in the field of natural medicine. It is widespread in northern temperate zones where it grows in clusters at the base of trees or stumps, especially oak trees. Recently, *Armillaria mellea* has been divided into various species that are identified by unique features, geographic distributions, or DNA analysis.

While primarily known for their medicinal properties, honey mushrooms also find a place in culinary traditions across the globe. The caps of the mature mushrooms are edible and are appreciated for their unique flavor. Rich in protein, fiber, and various essential minerals, honey mushrooms contribute to a well-balanced diet. However, it is crucial to note that proper identification is essential to avoid potential toxicity, as some *Armillaria* species can be confused with toxic varieties, such as the jack-o'-lantern mushroom (*Omphalotus illudens*) and the straw-colored fiber head mushroom (*Inocybe rimosa*, formerly *I. fastigiata*).

The medicinal value of honey mushrooms stems from the presence of bioactive compounds that exhibit various pharmacological properties. Rich in beta-glucans and polysaccharides known for their immune-modulating effects, honey mushrooms may enhance immune system function, making them a subject of interest in the field of immunotherapy. Additionally, honey mushrooms contain antioxidants, such as phenolic compounds, which play a crucial role in neutralizing free radicals in the body. Free radicals are implicated in various diseases and the aging process, and antioxidants help combat their harmful effects.

The immunomodulatory properties of honey mushrooms have been explored in the context of cancer therapy. While more research is needed, early studies suggest that certain compounds in honey mushrooms may exhibit anti-tumor activities and could potentially be integrated into cancer treatment protocols.

Traditional medicine has often turned to mushrooms for their antimicrobial properties, and honey mushrooms are no exception. Studies have shown that extracts from honey mushrooms possess antibacterial and antifungal activities. These properties open avenues for exploring the development of novel antimicrobial agents derived from honey mushrooms, which could be particularly valuable in the face of increasing antibiotic resistance.

Chronic inflammation is a key driving factor in various health conditions, from arthritis to cardiovascular diseases and depression to neurodegenerative disorders. Honey mushrooms contain compounds that exhibit anti-inflammatory properties, potentially offering a natural remedy for inflammatory disorders. Research in this area is ongoing, with a focus on understanding the mechanisms through which honey mushrooms modulate inflammatory responses.

Beyond scientific research, honey mushrooms have a history of traditional use in folk medicine. Indigenous cultures in different parts of the world have employed these mushrooms for various health purposes. From boosting the immune system to addressing respiratory conditions, the traditional knowledge surrounding honey mushrooms provides a valuable foundation for modern scientific exploration.

As the scientific community continues to unveil the value of honey mushrooms, there is growing interest in their potential applications in mainstream medicine. The development of standardized extracts or formulations derived from honey mushrooms could pave the way for the integration of these mushrooms into conventional medicine.

Honey mushrooms have value as natural solutions due to their emerging medicinal potential. From immunomodulatory effects to antioxidant and anti-inflammatory properties, the compounds found in honey mushrooms offer a diverse array of health benefits. As research in this field progresses, we may witness the integration of honey mushrooms into mainstream medicine, providing a natural and holistic approach to health and wellness.

NOTABLE COMPOUNDS: Polysaccharides, beta-glucans, phenolics, triterpenoids, sesquiterpenoids, protoilludane sesquiterpenoid aromatic esters, armillarikin, armillarin, amillaridin, armillaric acid, galactitol, arnamial, melleolides, tryptamine, L-tryptophan, serotonin

BENEFITS ACCORDING TO PRECLINICAL RESEARCH:

- Anticancer (liver)[1371,1372,1373]
- Anticancer (lung)[1374]
- Anticancer (breast)[1375]
- Anticancer (cervical)[1376]
- Anticancer (lymphoblastic leukemia. T cell leukemia, myelogenous leukemia)[1377,1378,1379]
- Anticancer (colorectal)[1380]
- Anticancer (esophageal; also enhances radiation effectiveness)[1381]
- Protects against damage caused by cyclophosphamide[1382]
- Improves the gut microbiome (increases the relative abundance of Lachnospiraceae, Ruminococcaceae, and Saccharimonadaceae)[1383,1384]

- 🍄 Enhances memory and learning[1385]
- 🍄 Neuroprotective[1386,1387,1388]
- 🍄 Mitigates neuroinflammation[1389]
- 🍄 Alleviates depression[1390,1391]
- 🍄 Improves sleep or relieves insomnia[1392,1393]
- 🍄 Stimulates immune function[1394,1395.1396]
- 🍄 Balances immune function (acts as a biological response modifier in inflammatory conditions)[1397]
- 🍄 Antidiabetic[1398,1399,1400]
- 🍄 Ameliorates liver fibrosis[1401]
- 🍄 Anti-inflammatory[1402]
- 🍄 Alleviates swelling[1403]
- 🍄 Reduces uric acid levels (fights gout)[1404,1405]
- 🍄 Enhances internal antioxidant defenses (glutathione peroxidase and superoxide dismutase)[1406]
- 🍄 Antioxidant[1407-1415]
- 🍄 Antimicrobial[1416,1417,1418]
- 🍄 Biodegrades pharmaceuticals, especially cardiovascular drugs and sulfamethoxazole[1419]

BENEFITS ACCORDING TO CLINICAL RESEARCH:

- ➢ None found.

THERAPEUTIC POTENTIAL: Insomnia, gout

CLINICAL DOSAGES: Unknown; typically used as part of a mushroom complex

POTENTIAL ADVERSE EFFECTS: Stomach upset, nausea/vomiting, diarrhea

CAUTIONS AND CONTRAINDICATIONS: Pregnancy, lactation, honey mushroom allergy

KING OYSTER
(Pleurotus eryngii)

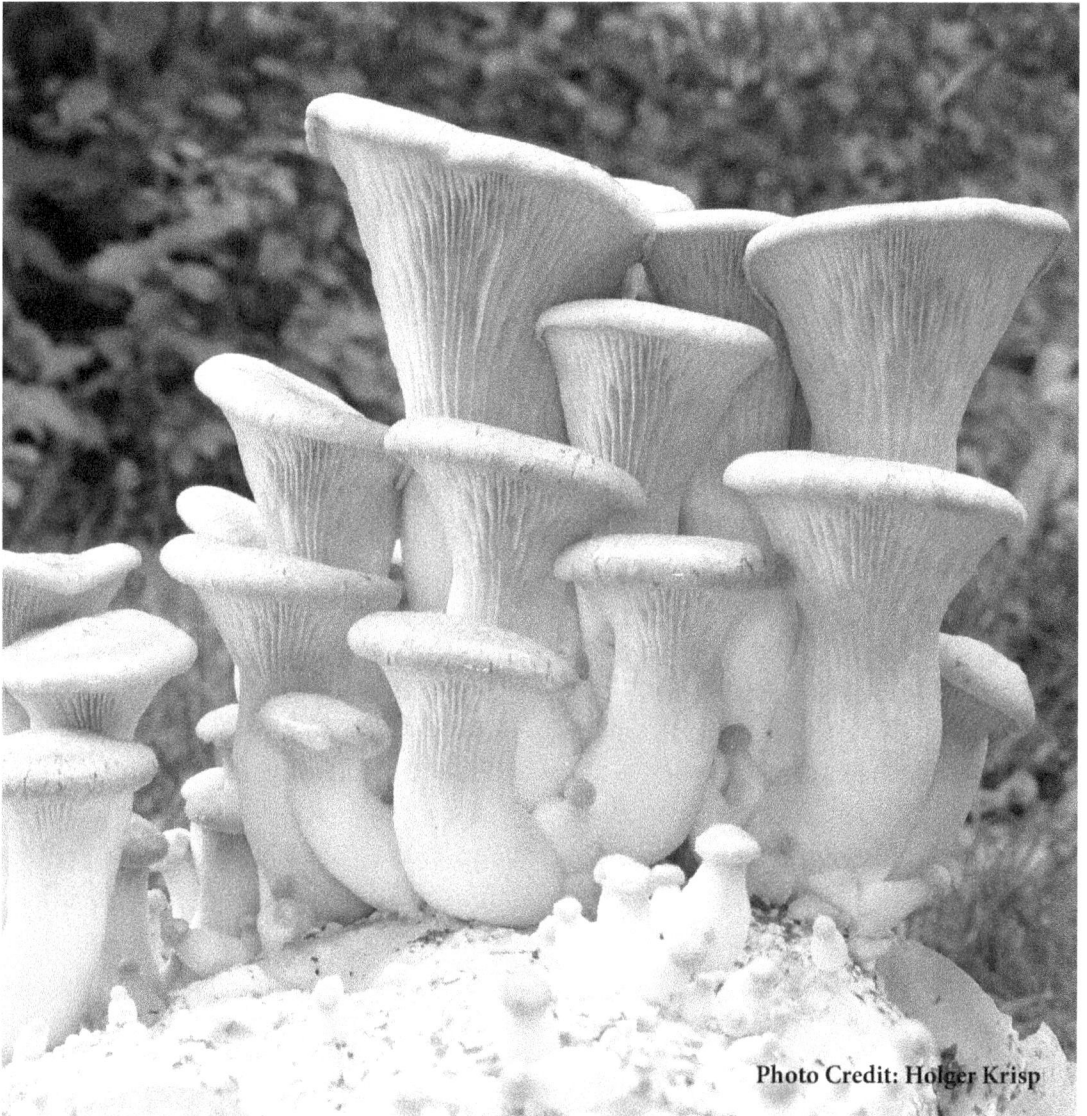

Photo Credit: Holger Krisp

Kingdom: Fungi
Phylum: Basidiomycota
Class: Agaricomycetes
Order: Agaricales
Family: Pleurotaceae
Genus: Pleurotus
Species: eryngii
Native Habitat: Mediterranean regions of Europe, the Middle East, and North Africa

Commonly known as the king trumpet mushroom, French horn mushroom, eringi, or king oyster mushroom, *Pleurotus eryngii* has gained popularity not only for its culinary usage but also for its significant medicinal potential. The king oyster mushroom belongs to the fungal family Pleurotaceae and the genus Pleurotus. This mushroom is native to Mediterranean regions of Europe, the Middle East, and parts of North Africa but is now widely cultivated around the world. Its natural habitat includes grassy areas, particularly near the base of wild thistles and other plants in the Apiaceae family, such as wild carrot (*Daucus carota*) and sea holly (*Eryngium campestre*). In the wild, *Pleurotus eryngii* can be found growing in clusters on the ground, often appearing after rain during the autumn and winter months.

King oyster mushrooms have distinctive physical characteristics that make them easily recognizable. The fruiting body, which is the part of the mushroom that is typically harvested for consumption, consists of a thick, meaty stem and a large, flattened cap. The cap can measure up to 10 to 20 centimeters in diameter and ranges in color from creamy white to pale brown. The stem is often cylindrical, stout, and can grow up to 10 to 15 centimeters long and 2 to 4 centimeters in diameter. These features give the mushroom its alternative name, the king trumpet mushroom, as the stout stem and wide cap resemble the shape of a trumpet.

King oysters are highly regarded for their nutritional content. They are a low-calorie, fat-free, and cholesterol-free food, making them an excellent addition to a healthy diet. They are an excellent source of protein—containing all the essential amino acids, causing them to be a valuable choice for vegetarians and vegans. These mushrooms are rich in dietary fiber, which aids in digestion and helps maintain a healthy digestive system. King oyster mushrooms are also a good source of B vitamins, particularly vitamin B3 (niacin) and vitamin B5 (pantothenic acid). They also contain modest amounts of vitamins B1 (thiamine) and B2 (riboflavin). They are rich in minerals like potassium, phosphorus, and copper, and contain smaller amounts of iron, selenium, and zinc.

King oyster mushrooms gained recognition and popularity in the culinary world for their unique flavor, meaty texture, and versatility. Its culinary uses span a wide range of dishes, including soups, stir-fries, salads, and more.

Beyond its culinary appeal, king oyster mushrooms offer myriad potential health benefits, making them an attractive subject for scientific research. The medicinal properties associated with this mushroom are primarily attributed to its bioactive compounds, including polysaccharides, antioxidants, and other unique compounds. The polysaccharides in king oyster mushrooms have been shown to have immunomodulatory effects, meaning they may enhance immune responses and help protect against infections. They contain antioxidants that can neutralize harmful free radicals and reduce oxidative stress, potentially reducing the risk of chronic diseases. Some research suggests that king oyster mushroom extracts may possess anti-inflammatory properties, while other research shows they possess antimicrobial activity. The king oyster mushroom may aid cardiovascular function because of its effects on blood pressure and cholesterol levels. Like many other mushrooms, their anticancer activity has also been investigated. Moreover, there is evidence to suggest that certain components of these mushrooms have neuroprotective properties and could potentially play a role in conditions related to neurodegeneration. Some studies indicate that king oyster mushrooms may help regulate blood sugar levels and could be beneficial for individuals with diabetes. Finally, the mushroom may support liver health by promoting detoxification and protecting the liver from damage.

The long list of medicinal properties of king oyster mushrooms have piqued the interest of researchers and scientists. Numerous studies have been conducted to better understand the potential health benefits of this mushroom, with current findings showing immunomodulatory, antioxidant, anticancer, anti-inflammatory, neuroprotective, cardioprotective, liver protective, antidiabetic, and bone strengthening properties.

The king oyster mushroom has not been researched as widely as its cousin the oyster mushroom (*Pleurotus ostreatus*), but its currently discovered properties and historical usage show it has remarkable medicinal value. Scientific research on this unique mushroom is continually expanding, shedding light on the various ways in which this mushroom may support health and well-being. As we continue to explore its potential, more will be revealed about this valuable member of the fungal kingdom's purpose in human health.

NOTABLE COMPOUNDS: Ergothioneine, polysaccharides, beta-glucans, bisabolane-type sesquiterpenes, rhamnose, arabinose, mannose, xylose, galactose, polypeptides, sterols, ubiquinone-9, pleurone, ergosterol peroxide, glutathione

BENEFITS ACCORDING TO PRECLINICAL RESEARCH:

- 🍄 Anticancer (liver)[1420,1421,1422,1423]
- 🍄 Anticancer (stomach adenocarcinoma)[1424,1425]
- 🍄 Anticancer (gastric)[1426,1427]
- 🍄 Anticancer (colorectal)[1428,1429,1430]
- 🍄 Anticancer (lung)[1431]
- 🍄 Anticancer (kidney)[1432]
- 🍄 Anticancer (cervical)[1433,1434]
- 🍄 Anticancer (acute myeloid leukemia)[1435]
- 🍄 Anticancer (breast)[1436,1437,1438]

- ☙ Blocks the activity of aromatase to lower estrogen levels—often used to treat breast cancer on postmenopausal women and gynecomastia in men[1439]
- ☙ Inhibits angiogenesis[1440]
- ☙ Maintains genome integrity—preserves the function of embryonic stem cells, which is a key to reducing the risk of cancer[1441]
- ☙ Ameliorates lung toxicity caused by doxorubicin[1442]
- ☙ Protects against testicular damage caused by doxorubicin[1443]
- ☙ Anticancer (rodent colorectal)[1444]
- ☙ Anticancer (rodent melanoma)[1445]
- ☙ Anticancer (rodent sarcoma)[1446]
- ☙ Improves gut microbiome (increases abundance of *Lactobacilli, Bifidobacteria, Lachnospiraceae, Porphyromonadaceae, Bacteroidaceae,* and *Rikenellaceae,* slightly increases abundance of Firmicutes, enhances short-chain fatty acid production)[1447-1453]
- ☙ Increases bile acid secretion[1454]
- ☙ Maintains intestinal integrity (reduces leaky gut)[1455]
- ☙ Enhances intestinal immunity, as well as expression of digestion and absorption proteins in the GI tract[1456]
- ☙ Ameliorates ulcerative colitis[1457,1458]
- ☙ Relieves inflammatory bowel disease[1459]
- ☙ Antidepressant[1460,1461]
- ☙ Preserves cognitive function (promotes neurite outgrowth, reduces neuroinflammation, normalizes zinc signaling, and protects neurons)[1462,1463]
- ☙ Alleviates memory and learning deficits (Alzheimer's disease)[1464,1465]
- ☙ Exerts antiplatelet effects (may help prevent or manage cardiovascular diseases)[1466]
- ☙ Prevents atherosclerosis[1467]
- ☙ Lowers high cholesterol[1468-1479]
- ☙ Alleviates fatty liver[1480]
- ☙ Combats obesity[1481,1482,1483,1484,1485]
- ☙ Alleviates insulin resistance[1486]
- ☙ Antidiabetic[1487,1488,1489,1490]
- ☙ Protects against diabetic-related kidney damage (diabetic nephropathy)[1491]
- ☙ Guards against organ damage caused by diabetes[1492]
- ☙ Stimulates or enhances immune function[1493-1506]
- ☙ Manages heart failure and reduces high blood pressure (inhibits angiotensin-I-converting enzyme)[1507]
- ☙ Normalizes skeletal development and growth during childhood despite an unbalanced diet[1508]

- ☂ Prevents osteoporosis[1509]
- ☂ Preserves bone density postmenopause related to estrogen deficiency (conflicting research)[1510,1511,1512]
- ☂ Antiallergic[1513]
- ☂ Mitigates multiple sclerosis (improves motor dysfunction and suppresses demyelination)[1514]
- ☂ Anti-inflammatory[1515,1516,1517,1518,1519,1520]
- ☂ Decrease lung inflammation[1521]
- ☂ Liver protective[1522,1523]
- ☂ Enhances antioxidant activity in aged subjects to potentially limit damage to multiple organs and reduce the risk of age-related conditions[1524]
- ☂ Mitigates oxidative stress and associated damage[1525,1526,1527]
- ☂ Antioxidant[1528-1547]
- ☂ Prevents or relieves eczema[1548]
- ☂ Preserves skin elasticity[1549]
- ☂ Antiviral (influenza H1N1)[1550]
- ☂ Antimicrobial[1551,1552,1553,1554,1555]
- ☂ Inhibits *H. pylori*, which could prevent gastric ulcers and gastric cancer[1556]
- ☂ Anthelmintic[1557]
- ☂ Detoxifies and degrades mycotoxins (aflatoxin B1)[1558,1559,1560]
- ☂ Remediates or biodegrades harmful chemicals[1561-1569]

BENEFITS ACCORDING TO CLINICAL RESEARCH:

- ➢ Manages metabolic disorders in metabolically unhealthy people[1570]
  - A snack with irradiated sliced mushrooms to enhance vitamin D content
- ➢ Improves postprandial (after-meal) blood sugar levels, promotes feelings of fullness and reduces hunger, and enhances ghrelin suppression (which reduces appetite) in obese individuals who are metabolically unhealthy[1571]
  - A meal with whole sliced mushrooms

THERAPEUTIC POTENTIAL: Diabetes, metabolic syndrome, high cholesterol, dysbiosis, infections

CLINICAL DOSAGES: Whole mushrooms incorporated into the diet; typical doses: 1,000 mg up to three times daily

POTENTIAL ADVERSE EFFECTS: Stomach upset, airway constriction or lung diseases if inhaled

CAUTIONS AND CONTRAINDICATIONS: Pregnancy, lactation, king oyster mushroom allergy; antidiabetic drugs, cholesterol-lowering drugs, drugs that affect blood pressure, immunosuppressants

LION'S MANE

(Hericium erinaceus)

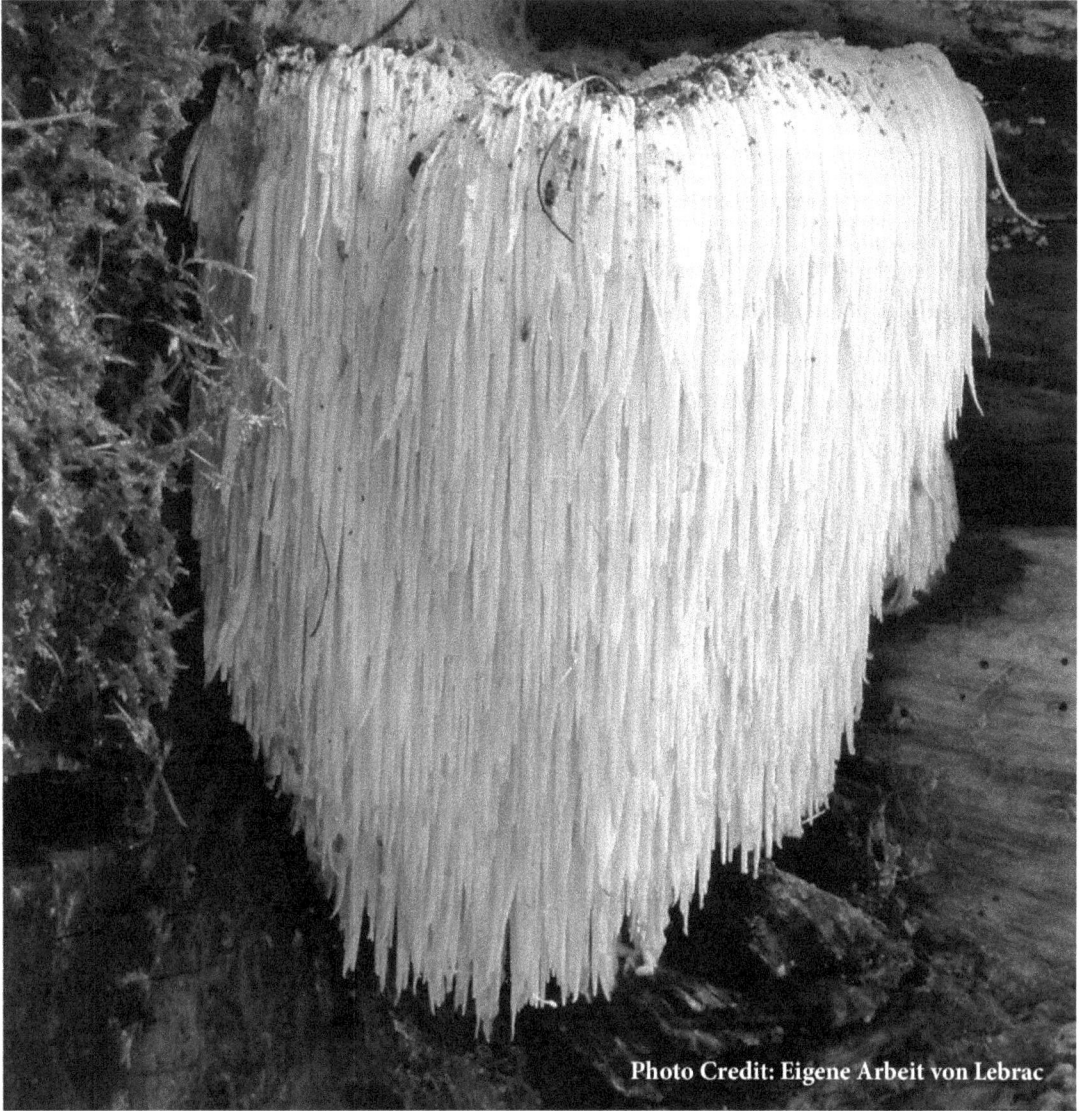

Photo Credit: Eigene Arbeit von Lebrac

Kingdom: Fungi
Phylum: Basidiomycota
Class: Agaricomycetes
Order: Russulales
Family: Hericiaceae
Genus: Hericium
Species: erinaceus
Native Habitat: North America, Europe, and Asia

With a striking resemblance to a lion's mane and the potential to boost brain health, support cognitive function, and enhance overall well-being, lion's mane mushroom (*Hericium erinaceus*) is a uniquely intriguing fungus with an impressive range of health benefits. Also known as "yamabushitake" in Japan, "monkey head mushroom" in China, and "pom pom blanc" in France, lion's mane grows on hardwood trees, particularly oak and beech trees. Lion's Mane is naturally found in temperate regions of North America, Europe, and Asia. Lion's Mane boasts cascading, white, hair-like spines that bear a striking resemblance to a lion's mane, hence its name. These spines can grow in clusters, forming impressive and eye-catching specimens in the wild.

Like most mushrooms, the origin of lion's mane mushroom's medicinal use begins in Asia, particularly in China, Japan, and Korea. It was revered for its potential health benefits and was traditionally used to address a variety of ailments. Lion's mane is probably best known for its cognitive benefits. It was historically believed to enhance mental clarity and brain power, and frequently used to improve memory and concentration—traditional uses that have been confirmed by modern research. Lion's mane was also used traditionally to promote digestive comfort, calm the nervous system during periods of stress and anxiety, boost immune function, reduce inflammation, and accelerate wound healing.

The resurgence of interest in natural remedies and traditional medicine has led to extensive scientific research into lion's mane, particularly since scientists are looking for novel ways to preserve or improve memory and thinking. Modern studies have provided valuable insights into the active compounds and potential health benefits associated with this noteworthy fungus. One of the most important findings is its neurotrophic properties. Lion's mane contains compounds called hericenones and erinacines that stimulate the production of nerve growth factor (NGF). NGF plays a crucial role in the growth, maintenance, and repair of neurons, making lion's mane a potential ally in supporting brain health and cognitive function. Because of this, lion's mane has massive potential to improve memory, concentration, and overall cognitive function. Today, it is a popular natural remedy for age-related cognitive decline and neurodegenerative conditions like Alzheimer's disease.

In addition, some studies indicate that lion's mane may promote nerve regeneration, which could have implications for individuals recovering from nerve injuries or conditions affecting the nervous system like neuropathy. It also possesses anti-inflammatory and antioxidant properties, which creates further interest in it to alleviate age-related conditions. Lastly, lion's mane has the potential to combat certain types of cancer.

In recent years, Lion's mane mushroom has experienced a surge in popularity as a natural supplement and functional food. Its adaptogenic and nootropic properties have shined a spotlight on not just lion's mane but mushrooms in general as excellent natural solutions for human health. If your goal is to maintain cognitive and memory function throughout the aging process—and who isn't striving for this?—you need to become familiar with lion's mane mushroom.

NOTABLE COMPOUNDS: Hericenones (A, B, I, O, P, Q, R), erinacines (erinacine A and S), beta-glucans, erinacine A, polysaccharides, erinarol K, phenols (erinaphenol A), erinachromanes A and B, flavonoids, isoindolinones (hericerin, isohericerinol A, N-de-phenylethyl isohericerin, and corallocin A), isolectins, ergosterol perozide, ursolic acid, sesquiterpene lactones, cerebrosides

BENEFITS ACCORDING TO PRECLINICAL RESEARCH:

- Anticancer (lung)[1572,1573]
- Anticancer (gastric)[1574,1575,1576,1577]
- Destroys precancerous gastric cells[1578]
- Anticancer (glioblastoma)[1579]
- Anticancer (cardiovascular)[1580]
- Anticancer (colorectal)[1581-1586]
- Anticancer (liver)[1587,1588]
- Prevents liver cancer[1589]
- Anticancer (acute myeloid leukemia)[1590]
- Anticancer (prevents metastasis: colon to lung)[1591]
- Anticancer (lung, prevents metastasis)[1592]
- Anticancer (liver, enhances doxorubicin activity)[1593]
- Anticancer (improves 5-fluorouracil activity by altering the gut microbiome)[1594]
- Reduces kidney toxicity caused by cisplatin[1595]
- Relieves neuropathic pain (eranicine S)[1596]
- Alleviates chronic pain, prevents morphine tolerance[1597,1598]
- Promotes neurite outgrowth, the creation of nerve growth factor (vital for the survival, growth, and maintenance of neurons), and the creation and survival of nerve cells (neurotrophic)[1599-1610]
- Stimulates nerve myelination (oligodendrocytes maturation, regulates myelin creation)[1611,1612]
- Promotes nerve regeneration and healing after injury[1613,1614,1615,1616]
- Encourages nerve regeneration (increase neurosteroid accumulation in nerve cells)[1617]
- Neuroprotective[1618-1635]
- Protects brain cells during and after seizure[1636]
- Repairs brain cells[1637]

- Preserves or improves cognitive and memory function[1638-1644]
- Reduces neuroinflammation[1645,1646,1647,1648,1649,1650]
- Alleviates Alzheimer's disease (improves memory, reduces behavioral alterations) [1651-1658]
- Mitigates delayed sleep phase syndrome associated with Alzheimer's disease[1659]
- Delays progression of age-related cognitive decline[1660]
- Prevents the progression of traumatic brain injury to Parkinson's disease[1661]
- Reduces symptoms of and neurotoxicity caused by Parkinson's disease[1662,1663]
- Antidepressant[1664,1665,1666,1667]
- Relieves anxiety[1668,1669]
- Alleviates anxiety caused by chronic sleep disturbance[1670]
- Improves gut microbiome (increases short-chain fatty acids, *Bifidobacterium, Faecalibacterium, Blautia, Butyricicoccus*, and *Lactobacillus*; reduces pathogenic bacteria: *Escherichia-Shigella, Klebsiella*, and *Enterobacter*)[1671-1677]
- Protects against age-related alterations in gut microbiome[1678]
- Enhances gut integrity, reduces leaky gut[1679,1680]
- Restores intestinal mucosal immunity and barrier function after damage by viral infection[1681,1682]
- Stomach protective, includes anti-*H. pylori* activity and protection of gastric cells[1683-1692]
- Protects against stomach damage caused by alcohol[1693,1694,1695,1696]
- Prevents mucosal injury in the colon/intestines[1697,1698]
- Ameliorates chronic atrophic gastritis[1699]
- Improves ulcerative colitis[1700,1701,1702,1703,1704,1705]
- Relieves inflammatory bowel disease[1706,1707]
- Promotes a healthy lifespan and longevity[1708,1709,1710]
- Liver protective[1711,1712,1713,1714]
- Shields against liver damage caused by alcohol[1715]
- Slows the progression of osteoarthritis[1716]
- Anti-inflammatory[1717,1718,1719,1720]
- Stimulates immune function (largely driven by regulating intestinal immune function)[1721-1740]
- Restores balanced immune function[1741]
- Reduces starch digestion (reduces blood sugar)[1742]
- Antidiabetic[1743-1750]
- Minimizes metabolic dysfunction and neurodegeneration caused by obesity[1751]
- Shields against diabetic-related organ (kidney, pancreas, liver) damage[1752,1753]
- Improves lipid metabolism[1754]
- Reduces high cholesterol[1755,1756]

- 🍄 Inhibits oxidation of cholesterol[1757]
- 🍄 Combats obesity[1758]
- 🍄 Diminishes inflammation associated with obesity[1759]
- 🍄 May prevent blood clots (antiplatelet)[1760]
- 🍄 Reduces fatigue[1761]
- 🍄 Enhances muscular endurance[1762]
- 🍄 Shields against damage caused by exposure to UV-A[1763]
- 🍄 Enhances wound healing[1764]
- 🍄 Diminishes inflammation after dengue infection[1765]
- 🍄 Antiviral (dengue virus serotype 2)[1766]
- 🍄 Antimicrobial[1767,1768,1769,1770]
- 🍄 Antioxidant[1771-1785]
- 🍄 Protects against oxidative stress damages[1786]
- 🍄 Prevents DNA mutations[1787]

BENEFITS ACCORDING TO CLINICAL RESEARCH:

- ➢ Improves cognitive function in healthy individuals over the age of fifty[1788]
  - 800 mg, four times daily for twelve weeks
- ➢ Reverses mild cognitive impairment in people aged fifty to eighty years old[1789]
  - 1,000 mg, three times daily for sixteen weeks
- ➢ Slows early Alzheimer's disease development in individuals older than fifty with a diagnosis of probable Alzheimer's disease[1790]
  - 350 mg capsules (standardized to 5mg/g erinacine A), three times daily for forty-nine weeks
- ➢ Reduces depression and anxiety[1791]
  - Consumption of four cookies daily containing 500 mg of lion's mane per cookie for four weeks
- ➢ Improves mood (reduced depression and anxiety) and sleep disorders in people who are overweight or obese, when combined with a low-calorie diet (1,400 calories for women and 1,700 calories for men)[1792]
  - 500 mg, three times daily for eight weeks
- ➢ Improves sleep quality and subjective well-being (elevated mood and decreased anxiety) among female college students
  - 650 mg (standardized to 6% amyloban; Amyloban 3399), three times daily for four weeks[1793]
- ➢ Improves the gut microbiome in healthy individuals (increases alpha diversity and short-chain fatty acid producing bacteria—Kineothrix alysoides, Gemmiger formicilis, Fusicatenibacter saccharivorans, Eubacterium rectale, Faecalibacterium prausnitzii—and reduces pathogenic bacteria, leading to

69

improved biomarkers—liver enzymes, LDL cholesterol, uric acid, and creatinine)[1794]
- 1,000 mg, three times daily for seven days
➤ Relieves chronic atrophic gastritis (abdominal discomfort, dyspepsia, and inflammatory infiltration)[1795]
- Article in Chinese, dose unknown

THERAPEUTIC POTENTIAL: Dementia/Alzheimer's disease prevention, cognitive function, depression, dysbiosis, gastritis, insomnia

CLINICAL DOSAGES: 350 to 1,000 mg, three times daily

POTENTIAL ADVERSE EFFECTS: Gastrointestinal discomfort, nausea, skin rash

CAUTIONS AND CONTRAINDICATIONS: Pregnancy, lactation, lion's mane mushroom allergy; diabetic medications, drugs that lower blood pressure

MAITAKE

(Grifola frondosa)

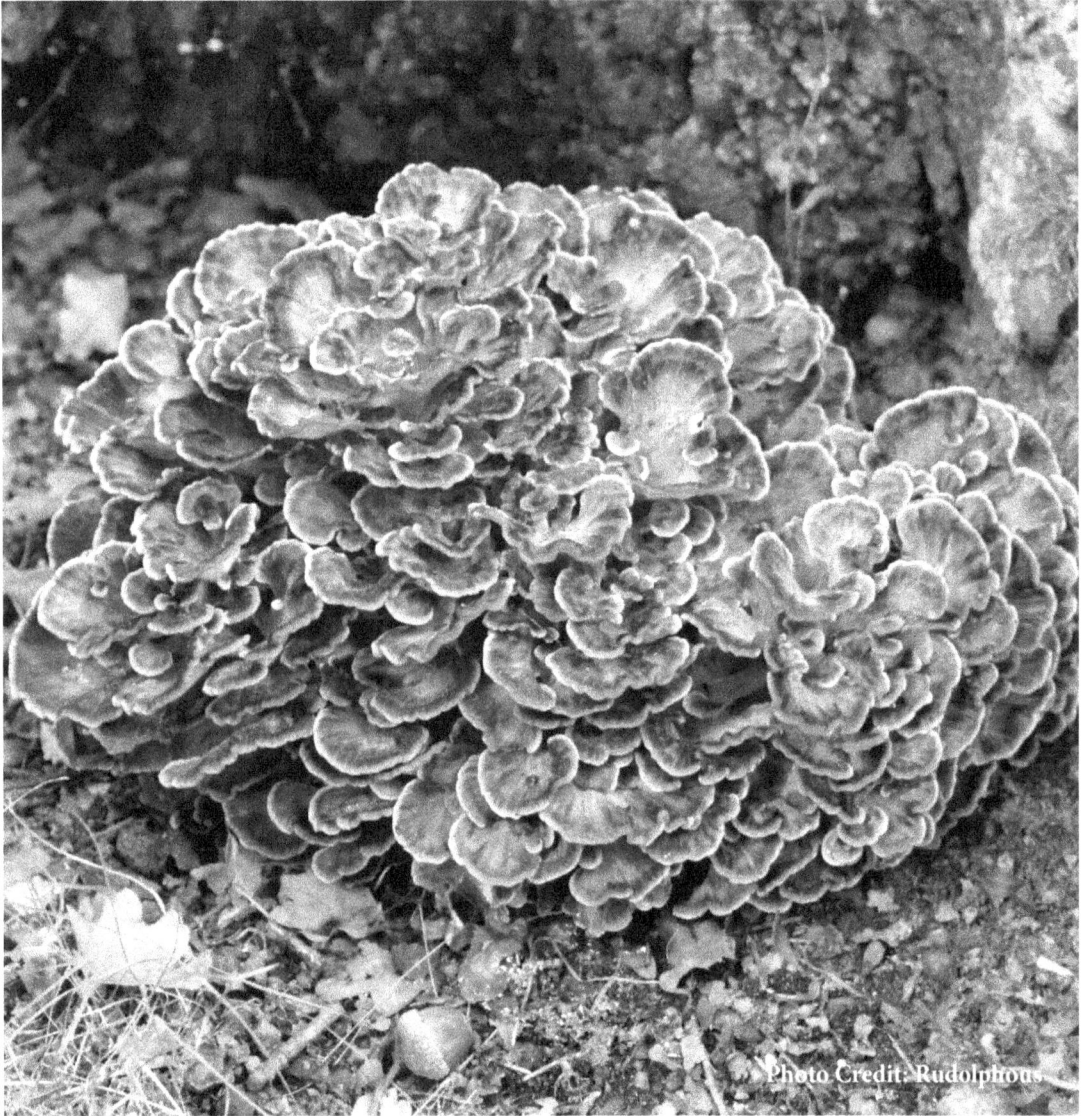

Photo Credit: Rudolphous

Kingdom: Fungi
Phylum: Basidiomycota
Class: Agaricomycetes
Order: Polyporales
Family: Meripilaceae
Genus: Grifola
Species: frondosa
Native Habitat: China, Europe, and North America

Both a culinary and medicinal mushroom, maitake is also called "Hen of the Woods" because of its distinctive appearance. Maitake mushrooms were first used in East Asia and have a rich history of medicinal use. They are native to the temperate forests of Asia, including Japan and China, and North America, forming large clumps at the base of stumps and on the roots of trees like oak, elm, maple, and persimmon. The mushrooms can vary in size, with some reaching substantial weights, resembling the plumage of a nesting hen. They have been admired in traditional Chinese and Japanese medicine for centuries for their potential health benefits.

Maitake mushrooms are not only known for their rich umami flavor but also for their impressive nutritional content. They are a valuable source of essential nutrients and bioactive compounds such as protein, vitamins—including niacin (B3), riboflavin (B2), and pantothenic acid (B5), minerals—like potassium, phosphorus, and selenium—and dietary fiber. Maitake mushrooms are prized in culinary circles for their rich, earthy flavor and distinctive texture. They can be prepared in various ways and add depth and complexity to a wide range of dishes.

Maitake mushrooms have a long history of use in traditional medicine, and their use in modern alternative medicine is increasing as science reveals their potential health benefits. One of the most common reasons maitake mushrooms are used medicinally is for immune support. The beta-glucans found in maitake mushrooms stimulate the activity of immune cells, enhancing the body's defense against infections and diseases. They also possess antioxidant properties to help combat damage caused by oxidative stress. Some studies suggest that maitake mushrooms may help regulate blood sugar levels, making them a potential adjunctive therapy in managing diabetes. They may also support healthy blood pressure and healthy cholesterol levels. While further research is needed, preliminary studies suggest that maitake mushrooms have anticancer properties, particularly specific fractions of the mushrooms like maitake D-fraction—a polysaccharide fraction of maitake mushroom consisting of beta-glucan branched with glucosides. Not surprisingly, maitake's influence on the gut microbiome is frequently credited as the reason for its biological activity.

In recent years, maitake supplements have gained popularity as individuals seek to harness the potential health benefits of these mushrooms. Maitake supplements are available in various forms, including capsules, tinctures, and powders, making it convenient for those who want to incorporate them into their daily wellness routines. These supplements are often standardized to contain specific bioactive compounds like beta-glucans. Most commonly, maitake supplements are used to support immune health, regulate blood sugar, and promote overall well-being.

Maitake mushrooms are a versatile and health-promoting member of the fungal kingdom. With their potential medicinal properties, they have earned their place as an important tool in traditional and modern wellness practices. As scientific research continues to uncover their potential, maitake mushrooms will become a more prominent natural solution in holistic health.

NOTABLE COMPOUNDS: Ergosterol, ergosterol peroxide, glycoproteins, polysaccharides, beta-glucans, alpha-glucan, o-orsellinaldehyde, vitamins, minerals, glycerides (1 and 2), sterols, glucosylceramide, D-fraction, SX-fraction, proteolytic enzymes

BENEFITS ACCORDING TO PRECLINICAL RESEARCH:

- Anticancer (breast)[1796-1802]
- Anticancer (colorectal)[1803]
- Anticancer (liver)[1804-1813]
- Anticancer (gastric)[1814,1815,1816,1817]
- Anticancer (monocytic leukemia)[1818]
- Anticancer (lung)[1819]
- Anticancer (laryngeal)[1820]
- Anticancer (liver, synergistic activity with vitamin C)[1821]
- Anticancer (enhances 5-fluorouracil activity against liver cancer)[1822]
- Anticancer (enhances therapeutic effect and reduces kidney toxicity and myelosuppression of cisplatin)[1823]
- Reverses white blood cell dysfunction and promotes maturation of hematopoietic progenitor cells to myeloid cells after chemotherapy-induced bone marrow injury[1824]
- Anticancer (rodent liver)[1825]
- Anticancer (rodent colorectal)[1826,1827,1828]
- Anticancer (rodent melanoma)[1829]
- Anticancer (rodent lymphoma)[1830]
- Anticancer (rodent liver; enhances cyclophosphamide activity)[1831]
- Anticancer (rodent sarcoma)[1832-1841]
- Inhibits angiogenesis (the growth of blood vessels, which its inhibition is important to fight cancer, prevent diabetic nephropathy, combat autoimmune and cardiovascular conditions, and prevent delayed wound healing)[1842,1843,1844]
- Protects against bone marrow cell damage caused by doxorubicin[1845]
- Shifts Th-2 dominance caused by cancer to Th-1 dominance[1846,1847]
- Enhances bone-marrow dendritic cell-based immunotherapy against colorectal cancer[1848]
- Stimulates immune activity against tumors[1849-1857]

- 🍄 Reverses memory impairment[1858,1859]
- 🍄 Preserves cognition and brain cells[1860,1861,1862]
- 🍄 Promotes bone health (mineralization and bone development)[1863,1864]
- 🍄 Alleviates colitis[1865]
- 🍄 Suppresses intestinal inflammation (beneficial to inflammatory bowel disease)[1866,1867]
- 🍄 Stimulates immune function and activity (including protecting against immunosuppression caused by cancer chemotherapy treatment)[1868-1901]
- 🍄 Balances immune function[1902]
- 🍄 Protects against immune dysfunction caused by arsenic exposure[1903]
- 🍄 Combats obesity[1904-1910]
- 🍄 Improves insulin resistance[1911,1912,1913]
- 🍄 Antidiabetic[1914-1937]
- 🍄 Ameliorates diabetic kidney damage (diabetic nephropathy)[1938,1939,1940]
- 🍄 Reverses immune dysfunction caused by diabetes[1941]
- 🍄 Reduces high cholesterol, improves lipid metabolism (inhibits liver and blood lipids)[1942-1954]
- 🍄 Prevents atherosclerosis[1955]
- 🍄 Lowers blood pressure[1956]
- 🍄 Protects against cardiovascular disease (inhibits adhesion molecule expression and binding of monocytes to the endothelium during an inflammatory response)[1957]
- 🍄 Improves gut microbiome (production of short-chain fatty acids, positively modifies microbiome diversity and numbers)[1958-1967]
- 🍄 Antiallergic[1968,1969]
- 🍄 Alleviates pain[1970]
- 🍄 Anti-inflammatory[1971-1978]
- 🍄 Relieves arthritis[1979]
- 🍄 Enhances healthy lifespan and longevity[1980,1981]
- 🍄 Protects against chemical-induced skin inflammation[1982]
- 🍄 Liver protective[1983,1984]
- 🍄 Ameliorates nonalcoholic fatty liver disease, liver fibrosis[1985,1986,1987]
- 🍄 Protects against cardiovascular disease (inhibits adhesion molecule expression and binding of monocytes to the endothelium during an inflammatory response)[1988]
- 🍄 Relieves atopic dermatitis (eczema)[1989]
- 🍄 Reduces dry skin by augmenting sebaceous lipogenesis[1990]
- 🍄 Protects against skin photoaging caused by exposure to UVA light[1991]

- Enhances physical performance and endurance (increases fat utilization and delays the accumulation of lactate and ammonia in muscles)[1992]
- Accelerates the clearance of mercury from the bloodstream[1993]
- Alleviates oxidative stress and associated damage[1994,1995]
- Antioxidant[1996-2004]
- Antiviral (enterovirus 71—a causative agent of hand, foot, and mouth disease in children and neurological disease epidemics)[2005]
- Antiviral (hepatitis B; also synergizes interferon alpha-2b therapy)[2006]
- Antiviral (HSV-1)[2007]
- Antiviral (influenza A/Aichi/2/68 virus)[2008]
- Combats leishmaniasis[2009]
- Antimicrobial[2010,2011]

BENEFITS ACCORDING TO CLINICAL RESEARCH:

- Stimulated and suppressed certain immune functions in women with breast cancer[2012]
  - 0.1–5.0 mg/kg body weight, twice daily
- Triggered remission of invasive bladder cancer in eighty-seven-year-old male (followed for two years after treatment)[2013]
  - 600 mg maitake mushroom powder with 40 mg Maitake PD-fraction, and 2,000 mg vitamin C daily
- Stimulates immune system (NK cell activity) to reduce cancer progression and tumor activity in people with stage 2–4 lung, lingual, breast, liver, or gastric cancer[2014]
  - 120 mg to 225 mg of Maitake D-Fraction daily divided into two doses morning and evening for 1 to 63 months; dose was divided as 40 mg morning and 80 mg evening, 50 mg morning and 100 mg evening, or 75 mg morning and 150 mg evening
- As adjunct treatment with concurrent chemoradiotherapy for advanced head and neck squamous carcinoma[2015]
  - 1,000 mg capsules containing Maitake D-Fraction, three times daily, one hour prior to a meal
- Triggers ovulation in women with polycystic ovary syndrome (PCOS) after failure to respond to clomiphene citrate[2016]
  - Three tablets containing 250 mg maitake powder plus 18 mg SX-fraction (a glycoprotein-rich extract), three times daily between meals beginning at the first day of menses

THERAPEUTIC POTENTIAL: Obesity, cancer, dysbiosis, high cholesterol, diabetes, improve fertility with PCOS, diabetes

CLINICAL DOSAGES: 250 mg to 1,000 mg, up to three times daily; Maitake D-Fraction—supplement providing 40 to 225 mg daily; best taken in the morning or early afternoon

POTENTIAL ADVERSE EFFECTS: Diarrhea, stomachache, skin rash

CAUTIONS AND CONTRAINDICATIONS: Pregnancy, lactation, maitake mushroom allergy, prior to surgery; drugs that lower blood pressure, diabetic medications

MESIMA

(Phellinus linteus)

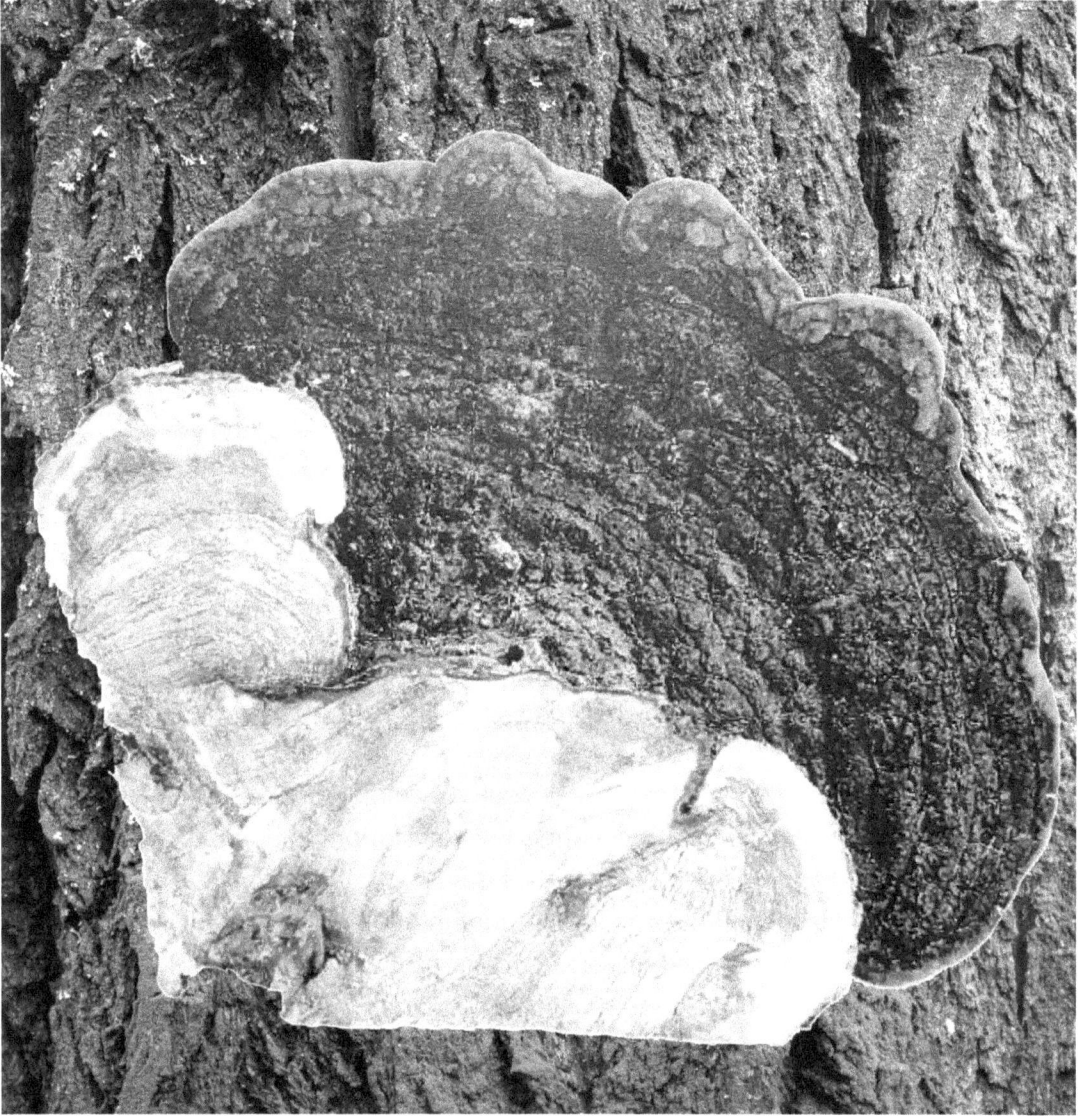

Kingdom: Fungi
Phylum: Basidiomycota
Class: Agaricomycetes
Order: Hymenochaetales
Family: Hymenochaetaceae
Genus: Phellinus
Species: linteus
Native Habitat: East Asia

Predominantly found in Asia, mesima mushrooms boast a rich history of medicinal use and an impressive range of potential health benefits. Mesima is a bracket fungus that grows on hardwood trees, particularly mulberry and oak, in temperate regions of Asia. It has been used in traditional Chinese, Japanese, and Korean medicine for centuries and is sometimes referred to as the "mushroom of immortality" because of its perceived health-enhancing and longevity-promoting properties.

The fruiting body of mesima appears as a woody, hoof-shaped bracket with a reddish-brown to dark brown surface, which is why it may also be called the black hoof mushroom. The underside typically features a layer of tiny pores where spores are produced. Its appearance is distinctive and differs from the typical mushroom cap-and-stem structure.

Many Asian medicine systems have relied upon this medicinal mushroom for centuries. In traditional Chinese medicine, mesima is known as *Sanghuang* and has been used for centuries to strengthen the body, enhance vitality, and support overall well-being. Like many medicinal mushrooms, it is believed to have adaptogenic properties, helping the body adapt to stress and maintain balance and homeostasis. In Korean traditional medicine, this mushroom is known as *Meshimakobu* and is used to support the immune system, promote longevity, and improve overall health. It is often prepared as a tea or tincture. Japanese folk medicine also utilizes mesima as a tonic and to promote longevity and vitality.

Mesima contains a diverse array of bioactive compounds, many of which are responsible for its potential health benefits. This mushroom is rich in polysaccharides, particularly beta-glucans, which enhance the body's immune defenses against illness. It also has various triterpenoids, including inotodiol and trametenolic acid. These compounds have demonstrated anti-inflammatory and antioxidant activities. The phenolic compounds found in mesima, such as flavonoids and phenolic acids, contribute to its antioxidant properties and potential health benefits. Adenosine is a nucleoside found in mesima that may have anti-inflammatory and immunomodulatory effects. Mesima has great potential to improve human health because of its impressive diversity of bioactive compounds.

Mesima has gained significant attention in recent years because of the scientific discovery of its many potential health benefits. The beta-glucans and other immune-stimulating compounds it contains have been extensively studied for their ability to enhance immune function. Triterpenoids and other compounds in this mushroom have shown anti-inflammatory properties, which is important not only for inflammatory conditions but also for overall well-being. It has also been explored for its anticancer potential, demonstrating the ability to inhibit the growth of cancer cells and enhance the body's natural defenses against cancer. Mesima may also play a role in managing metabolic conditions like diabetes and obesity by improving insulin sensitivity and regulating blood sugar levels. Lastly, this mushroom may support liver health by promoting detoxification and protecting liver cells from damage.

Mesima is not commonly used in culinary applications because of its tough and woody texture. Instead, it is typically consumed in the form of extracts, teas, tinctures, capsules, or powders. With its rich history in traditional medicine and its emerging role in modern health research, mesima is a mushroom of great interest. Its bioactive compounds, including beta-glucans, triterpenoids, and phenolic compounds, hold promise in various areas of health and wellness, from immune support and cancer research to anti-inflammatory and antioxidant effects.

As scientific research continues to unveil the potential of mesima, it is likely to find a more prominent place in nutraceuticals and complementary medicine. The future holds exciting possibilities as researchers uncover more about the therapeutic potential of this remarkable mushroom.

NOTABLE COMPOUNDS: Polysaccharides, beta-glucans, triterpenoids, inotodiol, trametenolic acid, adenosine, styrylpyrones, meshimakobnol A, hypholomine B, hispidins 1 and 2, inoscavin A, inotilone, 4-(3,4-dihydroxyphenyl)-3-buten-2-one, phellilane H, hispolin, sesquiterpenoids, ergosterol, phellinstatin

BENEFITS ACCORDING TO PRECLINICAL RESEARCH:

- 🍄 Anticancer (prostate)[2017,2018]
- 🍄 Anticancer (sensitizes androgen-sensitive prostate cancer cells to doxorubicin)[2019]
- 🍄 Anticancer (thyroid)[2020]
- 🍄 Anticancer (breast)[2021,2022,2023,2024]
- 🍄 Anticancer (synergizes 5-fluorouracil against breast cancer cells)[2025,2026]
- 🍄 Anticancer (cervical)[2027]
- 🍄 Anticancer (bladder)[2028,2029,2030]
- 🍄 Anticancer (prostate)[2031]
- 🍄 Anticancer (acute promyelocytic leukemia)[2032]
- 🍄 Anticancer (nasopharyngeal)[2033,2034]
- 🍄 Anticancer (oral)[2035]
- 🍄 Anticancer (colorectal)[2036-2043]
- 🍄 Anticancer (colorectal, synergizes camptothecini11)[2044]
- 🍄 Anticancer (fibrosarcoma)[2045,2046]
- 🍄 Anticancer (liver)[2047,2048,2049,2050]

- Anticancer (liver—sensitizes cancer cells to radiotherapy)[2051]
- Prevents liver cancer[2052]
- Anticancer (lung)[2053,2054,2055,2056]
- Anticancer (glioblastoma)[2057,2058,2059]
- Anticancer (neuroblastoma)[2060]
- Anticancer (pancreatic; also sensitizes cancerous cells to gemcitabine)[2061]
- Anticancer (sensitizes human cancer cells to tumor necrosis factor-related apoptosis)[2062]
- Anticancer (inhibits angiogenesis)[2063]
- Anticancer (prevents metastasis)[2064,2065,2066]
- Protects healthy cells against damage caused by radiation therapy[2067]
- Anticancer (rodent sarcoma)[2068,2069,2070]
- Anticancer (rodent melanoma)[2071-2079]
- Anticancer (rodent liver)[2080]
- Anticancer (rodent colorectal)[2081]
- Anticancer (rodent colorectal; enhances sensitivity to cetuximab)[2082]
- Improves insulin resistance[2083,2084]
- Antidiabetic[2085-2091]
- Inhibits ferroptosis in pancreatic beta-cells[2092]
- Protects against damage caused by diabetes[2093]
- Reduces high cholesterol, maintains cholesterol homeostasis[2094,2095,2096]
- Improves the gut microbiome (elevates short-chain fatty acids production, promotes the proliferation of beneficial bacteria and prevents the growth of pathogenic bacteria)[2097,2098]
- Aids intestinal immune function[2099]
- Neuroprotective[2100,2101,2102,2103]
- Decreases neuroinflammation[2104]
- Preserves cognitive function[2105]
- Lowers blood pressure (vasodilator, increases urinary sodium excretion)[2106,2107]
- Protects the heart during ischemia-reperfusion injury (a lack of oxygen to tissues followed by a subsequent return of oxygenation resulting in tissue damage)[2108]
- Heart protective[2109]
- Protects against liver damage caused by acetaminophen[2110,2111]
- Liver protective[2112,2113,2114,2115]
- Alleviates nonalcoholic fatty liver disease[2116,2117]
- Prevents liver fibrosis[2118,2119]
- Kidney protective[2120,2121]
- Lung protective[2122,2123]
- Prevents ulcers caused by NSAIDs (naproxen) or alcohol[2124,2125]

- Inhibits hemolysis of red blood cells[2126]
- Combats asthma[2127]
- Reduces allergies[2128,2129,2130,2131,2132,2133]
- Stimulates immune function (including reversing immunodeficiency and increasing cancer surveillance and destruction)[2134-2144]
- Balances immune function (regulates Th1/Th2 balance; restores IL-6/IL-10 balance)[2145,2146,2147,2148]
- Alleviates septic shock[2149]
- Prevents peritonitis (inflammation of the inner lining of the inner wall of the abdomen and the cover of the abdominal organs) and the subsequent adhesions and abscesses[2150,2151]
- Relieves pain[2152]
- Anti-inflammatory[2153-2166]
- Prevents and treats autoimmune arthritic conditions involving joint inflammation[2167]
- Protects against development of osteoarthritis and osteoporosis[2168,2169]
- Decreases prostate size in benign prostatic hyperplasia model[2170] (Note: other research suggests it may enlarge the prostate)[2171]
- Enhances endurance exercise performance[2172]
- Ameliorates age-related cataracts[2173]
- Antiobesity (inhibits lipase)[2174,2175]
- Antiviral (inhibits neuraminidase activity, which blocks the reproduction of viruses; particularly used for influenza)[2176,2177]
- Antimicrobial[2178,2179,2180,2181,2182]
- Alleviates allergic skin disease (eczema)[2183]
- Delays skin aging caused by ultraviolet rays[2184]
- Reduces hyperpigmentation of skin, skin brightening[2185,2186]
- Prevents the loss of elastin and subsequent skin aging and loss of skin elasticity[2187]
- Inhibits the activation of the aryl hydrocarbon receptor (a receptor that integrates environmental, dietary, microbial, and metabolic information and plays a vital role in cardiovascular, reproductive, immune, and red blood cell homeostasis—which when inhibited helps prevent several diseases)[2188]
- Prevents protein glycation[2189]
- Protects against damage caused by oxidative stress[2190,2191,2192,2193,2194]
- Prevents DNA mutations[2195]
- Antioxidant[2196-2203]

BENEFITS ACCORDING TO CLINICAL RESEARCH:

- ➢ Improves immune function (significantly increases NK cell activity) in individuals aged twenty to sixty-five with normal white blood cell counts[2204]
  - 500 mg mesima twice daily for eight weeks
- ➢ Improves symptoms of knee osteoarthritis in people aged forty to seventy-five years with knee pain for six months or longer[2205]
  - 750 mg mesima and 750 mg dextrin, twice daily for eight weeks
- ➢ Produced remission of hormone refractory prostate cancer in a sixty-eight-year-old male[2206]
  - No dosing reported in the case study
- ➢ Remission of liver cancer with multiple lung metastases in a seventy-nine-year-old male[2207]
  - Dose not reported but the mesima mushroom supplement was taken for one month
- ➢ Regression of liver cancer with skull metastasis in a sixty-five-year-old male in conjunction with radiotherapy
  - Dose not reported in case study
- ➢ Increases adherence to postoperative chemotherapy after surgical resection of pancreatic cancer[2208]
  - 1,100 mg, three times daily

THERAPEUTIC POTENTIAL: Improve immune function, rheumatoid arthritis, cancer

CLINICAL DOSAGES: 500 to 1,100 mg, up to three times daily

POTENTIAL ADVERSE EFFECTS: Upset stomach, diarrhea, prostate enlargement

CAUTIONS AND CONTRAINDICATIONS: Pregnancy, lactation, benign prostatic hyperplasia, mesima mushroom allergy; immunosuppressive medications, drugs metabolized by CYP2E1

OYSTER

(Pleurotus ostreatus)

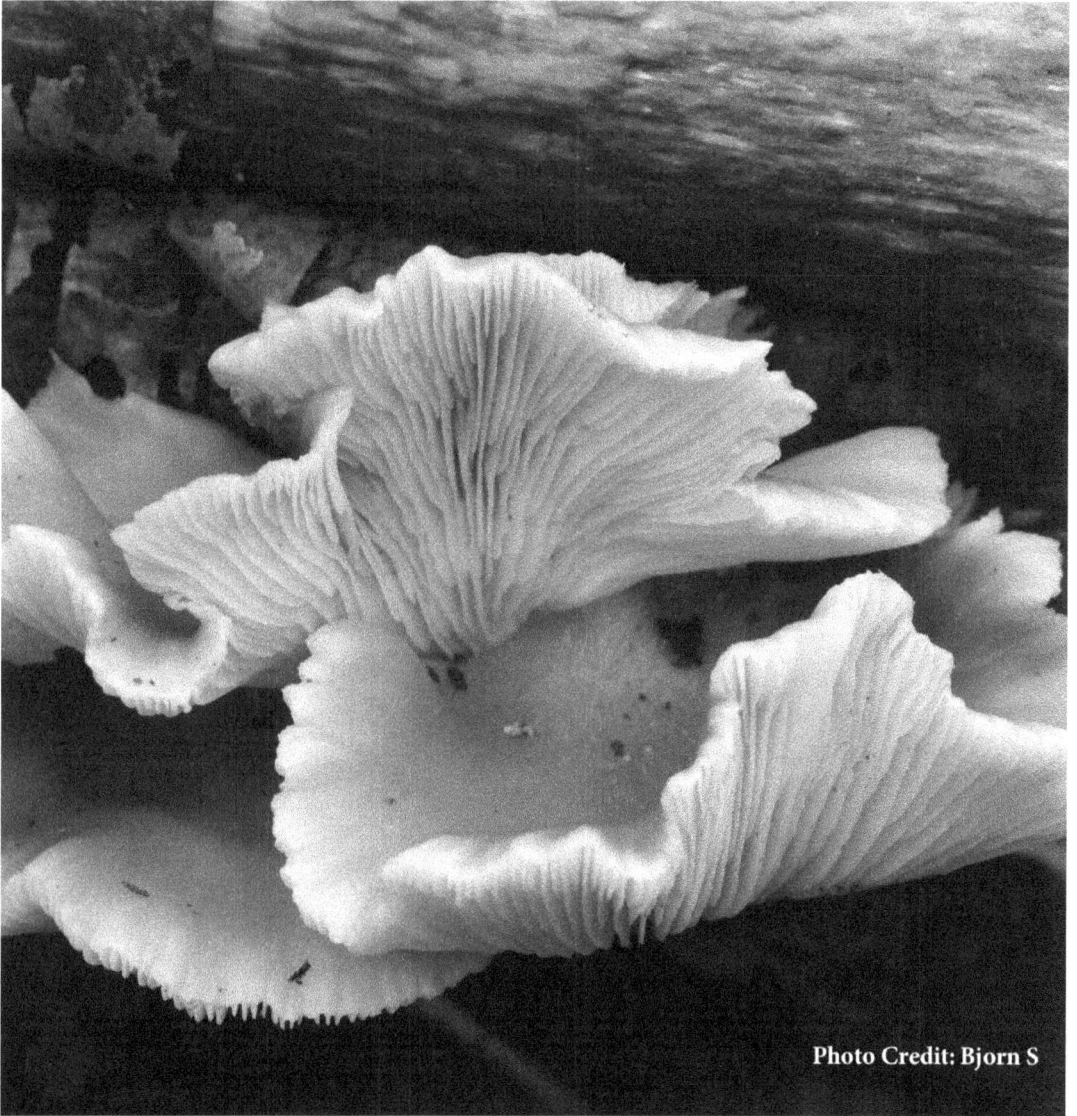

Photo Credit: Bjorn S

Kingdom: Fungi
Phylum: Basidiomycota
Class: Agaricomycetes
Order: Agaricales
Family: Pleurotaceae
Genus: Pleurotus
Species: ostreatus
Native Habitat: Temperate and subtropical forests throughout the world (absent from the Pacific Northwest and North America)

A versatile mushroom used for both culinary and medicinal purposes, the oyster mushroom is a sought-after choice among mycophiles and culinary enthusiasts. It has a distinct appearance with a fan-shaped or oyster-shell-like cap, typically measuring 5 to 25 centimeters (2 to 10 inches) across. It ranges in color from white to grayish-brown, with a smooth to slightly wrinkled surface. Unlike many mushrooms with downward-hanging gills, oyster mushrooms have gills that attach to the stalk. These gills are white to pale gray and are closely spaced. The stalk is short, thick, and off-center, often resembling a stem. It is white and smooth, with no ring or volva.

The oyster mushroom is highly prized in culinary circles for its mild, delicate flavor and firm texture. It can be used in a variety of culinary applications, such as sautéed or stir-fried, grilled or roasted, soups and stews, and vegetarian and vegan dishes. It may also be dried and powdered and used as a seasoning or flavor enhancer in various dishes.

The oyster mushroom is not only delectable but also nutritious, offering a range of vitamins, minerals, and other essential nutrients. It is a source of high-quality protein, dietary fiber, vitamins B3, B2, B5, and D, minerals (potassium, phosphorus, selenium, and iron), and antioxidants like ergothioneine.

Beyond its edible and culinary uses, the oyster mushroom also boasts several medicinal properties. Like many other medicinal mushrooms, they contain beta-glucans, which have immune-boosting properties. The antioxidants present in oyster mushrooms help protect cells from oxidative damage caused by free radicals, potentially reducing the risk of chronic diseases. Some research shows that oyster mushrooms help support a healthy inflammatory response, reduce cholesterol, balances blood sugar, and aids digestion. One of the most interesting properties of oyster mushroom is its ability to aid the detoxification of pharmaceuticals and chemicals in both the body and the environment, many of which are significantly harmful to both humans and environmental health.

The oyster mushroom is a culinary delight and a nutritional powerhouse with great versatility from the kitchen to the medicine cabinet. If you're seeking a natural solution to support immune or heart health, the oyster mushroom may be for you.

NOTABLE COMPOUNDS: Ergothioneine, ergosterol peroxide, polysaccharides, beta-glucans, pleuran, phenolic compounds, terpenoids, lectins, flavonoids, dipeptides, laccase, sterols, ostreopexin, sesquiterpenes, anthraquinone, lectins

BENEFITS ACCORDING TO PRECLINICAL RESEARCH:

- 🍄 Anticancer (breast)[2209,2210,2211,2212,2213,2214]
- 🍄 Anticancer (prostate)[2215]

- ♟ Anticancer (androgen-independent prostate)[2216]
- ♟ Anticancer (endometrial)[2217]
- ♟ Anticancer (liver)[2218]
- ♟ Anticancer (kidney)[2219]
- ♟ Anticancer (colorectal, cecum)[2220-2228]
- ♟ Prevents colorectal cancer[2229,2230]
- ♟ Anticancer (cervical)[2231,2232,2233]
- ♟ Anticancer (cervical, increases sensitivity to radiation therapy)[2234]
- ♟ Anticancer (gastric)[2235]
- ♟ Anticancer (larynx)[2236]
- ♟ Anticancer (neuroblastoma)[2237]
- ♟ Anticancer (promyelocytic leukemia)[2238]
- ♟ Anticancer (acute myeloid leukemia)[2239,2240]
- ♟ Anticancer (monocytic leukemia)[2241]
- ♟ Anticancer (leukemia, suppresses growth, preserves healthy production of white blood cells in bone marrow, and enhances immunity)[2242]
- ♟ Anticancer (inhibits telomerase, which cancer cells use to achieve cellular immortality)[2243]
- ♟ Anticancer (rodent liver)[2244,2245]
- ♟ Anticancer (rodent sarcoma)[2264-2252]
- ♟ Anticancer (rodent lymphoma)[2253,2254,2255]
- ♟ Anticancer (rodent breast)[2256]
- ♟ Anticancer (rodent liver)[2257]
- ♟ Anticancer (rodent mastocytoma)[2258]
- ♟ Anticancer (rodent melanoma)[2259]
- ♟ Alleviates cognitive impairment, protects neurons to preserve cognitive function[2260,2261,2262,2263]
- ♟ Preserves nervous cells and tissue to treat Parkinson's disease[2264]
- ♟ Protects blood cells and plasma against damage caused by radiation[2265]
- ♟ Enhances the gut microbiome (maintains healthy balance of microbes, increases *Lactobacillus* and *Bifidobacterium*, decreases *Bacteroides* and *Roseburia*, enhances short-chain fatty acid production)[2266,2267,2268,2269,2270,2271]
- ♟ Antidiabetic (comparable to metformin and glibenclamide)[2272,2273,2274,2275,2276]
- ♟ Stimulates or enhances immune function[2277-2288]
- ♟ Enhances immune and nutritional recovery in malnourished subjects[2289]
- ♟ Liver protective[2290,2291,2292]
- ♟ Liver protective (protects against mitochondrial dysfunction and oxidative stress after acetaminophen overdose)[2293]
- ♟ Ameliorates alcohol-related fatty liver[2294]

- Alleviates nonalcoholic fatty liver disease[2295]
- Kidney protective[2296,2297]
- Protects the colon and GI tract[2298,2299,2300]
- Restores healthy iron levels in anemic subjects[2301]
- Protects against cardiovascular disease (inhibits adhesion molecule expression and binding of monocytes to the endothelium during an inflammatory response)[2302]
- Reduces high blood pressure[2303,2304]
- Lowers high cholesterol, improves lipid profiles (inhibits oxidation, reduces cholesterol absorption, and increases cholesterol removal)[2305-2326]
- Modulates genes associated with fatty acid oxidation and lipid metabolism[2327,2328]
- Prevents the development of atherosclerosis[2329,2330,2331]
- Ameliorates ulcerative colitis[2332,2333]
- Combats obesity[2334,2335,2336,2337]
- Anti-inflammatory[2338,2339,2340,2341,2342,2343]
- Alleviates gout (reduces uric acid levels)[2344]
- Relieves arthritis[2345,2346]
- Antiarthritic (improves the efficacy of methotrexate treatment)[2347]
- Prevents cataracts[2348]
- Helps maintain healthy intraocular pressure[2349]
- Enhances wound healing[2350,2351]
- Protects skin against skin aging and damage caused by UV-A[2352,2353]
- Skin brightening[2354,2355]
- Increases protein digestibility[2356]
- Triggers creation of B vitamins[2357]
- Combats damage caused by oxidative stress[2358,2359]
- Prevents gene mutations[2360]
- Antioxidant[2361-2386]
- Improves antioxidant status during aging, which may help prevent age-associated disorders that involve free radicals[2387,2388,2389,2390]
- Antiviral (SARS-CoV-2)[2391]
- Antiviral (hepatitis B virus, stimulates innate immune response during hepatitis B virus tolerance stage)[2392]
- Antiviral (hepatitis C)[2393]
- Antiviral (adenovirus)[2394]
- Antiviral (increases survivability after HSV-2 infection)[2395]
- Antiviral (HIV-1)[2396]
- Antiviral (influenza H1N1)[2397]

- 🍄 Antimicrobial[2398-2414]
- 🍄 Trypanocidal (*T. cruzi*)[2415]
- 🍄 Acaricidal (*Rh. microplus*)[2416]
- 🍄 Amoebicidal[2417]
- 🍄 Antinematode[2418,2419]
- 🍄 Antiplasmodial (potential to manage malaria)[2420]
- 🍄 Antiprotozoal[2421,2422]
- 🍄 Aids detoxification and biodegradation of toxins (ochratoxin A, aflatoxin B) and protects against damage caused by harmful chemicals (acrylamide)[2423,2424,2425,2426,2427,2428]
- 🍄 Promotes biodegradation, remediation, and biosorption of pharmaceuticals, chemicals, pollutants, and products in the environment—soil, water, and air, acts as a biofilter[2429-2480]

BENEFITS ACCORDING TO CLINICAL RESEARCH:

- ➢ Lowers total cholesterol and triglycerides and stabilizes HDL cholesterol in people with dyslipidemia[2481]
  - 10 g of lyophilized powder daily for six weeks
- ➢ Improves lipid profile and reduced oxidized LDL cholesterol in individuals with moderate untreated high cholesterol[2482]
  - 30 g daily added to a soup consumed between 6:00–7:00 p.m.
- ➢ Reduces fasting and postprandial (after-meal) blood glucose levels in healthy individuals and postprandial glucose levels in people with type 2 diabetes[2483]
  - 50 mg/kg/bw of freeze-dried powdered oyster mushroom daily for two weeks
- ➢ Improves glucose tolerance and increases glucagon-like peptide-1 levels after a meal in people with impaired glucose tolerance[2484]
  - Consumption of a smoothie or soup enriched with 20 g of oven-dried mushroom powder (corresponding to 200 g or fresh mushroom powder)
- ➢ Improves glucose metabolism, lipids levels, and blood pressure in people with type 2 diabetes[2485]
  - 150 g daily as part of a meal for seven days
- ➢ Decreases fasting blood glucose, blood pressure, and HbA1c in men with high blood pressure and type 2 diabetes[2486]
  - 1,000 mg in a capsule three times daily for three months
- ➢ Lowers lipids (triglycerides, LDL cholesterol) in obese men with high blood pressure and no diabetes[2487]
  - 1,000 mg in a capsule three times daily for three months

- Decreases blood sugar, cholesterol, and triglycerides levels in women with type 2 diabetes[2488]
  - 200 g daily
- Reduces allergic responses and inflammation—stabilized IgE levels, reduced peripheral blood eosinophilia—in children aged two to ten with recurrent respiratory tract infections[2489]
  - 1 mL/5 kg/bw of Imunoglukan P4HW syrup (containing 10 mg pleuran and 10 mg vitamin C per 1 mL syrup) every morning on an empty stomach for six months
- Prevents recurrent respiratory tract infections in children aged one to twelve years old[2490,2491]
  - 1 mL/5 kg/bw of Imunoglukan P4HW syrup (containing 10 mg pleuran and 10 mg vitamin C per 1 mL syrup) every morning on an empty stomach for six months
- Decreases the occurrence and duration of bacterial exacerbations—acute events characterized by worsening of respiratory symptoms that is beyond normal day-to-day variations leading to a change in medications—in people with COPD[2492]
  - 100 mg pleuran with 60 mg vitamin C and 5 mg zinc, once daily, for three months
- Reduces the duration and severity of herpes simplex virus type 1 infection symptoms in individuals aged six or older with herpes simplex facialis/labialis in one of the first three stages (prodromal/tingle stage, blister stage, or weeping stage)[2493]
  - During acute treatment: 300 mg pleuran with 160 mg vitamin C and 10 mg zinc (Immunoglukan P4H ACUTE!) every morning on an empty stomach for ten days along with any recommended antiherpetic treatment (topical antiviral agents, analgesics, wound healing creams, or herpes patches); during preventive stage: Imunoglukan PH4 containing 100 mg insoluble beta-glucan (pleuran) and 100 mg vitamin C, every morning on an empty stomach for 120 days
- Decreases triglycerides, blood sugar, visceral fat, and cholesterol in women and blood glucose and triglycerides in men [2494]
  - 250 mg of whole mushrooms incorporated into a healthy diet of regional Mexican foods, four times weekly, for three months
- Protects athletes against upper respiratory tract infections[2495]
  - Imunoglukan—200 mg daily for three months
- Regulates exercise-induced changes in immune system function (natural killer cell activity) in athletes[2496]
  - 100 mg Imunoglukan, once daily for two months

- Restores cellular antitumor immune function in women with endocrine-dependent breast cancer (clinical stages I-II) in remission[2497]
  - High dose: 700 mg daily; low dose: 100mg to 200 mg daily, for twelve months
- Relieves eczema (severity, itching)[2498]
  - Topical application of Imunoglukan P4H cream
- Protects the skin against UV light damage, soothes and improves the skin[2499]
  - Topical application of a cream containing beta-D-glucans from oyster mushroom

THERAPEUTIC POTENTIAL: High cholesterol, detoxification, prevention and treatment of respiratory tract infections, eczema, diabetes

CLINICAL DOSAGES: 100 mg to 200 g daily; most commonly 1,000 mg, up to three times daily

POTENTIAL ADVERSE EFFECTS: Stomach upset, airway constriction or lung diseases if inhaled

CAUTIONS AND CONTRAINDICATIONS: Pregnancy, lactation, oyster mushroom allergy; Antidiabetic drugs, cholesterol-lowering drugs, drugs that affect blood pressure, immunosuppressants

PINK OYSTER

(Pleurotus djamor)

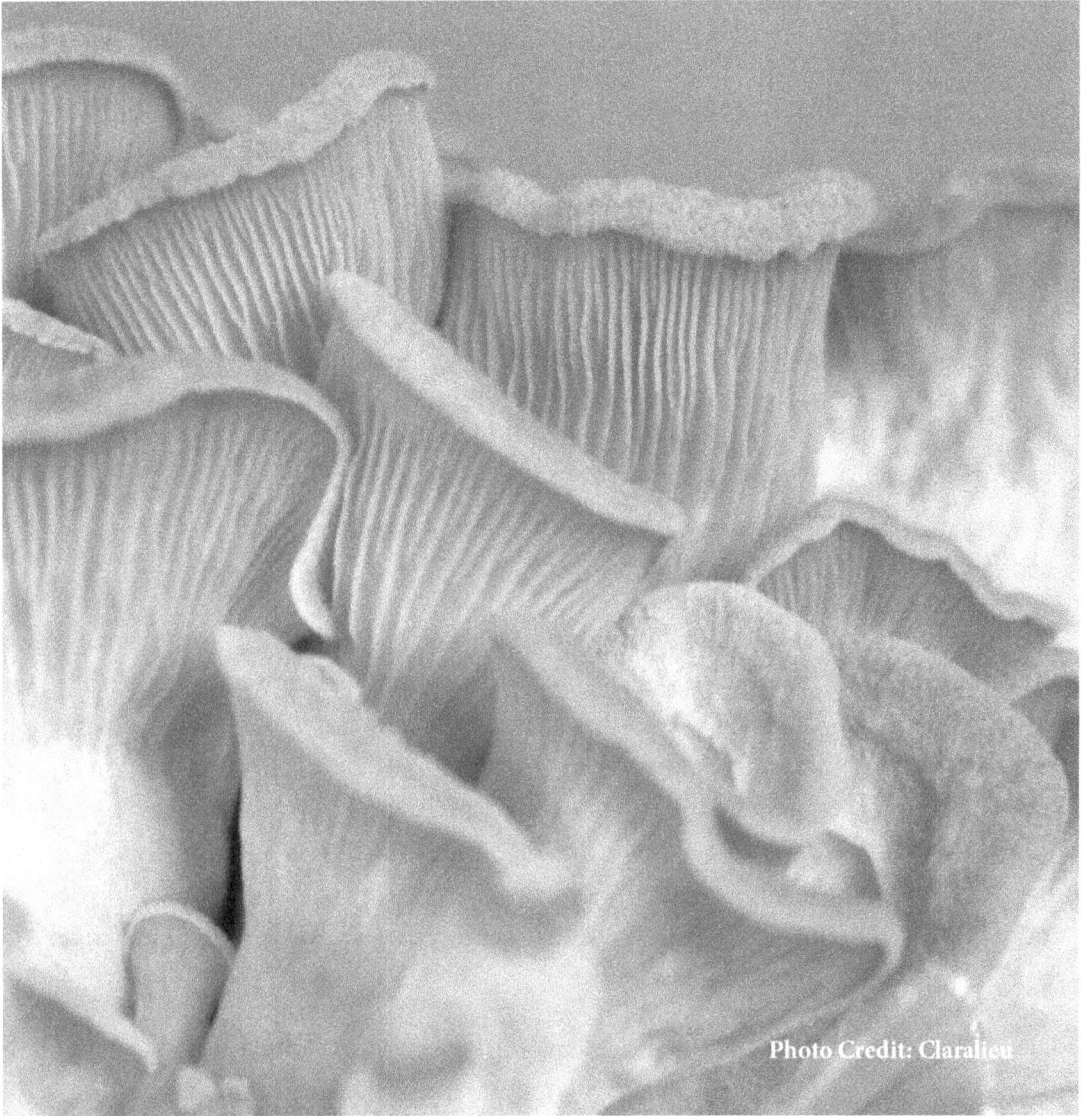

Photo Credit: Claralicu

Kingdom: Fungi
Phylum: Basidiomycota
Class: Agaricomycetes
Order: Agaricales
Family: Pleurotaceae
Genus: Pleurotus
Species: djamor
Native Habitat: Widespread in the tropics and subtropics of America and Asia

Like the oyster mushroom, the pink oyster mushroom is commonly used in culinary dishes and popularly grown because it is an easy species to cultivate. They grow in clusters on hardwood trees and release a strong woodsy and smoky aroma. They are tougher in texture than other oyster mushrooms. Pink oyster mushrooms are high in protein and fiber, a rich source of B vitamins, potassium, copper, selenium, and folate. Although most known for their eye-catching pinkish caps, they also have therapeutic potential because of the bioactive compounds they contain.

Within the genus Pleurotus, which includes various oyster mushroom species, *Pleurotus djamor* is eye-catching for its unique and vibrant pink or reddish-pink hue. The cap of the pink oyster mushroom is fan-shaped, with a distinctive pink to reddish-pink coloration that measures anywhere from 5 to 15 centimeters (2 to 6 inches) across and has a smooth to slightly wrinkled surface. Unlike traditional oyster mushrooms, pink oyster mushrooms exhibit a decurrent gill attachment, meaning the gills extend slightly down the stalk. These gills are close, crowded, and often a lighter pink color than the cap. The stalk of the pink oyster mushroom is thick, stubby, and generally eccentrically attached, meaning it is not centered under the cap. It shares the same pink hue as the cap.

The pink oyster mushroom's texture and mild, slightly sweet flavor make it an excellent choice for stir-fries and sautéed dishes. It absorbs flavors well and pairs beautifully with garlic, ginger, and a variety of sauces. They can be served raw in salads for their crispness and vibrant color, adding both visual appeal and a subtle mushroom flavor. They are frequently used as a meat substitute in vegetarian or vegan dishes because of their meaty texture and umami-rich taste. The pink oyster mushroom's ability to hold its shape and flavor in soups and stews makes it a preferred choice for enriching broths and adding a delightful depth of taste. Pink oyster mushrooms can be considered a functional food because of their nutritional and medicinal value.

The pink oyster mushroom is associated with several potential medicinal benefits, including antioxidant benefits, immune support, anti-inflammatory effects, cholesterol-lowering benefits, anticancer potential, and antimicrobial activity. Oyster mushrooms in general have a lot of medicinal potential, most of which is still untapped and waiting to be discovered.

The pink oyster mushroom may be a hidden gem in the fungal world. Its unique vibrant color, delightful flavor, and potential medicinal properties make it a valuable addition to both culinary creations, health-conscious diets, and your natural health toolbox.

NOTABLE COMPOUNDS: Ergothioneine, tannins, flavonoids, terpenoids, cardiac glycosides, and saponins, polysaccharides, sterols, beta-glucans

BENEFITS ACCORDING TO PRECLINICAL RESEARCH:

- ♟ Anticancer (breast)[2500, 2501]
- ♟ Anticancer (ovarian)[2502]
- ♟ Anticancer (rodent lymphoma)[2503]
- ♟ Anticancer (rodent sarcoma)[2504]
- ♟ Antidiabetic[2505]
- ♟ Protects against diabetic-related organ damage[2506]
- ♟ Alleviates chronic renal failure[2507]
- ♟ Liver protective[2508]
- ♟ Promotes healthy lifespan[2509]
- ♟ Mitigates age-related conditions associated with oxidative stress[2510]
- ♟ Antioxidant[2511-2517]
- ♟ DNA protective (UV-induced damage)[2518]
- ♟ Antimicrobial[2519,2520]
- ♟ Nematicidal[2521,2522,2523]
- ♟ Biodegrades harmful chemicals and pharmaceuticals[2524]

BENEFITS ACCORDING TO CLINICAL RESEARCH:

- ➢ None found.

THERAPEUTIC POTENTIAL: Antioxidant, diabetes

CLINICAL DOSAGES: Unknown.

POTENTIAL ADVERSE EFFECTS: Stomach upset, airway constriction or lung diseases if inhaled

CAUTIONS AND CONTRAINDICATIONS: Pregnancy, lactation, pink oyster mushroom allergy; antidiabetic drugs

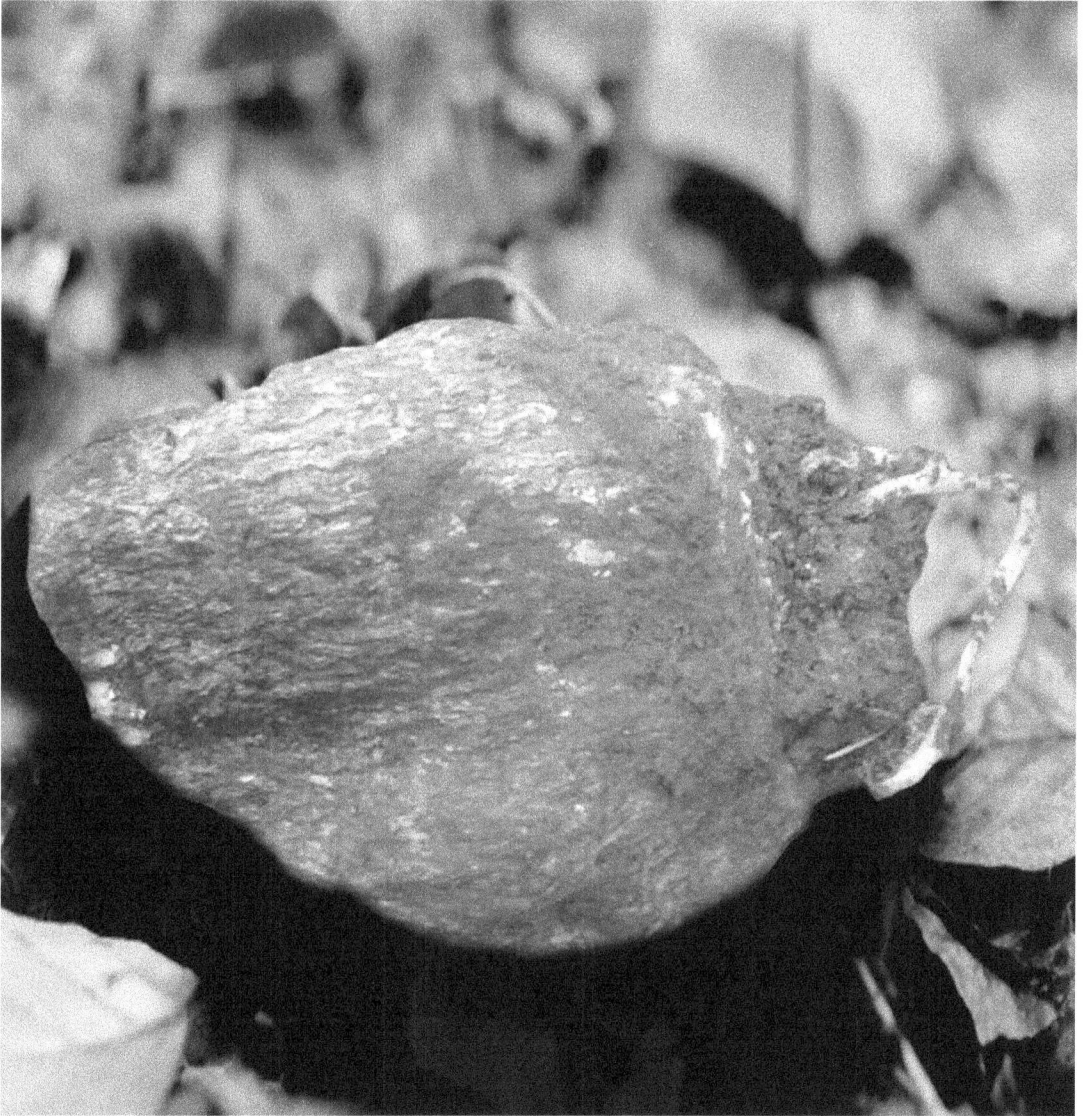

Kingdom: Fungi
Phylum: Basidiomycota
Class: Agaricomycetes
Order: Polyporales
Family: Polyporaceae Polyporaceae | Polyporaceae | Fomitopsidaceae
Genus: Wolfiporia | Poria | Wolfiporia | Pachyma
Species: extensa | cocos | cocos | cocos
Native Habitat: East Asia

Among the numerous fungi with therapeutic potential, poria stands out as a remarkable and multifaceted healing agent. This mushroom has been used for centuries in traditional Chinese medicine (TCM) for its various health benefits. Native to East Asia, particularly China and Japan, it is known by various names, including "Fu Ling" in Chinese, "Bak Fu Ling" in Cantonese, and "Tuckahoe" in English. Although recent research—phylogenetic analyses and morphological examination—has brought into dispute the connection between North American *Poria cocos* and Asian Fu Ling (*Pachyma hoelen*).[2525] These analyses show that they are related but distinct species and should no longer be commingled as they are currently in the literature. Resembling a small coconut, it is a wood-decay fungus with a subterranean growth habitat.

Poria is a unique-looking mushroom, unlike the classic cap-and-stem shape of most edible fungi. It grows as a sclerotium, which is a compact mass of mycelium and other fungal tissues. The outer appearance of poria is a hard, woody structure with a brown to reddish-brown color. This woody structure can vary in size and shape, ranging from small, spherical lumps to larger, irregular formations. The interior of poria is spongy, with small pores that can be seen upon cutting it open.

Poria primarily grows on the roots of pine trees and other conifers. It forms a mutualistic relationship with these trees, deriving nutrients from them while aiding in the tree's nutrient uptake. To cultivate poria, a similar environment can be replicated, with the mushroom's mycelium growing on a substrate of pine sawdust or other suitable materials. However, it should be noted that poria is slow-growing, taking several months or even years to reach maturity.

Poria has a rich history of use in ancient Asian medicinal systems, dating back over 2,000 years. It is often mentioned in ancient Chinese texts like the *Shennong Ben Cao Jing* and *Ben Cao Gang Mu* as a valuable medicinal fungus. In TCM, it is categorized as a Qi-invigorating herb, believed to strengthen the body's vital energy, or Qi, and promote overall well-being. Poria has been used to address various health issues, from digestive problems to emotional imbalances.

A variety of bioactive compounds contribute to the medicinal properties of poria including polysaccharides, triterpenes, ergosterol, and beta-glucans. It offers a wide range of potential health benefits because of these compounds, making it a valuable addition to holistic wellness practices. Poria is renowned for its immunomodulatory properties. The polysaccharides and beta-glucans in the mushroom can help stimulate the immune system, making it more effective at fighting off infections and illnesses. Inflammation is a major factor in many chronic conditions. Poria contains triterpenes, such as poricoic acids, with notable anti-inflammatory properties, making it valuable for arthritis, asthma, and other inflammatory disorders. Oxidative stress is a leading contributor to aging and various health problems. Poria contains antioxidant compounds that can neutralize harmful free radicals, protecting cells from damage and supporting overall health. This can potentially slow the aging process and reduce the risk of chronic diseases. In TCM, poria is often used to address digestive issues. It is believed to have a calming effect on the digestive system, so it is often used for treating diarrhea, indigestion, and other gastrointestinal disorders. Like other mushrooms, poria may support gut microbiome homeostasis. Some studies suggest that poria may have a positive impact on heart health because of its ability to decrease inflammation and lower blood pressure. This activity may reduce the risk of cardiovascular diseases, including heart attacks and strokes. As an adaptogen, it is believed to have a calming effect on the mind and can be used to alleviate symptoms of anxiety and improve sleep quality. Lastly, the triterpenes in poria have shown promise in laboratory studies as potential anticancer agents. From the mounting scientific evidence, it is clear why ancient cultures prized this powerful medicinal mushroom and why modern-day scientists should pay greater attention to discovering its medicinal properties.

Poria can be consumed in various forms to harness its medicinal benefits. In TCM, it is often simmered for a long time to create a decoction, which is a concentrated herbal tea. Poria is available in supplement form, such as capsules, tablets, or tinctures. This provides a convenient way to incorporate it into your daily routine. It is also available as a powder, which can be added to smoothies, soups, or other foods and beverages. Poria is a common ingredient in traditional Chinese dishes, especially in herbal soups and broths. It is often combined with other medicinal herbs and ingredients to create nourishing, health-promoting meals.

Poria is an intriguing and versatile medicinal mushroom with potential to boost the immune system, reduce inflammation, and support overall well-being. It deserves a place in the realm of holistic health and alternative medicine to support optimum wellness.

NOTABLE COMPOUNDS: Polysaccharides, triterpenes, beta-glucans, alpha-glucans, triterpene acids, poricoic acid B, poricoic acid G, poricoic acid H, polyporenic acid C, pachymic acid, pachymaran, dehydrotumulosic acid, dehydrotrametenolic acid, steroids, choline, histidine, lanostanoids, hoelen

BENEFITS ACCORDING TO PRECLINICAL RESEARCH:

- 🍄 Anticancer (breast)[2526-2534]
- 🍄 Impairs breast cancer cell invasion[2535]
- 🍄 Enhances the activity of doxorubicin against multidrug-resistant breast cancer[2536]
- 🍄 Anticancer (gastric)[2537,2538,2539]

- Anticancer (prevents invasion and metastasis of gastric cancer)[2540]
- Anticancer (acute promyelocytic leukemia)[2541]
- Anticancer (lung)[2542-2549]
- Anticancer (metastatic lung)[2550]
- Anticancer (liver)[2551,2552,2553,2554]
- Anticancer (leukemia)[2555,2556,2557,2558,2559,2560]
- Anticancer (colorectal)[2561,2562]
- Anticancer (pancreatic)[2563,2564]
- Anticancer (prostate)[2565,2566]
- Anticancer (ovarian)[2567]
- Anticancer (osteosarcoma)[2568]
- Anticancer (bladder)[2569]
- Anticancer (skin)[2570,2571]
- Prevents skin cancer[2572]
- Inhibits aberrant expression of cell division cycle 20 in metastatic breast and chemoresistant pancreatic cells, which can improve prognosis and reduce malignant progression[2573]
- Inhibits the expression of the proto-oncogene H-ras[2574]
- Anticancer (enhances the anticancer effect of 5-fluorouracil and reduces its side effects)[2575]
- Protects against cisplatin-induced kidney toxicity[2576]
- Reduces colon injuries caused by 5-fluorouracil[2577]
- Anticancer (rodent sarcoma)[2578,2579,2580,2581,2582]
- Improves gut dysbiosis (increasing the beneficial bacteria *Lactobacillus, Bifidobacterium, Erysipelotrichaceae*, and *Prevotellaceae*, and decreasing the sulfate-reducing bacteria *Desulfovibrio* and inflammatory associated bacteria *Proteobacteria, Cyanobacteria, Ruminococcaceae, Helicobacteraceae, Mucispirillum*, S24-7, and *Staphylococcus*)[2583-2591]
- Strengthens and preserves intestinal barrier function (reduces leaky gut)[2592-2598]
- Relieves ulcerative colitis[2599,2600]
- Shields against inflammatory bowel disease[2601]
- Ameliorates antibiotic-caused diarrhea[2602,2603]
- Relieves functional dyspepsia—upset stomach with no known cause (promotes repair of gastrointestinal mucosa, balances immune responses, regulates brain-gut peptides)[2604]
- Alleviates or prevents Alzheimer's disease (aids clearance of beta-amyloid, inhibits acetylcholinesterase)[2605,2606,2607,2608,2609,2610]
- Aids cognition[2611]
- Neuroprotective after ischemia/reperfusion (I/R) injury[2612]

- Antidiabetic[2613-2618]
- Protects against diabetic-associated kidney damage (diabetic nephropathy)[2619,2620]
- Antidepressant[2621,2622,2623,2624]
- Relieves anxiety[2625,2626]
- Alleviates insomnia[2627,2628]
- Enhances the sedating effects of pentobarbital[2629]
- Prevents arteriosclerosis/atherosclerosis[2630,2631]
- Aids bone strength, prevents or treats osteoporosis[2632,2633,2634]
- Relieves chronic nonbacterial prostatitis[2635,2636]
- Anti-inflammatory[2637-2649]
- Suppresses the progression and inflammation of osteoarthritis[2650]
- Relieves gout (lowers uric acid)[2651]
- Stimulates immune function, including restoring immune function after suppression[2652-2664]
- Balances immune function (polysaccharide dependent)[2665,2666,2667,2668,2669]
- Prevents rejection after cardiac allograft implantation or kidney transplant[2670,2671]
- Alleviates allergic asthma[2672]
- Mitigates food allergies/intolerances[2673]
- Kidney protective[2674-2689]
- Ameliorates chronic kidney disease/injury[2690,2691]
- Prevents the transition from acute kidney injury to chronic kidney disease[2692]
- Ameliorates acute pancreatitis and associated kidney damage[2693]
- Prevents kidney stones (calcium-oxalate stones)[2694,2695]
- Alleviates cystitis glandularis[2696]
- Liver protective[2697,2698,2699]
- Protects liver against damage caused by alcohol[2700]
- Protects against acetaminophen caused liver damage[2701,2702]
- Alleviates nonalcoholic fatty liver disease[2703-2710]
- Improves alcoholic fatty liver disease[2711]
- Cardioprotective[2712]
- Protects blood cells (inhibits free radical-induced lysis)[2713]
- Improves cardiac function and acts as a diuretic (beneficial for chronic heart failure)[2714,2715,2716,2717]
- Lowers high cholesterol, improves lipid profiles[2718,2719,2720,2721,2722,2723]
- Ameliorates glucolipid metabolism disorders[2724]
- Combats obesity[2725,2726]
- Mitigates peritonitis-induced sepsis[2727]

- ♈ Improves anemia (polysaccharide iron complex)[2728]
- ♈ Protects against lung fibrosis[2729]
- ♈ Shields against lung injury during immunosuppression by altering the lung and gut microbiome[2730]
- ♈ Mitigates pneumonia by reducing inflammation and respiratory cellular death[2731]
- ♈ Protects against ear toxicity caused by kanamycin[2732]
- ♈ Stimulates autophagy in aged cells—autophagy is a fundamental cellular process that eliminates molecules and subcellular elements, thereby maintaining energy homeostasis and the renewal of organelles, which plays a key role in aging and age-related conditions[2733]
- ♈ Antiepileptic[2734]
- ♈ Antiviral (SARS-CoV-2, inhibits Mpro)[2735]
- ♈ Antiviral (Epstein-Barr virus early antigen)[2736,2737]
- ♈ Antibacterial[2738,2739,2740]
- ♈ Antioxidant[2741-2752]
- ♈ Alleviates eczema[2753]
- ♈ Relieves delayed hypersensitivity reaction (contact dermatitis)[2754,2755]
- ♈ Brightens the skin[2756,2757,2758]
- ♈ Moisturizes the skin and improves skin barrier function[2759,2760]
- ♈ Reduces skin aging[2761]
- ♈ Protects skin against UV damage[2762]
- ♈ Alleviates chronic skin inflammation[2763]
- ♈ Improves sperm quality[2764]
- ♈ Reduces nausea and vomiting[2765]
- ♈ Nematocidal[2766]
- ♈ Trypanocidal[2767]

BENEFITS ACCORDING TO CLINICAL RESEARCH:

- ➤ Improves clinical response to and side effects of chemotherapy in women with ovarian cancer[2768]
  - Chinese multiherbal formula containing poria
- ➤ Reduces fasting blood glucose, postprandial (after-meal) blood glucose spikes, and HbA1c in people with type 2 diabetes when used with conventional drugs[2769]
  - Chinese multiherbal formula containing poria

THERAPEUTIC POTENTIAL: Leaky gut, dysbiosis, nonalcoholic fatty liver disease, insomnia, anxiety, kidney stones

CLINICAL DOSAGES: Used as an ingredient in multiherbal formulas; capsules: 500 mg, up to three times daily; tincture: 970 mg up to four times daily

POTENTIAL ADVERSE EFFECTS: Vomiting, diarrhea

CAUTIONS AND CONTRAINDICATIONS: Pregnancy, lactation, poria mushroom allergy; sedative drugs (e.g., barbiturates), cholesterol-lowering drugs, antidiabetic meds

PSILOCYBE

(*Psilocybe azurescens, Psilocybe semilanceata, Psilocybe cyanescens, Psilocybe cubensis, Psilocybe bohemica* (syn. *P. serbica*), *Psilocybe baeocystis, Psilocybe tampanensis, Psilocybe weilii, Psilocybe hoogshagenii, Psilocybe* spp.)

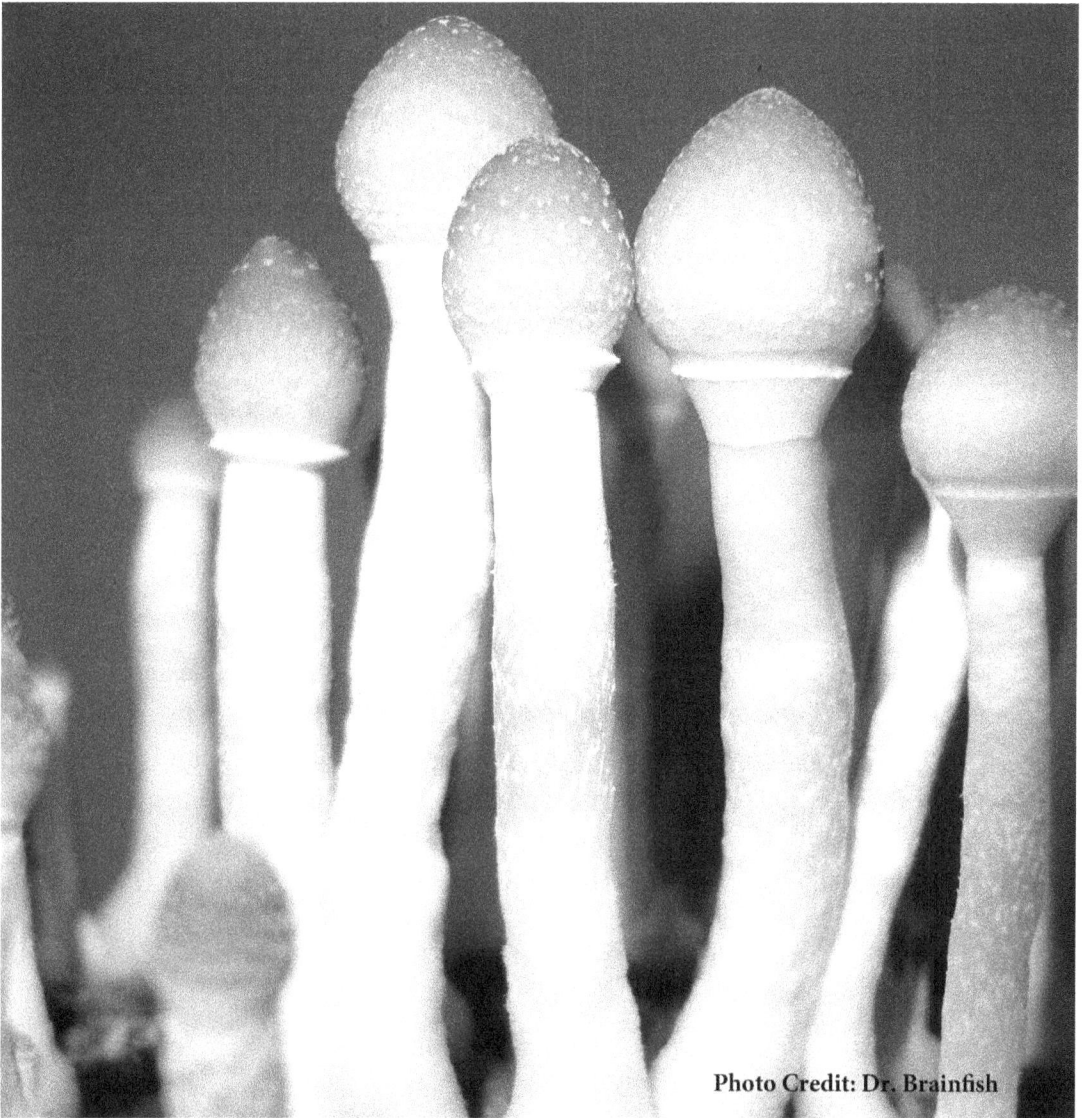

Photo Credit: Dr. Brainfish

Kingdom: Fungi
Phylum: Basidiomycota
Class: Agaricomycetes
Order: Agaricales
Family: Hymenogastraceae
Genus: Psilocybe

Species: azurescens | semilanceata | cyanescens | cubensis | bohemica | baeocystis | tampanensis | weilii | hoogshagenii

Native Habitat: Germany, Netherlands, New Zealand, United Kingdom, United States | Northern Hemisphere, particularly Europe, and the Southern Hemisphere | Northwestern United States | Cuba, Central America, and South America | Europe | Pacific Northwest United States | Southeast United States | North America, particularly the Pacific Northwest | Mexico and South America

This book would be incomplete without a mention of the *Psilocybe* family of mushrooms despite their current classification in the United States and many other countries as a controlled substance. Affectionately known as "magic mushrooms," these mushrooms contain the naturally occurring psychedelic prodrug compound psilocybin, which is produced by over two hundred species of fungi. Although psylocibin has a hallucinogenic and mind-altering effect at higher doses, microdoses of psylocibin, or mushrooms that contain psylocibin, have massive potential to improve human health. A microdose should not produce any significant psychoactive response, predominantly triggering a subtle shift in mood and perception and possibly an increase in creativity and focus. Research suggests that most people perceive a dose of 45 mcg/kg of body weight as psychoactive, suggesting 3.15 mg of psilocybin in the average person (70 kg; 154 lbs.) may be psychoactive.[2770] Some suggest that doses of 0.25 to 1.25 mg of psilocybin are imperceptible. What constitutes a microdose is hotly debated, but it generally is considered to be between 0.1 and 0.5 grams of dried mushroom—most commonly 0.1 to 0.3 grams—which would provide between 0.9 to 4.5 mg of psilocybin. Noting that 3.15 mg is perceived as psychoactive, it may be best to limit your dose to 2.5 mg to limit the possibility of a psychoactive response. Hopefully, the evolving legal landscape and emerging research demonstrating the safety of psylocibin will eventually move these important mushrooms from the prohibited and banned list to allowance for medicinal purposes similar to what is occurring for cannabis medicines.

The use of Psilocybe mushrooms dates back centuries, with a rich history of indigenous use in various cultures. These mushrooms have played significant roles in spiritual, shamanic, and medicinal practices. Psilocybe mushrooms were used by indigenous peoples in Mesoamerica, with evidence dating back thousands of years. The Aztecs referred to them as *teonanácatl*, meaning "flesh of the gods," highlighting their spiritual significance. Some indigenous peoples of the American continent have incorporated Psilocybe mushrooms into their rituals and ceremonies, considering them as a means of communicating with the spiritual world. Today, shamanic traditions in various parts of the world continue to utilize Psilocybe mushrooms as tools for healing and spiritual insight.

The primary psychoactive compounds in Psilocybe mushrooms are the tryptamine alkaloids psilocybin and psilocin. In addition to psilocybin and psilocin, Psilocybe mushrooms contain various amounts of other analogs such as baeocystin, norbaeocystin, aeruginascin, and bufotenine. Psylocibin is itself biologically inactive, but the body rapidly converts it to psilocin, which has biological activity when ingested. Essentially, psilocin mimics serotonin and binds to serotonin receptors, therefore activating them. In addition, these alkaloids can increase brain-derived neurotrophic factor (BDNF), which triggers the growth of new synapses and neurons. When sufficient doses are ingested, people may experience altered perception, visual and auditory distortions, elevated mood, feelings of euphoria, enhanced creativity, profound mystical and spiritual experiences, increased empathy, challenging experiences, and an expanded interconnection with nature.

While the recreational use of Psilocybe mushrooms is well-documented, scientific research over the last few decades has shed light on the potential health benefits associated with their controlled and responsible use at microdoses—subperceptual doses that do not produce a psychedelic effect—and low doses, which can produce a mild psychedelic effect along with the therapeutic effect. Psilocybin-assisted therapy has shown promise in the treatment of mood disorders like depression, PTSD, and anxiety. Clinical trials have demonstrated that a single dose of psilocybin, when administered in a therapeutic setting, can lead to lasting reductions in depressive symptoms. Ironically, psilocybin has been investigated as a potential treatment for substance use disorders, including alcohol and tobacco addiction. It is believed to work by disrupting addictive patterns and promoting introspection and self-reflection. Research suggests that psilocybin therapy can help individuals with life-threatening illnesses cope with end-of-life anxiety and existential distress. It can lead to a more peaceful acceptance of mortality. They can also be helpful for hard-to-treat painful conditions like migraines and neuropathy. Some individuals report long-lasting improvements in mood, well-being, and quality of life following a psychedelic experience with Psilocybe mushrooms. Finally, Psilocybe mushrooms may boost creativity, cognitive function, and problem-solving abilities, potentially aiding in personal growth and professional development.

An interesting aspect of psilocybin use is emerging research suggesting that men and women respond differently to it. This can be at least partly explained by the fact that estrogen affects serotonin transmission, binding, and metabolism—serotonin sites are a major target of psilocin. Since estrogen levels fluctuate throughout a woman's monthly cycle and lifetime, this influences a woman's response to psylocibin. Some indigenous wisdom experts suggest women take psilocybin around the ovulation period rather than closer to menstruation for best results. Not surprisingly, taking psylocibin may cause the menstrual cycle to come a little early and has therapeutic potential to restore menstruation when it is absent or reestablish regularity in the menstrual cycle.

One Mechanism of Microdosing

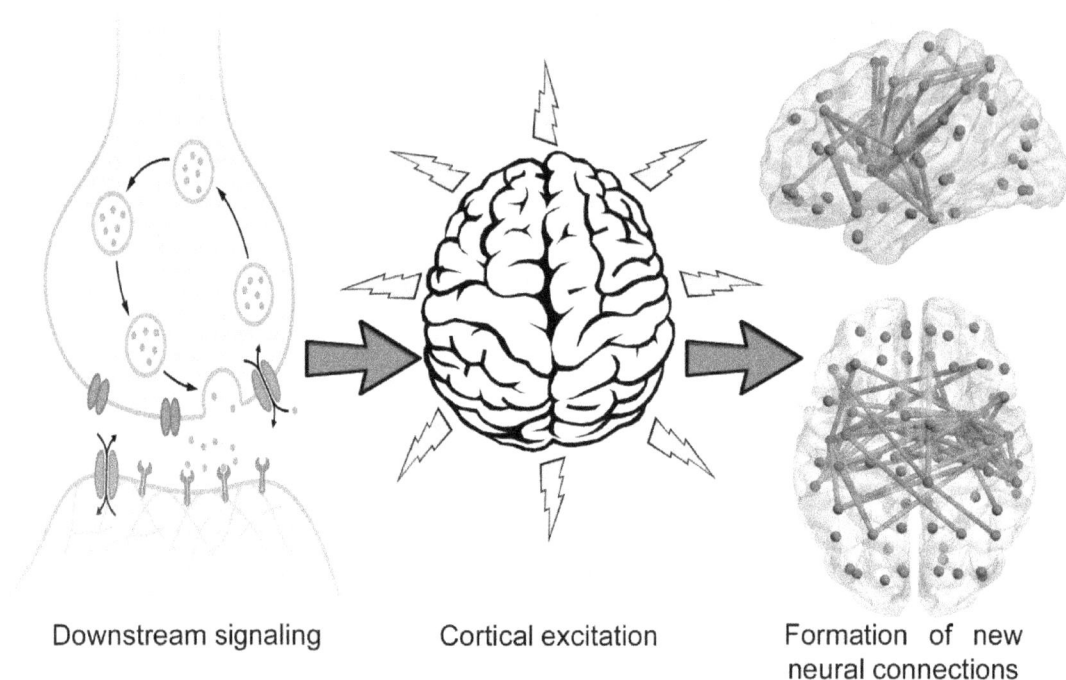

| Downstream signaling | Cortical excitation | Formation of new neural connections |

Notable strains of *Psilocybe cubensis* mushrooms include:

Penis Envy. If you can get past the middle school giggles produced by this strain's name, penis envy is a highly sought-after potent strain. It earned its name because of its distinct appearance with a thick bulbous cap and short stem that resembles a circumcised penis. It is prized for its consistently high levels of psilocybin, reported to be as high as 2.95 percent. Taking more than microdoses of this strain is linked to intense hallucinations accompanied by a deep sense of introspection.

B+ Strain. Known for its large meaty caps and thick stems, the B+ strain is a potent strain known for producing intense visuals and strong senses of euphoria when taken above microdoses. Use of this strain is associated with enhanced mental clarity and sharpened focus.

Golden Teacher. Highly regarded as one of the most potent strains, golden teacher can produce significant mystical experiences that are useful for self-growth and inner healing. It is popular among beginners because it is relatively easy to grow.

Tidal Wave. Known for its fast growth and intense euphoric effects, tidal wave is a potent Psilocybe strain, which boasts the ability to produce very high total tryptamine content. It is actually a hybrid of the penis envy and B+ strains. People who use this strain report strong visuals, enhanced mental clarity, and an overall feel-good sensation.

Mazatapec. Native to Mexico and named after the Mazatec people, this strain is known for its mild yet euphoric effects and ability to fabricate a deep meditative state. It is considered to be less potent on average than other *P. cubensis* strains.

The use of Psilocybe mushrooms, particularly for therapeutic purposes, raises important ethical and legal considerations, including respecting individual autonomy and promoting their safe use to minimize the risks associated with psychedelic experiences. Psilocybe mushrooms, with their psychoactive properties and potential health benefits, offer a fascinating and complex subject for exploration. While they have a long history of use in indigenous cultures and have been associated with profound spiritual experiences, scientific research is shedding new light on their therapeutic potential. Encouragingly, there is increasing evidence of safety emerging from clinical trials and emergency room data with primarily mild and transient adverse effects reported. One study found that out of over 9,200 Psilocybe mushroom users, only 0.2 percent reported seeking emergency medical treatment for an adverse event, with the most common symptoms being anxiety/panic attack and paranoia.[2771] As research continues, it is crucial to balance the pursuit of knowledge with ethical and legal considerations to ensure that the benefits of Psilocybe mushrooms can be harnessed safely and responsibly. Psilocybe mushrooms have massive potential to help millions of people with conditions very difficult to treat with current chemical medicines, such as chronic pain, chronic inflammation, and mental health conditions. One need only review the clinical research and the countless lives that have been improved by these mushrooms to realize that there is an urgent need to create a path whereby people have access to these remarkably medicinal mushrooms and their active compounds. We can no longer deny people access to life-altering and potentially lifesaving medicinal mushrooms in the Psilocybe family.

The possession, consumption, or distribution of psilocybin or Psilocybe mushrooms may carry heavy prison sentences and fines in many countries. This book and the author do not propose their use until legislation permits. Some states and municipalities have decriminalized the person use of psylocibin, but that doesn't mean you won't be subject to criminal prosecution or legal consequences. Check with your local authorities and consult an attorney to determine your legal risks. Also note that the risks are significantly elevated if you share psilocybin-containing products with others.

AVERAGE ALKALOIDAL CONTENT BY PSILOCYBE SPECIES:[2772-2780]

Species	Psilocybin	Psilocin	Baeocystin
P. semilanceata	0.01%–1.96%	tr–0.90%	0.07%–0.45%
P. subaeruginosa	0.01%–1.93%	0.0%–0.17%	tr
P. azurescens	1.70%–1.78%	0.38%	0.35%
P. serbica	tr–1.55%	tr–0.79%	0.00%–0.34%
P. cyanescens	0.23%–1.38%	0.04%–1.00%	0.02%–0.29%
P. bohemica	0.60%–1.34%	0.11%–0.28%	0.00%–0.04%
P. cubensis	0.00%–1.10%	0.01%–0.60%	0.01%–0.09%
P. zapotecorum	0.90%–0.97%	0.03%–0.04%	0.04%–0.05%
P. samuiensis	0.02%–0.90%	0.05%–0.81%	0.01%–0.05%
P. baeocystis	0.85%	0.59%	0.10%
P. subcubensis	0.80%	0.02%	0.00%
P. ovoideocystidiata	0.09%–0.72%	tr–0.55%	0.02%–0.07%
P. tampanensis	0.00%–0.68%	0.01%–0.32%	0.00%
P. weilii	0.61%	0.27%	0.05%
P. hoogshagenii	0.60%	0.10%	0.00%
P. caerlipes	0.22%–0.57%	0.05%–0.28%	tr–0.01%
P. subcaerulipes	tr–0.55%	–	–
P. mexicana	0.33%–0.39%	0.19%–0.20%	0.03%
P. stuntzii	0.36%	0.12%	0.02%
P. semperviva	0.30%	0.07%	0.00%
P. cyanofibrillosa	0.21%	0.04%	0.00%
P. liniformans	0.16%	0.00%	tr
P. pelliculosa	0.12%	0.00%	0.00%
P. medulossa	0.01%–0.10%	0.00–tr	tr–0.04%
P. caerulescens	0.02%–0.03%	0.03%–0.04%	tr–0.01%
Average	0.90%	0.28%	0.09%

AVERAGE ALKALOIDAL CONTENT OF NON-PSILOCYBE SPECIES:[2781,2782,2783,2784]

Species	Psilocybin	Psilocin	Baeocystin
Pluteus salicinus	1.20%	0.00%	0.00%
Panaeolus cyanescens	tr–1.15%	0.09%–0.90%	0.00%–0.02%
Conocybe cyanopus	0.33%–0.93%	tr–0.70%	0.00%–0.03%
Agrocybe praecox	0.80%	0.00%	0.00%
Pluteus salicinus	0.35%	0.01%	–
Gymnopilus purpuratus	0.24%–0.34%	0.29%–0.35%	0.01%–0.05%
Inocybe aeruginascens	0.16%–0.32%	0.05%–0.11%	0.15%–0.20%
Copelandia cambodginiensis			
Pluteus americanus	0.12%–0.24%	0.01%–0.04%	0.02%–0.04%
Panaeolus cinctulus	0.01%–0.16%	tr–0.03%	0.01%–0.15%
Panaeolus subbalteatus	0.16%	0.00%	0.08%
Panaeolus semiovatus var. *semiovatus*	0.11%	0.14%	–
Inocybe corydalina	tr–0.03%	tr	0.05%–0.10%

NOTABLE COMPOUNDS: Psylocibin, psilocin, baeocystin, norbaeocystin, norpsilocin, aeruginascin, tryptamine, beta-carbolines, polysaccharides, sesquiterpenoids, alkaloids, flavonoids, tannins, saponins

BENEFITS ACCORDING TO PRECLINICAL RESEARCH:

- 🍄 Antidepressant[2785-2792]
- 🍄 Alters sleep-wake architecture, local sleep homeostasis, and cortical brain activity, which may reduce depression[2793]
- 🍄 Diminishes obsessive-compulsive disorder (taking with buspirone may reduce psychedelic effects without diminishing reductions in OCD)[2794,2795,2796]
- 🍄 Increases resilience to stress and diminishes compulsive actions[2797]
- 🍄 Reduces anxiety[2798]
- 🍄 Alters brain activity and function (reduced spike activity in hippocampal CA1 pyramidal neurons, suppressed glutamate transmission, brain metabolism changes, desyncing of cerebral hemisphere, enhances neuroplasticity, increases synaptic density, acts as an agonist for 5HT receptors, increases cortical activities, elevates c-Fos expression, binds to TrkB (the receptor for BDNF), increases central amygdala activity in males and females and stimulus specific central amygdala activity only in females)[2799-2818]
- 🍄 Modifies neurotransmitters levels (serotonin and dopamine)[2819,2820,2821,2822]
- 🍄 Ameliorates stress-related behavioral deficits and promotes synaptic rewiring of the cortex[2823]
- 🍄 Enhances cognitive flexibility[2824]
- 🍄 Mitigates cognitive deficits associated with Fragile X syndrome[2825]
- 🍄 Does not impair decision-making or motivation[2826]
- 🍄 Facilitates fear extinction (diminishment of a learned or conditioned fear behavior, which is important for PTSD)[2827,2828]
- 🍄 Decreases startling (high doses) or increases startling (low doses)[2829]
- 🍄 Regulates meth-induced behavioral alterations[2830]
- 🍄 Reduces nicotine addiction[2831]
- 🍄 Diminishes alcohol consumption in males but not females[2832]
- 🍄 Reduces the resumption of alcohol seeking after a memory retrieval-reconsolidation of alcohol-related memories[2833]
- 🍄 Reduces alcohol consumption and relapse by restoring mGluR2 expression (reduced prefrontal mGluR2 expression and function combined with impaired executive function is linked to alcohol craving)[2834]
- 🍄 Decreases consumption of high-calorie foods and lowers body weight[2835]
- 🍄 Reduces sugar preference, but not binge-like eating (single high dose)[2836]

- 🍄 Anti-inflammatory[2837,2838,2839,2840]
- 🍄 Reduces brain inflammation when combined with eugenol[2841]
- 🍄 Alleviates epilepsy[2842]
- 🍄 Regulates immunological pathways and the expression of immune-related genes[2843]
- 🍄 Increases prolactin levels[2844]
- 🍄 Antioxidant[2845]
- 🍄 Antiviral (SARS-CoV-2)[2846]
- 🍄 Antibacterial[2847,2848]
- 🍄 Mosquito larvicidal[2849]

BENEFITS ACCORDING TO CLINICAL RESEARCH:

- ➢ Significantly improves depression in people with long-lasting moderate-to-severe major depressive disorder aged eighteen to eighty better than the SSRI escitalopram (Lexapro, Cipralex)—subjects were monitored for six months after the two doses[2850]
  - 25 mg psilocybin three days apart (total of two doses)
- ➢ Substantially improves depression in people with moderate-to-severe major depressive disorder aged twenty-one to seventy-five[2851]
  - Two doses of 20 mg/70 kg/bw and 30 mg/70 kg/bw spaced two weeks apart
- ➢ Significantly improves depression in people with potentially life-threatening cancer[2852]
  - 22–30 mg/70 kg/bw administered twice about five weeks apart
- ➢ Significantly improves depression in people with potentially life-threatening cancer[2853]
  - Single dose of 0.3 mg/kg/bw psilocybin
- ➢ Persistently (about two months) improves depression[2854]
  - Single dose of 0.3 mg/kg body weight psilocybin
- ➢ Improves psycho-social-spiritual well-being in people with cancer and major depressive disorder
  - Single dose of 25 mg of psilocybin
- ➢ Reduces depression in people with cancer[2855]
  - Single dose of 25 mg of psilocybin
- ➢ Significantly reduces anxiety in people diagnosed with cancer[2856]
  - Single dose of 0.2 mg/kg/bw psilocybin
- ➢ Increases global integration in the brain to reduce depression in people with major depressive disorder[2857]
  - 10 mg and 25 mg psilocybin, seven days apart; or 25 mg psilocybin, three weeks apart

- Improves depression in females with severe, unipolar, treatment-resistant major depression, which benefits persist for six months[2858]
  - 10 mg and 25 mg psilocybin, seven days apart
- Revives emotional responsiveness in people with mild-to-severe treatment-resistant depression[2859]
  - 10 mg psilocybin, followed by 25 mg one week later
- Reduces depressive symptoms, sustaining these effects for at least two weeks as evidenced by EEG reading showing an increase in theta power[2860]
  - Single dose of 0.3 mg/kg/bw psilocybin
- Improves major depressive disorder[2861]
  - 20 mg/70 kg/bw followed by 30 mg/70 kg/bw 1.6 weeks later
- Promotes neuroplasticity and relieves depression by desynchronizing brain activity across spatial scales (area, network, whole brain)—threefold greater acute changes in functional networks than methylphenidate[2862]
  - Single dose of 25 mg psilocybin
- Alleviates major depressive disorder[2863]
  - Single dose of 25 mg psilocybin—a single dose of 10 mg was considered ineffective
- Positively changes personality (reduces neuroticism and increases extraversion) in individuals with treatment-resistant depression[2864]
  - 10 mg psilocybin, followed by 25 mg one week later
- Enhances processing of emotional faces in people with treatment-resistant depression—people who are depressed frequently exhibit biases in emotional processing[2865]
  - 10 mg psilocybin, followed by 25 mg one week later
- Improves treatment-resistant depression by triggering a "reset" that involves the reintegration and resumption of normal brain functioning[2866]
  - 10 mg psilocybin, followed by 25 mg one week later
- Reduces depression and anxiety and improves quality of life in people with treatment-resistant major depressive disorder[2867]
  - A single dose of either 10 mg or 25 mg of psilocybin, with 25 mg producing greater effects
- Promotes sustained reduction in depressive symptoms and functional disability in people with major depressive disorder[2868]
  - Single dose of 25 mg psilocybin
- Promotes positive personality changes—reduced neuroticism, introversion, disagreeableness, and impulsivity, with increases in conscientiousness, openness, and absorption—in people with depression
  - 25 mg of psilocybin followed by another 25 mg of psilocybin three weeks later

- Elevates responsiveness to music in people with depression[2869,2870]
  - 10 mg psilocybin, followed by 25 mg one week later
- Improves mood and lessens biases toward negative facial expressions in healthy people[2871]
  - Single dose of 215 mcg/kg/bw psilocybin
- Reduces associative, but concurrently increases sensory, brain-wide connectivity, which may alleviate depression and promote a balanced mood[2872]
  - Single dose of 0.2 mg/kg/bw psilocybin
- Alleviates depression and anxiety associated with Lyme disease that was unresponsive to antimicrobial and benzodiazepine drugs in a thirty-four-year-old male[2873]
  - 100 mg three times weekly, increased to 125 mg three times weekly after two weeks of use
- Increases cognitive flexibility and neural flexibility (depression can change a person's ability to think and decrease the ability to adapt to change) in people with major depressive disorder[2874]
  - 20 mg/70 kg/bw followed by 30 mg/70 kg/bw 1.6 weeks later
- Alleviates posttraumatic stress disorder (PTSD)[2875]
  - Up to three 10–25 mg doses psilocybin spaced weeks to months apart
- Increases connection to nature and decreases authoritarian political views in people with treatment-resistant depression[2876]
  - 10 mg psilocybin, followed by 25 mg one week later
- Profoundly reduces migraine headache intensity and vomiting in a thirty-three-year-old male with poor response to first-line migraine drugs[2877]
  - 1.2 g of dried fruiting body of *Psilocybe cubensis* mushroom along with 400 mg ibuprofen and 1,000 mg acetaminophen at the onset of migraine aura
- Suppresses migraine frequency in individuals who experience two or more migraines weekly[2878]
  - Single dose of 0.143 mg/kg/bw psilocybin
- Reduces cluster headache occurrence frequency[2879]
  - Three doses of 0.143 mg/kg/bw psilocybin, five days apart
- Immediately reduces proinflammatory TNF-alpha in healthy individuals, which returns to baseline seven days later, but IL-6 and CRP decreased at seven days, corresponding with mood improvements[2880]
  - Single dose of 0.17 mg/kg/bw psilocybin
- Diminishes chronic neuropathic pain[2881]
  - Case 1: Single dose of 5 g of dried Psilocybe mushroom (produced a psychedelic experience and 8 to10 hours of pain relief), dose was subsequently reduced to 250 mg, which provided 6 to 8 hours of pain relief;

Case 2: 500 mg of dried Psilocybe mushroom (3 to 4 hours of 80% pain relief), increased dosage to 750–1,000 mg and experienced 6 to 8 hours of 100% pain relief; Case 3: 1,000 mg of dried Psilocybe mushroom in a chocolate bar combined with home exercise routines performed while pain relief was experienced, resulting in increased mobility, which provided pain relief for two weeks, subject continued taking a dose every 6 to 8 weeks

➢ Reduced debilitating joint pain associated with lupus for twelve months in a sixty-seven-year-old male who failed to respond to hydroxychloroquine and NSAIDs[2882]

- Single dose of 6 g of *Psilocybe cubensis*

➢ Reduces alcohol dependence[2883]

- 0.3 and 0.4 mg/kg/bw psilocybin (two total doses weeks apart)

➢ Reduces alcohol dependence and improves cardiovascular safety when combined with viewing a nature-themed video[2884]

- Single dose of 25 mg psilocybin

➢ Diminishes number of heavy drinking days in alcoholics[2885]

- Single dose of 25 mg/70 kg/bw psilocybin, followed by 25–40 mg/70 kg/bw psilocybin four weeks later

➢ Reduces the subjective effects of alcohol[2886]

- Dosing not reported

➢ Promotes smoking cessation[2887,2888,2889]

- Single dose of 20–30 mg/70 kg/bw psilocybin

➢ Associated with a reduction in cannabis, opioid, or stimulant use[2890]

- Unknown usage (dosing not reported because of observational nature of research)

➢ Improves emotional and brain plasticity for about one month[2891]

- Single dose of 25 mg/70 kg/bw psilocybin

➢ Enhances emotional empathy in healthy individuals[2892]

- Single dose of 0.215 mg/kg/bw psilocybin

➢ Improves subjective sense of well-being and life satisfaction in healthy individuals with no history of psychiatric disorders[2893]

- Three escalating doses of oral psilocybin (0.3 mg/kg/bw; 0.45 mg/kg/bw; 0.6 mg/kg/bw) a minimum of four weeks apart in a supervised setting

➢ Promotes persistent improvements in mental health and well-being—reductions in anxiety, depression, neuroticism, burnout, and alcohol misuse and increases in cognitive flexibility, emotion regulation, spiritual well-being, and extraversion[2894]

- Average of 3.1 g of dried Psilocybe mushrooms

- Reduces subjective attachment anxiety in male long-term AIDS survivors with moderate-severe demoralization[2895,2896]
  - Single dose of 0.3–0.36 mg/kg/bw psilocybin sandwiched between multiple group therapy sessions
- Encourages a positive mood despite negative stimuli in healthy individuals[2897]
  - Single dose of 0.16 mg/kg/bw psilocybin
- Markedly decreases symptoms of obsessive-compulsive disorder[2898]
  - Dose escalation: 25, 100, 200, and 300 mcg/kg/bw once weekly
- Improves SSRI-resistant body dysmorphic disorder, with results lasting through week twelve of observation[2899]
  - Single dose of 25 mg of psilocybin
- Promotes rapid and persistent reductions in anxiety in people with subclinical anxiety[2900]
  - Average of 27.1 mg psilocybin consumption as a single dose
- Produces a long-lasting increase in mindfulness[2901,2902,2903,2904]
  - Single dose of 0.2–0.3 mg/kg/bw psilocybin; or single dose of 315 mcg/kg/bw psilocybin
- Enhances creative thinking, empathy, and subjective well-being in healthy individuals[2905,2906]
  - Consumption of varying numbers of 15 g truffles containing 1.9 mg psilocybin and 10.5 mg psilocin (average consumption of 34.2 g of truffles—4.33 mg psilocybin and 23.94 psilocin); or single dose of 0.17 mg/kg/bw psilocybin
- Improves working memory in females with a history of hallucinogen use[2907]
  - 10, 20, and 30 mg/70 kg/bw psilocybin
- Alters subjective arousal and attention by significantly reducing the rate of binocular rivalry switching in healthy individuals[2908]
  - Single dose of 215 mcg/kg/bw psilocybin
- Significantly increases feelings of openness[2909]
  - Session providing a single dose of 30 mg/70 kg/bw psilocybin
- Enhances feelings of awe in response to videos[2910]
  - Capsules supplying about 1.5 mg of psilocybin five to seven times over the course of three weeks
- Enhances insights into life and existence and encourages spiritual experiences[2911]
  - Single dose of 170–215 mcg/kg/bw psilocybin
- Does not negatively alter memory consolidation or cognition in healthy people[2912,2913]
  - Single dose of 1 mg/5 kg/bw psilocybin; or a single dose of 10 or 25 mg psilocybin

- Microdosers exhibit lower levels of depression, anxiety, and stress across gender
  - Chronic use (dosing not reported because of observational nature of research)[2914]
- A systemic review and dose-response meta-analysis of human studies concluded that effective therapeutic doses of psilocybin for depression are 8.92 mg/70 kg/bw (secondary depression), 24.68 mg/70 kg/bw (primary depression), and 36.08 mg/70 kg/bw (subgroups: major depressive disorder or cancer-related depression).[2915]
- Associated with pain relief among people with fibromyalgia, arthritis, migraine, tension-type headache, but not sciatica[2916]
  - Microdoses (dosing not reported because of observational nature of research)
- Associated with a lower risk of cardiovascular disease and diabetes[2917]
  - At least one use of psychedelics during lifetime (dosing not reported because of observational nature of research)
- Associated with reduced suicidal ideation, planning, and attempts[2918,2919]
  - Chronic use (dosing not reported because of observational nature of research)
- Associated with an increased ability to quit smoking and maintain abstinence in people who smoked on average fourteen cigarettes daily for eight years and had tried to quit five times previously[2920]
  - Dosing not reported because of observational nature of research
- Associated with a decreased odd of crime arrests[2921]
  - Chronic use (dosing not reported because of observational nature of research)

THERAPEUTIC POTENTIAL: Depression, anxiety, PTSD, mood stabilization, ADHD, OCD, substance use disorders, traumatic brain injury, pain, autism spectrum disorder, cluster headaches or migraines, performance and creativity enhancement

CLINICAL DOSAGES: A microdose is considered 100 to 500 mg of dried mushrooms (average of 0.9 mg to 4.5 mg of psilocybin), taken every three to four days, although staying under 3 mg of psylocibin may be necessary to avoid a psychoactive response; a low dose 501 to 1,500 mg of dried mushroom (average of 4.5 mg to 13.5 mg of psilocybin), which is usually taken after two months of microdosing; a medium dose 1,501 to 3,000 mg of dried mushroom (average 13.5 mg to 27 mg psilocybin); a high dose 3,501 to 5,000 mg of dried mushroom (average 31.5 mg to 45 mg psilocybin); and a heroic dose 5,001 to 10,000 mg (average of 45 mg to 90 mg psilocybin); *Typical therapeutic dose*: 10 mg to 35 mg* on an empty stomach, preferably in the morning, which can be taken every seven to twenty-one days depending on your personal response; the most common dosage is 25 mg, or a weight-adjusted dose of 0.3 mg/kg/bw, although some research suggests that body weight isn't a significant factor in benefits; as little as 3 to 5 mg every three to four days may be effective, producing perceptible changes, and has a lower risk of adverse effects; *Therapeutic dose of whole dried Psilocybe mushrooms*: 1–4 grams dried mushroom/70 kg/bw (depending on species this would supply from 6 mg to 17 mg—average 9 mg—of psilocybin per gram of dried mushroom), every seven to twenty-one days, with a goal to target about 25 mg of psilocybin per dose; it is highly recommended to start with a lower dose (the lower end of microdosing) and adjust as necessary or recommended by your psilocybin-aware health-care professional

* In addition, doses on the higher end may be more stimulating while lower doses are less stimulating. Unlike medications and supplements, psilocybin does not need to be taken daily to experience the ideal effects, despite it having a short half-life. An "ideal effect" is achieved when you feel good, work effectively, and frankly forget you have taken something.

PSILOCYBIN EXPERIENCES BY DOSAGE

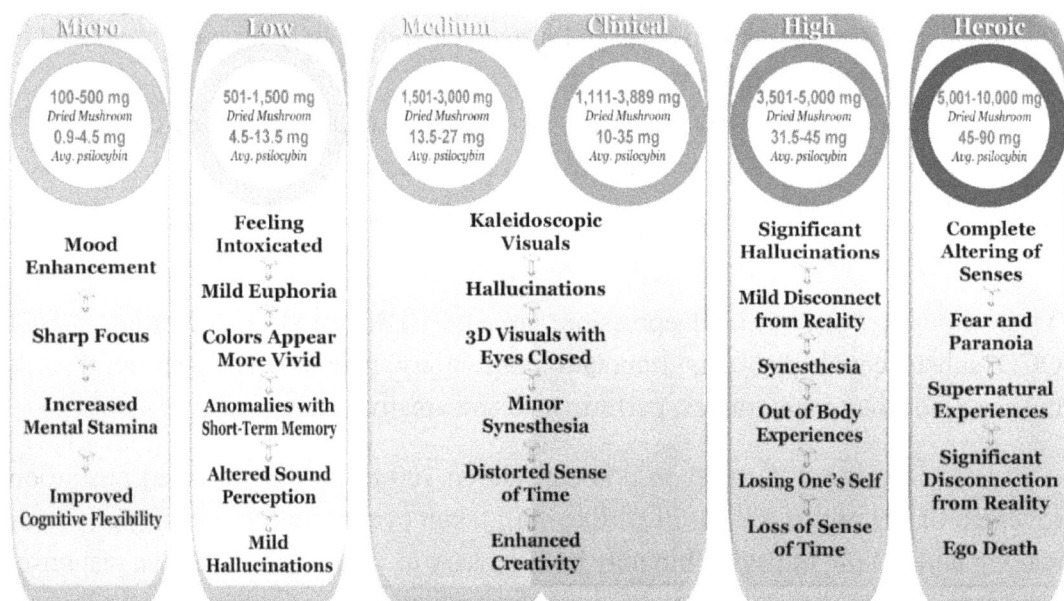

Micro	Low	Medium	Clinical	High	Heroic
100-500 mg Dried Mushroom 0.9-4.5 mg Avg. psilocybin	501-1,500 mg Dried Mushroom 4.5-13.5 mg Avg. psilocybin	1,501-3,000 mg Dried Mushroom 13.5-27 mg Avg. psilocybin	1,111-3,889 mg Dried Mushroom 10-35 mg Avg. psilocybin	3,501-5,000 mg Dried Mushroom 31.5-45 mg Avg. psilocybin	5,001-10,000 mg Dried Mushroom 45-90 mg Avg. psilocybin
Mood Enhancement	Feeling Intoxicated	Kaleidoscopic Visuals		Significant Hallucinations	Complete Altering of Senses
Sharp Focus	Mild Euphoria	Hallucinations		Mild Disconnect from Reality	Fear and Paranoia
Increased Mental Stamina	Colors Appear More Vivid	3D Visuals with Eyes Closed		Synesthesia	Supernatural Experiences
Improved Cognitive Flexibility	Anomalies with Short-Term Memory	Minor Synesthesia		Out of Body Experiences	Significant Disconnection from Reality
	Altered Sound Perception	Distorted Sense of Time		Losing One's Self	Ego Death
	Mild Hallucinations	Enhanced Creativity		Loss of Sense of Time	

Depending on the amount taken, form it is taken in, and your individual biology, you should feel the acute effects of psilocybin approximately 30 to 45 minutes after ingestion, with these acute effects peaking two to three hours later and lasting around four to six hours.

A full psychedelic dose—a dose sufficient to produce significantly altered perception (hallucinations, light sensitivity, color enhancement, pulsation of light or objects, kaleidoscopic and geometric patterns, hearing sounds, and warping or swirling of objects) and mystical-type experiences—is estimated to be 20 to 30 mg of psilocybin for the average person, but it may be lower for you depending on various factors. There is no on-size-fits-all dose.

It should be noted that if you are taking dried psilocybe mushrooms, the amount of psilocybin can vary dramatically from species to species and even among the same species depending on multiple factors, which makes it difficult to determine exactly how much psilocybin you are actually taking. QTests are one way to quantify the potency of psilocybin-containing mushrooms in milligrams or as a percentage.

Research shows that your emotions and brain function are positively altered for up to one month following a single dose of 25 mg/70 kg/bw psilocybin, suggesting that psilocybin can have long-lasting positive effects on mood and thinking.[2922]

Tips to use microdose psilocybin safely:

1. Begin with a low dose and gradually adjust (titrate) until you determine how you will respond. Start with 0.1 grams of psilocybe mushrooms on day one. Assess the effects, and if the desired result were not achieved, increase the dosage by 0.05 grams each microdosing day until you reach your ideal response. In some cases, it may take several weeks of microdosing to feel the effects because people experience psychedelics differently. Some possible reasons why this may occur include: 1) impact of the environment you take the psychedelics in, 2) an inability to "let go" and trust in the experience, 3) potential drug interactions, 4) an adulterated or weak product, and 5) you've developed a tolerance to psilocybin.
2. Take your dose in a safe and comfortable environment where you can be related.
3. Have a trusted friend or health-care professional present for support and to ensure your safety and well-being.
4. Stay hydrated by drinking water before, with, and during your psilocybin session.
5. Be aware of contraindications and potential drug interactions.
6. Do not take psilocybin with other substances like alcohol or cannabis.
7. Avoid taking psilocybin too frequently. It is not only unnecessary, but increases the risk of adverse effects.
8. Don't drive or operate heavy machinery until the effects of the psilocybin have worn off (approximately four to eight hours depending on individual factors such as metabolism, weight, and tolerance).
9. Seek professional help immediately if you experience any serious negative or unexpected effects.

POTENTIAL ADVERSE EFFECTS: Mood changes, anxiety, fatigue, fear or paranoia, hallucinations (higher doses), headache (higher doses are most likely to cause headache), high blood pressure, nausea, irregular heartbeat, body tingling sensations, hyperactivity, sweating, loss of appetite, sleep disturbance, heart attack (case reports showing an association with indole concentrations in Psilocybe mushrooms and the risk of adverse CNS and cardiovascular effects); the most common side effects of therapeutic doses of psilocybin are fatigue and headache days after use, with dose-response association with rare adverse events such as physical discomfort, increased blood pressure, nausea/vomiting, or prolonged psychosis-like symptoms

CAUTIONS AND CONTRAINDICATIONS: Pregnancy, lactation, bipolar disorder, schizophrenia, irritable bowel syndrome, cardiac disorders, Psilocybe mushroom allergy; stimulant drugs, caffeine, tricyclic antidepressants, MAOI inhibitors, Remeron (mirtazapine), antipsychotics, anxiety medications, buspirone, gabapentin, opiate drugs, lithium, valproic acid, adrenergic agents

REISHI

(Ganoderma lucidum)

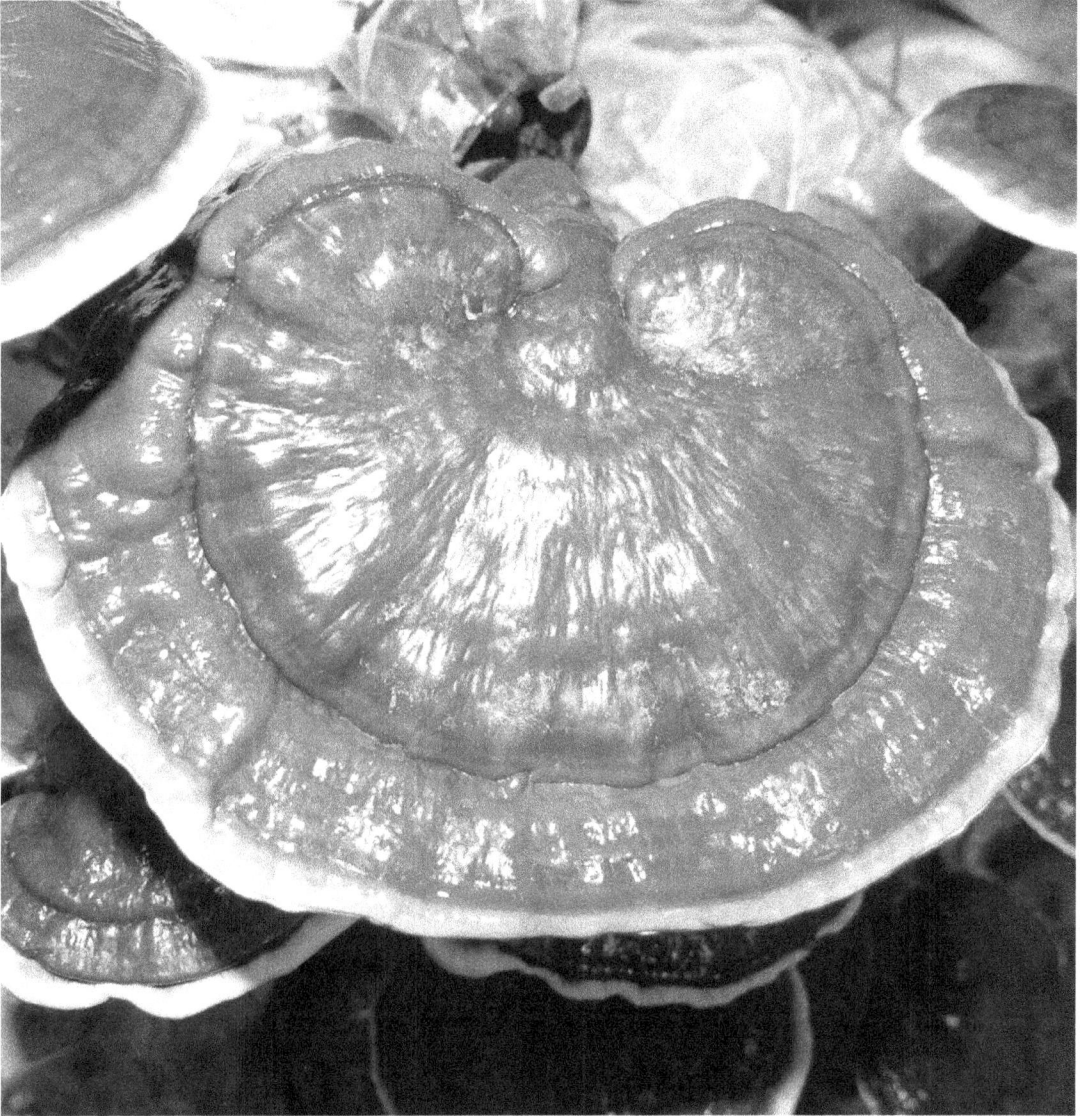

Kingdom: Fungi
Phylum: Basidiomycota
Class: Agaricomycetes
Order: Polyporales
Family: Ganodermataceae
Genus: Ganoderma
Species: lucidum
Native Habitat: Europe, North America, and Asia

Among the enormous fungal kingdom, reishi shines as one of the most widely used mushrooms in history. It has a long history of use in traditional medicine and a reputation as a symbol of longevity and vitality. It is one of the most well-known and extensively studied species because of its historical significance and demonstrated therapeutic properties.

Reishi is renowned for its distinctive appearance. The cap of the mushroom is usually kidney-shaped or semicircular, with a smooth, shiny surface. It typically ranges in color from reddish-brown to dark brown. The underside of the cap features tiny pores rather than the gills seen in many other mushroom species. Its stalk is short and centrally attached to the cap. It is often dark brown and has a woody texture. The mushroom has a tough and leathery texture, making it inedible in its raw form. To harness its medicinal benefits, it is typically prepared as a tea, extract, or supplement.

Reishi has a rich history of use in traditional Chinese medicine (TCM), where it is called "Lingzhi" and that tradition is continued in the modern day. In TCM, it is considered the "mushroom of immortality" and has been used for thousands of years to promote health, longevity, and vitality. It is often associated with the idea of balancing the body's vital energies, known as "Qi" in TCM. Moreover, it is a symbol of good luck, prosperity, and longevity in Chinese culture. Its image is frequently seen on artwork, clothing, and various decorative items. It is also a common motif in TCM clinics and pharmacies.

With its long history of use and hundreds of scientific studies, a vast array of therapeutic properties has been discovered about this mushroom. One of the most well-researched aspects of reishi is its ability to modulate the immune system. It contains bioactive compounds, including beta-glucans and other polysaccharides, that stimulate and strengthen the immune response. This makes it valuable in supporting overall immune health and potentially enhancing the body's ability to fight infections and diseases. It is a rich source of antioxidants, such as triterpenoids and polyphenols, which combat oxidative stress and reduce the risk of chronic diseases associated with free radical damage. Its anti-inflammatory properties make it useful for a variety of inflammatory conditions, particularly chronic inflammatory conditions. Of course, reishi possesses adaptogenic qualities that help one better cope with stress and maintain balance in key body functions. This can contribute to better overall well-being. Some studies suggest that reishi may have a positive impact on cardiovascular health by promoting healthy blood pressure and cholesterol levels. It is also protective of the liver and nervous system and has been explored for its anticancer activity.

As a supplement, it is most commonly consumed as a tea, extract, powder, or capsule. It is frequently combined with other herbs or mushrooms for specific health purposes in TCM.

Reishi is a revered and symbolically significant mushroom with a rich history of use in traditional medicine. Its potential therapeutic properties, including immune modulation, antioxidant effects, and anti-inflammatory qualities, have garnered attention in the world of modern scientific research. While more studies are needed to fully understand its mechanisms of action and applications, reishi continues to be a highly valuable natural solution in the realm of natural health and wellness.

NOTABLE COMPOUNDS: Polysaccharides, oligosaccharides, beta-glucans, heteroglycans, lanostane triterpenoids, ganodertepene A, adenosine, sterols, ganoderol B, ganoderone A, ganodermanondiol, ganoderiol F, fucoxylomannan, ergosterols, lucidumol A, galactose, mannose, polyphenols, hesperidin, quercetin, kaempferol, naringenin, resveratrol, lucidimines B and C, glucuronic acid, ganoderic acids A, B, C2, G, H, and I, ganoderenic acid D, proteoglycans, ganodermasides C and D

BENEFITS ACCORDING TO PRECLINICAL RESEARCH:

- Anticancer (liver)[2923-2953]
- Anticancer (lung)[2954-2982]
- Antagonizes the release of mediators—PGE2, TGF-β, IL-10, and VEGF—that suppress immune function by lung cancer cells[2983]
- Prevents lung cancer caused by tobacco smoke and other chemicals[2984,2985]
- Anticancer (prostate)[2986-2998]
- Anticancer (ovarian)[2999,3000,3001]
- Anticancer (cervical)[3002-3017]
- Anticancer (breast)[3018-3051]
- Anticancer (inflammatory breast cancer)[3052,3053,3054,3055]
- Prevents breast cancer, impairs breast cancer stem cells[3056,3057]
- Suppresses breast-to-lung cancer metastasis[3058,3059]
- Anticancer (esophageal squamous cell carcinoma)[3060,3061]
- Anticancer (lymphoma)[3062-3068]
- Anticancer (acute myelocytic leukemia)[3069-3082]
- Anticancer (multiple myeloma)[3083]
- Anticancer (pancreatic)[3084,3085]
- Anticancer (osteosarcoma)[3086,3087,3088,3089]
- Anticancer (fibrosarcoma)[3090]
- Anticancer (hematologic malignant)[3091]
- Anticancer (melanoma)[3092,3093,3094,3095]
- Anticancer (prevents melanoma metastasis)[3096]
- Anticancer (skin, epidermoid carcinoma)[3097]
- Prevents skin cancer, possibly by reducing UV-induced immune suppression[3098]

- Anticancer (nasopharyngeal)[3099,3100]
- Anticancer (laryngeal)[3101]
- Anticancer (esophageal squamous cell carcinoma)[3102]
- Anticancer (oral)[3103,3104]
- Anticancer (tongue)[3105,3106]
- Anticancer (cholangiocarcinoma)[3107]
- Anticancer (glioma)[3108,3109]
- Anticancer (glioblastoma)[3110,3111]
- Anticancer (neuroblastoma)[3112,3113]
- Anticancer (meningioma)[3114]
- Anticancer (bladder)[3115]
- Anticancer (gastric)[3116-3123]
- Works synergistically with quercetin against Epstein-Barr virus-associated gastric cancer[3124]
- Anticancer (colorectal)[3125-3150]
- Prevents the formation of tumors in the colon[3151,3152,3153,3154,3155,3156]
- Suppresses the progression of premalignant urothelial cells to bladder cancer and improves the clearance of high-risk urothelial cells[3157,3158,3159]
- Suppresses aggressive cancer cells that typically contribute to cancer recurrence after chemotherapy by overcoming drug resistance conferred by miR-378 (a small noncoding RNA molecule that helps cancer cells survive, form colonies, and become more drug resistant)[3160]
- Enhances photothermal therapy against liver cancer[3161]
- Reverses resistance to doxorubicin of oral epidermoid carcinoma tumor cells[3162]
- Reverses resistance of multidrug-resistant leukemia cells to doxorubicin[3163]
- Reverses multidrug-resistance of liver cancer cells to chemotherapy[3164]
- Potentiates the activity of radiotherapy against leukemia cells[3165]
- Enhances the sensitivity of ovarian and cervical cancer cells to cisplatin[3166,3167,3168]
- Improves the sensitivity of cervical cancer cells to radiotherapy[3169]
- Potentiates the activity of cisplatin against lung cancer[3170]
- Enhances the sensitivity of liver cancer cells to radiotherapy or cisplatin[3171,3172]
- Potentiates the activity of 5-fluorouracil against colorectal cancer[3173]
- Ameliorates neutropenia—abnormally low neutrophil levels in the blood—caused by chemotherapy[3174]
- Mitigates leukopenia—a decrease in the number of white blood cells—caused by cyclophosphamide and improves overall immune function[3175]
- Improves immune responses and reverses immunosuppression caused by cyclophosphamide[3176]

- Protects against cardiac and kidney toxicity caused by doxorubicin[3177,3178,3179,3180]
- Shields against cachectic myopathy—a debilitating multifactorial wasting syndrome characterized by severe skeletal muscle wasting and dysfunction—caused by cisplatin and docetaxel[3181]
- Protects against liver or kidney injury caused by cisplatin[3182,3183,3184]
- Attenuates intestinal damage caused by 5-florouracil or methotrexate[3185,3186]
- Improves cognitive function reduced by 5-florouracil[3187]
- Ameliorates intestinal barrier injury caused by paclitaxel[3188]
- Decreases nausea and vomiting because of chemotherapy[3189]
- Diminishes chemotherapy-related fatigue[3190]
- Blocks angiogenesis (the growth of blood vessels to support tumor growth), which supports an antitumor effect[3191,3192]
- Stabilizes G-quadruplex structures, which could inhibit telomerase or downregulate oncogenes to reduce the risk of cancer[3193]
- Anticancer (rodent sarcoma)[3194-3206]
- Anticancer (rodent liver)[3207,3208,3209,3210,3211]
- Anticancer (rodent breast)[3212,3213,3214]
- Anticancer (rodent cervical)[3215]
- Anticancer (rodent bladder)[3216]
- Anticancer (rodent lung)[3217]
- Anticancer (rodent reticulocyte sarcoma)[3218,3219]
- Anticancer (rodent lymphoma or leukemia)[3220,3221,3222,3223]
- Anticancer (rodent melanoma)[3224-3231]
- Anticancer (rodent skin)[3232]
- Kills papilloma cells and prevents the progression of HPV transformed cells to cervical cancer[3233,3234]
- Neuroprotective[3235-3250]
- Decreases neuroinflammation and the subsequent death of neurons, including inhibiting fatty acid amide hydrolase (FAAH), which increases endocannabinoids concentration and is a therapeutic target for neurodegeneration[3251-3261]
- Mitigates age-associated brain physiological dysfunction by improving sphingolipid metabolism (plays an important role in neurodegeneration, neuroinflammation, and mental health disorders), prolonging telomere length (maintains youthful function of cells), and enhancing autophagy (allowing for the removal of pathological metabolites)[3262]
- Neurotrophic, promotes neurite outgrowth, stimulates nerve growth factor, enhances mitochondrial biogenesis in neurons[3263,3264,3265,3266]

- Mitigates multiple sclerosis (improves motor dysfunction, suppresses demyelination, and reduces MS-related weight loss)[3267]
- Preserves healthy cognitive function and memory (inhibits acetylcholinesterase)[3268,3269,3270,3271]
- Delays cognitive impairment or the development of Alzheimer's disease[3272,3273,3274]
- Alleviates cognitive impairment[3275]
- Improves mitochondrial function in aged brains, which may protect against age-related neurodegeneration[3276]
- Reverses Alzheimer's disease (dissolves or reduces senile plaques and neurofibrillary tangles in the brain, positively alters protein and gene expression, promotes neural progenitor proliferation, protects brain cells from premature death)[3277-3284]
- Alleviates Parkinson's disease by inhibiting leucine-rich repeat kinase 2 (LRRK2)—a key factor in the development of Parkinson's disease, reducing neuroinflammation, preserving dopamine-producing neurons, and suppressing the inflammatory response and oxidative stress[3285,3286,3287,3288,3289,3290]
- Ameliorates damage caused by traumatic brain injury[3291]
- Mitigates behavioral alterations caused by binge drinking alcohol in a model evaluating motor, cognitive, and psychiatric disorders[3292]
- Improves energy supply to the brain, protects the liver, and decreases the prevalence of inhibitory neurotransmitters that are characteristic of moderate alcohol consumption[3293]
- Prevents memory deficits caused by hypoxia[3294]
- Anticonvulsive, antiepileptic[3295,3296,3297,3298]
- Mitigates amnesia[3299]
- Antidepressant (works partly by upregulating BDNF and modulating Dectin-1 and the innate immune system)[3300,3301,3302,3303,3304,3305]
- Relieves anxiety[3306,3307]
- Reduces stress-induced anxiety[3308]
- Alleviates anxiety and depression associated with maternal separation[3309]
- Improves the gut microbiome (promotes healthy flora, increases the relative abundance of beneficial bacteria such as *Lactobacillaceae*, *Roseburia*, *Adlercreutzia*, *Prevotella*, *Desulfovibrionaceae*, and *Lachnospiraceae*, reduces proportion of *Blautia*, protects *Lactobacillus* against destruction by gastric juices, increases short-chain fatty acids production, reduces endotoxemia, increases production of antimicrobial peptides, reduces cancer risk genera: *Desulfovibrio* and *Odoribacter*)[3310-3319]
- Restores gut microbiome balance in non-hepatitis B virus-related liver cancer[3320]

- ☂ Boosts gut barrier function (reduces leaky gut)[3321,3322,3323,3324]
- ☂ Repairs the intestinal mucosa after injury[3325]
- ☂ Alleviates chronic pancreatitis[3326,3327]
- ☂ Reduces intestinal inflammation[3328,3329,3330]
- ☂ Increases gut immune activity to reduce the risk of intestinal infection[3331]
- ☂ Anti-inflammatory[3332-3363]
- ☂ Antirheumatic (suppresses rheumatoid arthritis synovial fibroblast proliferation and migration, balances inflammatory pathways, inactivates NF-κB and MPAK signaling pathways, reduces the production of proinflammatory cytokines by synovial fibroblasts, and balances humoral and cellular immunity)[3364,3365,3366,3367]
- ☂ Reduces periodontal inflammation[3368]
- ☂ Diminishes high uric acid levels (relieves gout)[3369,3370]
- ☂ Relieves pain[3371,3372,3373]
- ☂ Significantly inhibits testosterone-induced growth of the prostate (alleviates benign prostatic hyperplasia, inhibits 5alpha-reductase)[3374-3380]
- ☂ Stimulates immune function (activity of white blood cells, release of cytokines and nitric oxide), including preventing drug-induced immunosuppression and enhancing activity against cancer cells[3381-3469]
- ☂ Balances immune function or alleviates autoimmunity[3470,3471,3472,3473,3474,3475]
- ☂ Restores immune function after intense exercise[3476]
- ☂ Water extracts may enhance NK cell activity against cancer cells and stimulate overall immune function, whereas ethanol extracts reduce these activities[3477]
- ☂ Modulates the expression of multiple cell adhesion molecules—dysfunction of cell adhesion molecules is a factor in the development of a wide range of conditions, including cancer, autoimmunity, neurological disorders, cardiovascular disease, inflammatory bowel disease, and asthma[3478,3479]
- ☂ Relieves allergies[3480,3481,3482,3483,3484]
- ☂ Alleviates itching[3485]
- ☂ Suppresses mosquito allergy-induced itching[3486]
- ☂ Reduces neural tube defects[3487]
- ☂ Antidiabetic[3488-3535]
- ☂ Prevents diabetes and associated lipid disorders in prediabetic subjects[3536]
- ☂ Improves insulin release from pancreatic beta-cells and cellular glucose uptake[3537,3538,3539,3540,3541]
- ☂ Decreases insulin resistance[3542,3543]
- ☂ Protects pancreatic beta-cells against premature cell death[3544,3545,3546]
- ☂ Reduces metabolic diseases[3547,3548]

- ❦ Mitigates gestational diabetes (improves glucose metabolism, reduces lipid peroxidation, protects fetuses against damage)[3549]
- ❦ Shields the brain against diabetic-related damage[3550]
- ❦ Diminishes diabetes-related muscle atrophy[3551]
- ❦ Protects against diabetes-related kidney damage (diabetic nephropathy)[3552,3553,3554,3555,3556,3557]
- ❦ Promotes healing of nonhealing diabetic wounds[3558]
- ❦ Improves galactosemia—a rare genetic metabolic disorder that affects the ability to metabolize the sugar galactose—by inhibiting aldose reductase; aldose reductase inhibitors are also used to prevent eye and nerve damage in people with diabetes[3559,3560,3561,3562,3563,3564]
- ❦ Alleviates diabetic cardiomyopathy and cardiovascular dysfunction, promotes vascular repair in diabetic model[3565,3566,3567]
- ❦ Corrects harmful lipid profiles in subjects with diabetes[3568,3569,3570]
- ❦ Protects against diabetes-related testicular damage[3571,3572,3573]
- ❦ Restores a healthy gut microbiome in subjects with diabetes[3574]
- ❦ Mitigates diabetes-related erectile dysfunction[3575]
- ❦ Lowers high cholesterol, reduces its creation in the body, and prevents its oxidation[3576-3596]
- ❦ Promotes weight loss[3597]
- ❦ Combats obesity and obesity-related inflammation[3598-3606]
- ❦ Inhibits lipase activity (decreases the absorption of fats in the GI tract)[3607]
- ❦ Reduces metabolic disorder-related obesity[3608]
- ❦ Diminishes obesity-related inflammation of the salivary glands[3609]
- ❦ Cardioprotective[3610-3618]
- ❦ Reduces progression of or alleviates atherosclerosis[3619-3627]
- ❦ Protects heart mitochondrial function during a heart attack[3628]
- ❦ Preserves cardiac function during sepsis[3629]
- ❦ Decreases high blood pressure[3630,3631,3632,3633]
- ❦ Downregulates the expression of advanced glycation end products (AGEs), which could protect aortal tissue and lower blood pressure[3634]
- ❦ Inhibits angiotensin-I-converting enzyme (ACE; lowers blood pressure and treats heart failure)[3635,3636]
- ❦ Antiplatelet or antithrombotic activity[3637,3638,3639,3640,3641]
- ❦ Ameliorates hypertrophic cardiomyopathy (thickening of the heart muscle) and heart failure[3642]
- ❦ Liver protective[3643-3673]
- ❦ Promotes liver healing after monopolar electrosurgery[3674]
- ❦ Ameliorates nonalcoholic fatty liver disease[3675,3676,3677,3678]

- 🍄 Prevents or relieves liver fibrosis[3679,3680,3681,3682]
- 🍄 Kidney protective[3683,3684,3685,3686,3687]
- 🍄 Inhibits kidney fibrosis[3688,3689]
- 🍄 Mitigates proteinuria (protein in the urine)-induced renal disease[3690,3691,3692]
- 🍄 Slows the development of kidney cysts, useful for autosomal dominant polycystic kidney disease[3693]
- 🍄 Protects against anemia by reducing hemolysis—the rupturing and destruction of red blood cells[3694,3695,3696]
- 🍄 Spleen protective[3697]
- 🍄 Lung protective (restores mitochondrial function, protects cells after injury)[3698]
- 🍄 Protects against pulmonary fibrosis[3699]
- 🍄 Ameliorates tuberculosis in a spontaneous latent model of tuberculosis infection[3700]
- 🍄 Reduces asthma-related lung inflammation[3701,3702]
- 🍄 Improves acute pneumonia[3703]
- 🍄 Preserves bone health and strength, reverses osteoporotic bone loss[3704,3705,3706,3707,3708,3709]
- 🍄 Mitigates calvarial bone defects (a rare group of disorders that affect the skull)[3710]
- 🍄 Shields against testicular damage caused by lithium carbonate or cadmium[3711,3712]
- 🍄 Preserves healthy testicular structure and function during aging[3713]
- 🍄 Maintains healthy salivary gland status and prevents salivary secretion disorders during aging[3714]
- 🍄 Promotes healthy aging and a healthy lifespan[3715,3716,3717,3718]
- 🍄 Combats recurrent oral ulcers[3719]
- 🍄 Protects against gastrointestinal injury, including ulcers caused by alcohol and NSAIDs[3720-3727]
- 🍄 Relieves ulcerative colitis[3728-3737]   [3737]
- 🍄 Protects against kidney damage caused by colitis[3738]
- 🍄 Prevents colitis-related cancer[3739]
- 🍄 Promotes healthy sleep[3740,3741,3742,3743]
- 🍄 Attenuates oxidative stress and its subsequent damage to cells, tissues, and organs, increases antioxidant enzyme activity[3744-3762]
- 🍄 Inhibits damage to genetic information (DNA)[3763-3769]
- 🍄 Protects against damage caused by X-ray or gamma-radiation[3770-3777]
- 🍄 Antioxidant[3778-3827]
- 🍄 Reduces age-related decline in antioxidant status[3828]
- 🍄 Protects cell membranes against oxidation[3829]

- ☻ Controls high-altitude-related maladies[3830]
- ☻ Increases tolerance to low oxygen environments[3831]
- ☻ Diminished muscle mass loss caused by hypobaric hypoxia through preventing oxidative stress and triggering the formation of skeletal muscle tissue[3832]
- ☻ Preserves cellular energy production ability during the aging process[3833]
- ☻ Promotes fatigue recovery and improves physical endurance[3834]
- ☻ Protects against testicular damage caused by a torsion-detorsion injury[3835]
- ☻ Reduces chemotherapy-related fatigue[3836]
- ☻ Suppresses eczema development and relieves existing eczema[3837,3838]
- ☻ Alleviates frostbite when applied as a nanogel[3839,3840]
- ☻ Protects against UV-induced DNA damage[3841]
- ☻ Shields against UV-induced skin damage[3842]
- ☻ Accelerates wound healing by protecting cells against free radicals, enhancing re-epithelialization, and upregulating expression of wound healing proteins[3843,3844,3845,3846]
- ☻ Promotes burn wound healing[3847,3848]
- ☻ Protects skin flaps against ischemia-reperfusion injury[3849]
- ☻ Prevents photoaging and age spots[3850,3851,3852,3853]
- ☻ Protects skin against oxidative damage[3854]
- ☻ Skin brightening[3855,3856,3857]
- ☻ Reduces cadmium toxicity[3858,3859,3860]
- ☻ Antiviral (Epstein-Barr virus)[3861,3862]
- ☻ Antiviral (dengue virus)[3863,3864]
- ☻ Antiviral (hepatitis B)[3865,3866,3867]
- ☻ Antiviral (SARS-CoV-2)[3868]
- ☻ Antiviral (herpes simplex virus 1 and 2; also synergizes the activity of antiviral drugs)[3869-3875]
- ☻ Antiviral (human immunodeficiency virus 1)[3876,3877,3878,3879]
- ☻ Antiviral (enterovirus 71)[3880,3881]
- ☻ Antiviral (simian acquired immune deficiency syndrome)[3882]
- ☻ Antiviral (vesicular stomatitis virus)[3883]
- ☻ Antiviral (porcine circovirus 2)[3884]
- ☻ Antiviral (Newcastle disease virus)[3885]
- ☻ Antiviral (general)[3886]
- ☻ Antimicrobial[3887-3907]
- ☻ Antiprotozoal[3908]
- ☻ Antiplasmodial/antimalarial[3909,3910,3911,3912,3913]
- ☻ Antitoxoplasmosis[3914]
- ☻ Antischistosomiasis[3915]
- ☻ Biodegrades or removes chemicals from the environment[3916,3917,3918,3919,3920,3921]

- ➢ Enhances immune activity in healthy individuals to bolster their defenses against infections[3922]
  - 200 mg of reishi beta-glucans daily before or during breakfast for eighty-four days
- ➢ Enhances immune function in asymptomatic children aged three to five years old, which suggests it could reduce the risk of infections[3923]
  - 350 mg of reishi beta-glucans consumed in yogurt daily for twelve weeks
- ➢ Improves physical fitness—endurance, lower body flexibility, and velocity—in women with fibromyalgia[3924]
  - 3,000 mg dissolved in warm water, twice daily for six weeks
- ➢ Produces trends toward greater levels of happiness and life satisfaction and reduced depression in women with fibromyalgia[3925]
  - 3,000 mg twice daily for six weeks
- ➢ Improves the clearance of human papillomavirus—HPV16 or HPV18 (88% clearance rate)[3926]
  - 400 mg of a combination of turkey tail and reishi daily for two months
- ➢ Improves lower urinary tract symptoms—urination problems—in men over the age of forty-nine with International Prostate Symptom Scores (IPSS) suggestive of benign prostatic hyperplasia; IPSS scores decreased an average of 2.1 points by the end of treatment[3927,3928]
  - Two tablets containing 6 mg (3 mg per tablet) of reishi (83.65% maltitol, 10% cornstarch, 3% vitamin C, 3% sucrose) once daily with a meal
- ➢ Preserves healthy immune function in athletes participating in endurance training[3929]
  - 5,000 mg per day for six weeks
- ➢ Protects against atherosclerosis in people with stable and high-risk angina by increasing antioxidant status and decreasing circulating endothelial cells and endothelial progenitor cells[3930]
  - 250 mg (containing 180 mg beta-D glucan) three times daily for ninety days while continuing previously prescribed medications
- ➢ Reduces endothelial injury and improves endothelial function in people with high-risk or stable angina[3931]
  - 250 mg three times daily in addition to regular medications
- ➢ Improves insulin resistance in people with mild high blood pressure and high cholesterol[3932]
  - 720 mg twice daily for twelve weeks
- ➢ Inhibits platelet aggregation in people with atherosclerosis and healthy individuals[3933]
  - 1,000 mg three times daily

- ➤ Reduces hepatitis B activity and improves liver function[3934]
  - 1,800 mg three times daily for twelve weeks
- ➤ Enhances immune responses in people with advanced-stage cancer[3935]
  - 1,800 mg Ganopoly three times daily before meals for twelve weeks
- ➤ Beneficially modulates immune system function in people with advanced colorectal cancer[3936]
  - 1,800 mg three times daily before meals for twelve weeks
- ➤ Achievement of stability of gynecological cancer in five women after at least two unsuccessful chemotherapy regimens[3937]
  - 1,000 mg reishi body fruit or spore extract and 200 mg vitamin C in 200 mL of distilled water one hour before a meal, twice daily, for two days, then increasing to 2,000 mg reishi plus 400 mg vitamin C in 200 mL of distilled water one hour before a meal, twice daily, during days three and four, with dosing being 3,000 mg reishi plus 600 mg vitamin C in 200 mL of distilled water one hour before a meal, twice daily, for twelve weeks
- ➤ Suppresses the development of colorectal adenoma polyps in people over age forty with colorectal adenoma polyps (demonstrates a colorectal cancer preventive effect)[3938]
  - 750 mg of reishi mycelia twice daily for twelve months
- ➤ Diminishes cancer-related fatigue, anxiety, and depression, and improves quality of life in women with breast cancer undergoing endocrine therapy[3939]
  - 1,000 mg three times daily for four weeks
- ➤ Improves the clinical symptoms of neurasthenia[3940]
  - 1,800 mg three times daily for eight weeks
- ➤ Treats acute mushroom poisoning with liver injury (reduces length of hospital stay, hospitalization costs, improves blood parameters, and increases survivability)[3941]
  - Unknown dose
- ➤ Curbs oxidative stress (enhances total antioxidant capacity, total thiols, and glutathione) and reverses mild fatty liver to normal in healthy individuals[3942]
  - 225 mg daily after lunch or dinner for six months
- ➤ Produces a nonstatistically significant reduction in lipids and uric acid and increases in total antioxidant capacity after short-term supplementation in healthy people[3943]
  - 720 mg day for ten days or 3,300 mg as a single dose
- ➤ Decreased postherpetic neuralgic pain dramatically in two individuals[3944]
  - 36–72 g dry weight/day of a hot-water-soluble extract
- ➤ Stabilized motor symptoms, increased mindfulness, maintained mood state, and reduced bodily discomfort in a fifty-year-old male with Parkinson's disease[3945]
  - 300 mg reishi plus 1,000 mg davon polysaccharide daily before noon (also took coQ10, *Mucuna pruriens*, and a multivitamin prior to beginning and concurrently with reishi supplementation)

> Treats myotonic dystrophy (a type of muscular dystrophy) according to a presentation of ten case studies[3946]
  - Dosing not reported

THERAPEUTIC POTENTIAL: Dysbiosis, leaky gut, angina, viral infections, infection prevention, diabetes and diabetes-related complications, metabolic syndrome, fibromyalgia, rheumatoid arthritis, colon cancer prevention, insomnia, benign prostatic hyperplasia

CLINICAL DOSAGES: 6 mg to 3,000 mg, up to three times daily; typically, 500 mg to 1,500 mg up to four times daily of extract; or 11.25 g to 18.75 g of fresh mushroom daily

POTENTIAL ADVERSE EFFECTS: Dizziness, dry mouth, rash, itching, nausea, upset stomach

CAUTIONS AND CONTRAINDICATIONS: Pregnancy, lactation, bleeding disorders, reishi mushroom allergy, prior to surgery; drugs that thin the blood, blood pressure-lowering drugs, antidiabetic drugs, pentobarbital or other barbiturates, antiviral drugs, trifluoperazine and other drugs metabolized through UGT1A4

SHIITAKE

(Lentinula edodes, formerly Lentinus edodes)

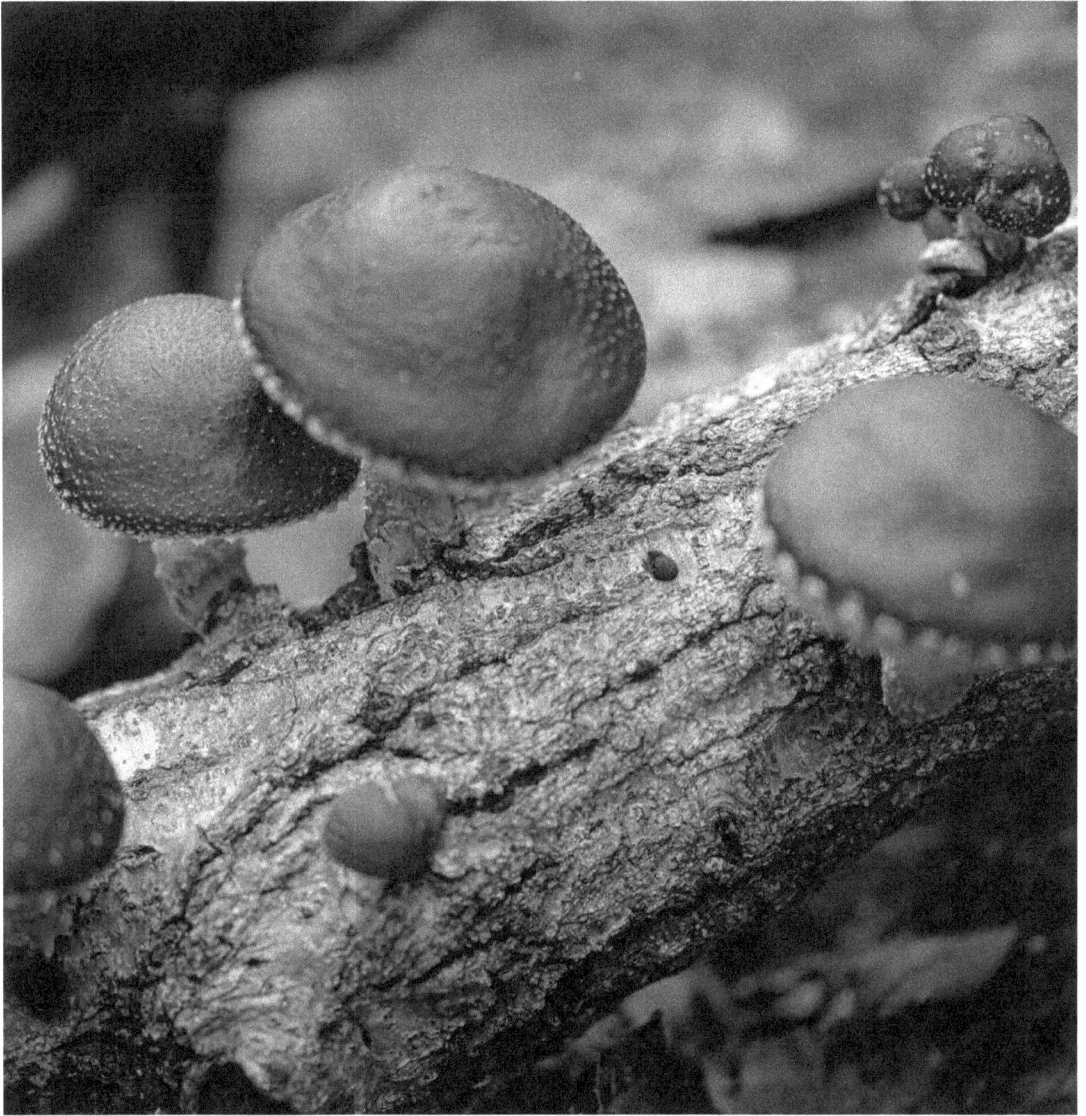

Kingdom: Fungi
Phylum: Basidiomycota
Class: Agaricomycetes
Order: Agaricales
Family: Marasmiaceae
Genus: Lentinula
Species: edodes
Native Habitat: East Asia

As Japan's most popular edible mushroom, few mushroom varieties have earned as much acclaim and respect as the shiitake mushroom. With its rich flavor, versatile culinary applications, and a wealth of therapeutic potential, the shiitake mushroom deserves significant attention from researchers, clinicians, and health enthusiasts alike.

The cap of the shitake mushrooms is broad, convex, and ranges in color from light to dark brown. It typically measures 5 to 10 centimeters (2 to 4 inches) in diameter and has a smooth, sometimes slightly wrinkled surface. Beneath the cap, shiitake mushrooms feature closely spaced, white to pale brown gills. These gills extend down the stem. The stem is thick, firm, and white or pale brown. It is often shorter in comparison to the cap and can be somewhat fibrous. Shiitake mushrooms have a meaty, substantial texture and are prized for their umami flavor.

Shiitake mushrooms are famous for their culinary versatility and robust flavor profile. They are widely used in various cuisines around the world, such as stir-fries, Asian dishes, to enhance the flavor of stocks, broths, and sauces, dried or dehydrated to concentrate the flavor, or grilled or pan-fried to add to dishes or eaten alone.

Shiitake mushrooms offer a range of essential nutrients and bioactive compounds. They are a good source of plant-based protein and a rich source of dietary fiber. Shiitake mushrooms provide vitamins, including B vitamins such as niacin (B3), riboflavin (B2), and pantothenic acid (B5). They are also one of the few natural sources of vitamin D when they are exposed to sunlight or ultraviolet (UV) light. They contain essential minerals like potassium, phosphorus, selenium, and copper. Additionally, shiitake mushrooms contain bioactive polysaccharides, including beta-glucans, and antioxidants like ergothioneine which can aid immune function and potentially reduce the risk of chronic diseases.

Shiitake mushrooms have been extensively evaluated in scientific research, revealing a host of therapeutic potential. The beta-glucans and other polysaccharides found in shiitake mushrooms have immune-enhancing properties. Shiitake mushrooms have been studied for their potential to inhibit the growth of many different types of cancer cells. Certain compounds, like lentinan, have shown promise in cancer therapy by enhancing the immune response and promoting apoptosis (cell death) in cancer cells. Some research suggests that shiitake mushrooms may help lower cholesterol levels and reduce the risk of heart disease by inhibiting cholesterol absorption in the gut. They may have a role in blood sugar control because they contain compounds that can improve insulin sensitivity and may be beneficial for individuals with diabetes or at risk of diabetes. Some studies also suggest that shiitake mushrooms can support liver function by promoting detoxification and protecting against liver damage.

Shiitake mushroom supplements, available in various forms—teas, powders, and capsules—can provide a concentrated dose of their beneficial compounds. Shiitake mushrooms are a culinary delight and a therapeutic treasure. Its rich umami flavor, versatile culinary applications, and potential therapeutic benefits make it a beloved ingredient in kitchens and an object of scientific interest to discover how to use it for improving human health. From immune support and cancer research to heart health and blood sugar management, shiitake mushrooms continue to unveil their healing potential. As we journey through the world of fungi, the shiitake stands as a remarkable example of how nature's bounty can enrich both our palates and our well-being.

NOTABLE COMPOUNDS: Polysaccharides, mannose, galactose, alpha-glucans, beta-glucans, quercetin, catechin, ergosterol, latcripin-3, latcripin-7A, latcripin-15, polyacetylenes, lentinan, lignosulfonic acid, syringic acid, amino acids, phenolics, pyrrole alkaloids, proteoglycans, chitins, eritadenine, lenthionine, sulfur compounds

BENEFITS ACCORDING TO PRECLINICAL RESEARCH:

- Anticancer (breast)[3947,3948,3949,3950]
- Anticancer (cervical)[3951,3952]
- Anticancer (prostate)[3953,3954]
- Anticancer (gastric)[3955,3956]
- Anticancer (colorectal)[3957,3958,3959,3960]
- Prevents intestinal polyp development, which may prevent colorectal cancer[3961]
- Anticancer (liver)[3962,3963,3964,3965]
- Anticancer (pancreatic)[3966]
- Anticancer (acute promyelocytic leukemia)[3967]
- Anticancer (lymphoma)[3968]
- Anticancer (lung)[3969,3970,3971,3972]
- Anticancer (enhances radiation therapy against lung cancer)[3973]
- Anticancer (melanoma)[3974,3975]
- Anticancer (skin)[3976]
- Alleviates cisplatin-induced kidney toxicity[3977]
- Anticancer (rodent skin)[3978]
- Restores antitumor immunity that has become impaired in old age[3979]
- Reduces hair loss caused by the chemotherapy drug cytarabine[3980]
- Protects against liver injury caused by the chemotherapy drugs 6-mercaptopurine and methotrexate[3981]
- Mitigates myelosuppression caused by therarubicin—a chemotherapy agent commonly associated with severe myelosuppression—by activating bone marrow-derived macrophages[3982]

- 🍄 Upregulates COX-2 expression in malignant progressive fibrosarcoma cancer cells (which may mean it is necessary to take a COX-2 inhibitor when using shiitake mushrooms with fibrosarcoma cancer treatment)[3983]
- 🍄 Prevents cognitive impairment[3984]
- 🍄 Modifies the gut microbiome (promotes the proliferation of *Lactobacillus rhamnosus* and *L. plantarum*, increases relative abundance of promote the production of Bacteroides, acts as a prebiotic)[3985,3986,3987,3988]
- 🍄 Preserves/restores intestinal barrier function (reduces leaky gut)[3989,3990]
- 🍄 Stimulates immune function[3991-3999]
- 🍄 Balances immune function (polysaccharide dependent, which is affected by extraction method, composition, molecular weight, branching degrees, and helical conformation)[4000,4001]
- 🍄 Suppresses immune function[4002]
- 🍄 Maintains healthy immune function despite tumor presence[4003]
- 🍄 Rejuvenates age-related deficient immune function by restoring age-related changes to the gut microbiome[4004]
- 🍄 Enhances immune response against and expels *Trichinella spiralis*—a parasitic roundworm responsible for trichinellosis—after infection[4005]
- 🍄 Increases survival and efficacy of amphotericin B after invasive pulmonary aspergillosis infection[4006]
- 🍄 Antidiabetic[4007,4008,4009,4010]
- 🍄 Alleviates ulcerative colitis[4011,4012,4013]
- 🍄 Relieves intestinal inflammation, making it useful for inflammatory bowel disease[4014]
- 🍄 Anti-inflammatory[4015-4023]
- 🍄 Promotes healthy blood pressure levels (acts as an angiotensin-I converting enzyme (ACE) inhibitor)[4024]
- 🍄 Prevents atherosclerosis[4025]
- 🍄 Lowers cholesterol[4026,4027,4028,4029,4030]
- 🍄 Increases blood pressure in subjects with hypotension[4031]
- 🍄 Combats obesity in postmenopausal subjects[4032]
- 🍄 Maintains bone health, regulates bone development[4033,4034]
- 🍄 Liver restorative/protective[4035,4036,4037,4038,4039,4040,4041,4042,4043]
- 🍄 Kidney protective[4044,4045]
- 🍄 Lung protective, reduces lung inflammation[4046,4047,4048]
- 🍄 Combats oxidative stress and subsequent damage[4049,4050,4051,4052]
- 🍄 Antioxidant[4053-4070]
- 🍄 Prevents DNA mutations[4071,4072,4073]
- 🍄 Decreases lactic acid levels[4074]

- Antiviral (SARS-CoV-2)[4075,4076]
- Antiviral (poliovirus type 1)[4077]
- Antiviral (hepatitis C)[4078]
- Antiviral (adenovirus)[4079]
- Antiviral (influenza A/Puerto Roco/8/34, A/WSN/33, and B/Shanghai/361/02)[4080]
- Antiviral (herpes simplex virus type 2)[4081,4082]
- Antiviral (West Nile virus)[4083]
- Antiviral (bovine herpes virus type 1)[4084]
- Antimicrobial[4085-4094]
- Inhibits the formation of sucrose-induced oral biofilms[4095]
- Reduces cavities (dental caries) risk[4096,4097]
- Inhibits periodontal pathogens (*Fusobacterium nucleatum, Aggregatibacter actinomycetemcomitans and Porphyromonas gingivalis*, and *Prevotella intermedia*)[4098]
- Antigingivitic because of its ability to reduce pathogenic oral bacteria without harming commensal (beneficial) oral bacteria[4099]
- Relieves eczema[4100]
- Promotes bioremediation or biodegradation of pharmaceuticals, chemicals, heavy metals, and endocrine disruptors[4101-4112]
- Nematocidal[4113]
- May chelate (bind to) essential minerals and elements at higher doses[4114]

BENEFITS ACCORDING TO CLINICAL RESEARCH:

- Supports immune activity to eliminate persistent high-risk human papillomavirus (HPV) infections (response rate of 58.8%)[4115]
  - 3,000 mg daily on an empty stomach for six months
- Improves the gut microbiome in individuals with mild untreated high cholesterol[4116]
  - 10.4 g/day of beta-D-glucan enriched shiitake mushroom extract (providing 3.5 g of beta-D-glucan daily)
- Improves immunity in healthy individuals[4117]
  - 5 or 10 g of whole mushrooms daily as part of the diet
- Enhances stress resilience and improves ability to fall asleep and stay asleep in chronically stressed individuals; also increases immune activity (natural killer cells)[4118]
  - 1,000 mg before breakfast, lunch, and dinner for five days
- Improves quality of life and promotes the efficacy of chemotherapy and radiation therapy for multiple cancers (lung, ovarian, cervical, nasopharyngeal,

colorectal) based on a review of 135 independent Chinese studies and over 9,400 cases[4119]

- Doses varied greatly

➢ Maintains quality of life and preserves immune function in women with breast cancer[4120,4121]

- 900 mg, twice daily, one dose in the morning and the other dose in the evening

➢ Enhances immune function and quality of life among women undergoing postoperative breast cancer hormone therapy[4122]

- 600 mg shiitake mycelia extract, three times daily for twelve weeks

➢ Improves quality of life and immune function in people undergoing postoperative chemotherapy for breast or gastrointestinal cancer, or receiving chemotherapy to prevent recurrence of gastrointestinal cancer[4123]

- 900 mg, twice daily, one dose in the morning and the other dose in the evening

➢ Improves nutritional status and immune function in people with resectable or borderline-resectable pancreatic cancer treated with neoadjuvant therapy[4124]

- 1,000 mg active hexose-correlated compound (AHCC; a standardized shiitake extract with 20% partly acylated alpha-1,4 glucans), three times daily, from the first day of neoadjuvant therapy (the administration of gemcitabine prior to surgery) continuing until the day before surgery

➢ Prevents cancer recurrence after liver resection (removal) in people in remission from liver cancer[4125]

- 1,000 mg, three times daily for two years

➢ Enhances immune activity against cancer and maintains quality of life in people undergoing cancer immunotherapy[4126,4127]

- 900 mg, twice daily, one dose in the morning and the other dose in the evening

➢ Prevents taste disorders in people with advanced pancreatic ductal adenocarcinoma who are receiving chemotherapy[4128]

- 6,000 mg daily of AHCC shiitake mushroom extract for eight to twelve weeks

➢ Improves survival and reduces severe adverse events in people with resectable pancreatic cancer undergoing neoadjuvant therapy[4129]

- 1,000 mg three times daily on an empty stomach

➢ Reduces side effects (nausea, abdominal pain) of chemotherapy in people with advanced metastatic gastrointestinal cancer undergoing chemotherapy; also improves immune markers[4130]

- 1,800 mg daily for four weeks

➢ Promotes greater overall well-being and quality of life in healthy individuals[4131]
  - 1–2 mL Lentinex (a shiitake mushroom extract standardized to beta-(1-3,1-6)-glucan), daily for four weeks

Note: many of the cancer studies used active hexose-correlated compound (AHCC).

THERAPEUTIC POTENTIAL: Chemotherapy side effects or to enhance chemotherapy agents' activity against cancer, viral infections, increase mental stress resilience, oral health

CLINICAL DOSAGES: 600 mg to 1,000 mg, up to three times daily

POTENTIAL ADVERSE EFFECTS: Abdominal discomfort, nausea, vomiting, diarrhea, dermatitis (rare), eosinophilia (large doses)

CAUTIONS AND CONTRAINDICATIONS: Pregnancy, lactation, eosinophilia, shiitake mushroom allergy; immunosuppressive drugs

STOUT CAMPHOR

(Antrodia camphorata, syn. Antrodia cinnamonea, Taiwanofungus camphoratus)

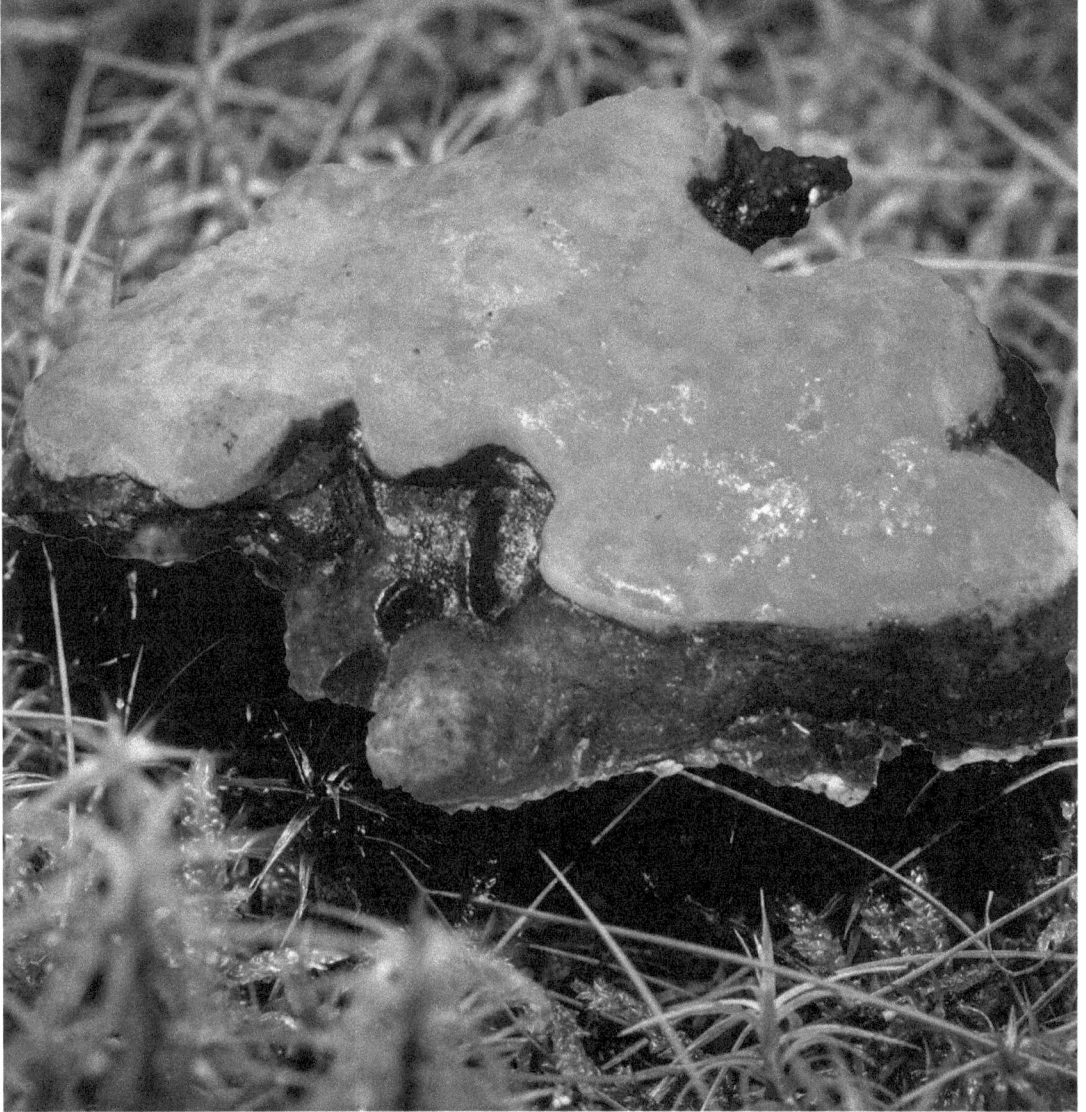

Kingdom: Fungi
Phylum: Basidiomycota
Class: Agaricomycetes
Order: Polyporales
Family: Fomitopsidaceae
Genus: Antrodia | Antrodia | Taiwanofungus
Species: camphorata | cinnamonea | camphoratus
Native Habitat: Taiwan

Deep within the forests of Taiwan, the stout camphor mushroom, often referred to as "Niu-Chang-Chih" in traditional Chinese medicine, thrives. For centuries, this elusive mushroom has remained a well-guarded secret among the indigenous people of Taiwan, who used it for a variety of medicinal purposes. Its remarkable medicinal properties have, however, propelled it into the spotlight in recent years, garnering the attention of scientists, herbalists, and health enthusiasts worldwide.

The stout camphor mushroom has a distinguished history deeply rooted in Taiwanese indigenous cultures. The indigenous people of Taiwan, such as the Bunun and the Truku, used the mushroom to address a wide range of health issues, from liver disorders to cancer. Traditional Chinese medicine also holds it in high regard, appreciating its unique characteristics and potential health benefits. However, it was only in recent decades that modern science began to unlock the mushroom's secrets and validate its medicinal value.

The stout camphor mushroom is rich in biologically active compounds, including polysaccharides, that are well-researched for their immune-boosting properties. They stimulate the immune system, enhancing the body's ability to ward off infections and diseases. Triterpenoids found in the mushroom have anti-inflammatory and antioxidant properties, which are valuable for reducing inflammation and protecting cells from oxidative damage. It is particularly renowned for its liver-protecting effects and anticancer properties.

In recent years, the therapeutic potential of this notable mushroom has attracted significant attention. Scientific research and clinical studies have begun to validate its traditional use and have uncovered new applications for modern medicine. Not surprisingly, the stout camphor mushroom is being studied for its ability to support liver detoxification and regeneration. Its polysaccharides stimulate the immune system, making it a valuable addition to immune-boosting formulations. As expected, its triterpenoids have demonstrated anti-inflammatory properties. Stout camphor's anticancer potential is a subject of ongoing research, and it is being explored as a complementary therapy for cancer patients. Some research indicates that it may have cardiovascular benefits, such as lowering blood pressure and improving blood lipid profiles.

Hundreds of scientific studies have been conducted to reveal its medicinal properties. These studies have provided valuable insights into the mushroom's potential therapeutic applications. There are several ways to harness the medicinal value of stout camphor, including dietary supplements or as part of herbal formulas tailored to individual health needs.

Stout camphor is another recently rediscovered natural solution, with a rich history and a burgeoning reputation for its remarkable medicinal value. Its traditional uses in indigenous cultures and traditional Chinese medicine are now being supported by scientific research, unveiling its potential as a healing solution. Whether you seek to support your liver, bolster your immune system, reduce inflammation, alleviate respiratory issues, or explore its potential in cancer treatment, stout camphor offers a wide array of health benefits that are worth exploring.

NOTABLE COMPOUNDS: Polysaccharides, terpenoids, beta-glucans, sterols, antrosterol, antrodin A, antrodin C, 4-acetylantroquinonol B, antcamphins A–L and Y, antcamphorols A–K, benzenoids, antroquinol, antroquinonol D, dehydroeburicoic acid, eburocoic acid, zhankuic acids, antcin A, antcin B, antcin K, ergostatrien-3β-ol, benzocamphorin F, 4-acetylantroquinonol B, methylantcinate A, coenzyme Q_0

BENEFITS ACCORDING TO PRECLINICAL RESEARCH:

- 🍄 Anticancer (colorectal)[4132-4140]
- 🍄 Prevents colon cancer and interferes with colon cancer stem cells[4141,4142]
- 🍄 Anticancer (ovarian)[4143,4144]
- 🍄 Anticancer (cervical)[4145]
- 🍄 Anticancer (breast)[4146-4159]
- 🍄 Anticancer (lung)[4160-4167]
- 🍄 Anticancer (liver)[4168-4178]
- 🍄 Prevents liver cancer cells by inhibiting tumorigenic liver progenitor cells[4179]
- 🍄 Anticancer (bladder)[4180,4181]
- 🍄 Anticancer (pancreatic)[4182,4183]
- 🍄 Anticancer (oral)[4184,4185,4186]
- 🍄 Anticancer (prostate)[4187,4188,4189,4190]
- 🍄 Anticancer (osteosarcoma)[4191]
- 🍄 Anticancer (promyelocytic leukemia)[4192-4200]
- 🍄 Anticancer (glioma)[4201]
- 🍄 Anticancer (glioblastoma)[4202,4203]
- 🍄 Anticancer (melanoma)[4204,4205,4206]
- 🍄 Anticancer (malignant melanoma)[4207]
- 🍄 Anticancer (squamous cell carcinoma)[4208]
- 🍄 Inhibits Ras, leading to activation of autophagy and cancer cell death[4209]
- 🍄 Potentiates the activity of chemotherapy drugs against liver cancer cells[4210,4211]
- 🍄 Enhances the activity of amphotericin B against colorectal cancer cells[4212]
- 🍄 Anticancer (rodent colorectal)[4213]
- 🍄 Prevents angiogenesis[4214]

- Induces DNA demethylation and recovers multiple tumor suppressor genes[4215]
- Inhibits aryl hydrocarbon receptor (a ligand-activated transcription factor that is a therapeutic target for cancer therapy)[4216]
- Neuroprotective[4217-4225]
- Improves Alzheimer's disease-related pathologies[4226,4227,4228]
- Decreases neuroinflammation[4229]
- Alleviates Parkinson's disease-related neuroinflammation and neuropathological changes[4230,4231]
- Liver protective and restorative, improves responses to liver injury and inflammation, speeds the metabolism and clearance of alcohol, promotes liver homeostasis[4232-4249]
- Inhibits liver fibrosis[4250-4256]
- Kidney protective[4257,4258,4259]
- Regulates immune function in severe lupus nephritis[4260]
- Bladder protective after obstructive bladder dysfunction[4261]
- Lung protective[4262]
- Enhances the gut microbiome (balances microbiome)[4263]
- Alleviates ulcerative colitis[4264]
- Lowers blood pressure in subjects with high blood pressure[4265]
- Relaxes blood vessels[4266]
- Reduces scar formation in the cardiovascular system and vascular smooth muscle cell migration (a factor in atherosclerosis)[4267]
- Ameliorates atherosclerosis[4268]
- Ameliorates thromboembolic diseases—when a blood clot forms and breaks loose traveling through the bloodstream to block another blood vessel[4269]
- Improves lipid profiles or shields against oxidation of cholesterol (LDL)[4270,4271,4272,4273,4274,4275]
- Antidiabetic[4276-4284]
- Stimulates immune function[4285,4286,4287,4288,4289]
- Relieves asthma[4290]
- Anti-inflammatory[4291-4318]
- Decreases the inflammatory response in late-stage sepsis[4319]
- Relieves pain[4320,4321]
- Reverses osteoporosis[4322]
- Prevents cigarette smoke-induced oxidative stress and diseases (e.g., atherosclerosis)[4323]
- Protects DNA against damage[4324]
- Antioxidant[4325,4326,4327,4328,4329,4330]
- Reduces physical fatigue or improves physical performance[4331,4332]

- 🍄 Relieves eczema (atopic dermatitis) and improves skin barrier function[4333]
- 🍄 Promotes wound healing[4334]
- 🍄 Shields against inflammation in and photoaging of skin[4335]
- 🍄 Antiviral (hepatitis B)[4336]
- 🍄 Antiviral (herpes simplex virus)[4337]
- 🍄 Inhibits *H. pylori*[4338]
- 🍄 Antimicrobial[4339]
- 🍄 Antischistosomiasis (improves immune activity during Schistosoma infection)[4340,4341]

BENEFITS ACCORDING TO CLINICAL RESEARCH:

- ➤ Restores liver function—as measured by liver enzyme tests—in people with elevated liver enzymes after alcoholic fatty liver disease[4342]
  - 300 mg daily for twelve weeks

THERAPEUTIC POTENTIAL: Liver health (fatty liver and fibrosis), preserve memory and cognition, inflammatory disorders

CLINICAL DOSAGES: 300 mg daily

POTENTIAL ADVERSE EFFECTS: Diarrhea, nausea, vomiting

CAUTIONS AND CONTRAINDICATIONS: Pregnancy, lactation, stout camphor mushroom allergy; antidiabetic medications

TURKEY TAIL

(Trametes versicolor, syn. Coriolus versicolor, Polyporous versicolor)

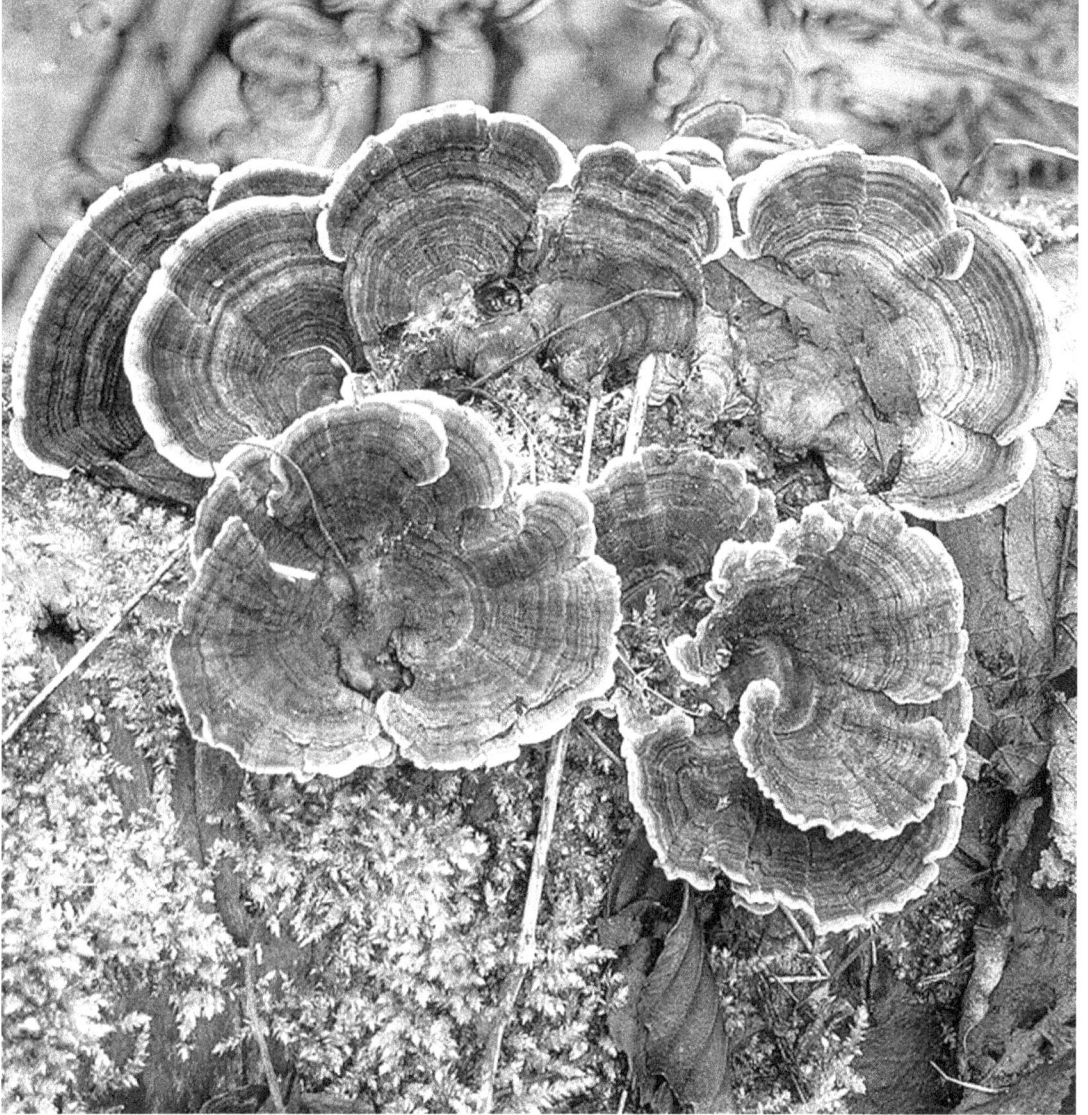

Kingdom: Fungi
Phylum: Basidiomycota
Class: Agaricomycetes
Order: Polyporales
Family: Polyporaceae
Genus: Trametes | Coriolus | Polyporous
Species: versicolor
Native Habitat: North America, China, and Europe

Few mushrooms have gained as much recognition for their medicinal value as the turkey tail mushroom. With its distinctive appearance resembling the multicolored tail feathers of a turkey, this mushroom has captured the attention of researchers, traditional healers, and health enthusiasts worldwide. Within the genus Trametes, various mushroom species exhibit similar fan-shaped fruiting bodies and decurrent (running down the stem) pores. However, turkey tail stands out because of its vibrant and varied colors.

The distinctive appearance of turkey tail mushrooms is characterized by a thin, flat, and fan-shaped cap, with concentric zones of varying colors that resemble the patterns on a turkey's tail feathers. These colors can range from shades of brown, tan, white, blue, green, and even red. The underside of the cap features numerous tiny pores instead of traditional gills, a common feature in polypore mushrooms. The size of turkey tail mushrooms varies but typically ranges from 3 to 8 centimeters (1.2 to 3.1 inches) in diameter. Its cap and stem are tough, leathery, and inedible in raw form.

Turkey tail mushrooms have been prized for their cultural and medicinal significance across different regions of the world. In TCM, turkey tail mushrooms are known as "Yun Zhi" and have been used for centuries to support overall health, particularly healthy immune system function. In Japan, these mushrooms are referred to as "Kawaratake" and have been consumed for their potential health benefits for centuries. They even have a history of traditional use among Natives of the American continent, where they were utilized medicinally and revered as symbols of longevity and wellness.

Today, turkey tail mushrooms continue to gain recognition for their medicinal properties and are widely studied for their potential health benefits. These mushrooms contain bioactive compounds, particularly polysaccharopeptides (PSP) and beta-glucans, which stimulate and modulate the immune system. They enhance the activity of immune cells, such as T cells and natural killer cells, potentially improving the body's ability to defend against infections and diseases. Turkey tail mushrooms are rich in antioxidants, including phenols and flavonoids. They have demonstrated antiviral properties and could be explored for their potential in viral infections. Turkey tail has been extensively researched for its potential role in cancer therapy. Compounds like PSP have shown promise in cancer treatment by enhancing the immune response, inhibiting tumor growth, and promoting apoptosis in cancer cells. These mushrooms may support digestive health by promoting a balanced gut microbiome, which can contribute to overall well-being and reverse many chronic health conditions. Turkey tail mushrooms have been investigated for their potential to protect the liver from damage and support detoxification processes. Moreover, these mushrooms support healthy respiratory function, making them useful for chronic obstructive pulmonary disease (COPD) and asthma.

Incorporating turkey tail mushrooms into your daily routine can have remarkable health benefits. They are available in various forms including teas, extracts, powders, and supplements.

The turkey tail mushroom provides robust evidence that mushrooms have massive medicinal value and remarkable potential to improve human health. With its rich cultural history, extensive scientific research, and a wide range of potential health benefits, turkey tail mushrooms have great value in natural medicine.

NOTABLE COMPOUNDS: Polysaccharides, beta-glucans, alpha-glucans, peptides, purified polysaccharopeptide (PSP), protein-bound polysaccharide-K (PSK; polysaccharide krestin), phenolics, vanillic acid, homogentisic acid, p-hydroxybenzoic acid, quinic acid, glycosides, sterols, triterpenoids, tramesan, baicalein, quercetin, catechin, musarin, nicotinamide, coriolan, ternatin

BENEFITS ACCORDING TO PRECLINICAL RESEARCH:

- ♣ Anticancer (breast)[4343-4351]
- ♣ Anticancer (cervical)[4352,4353,4354]
- ♣ Anticancer (prostate)[4355,4356]
- ♣ Prevents prostate cancer by targeting prostate cancer stem cell-like populations[4357]
- ♣ Anticancer (liver)[4358,4359,4360]
- ♣ Prevents liver cancer caused by the azobenzene dye methyl yellow (3-MDAB)[4361]
- ♣ Anticancer (colorectal)[4362,4363,4364,4365,4366]
- ♣ Anticancer (gastric)[4367]
- ♣ Anticancer (acute myeloid leukemia)[4368-4383]
- ♣ Anticancer (B-cell lymphoma)[4384]
- ♣ Anticancer (lung)[4385,4386,4387]
- ♣ Anticancer (glioblastoma)[4388]
- ♣ Anticancer (esophageal)[4389]
- ♣ Anticancer (pancreatic)[4390]
- ♣ Anticancer (fibrosarcoma)[4391]
- ♣ Anticancer (melanoma)[4392,4393]
- ♣ Anticancer (amelanotic melanoma)[4394,4395,4396]
- ♣ Anticancer (enhances docetaxel activity against prostate cancer)[4397]
- ♣ Anticancer (enhances cisplatin activity against liver and ovarian cancer)[4398]
- ♣ Anticancer (enhances doxorubicin and etoposide against breast cancer)[4399]
- ♣ Preserves immune function during radiotherapy for glioma tumors[4400]
- ♣ Inhibits tumor-promoting factors associated with inflammation[4401]

- Protects against biochemical serum changes and increases time to peak drug concentration of tamoxifen[4402]
- Anticancer (canine hemangiosarcoma)[4403]
- Anticancer (rodent melanoma)[4404]
- Anticancer (rodent breast)[4405, 4406,4407]
- Prolongs survival after breast cancer (rodent breast)[4408]
- Anticancer (rodent sarcoma)[4409,4410,4411]
- Anticancer (rodent liver)[4412]
- Enhances the gut microbiome (significantly increases levels of *Bifidobacterium* and *Lactobacillus*, reduces *Clostridium*, *Staphylococcus*, and *Enterococcus*)[4413]
- Antidepressant[4414]
- Promotes healthy cognition (inhibits acetylcholinesterase)[4415,4416]
- Anti-inflammatory[4417,4418,4419,4420,4421]
- Blocks the development of morphine dependence and withdrawal by upregulating cannabinoid type 2 (CB2) receptors and beta-endorphin while simultaneously reducing IL-1, inducible nitric oxide, and PGE2[4422]
- Relieves pain by activating IL-2[4423]
- Relieves pain in an acetylsalicylic acid-like manner[4424]
- Diminishes pain without affecting the female reproductive system or embryonic development[4425]
- Preserves bone strength[4426,4427]
- Stimulates immune function, activates multiple immune cells, regulates multiple immune pathways, enhances both humoral and cellular immunity, limits immunosuppression caused by cancerous tumors and potentiates immune activity against cancers[4428-4463]
- Stimulated immune function in subjects with endotoxin tolerance, such as sepsis, cystic fibrosis, or ischemia[4464]
- Enhances adaptive immunity against intracellular *Neisseria gonorrhoeae*, the causative bacteria of the sexually transmitted infection gonorrhea[4465]
- Restores healthy immune function after suppression by cyclophosphamide[4466]
- Balances immune function, which may be beneficial for autoimmune disorders (promotes th1/Th2 balance)[4467,4468,4469]
- Alleviates allergies[4470]
- Promotes healthy cholesterol levels[4471]
- Ameliorates ulcerative colitis[4472,4473]
- Suppresses inflammatory bowel disease[4474]
- Combats obesity[4475,4476]
- Alleviates metabolic syndrome[4477]
- Antidiabetic[4478-4486]

- Mitigates high cholesterol, fatty liver, oxidative stress, and high blood sugar in type 2 diabetic subjects[4487,4488]
- Alleviates diabetic cardiomyopathy by reducing cardiac fibrosis and inflammation[4489]
- Cardioprotective[4490]
- Ameliorates autoimmune myocarditis[4491]
- Suppressed paracetamol-induced liver damage[4492]
- Protects against nonalcoholic fatty liver disease[4493]
- Mitigates alcohol-induced liver injury[4494]
- Promotes neurogenesis (the formation of new neurons leading to brain growth in relation to organization)[4495]
- Neuroprotective, prevents the progression of neurodegenerative conditions[4496,4497,4498,4499]
- Reduces neuroinflammation[4500]
- Counteracts neuroinflammation and neurodegeneration caused by sepsis[4501]
- Suppresses Alzheimer's disease-related neuroinflammation and degeneration[4502]
- Restores spleen function after spleen injury caused by gamma-ray irradiation[4503]
- Improves physical performance and reduces fatigue[4504]
- Promotes healthy aging (augments SIRT1) and prolongs lifespan[4505,4506]
- Prevents gene mutations and DNA damage[4507,4508,4509]
- Antioxidant[4510-4527]
- Enhances superoxide dismutase (SOD) activity or mimics SOD activity[4528-4534]
- Improves glutathione peroxidase activity, including selenium-dependent glutathione peroxidase (SeGPx) and non-selenium-dependent glutathione peroxidase (non-SeGPx; also called glutathione S-transferase [GST])[4535,4536]
- Antiviral (influenza H9N2 avian, influenza A H1N1)[4537,4538]
- Antiviral (human immunodeficiency virus type 1—HIV-1)[4539,4540,4541]
- Antimicrobial[4542-4548]
- Antiparasitic (*Toxoplasma gondii*)[4549]
- Antileishmanial[4550]
- Skin brightening[4551]
- Prevents the production of, degrades, and removes mycotoxins[4552-4561]
- Bioremediates, biodegrades, bioconverts, or transforms heavy metals, pesticides, chemicals, micropollutants, and pharmaceuticals[4562-4617]

BENEFITS ACCORDING TO CLINICAL RESEARCH:

➤ Improves the clearance of human papillomavirus—HPV16 or HPV18 (88% clearance rate)[4618]
  - 400 mg of a combination of turkey tail and reishi daily for two months

- Reduces human papillomavirus (HPV) in women with cervical and uterine high-risk HPV infection (78.5% of women responded to treatment and 70.8% experienced HPV remission)[4619]
    - Use of turkey tail mushroom-based vaginal gel (Papilocare), one cannula per day for twenty-one consecutive days, followed by a seven-day rest, and then continuing with 1 cannula every other day during month two (except when menstruating)
- Enhances clearance of HPV and promotes healing of HPV-dependent cervical lesions in women with total and high-risk HPV[4620,4621]
    - Use of turkey tail mushroom-based vaginal gel (Papilocare), one cannula per day for twenty-one consecutive days (except when menstruating), followed by a seven-day rest, and then continuing with 1 cannula every other day during subsequent months (except when menstruating), with treatments lasting as long as twelve months
- Repairs low-degree HPV-related cervical lesions and enhances clearance of HPV in women older than forty years with HPV infection[4622]
    - Use of turkey tail mushroom-based vaginal gel (Papilocare), one cannula per day for twenty-one consecutive days (except when menstruating), followed by a seven-day rest period, continuing this pattern for one to three months before switching to application every other day for three to five months
- Promotes healing of the cervix and improves the vaginal microbiome and health in women infected with HPV exhibiting no symptoms[4623]
    - Application of a turkey tail mushroom-based gel (Palomacare) once during the day and at bedtime for twelve consecutive days between periods
- Positively modulates the gut microbiome[4624]
    - 1,200 mg, three times daily on an empty stomach for fourteen days
- Induces vitagenes (HO-1, Hsp70, Trx, SIRT-1, and γ-GC liase) in people with Meniere's disease to counteract oxidative stress, which could potentially reduce neuroinflammation and limit neurodegeneration[4625]
    - 1,500 mg every twelve hours for two months
- Reduces absolute five-year mortality in cancer patients by 9 percent, resulting in one additional person remaining alive per eleven people treated, in people with breast, gastric, or colorectal cancer treated with chemotherapy[4626]
    - Dosing not reported because of the nature of the study
- Recovers immune function in immunocompromised women after chemotherapy and radiation for breast cancer[4627]
    - Dose escalation from 1,500 mg twice daily to 3,000 mg twice daily to 3,000 mg three times daily

➤ Improves quality of life, but not time to progression or survival rates, in people with liver cancer and poor liver function who are unfit for standard therapy[4628]

- 2,400 mg daily for six to twelve weeks

➤ Improves three-year recurrence-free survival among people with stage II/III gastric cancer receiving postoperative chemotherapy[4629]

- 3,000 mg per day of PSK

➤ Enhances immune activity and improves chemotherapy in an eighty-three-year-old woman with advanced, metastatic inflammatory breast cancer (cancer free after following her for 3.5 years)[4630]

- 4,000 mg, twice daily in combination with chemotherapy

THERAPEUTIC POTENTIAL: HPV infection, viral infections, as an adjuvant solution during and after cancer treatment, gut dysbiosis

CLINICAL DOSAGES: 400–4,000 up to two or three times daily; typically, 1,000 mg up to three times daily

POTENTIAL ADVERSE EFFECTS: Gastrointestinal discomfort, heartburn, dark stool, darkening of fingernails

CAUTIONS AND CONTRAINDICATIONS: Pregnancy, lactation, turkey tail mushroom allergy, prior to surgery; antidiabetic drugs, tamoxifen, cyclophosphamide, antipyrine

WHITE JELLY
(Tremella fuciformis)

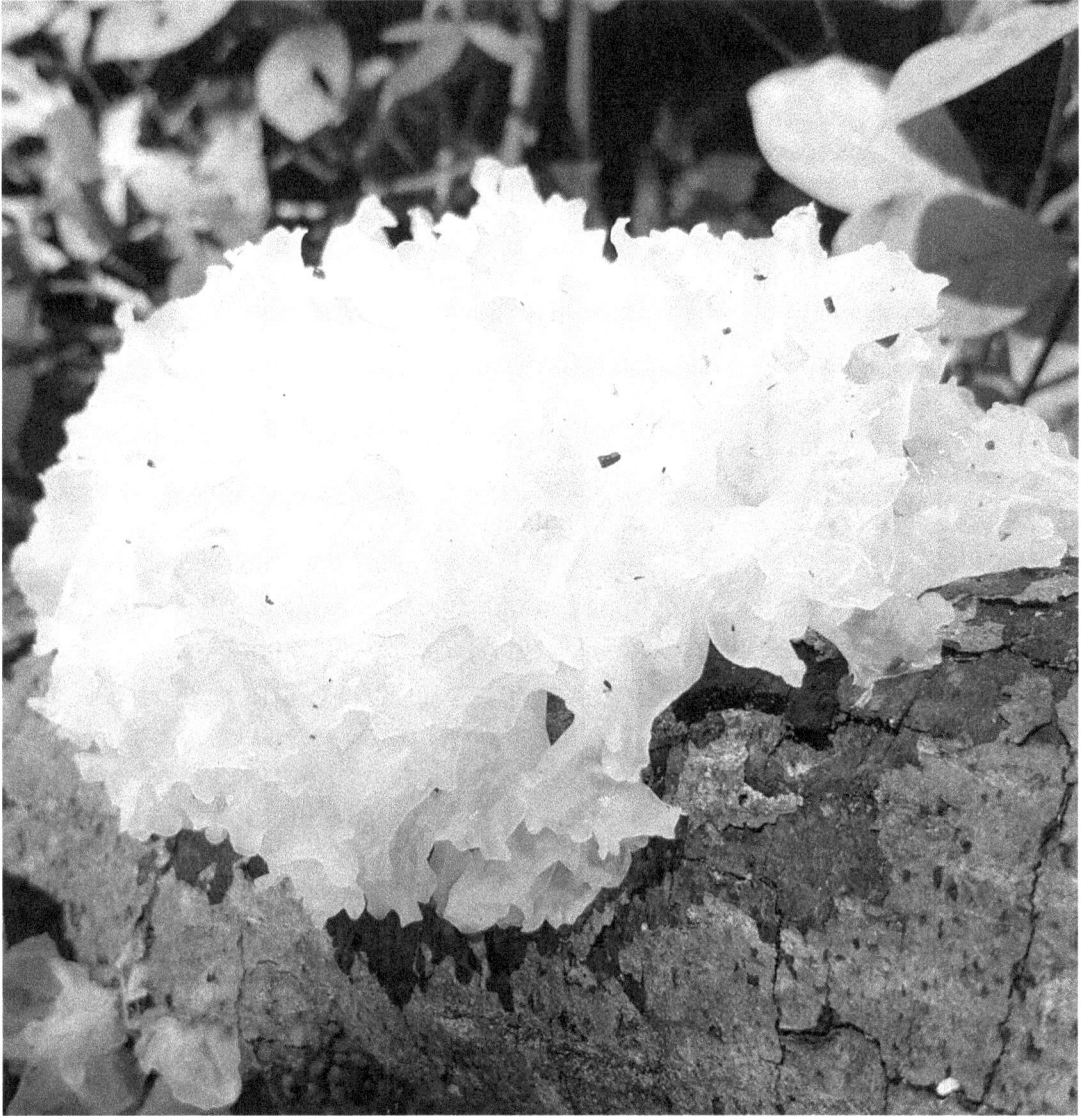

Kingdom: Fungi
Phylum: Basidiomycota
Class: Tremellomycetes
Order: Tremellales
Family: Tremellaceae
Genus: Tremella
Species: fuciformis
Native Habitat: China, Japan, Korea, Vietnam, Indonesia, Malaysia, Thailand

In the realm of traditional Chinese medicine (TCM) and beyond, the white jelly mushroom, also known as the snow mushroom, white fungus, or silver ear mushroom, has been revered for centuries for its potent medicinal properties. This unique and lesser-known mushroom, often prized for its gelatinous and translucent appearance, boasts a wide range of health benefits and has gained significant attention in recent years for its potential in modern wellness practices.

White jelly holds a special place in the annals of TCM with a history spanning over two thousand years. This mushroom was highly regarded by ancient herbalists for its legendary healing powers. Its history can be traced back to the Ming Dynasty (1368–1644 AD), where it was hailed as a "beauty mushroom" by Empress Yang Guifei, renowned for her stunning looks. Even then, it was believed that this mushroom could enhance one's appearance and vitality. Continuing its use for beauty today, white jelly extracts are often added to serums, creams, and masks to promote skin hydration, reduce fine lines and wrinkles, and rejuvenate the skin's appearance.

Like other mushrooms, white jelly contains an abundance of biologically active compounds, including polysaccharides and beta-glucans. The mushroom's high water content, combined with its ability to retain moisture, has made it a novel ingredient in skin-care products. Those who have used products with this unique-looking fungi can attest that it nourishes the skin, helps maintain hydration, and reduces the appearance of fine lines and wrinkles. White jelly contains a variety of antioxidants, such as ergosterol and mannitol, which help combat oxidative stress, reduce inflammation, and protect cells from damage. These properties are believed to contribute to its antiaging effects.

Over the years, the white jelly mushroom has found a place in modern medicine and wellness practices, thanks to emerging and ongoing scientific research that is beginning to reveal its potential health benefits. Some studies suggest that white jelly may help regulate cholesterol levels, lowering LDL cholesterol and promoting favorable lipid profiles. The polysaccharides found in white jelly stimulate the immune system, helping the body defend against infections and illnesses. These compounds also have anti-inflammatory properties, which can be beneficial in chronic inflammatory conditions, and for overall well-being. Additional research indicates that white jelly may have neuroprotective properties by safeguarding brain cells against oxidative stress and inflammation, potentially offering benefits in cognitive health.

Scientific interest in white jelly has been steadily growing, driven by the mushroom's promising medicinal properties. Researchers have conducted numerous studies to better understand its potential benefits and mechanisms of action. Its immunomodulatory, antioxidant, and skin-enhancing properties have all been validated by this research.

White jelly is available in various forms such as capsules, powders, and extracts. These supplements can provide a concentrated dose of its beneficial compounds. If you're looking to leverage its skin benefits, look for skin-care products that contain *Tremella fuciformis* extract or Tremella-derived ingredients. In Asian cuisine, white jelly is used in soups, stews, and desserts for its unique texture and mild flavor.

White jelly provides many health benefits and has potential applications in skin care, immune support, and more. While more studies are needed to fully reveal its potential, the mushroom's unique properties and centuries-old reputation make it a fascinating and promising subject of medicinal exploration. Whether used as a dietary supplement, a skin-care ingredient, or a culinary delight, white jelly has promise for its natural healing capabilities.

NOTABLE COMPOUNDS: Polysaccharides, heteroglycans, mannose, glucuronic acid, glucose, galactose, xylose, rhamnose, flavonoids, terpenoids, phenolic acids, 4-hydroxybenzoic acid, gentisic acid, 4-coumaric acid, 1,3-O-beta-D-glucopyranosyl-22E,24R-5alpha,8alpha-epidioxyergosta-6,22-diene

BENEFITS ACCORDING TO PRECLINICAL RESEARCH:

- Anticancer (prostate)[4631]
- Anticancer (melanoma)[4632]
- Anticancer (rodent sarcoma)[4633]
- Anticancer (rodent melanoma)[4634]
- Enhances the gut microbiome (promotes balance and diversity, improves the Firmicutes/Bacteroidetes ratio, increases the relative abundances of *Lactobacillus, Odoribacter, Helicobacter, Ruminococcaceae, Phascolarctobacterium, Lachnoclostridium,* and *Marinifilaceae,* increases production of short-chain fatty acids)[4635]
- Neuroprotective[4636,4637]
- Neurotrophic (promotes neurite outgrowth)[4638,4639,4640,4641]
- Reverses memory impairment[4642,4643]
- Antidiabetic[4644,4645,4646]
- Anti-inflammatory[4647,4648,4649]
- Stimulates or enhances immune system function[4650-4656]
- Balances immune function[4657,4658]
- Ameliorates ulcerative colitis[4659]
- Decreases intestinal inflammation[4660]
- Combats obesity[4661,4662]
- Lowers cholesterol[4663]
- Alleviates nonalcoholic fatty liver disease and associated inflammation[4664]

- ♣ Acts as a calcium channel blocker (helps lower blood pressure)[4665]
- ♣ Attenuates oxidative stress and its associated damage to cells, tissues, and organs[4666]
- ♣ Antioxidant[4667-4678]
- ♣ Shields against damage caused by gamma-radiation[4679]
- ♣ Relieves eczema (atopic dermatitis)[4680]
- ♣ Protects skin against UV-induced photodamage, oxidative stress, and premature aging[4681,4682,4683]
- ♣ Accelerates wound healing[4684]
- ♣ Brightens the skin[4685]
- ♣ Antiviral (hepatitis B)[4686]
- ♣ Antimicrobial[4687,4688]

BENEFITS ACCORDING TO CLINICAL RESEARCH:

- ➤ Enhances cognition—improves memory and executive function—and relieves subjective memory problems in people reporting they experience cognitive impairment[4689]
  - 200–400 mg three times per day for eight weeks

THERAPEUTIC POTENTIAL: Dysbiosis, cognitive health, skin care

CLINICAL DOSAGES: 200–400 mg three times daily

POTENTIAL ADVERSE EFFECTS: None currently known

CAUTIONS AND CONTRAINDICATIONS: Pregnancy, lactation, white jelly mushroom allergy

WOOD EAR
(*Auricularia auricula-judae*)

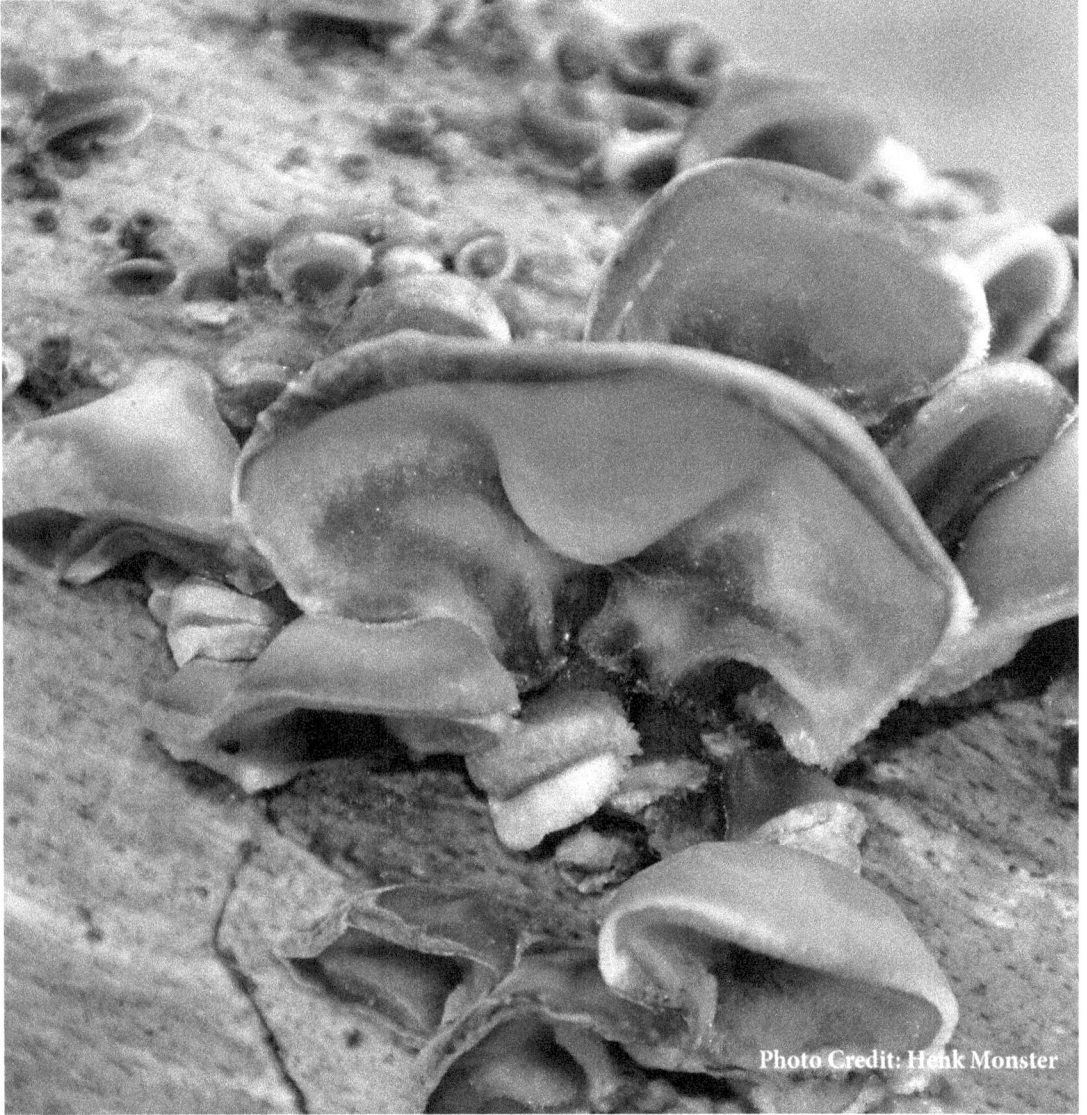

Photo Credit: Henk Monster

Kingdom: Fungi
Phylum: Basidiomycota
Class: Agaricomycetes
Order: Auriculariales
Family: Auriculariaceae
Genus: Auricularia
Species: auricula-judae
Native Habitat: Europe

Known as the wood ear mushroom, jelly ear mushroom, Judas's ear mushroom, or black fungus, this ear-shaped mushroom has gained prominence in the world of natural healing because of its history, nutritional content, and therapeutic applications in modern medicine. Found on wood, especially elder, it was once believed that wood ear mushrooms had a worldwide distribution, but modern analysis shows that non-European species are distinct. Similar mushrooms found in China and East Asia are actually *Auricularia heimuer* or *Auricularia villosula*, while North American wood ear mushrooms found on conifers are *Auricularia americana* and those on broadleaf trees *Auricularia angiospermarum.*[4690],[4691],[4692] These mushrooms were widely used as medicine through the nineteenth century but have only recently regained attention as a promising natural solution for a variety of ailments.

The use of wood ear varieties dates back thousands of years, and it has a rich history of use in traditional Chinese and Japanese medicine. It has been utilized in traditional remedies to treat a variety of health conditions, such as sore throats, eye problems, jaundice, and more. Wood ear boasts an impressive nutritional profile that contributes to its medicinal value. These mushrooms are an excellent source of important nutrients, like proteins, polysaccharides, vitamins, minerals, and fiber.

Studies suggest that regular consumption of these mushrooms may strengthen the immune system, which may be because of their polysaccharide content. They also contain compounds known for the antioxidant properties, such as ergosterol peroxide. Wood ear has a long history of use for inflammation, and modern research confirms this historical use, showing that it inhibits proinflammatory pathways. Wood ear also possesses antiviral and antimicrobial properties, making it useful for infectious illnesses. More recently, it has been used to reduce the risk of cardiovascular diseases and to manage metabolic disorders like diabetes. With the seemingly unceasing increases in overweight and obesity in modern society, wood ear mushrooms have also been investigated as a weight-loss aid. Lastly, traditional medicine systems use these mushrooms to accelerate the wound healing process and prevent wound infections.

The medicinal properties of wood ear have piqued the interest of modern science, leading to numerous studies exploring its potential therapeutic applications. Some noteworthy research findings suggest that the mushroom's bioactive compounds, especially polysaccharides, have antitumor properties. They may inhibit the growth of cancer cells and enhance the body's ability to fight cancer. This makes it a subject of interest in cancer research. Research indicates that extracts from wood ear exhibit antiviral effects, with potential applications in treating viral infections, including influenza and herpes. Preliminary studies have explored the use of wood ear extracts in wound healing, which demonstrate faster healing rates and reduced infection risk.

Other research suggests that the mushroom may be beneficial for gastrointestinal disorders, liver protection, and neurodegenerative diseases like Alzheimer's disease and Parkinson's.

Wood ear mushrooms are versatile and can be incorporated into various dishes. In Asian cuisine, they are often used in soups, stir-fries, and salads, adding a unique texture and flavor. Their ability to absorb the flavors of other ingredients makes them a valuable addition to culinary creations.

In traditional Chinese medicine, these mushrooms are prepared in herbal decoctions and tonics. These decoctions and tonics are then used for immune support, respiratory health, anemia, or other blood-related disorders, and to alleviate poor digestion or gastrointestinal discomfort.

Wood ear mushrooms have a long history of medicinal use, particularly in traditional Chinese and Japanese medicine. Their rich nutritional profile, which includes proteins, polysaccharides, vitamins, and minerals, makes them a valuable addition to a healthy diet. Modern research has revealed the diverse therapeutic properties of these mushrooms, including their immunomodulatory effects, antioxidant properties, anti-inflammatory benefits, and potential in preventing and managing various health conditions.

As the realm of mycology continues to expand, the potential of mushrooms like wood ear to improve human health becomes increasingly apparent. Further research and exploration may uncover additional applications for these remarkable fungi, reaffirming their status as a medicinal marvel in the world of natural remedies.

NOTABLE COMPOUNDS: Polysaccharides, beta-glucans, glucuronoxylogalactoglucomannan, melanin

BENEFITS ACCORDING TO PRECLINICAL RESEARCH:

- 🍄 Anticancer (liver)[4693]
- 🍄 Anticancer (gastric)[4694,4695]
- 🍄 Anticancer (bronchioalveolar)[4696,4697]
- 🍄 Anticancer (lymphoma)[4698]
- 🍄 Anticancer (tropomyosin receptor kinase B-positive cancers)[4699]
- 🍄 Anticancer (rodent sarcoma)[4700,4701,4702]
- 🍄 Anticancer (rodent lymphoma)[4703]
- 🍄 Enhances the gut microbiome (improves balance and diversity, promotes the proliferation of beneficial bacteria: *Lactobacillus, Roseburia, Faecalibaculum, Dubosiella, Alloprevotella,* and *Lachnospiraceae,* increases short-chain fatty

acid production, inhibits harmful bacteria—*Desulfovibrio, Enterorhabdus*, and *Helicobacter*, decreases the abundance of Firmicutes and increases that of Bacteroidetes, enhances production of B vitamins)[4704,4705]

- Improves intestinal barrier function (relieves leaky gut)[4706]
- Ameliorates sickle cell anemia by stabilizing red blood cell membrane integrity and structure[4707]
- Combats obesity[4708,4709,4710,4711]
- Antidiabetic[4712-4718]
- Improves lipid/cholesterol profiles[4719,4720,4721,4722]
- Liver protective[4723]
- Prevents or alleviates nonalcoholic fatty liver disease[4724,4725]
- Protects the stomach and liver against acute alcohol binge drinking[4726]
- Prolongs healthy lifespan[4727,4728,4729]
- Anti-inflammatory[4730,4731]
- Stimulates immune function[4732,4733,4734,4735]
- Reduces the risk of cardiovascular disease (anticomplement activity)[4736]
- Anticoagulant[4737]
- Antioxidant[4738-4751]
- Improves glucose utilization[4752]
- Accelerates wound healing and promotes collagen production[4753,4754]
- Antimicrobial[4755,4756]

BENEFITS ACCORDING TO CLINICAL RESEARCH:

➢ None found

THERAPEUTIC POTENTIAL: Gut microbiome support, sickle cell anemia

CLINICAL DOSAGES: Unknown; most commonly found as dried whole mushrooms

POTENTIAL ADVERSE EFFECTS: Digestive discomfort, bloating, gas

CAUTIONS AND CONTRAINDICATIONS: Pregnancy, lactation, wood ear mushroom allergy; drugs that thin the blood, antidiabetic drugs

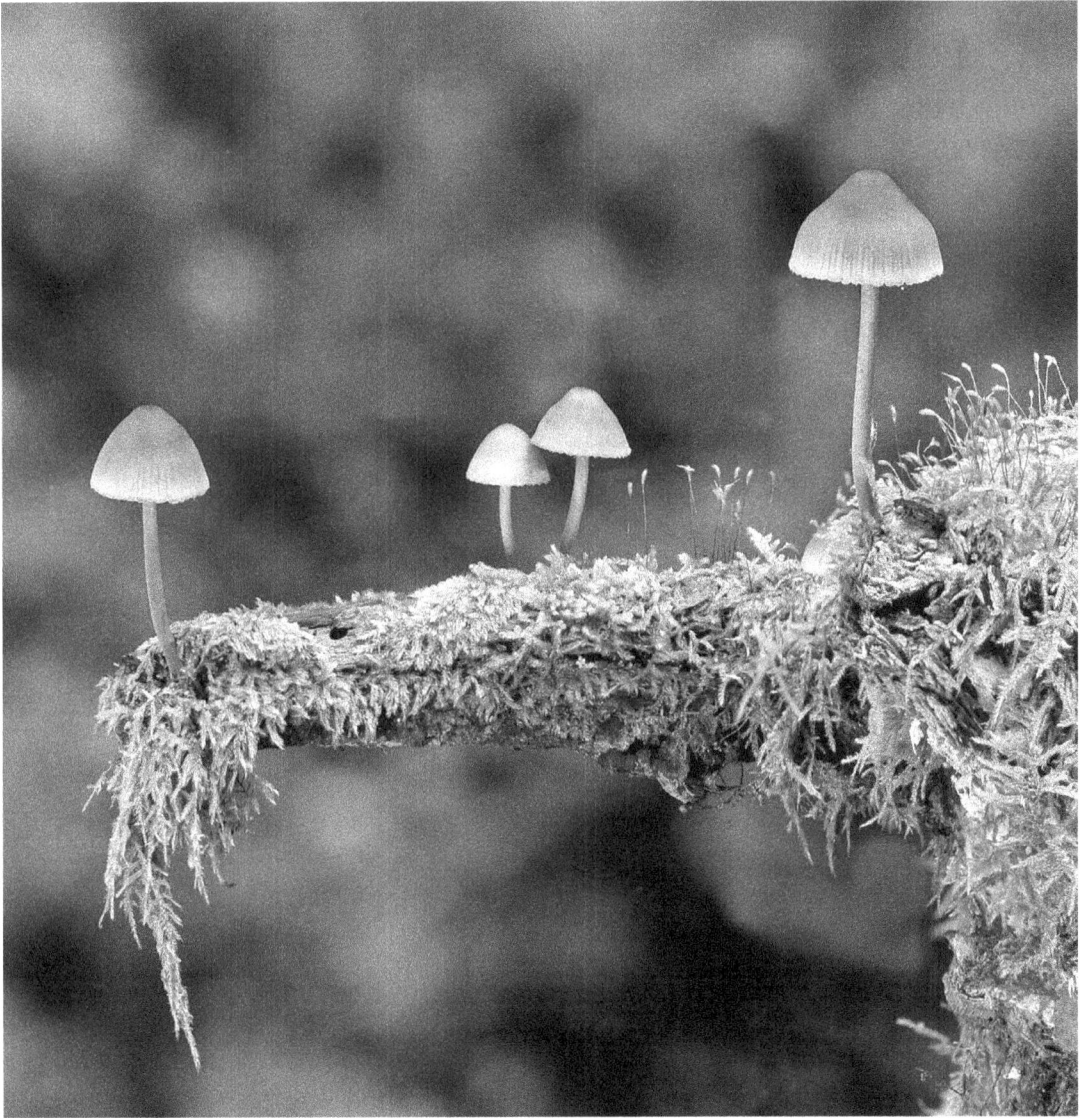

Given the massive amount of research emerging and the centuries-long history of the clinical use of medicinal mushrooms, their use as dietary supplements and natural solutions has gained popularity in recent years. While each mushroom has unique properties, it is clear that consuming mushrooms and their extracts has enormous potential to improve human health. Many of the mushrooms positively influence immune function, help maintain a healthy balance in the gut microbiome, balance blood sugar levels, and aid a healthy inflammatory response. Since health begins and ends in the gut and two of the most important factors to optimize your health are maintaining healthy blood sugar levels and inflammation, mushrooms can dramatically alter your health in a short period of time. With the mechanisms, cellular targets, and properties revealed in preclinical research and the clinical studies that validate these properties and determine effective doses, we are now ready to use them clinically to improve human health.

Medicinal mushrooms are available in many forms, including capsules, tinctures, powders, and teas. Capsules and tablets often provide a standardized dosage of the active compounds, making it convenient to achieve the therapeutic levels necessary for your health needs. Tinctures are liquid extracts of medicinal mushrooms and are usually added to another beverage to consume. They are known for their rapid absorption and are suitable for individuals who have difficulty swallowing capsules or tablets. Mushroom powders can be added to smoothies, soups, other foods, or a beverage. A more traditional method of consuming therapeutic quantities of medicinal mushrooms is in tea form. While they can be added to the diet, whole mushrooms are less concentrated than their extracts, requiring the consumption of several grams to realize their medicinal value.

Regardless of the form you choose, it's crucial that you use a pure, high-quality extract. Ensure you purchase mushroom supplements from reputable suppliers that are sustainably cultivated and harvested. If you plan to cultivate or wildcraft your own mushrooms, be sure you can readily identify the species. Look for supplements that are third-party tested to confirm their purity and potency, and to ensure they are free of contaminants. The way a mushroom is extracted can affect its efficacy. Look for products that use hot-water extraction, alcohol, or fermentation to maintain the bioactive compounds. Lastly, pay attention to the recommended dosage on the product label.

Mushrooms often work better when used together, as a mushroom complex, providing synergistic benefits and improved results. You don't have to find a mushroom complex with the exact recommended mushrooms for each condition, but the complex should contain as many of the recommended mushrooms as possible. If the supplement contains additional mushrooms not listed in the protocols, this is fine as well. The protocols in this chapter are based on current evidence and knowledge and designed for adults. You don't need to take all of the mushrooms, complementary supplements, or essential oils at the same time to get results. Always consult an integrative health-care professional knowledgeable in natural solutions before using the protocols.

When it comes to mushrooms, they have massive upside potential in preserving, promoting, and restoring human health. These organisms will continue to be a focus of scientific research, particularly among Asian researchers, and additional medicinal qualities will be revealed, making them even more highly sought-after in the future. You can typically expect results from high-quality mushroom supplements within a few weeks, maybe a few days if used intensively. Join the fungal frenzy and see how these neglected natural remedies can improve your health today.

Note: Psilocybin, or psilocybe mushroom recommendations are provided as a reference for those living within a jurisdiction where it is legal to possess and use them. Growing, possessing, and using psilocybe mushrooms or their alkaloids is a serious criminal offense in many states and countries and could lead to criminal prosecution, fines, and incarceration. Clinical and therapeutic doses should always be taken under the guidance of a healthcare professional. Always consult your own healthcare professional before using psilocybin or psilocybe mushrooms and before decreasing or stopping any medications you are currently taking.

Addiction (Alcohol, nicotine)

Recommended mushrooms: Psylocibin, reishi

Form/Dosage: 1–2.5 mg of psilocybin every three to four days, titrated up to 5 mg if necessary, for four to eight weeks, followed by a two-week rest, or two 20–30 mg doses spaced weeks apart under the care of an informed health-care professional; 500 mg to 1,500 reishi up to three times daily

Duration: As determined by a health professional

Complementary supplements: 500 mg of citicoline twice daily; 600 mg of n-Acetyl cysteine, two to three times daily; D-phenylalanine, L-glutamine, and L-5-hydroxytryptophan as instructed on the product label

Complementary essential oils: Inhale a combination of black pepper, clove, and grapefruit essential oils as needed

Allergies

Recommended mushrooms: Almond, Cordyceps militaris, enoki, mesima, reishi

Form/Dosage: Mushroom complex as instructed by the product label

Duration: As long as symptoms persist

Complementary supplements: Heal the gut through the strategies listed in *Heal the Gut, Heal the Immune System*; 300 mg of stinging nettle two to three times daily; 600 mg of n-Acetyl cysteine twice daily; bromelain and quercetin supplement as instructed on the product label

Complementary essential oils:	Take a capsule filled with 3 drops each of German chamomile and lavender, and 1 drop each of lemon and peppermint, morning and evening

Alzheimer's Disease

See Cognitive Function

Anemia, Sickle Cell

Recommended mushrooms:	Wood ear, reishi
Form/Dosage:	Mushroom complex containing wood ear and reishi as instructed on the product label
Duration:	As needed for symptoms
Complementary supplements:	n/a
Complementary essential oils:	Topical application of lemon and German chamomile essential oil diluted to 5% over the spleen area (upper left side of the abdomen)

Antiaging (limit age-related conditions)

Recommended mushrooms:	Cordyceps sinensis, Cordyceps militaris, enoki, reishi, turkey tail
Form/Dosage:	Mushroom complex as instructed on the product label
Duration:	Indefinitely
Complementary supplements:	250–1,000 mg MNM on an empty stomach daily (preferably with 250–500 mg of resveratrol)
Complementary essential oils:	1 to 2 drops of frankincense under the tongue each day

Anxiety

Recommended mushrooms:	Psilocybin
Form/Dosage:	1–2.5 mg of psilocybin every three to four days, titrated up to 5 mg if necessary, for four to eight weeks, followed by a two-week rest, or 15 mg under the guidance of a health-care professional as instructed
Duration:	As determined by health-care professional
Complementary supplements:	500 mg of chamomile extract (standardized to minimum 1.2% apigenin) once daily

| *Complementary essential oils*: | 80 mg of lavender essential oil in a capsule, twice daily; inhale a combination of lavender, sweet orange, and vanilla for acute anxiety |

Asthma

Recommended mushrooms:	Cordyceps sinensis, enoki
Form/Dosage:	1,200 mg of Corbin (cordyceps) three times daily; mushroom complex with cordyceps and enoki as instructed on the product label
Duration:	As long as symptoms persist
Complementary supplements:	50–75 mg of butterbur two or three times daily; 500 mg of Boswellia serrata extract one to three times daily
Complementary essential oils:	Inhale respiratory-supportive essential oils like eucalyptus, rosemary, myrtle, and ginger as needed

Atherosclerosis

Recommended mushrooms:	Reishi
Form/Dosage:	180 mg reishi beta-glucans three times daily
Duration:	90–120 days
Complementary supplements:	600 mg of aged garlic twice daily; fish oil supplying a minimum of 1,000 mg of combined EPA and DHA daily; 100–200 mg of ubiquinol (CoQ10) daily
Complementary essential oils:	Ingest 1 to 2 drops each of lemon, sweet orange, and lemongrass in a capsule, twice daily

Attention Deficit Hyperactivity Disorder (ADHD)

Recommended mushrooms:	Psylocibin
Form/Dosage:	1–2.5 mg of psilocybin every three to four days, titrated up to 5 mg if necessary, for four to eight weeks, followed by a two-week rest, or 25 mg under the guidance of a health-care professional
Duration:	As determined by health-care professional
Complementary supplements:	Fish oil supplying 500–2,000 mg of DHA and 250–1,250 mg of EPA daily; 200–300 mg of phosphatidylserine daily; 1 mg/kg body weight of zinc for hyperactive subtype
Complementary essential oils:	Dilute cedarwood, frankincense, lavender, and German chamomile, and vetiver to 5%–15% and apply on the back of the neck

Autism Spectrum Disorder

Recommended mushrooms: Psylocibin

Form/Dosage: 1–2.5 mg of psilocybin every three to four days, titrated up to 5 mg if necessary, for four to eight weeks, followed by a two-week rest, or 25 mg under the guidance of a health-care professional

Duration: As determined by health-care professional

Complementary supplements: Multistrain probiotic as instructed on the product label; 5,000 IU of vitamin D daily; 200 mg of magnesium citrate, bisglycinate, or complex daily; 50–100 mg of vitamin B6 daily; 1,000–5,000 mcg of sublingual methylcobalamin daily; 15 mg of L-methylfolate daily

Complementary essential oils: Create a roller bottle blend of 2 to 3 drops each of melissa, frankincense, ylang ylang, lavender, and vetiver, filling the rest of the bottle with carrier oil, and apply this blend to the base of the neck/skull, twice daily

Autoimmune Disorder

Recommended mushrooms: camphor   Agaricus, maitake, mesima, reishi, shiitake, stout

Form/Dosage: label   Mushroom complex as instructed on the product

Duration: Until significant improvements are experienced and then for an additional two months; may need to continue supplementation to keep autoimmunity in remission

Complementary supplements: Heal the gut using the strategies from *Heal the Gut, Heal the Immune System*; 2–6 mg/kg body weight CBD daily; 100–1,000 mg (depending on standardization) Boswellia extract daily; 500 mg turmeric up to three times daily

Complementary essential oils: 1 to 2 drops of copaiba or frankincense essential oil under the tongue, twice daily

Body Dysmorphic Disorder

Recommended mushrooms: Psylocibin

Form/Dosage: 1–2.5 mg of psilocybin every three to four days, titrated up to 5 mg if necessary, for four to eight weeks, followed by a two-week rest, or 25 mg under the guidance of a health-care professional

Duration: As determined by health-care professional

Complementary supplements: 150–250 mg of 5-HTP once or twice daily

Complementary essential oils: Inhale sweet orange oil as needed

Cancer

Recommended mushrooms: Maitake D-fraction, reishi, turkey tail, mesima

Form/Dosage: 40–150 mg of maitake D-fraction (MD-fraction) plus 4,000–6,000 mg of maitake supplements daily; 1,800–3,000 mg reishi supplements three times daily; mushroom complex containing some of the above mushrooms

Duration: As determined by a health-care professional

Complementary supplements: 1,000 mg vitamin C three times daily

Complementary essential oils: See chapter 6 of *Medicinal Essential Oils: The Science and Practice of Evidence-Based Essential Oil Therapy* (Second Edition)

Chemotherapy Side Effects

Recommended mushrooms: Mesima, reishi, shiitake, turkey tail

Form/Dosage: 1,000 mg reishi three times daily; 600–1,000 mg shiitake three times daily; 1,200–4,000 mg of turkey tail supplement twice daily; 1,100 mg of mesima supplement three times daily; mushroom complex as instructed on the product label

Duration: During and for four weeks after chemotherapy if physician approves

Complementary supplements: Multistrain probiotic as instructed on the product label or by an informed health-care professional; 5,000 mg of powdered L-glutamine on an empty stomach, once or twice daily

Complementary essential oils: See chapter 6 of *Medicinal Essential Oils: The Science and Practice of Evidence-Based Essential Oil Therapy* (Second Edition)

Chronic Obstructive Pulmonary Disease (COPD)

Recommended mushrooms:	Cordyceps sinensis, oyster
Form/Dosage:	100 mg oyster pleuran daily; mushroom complex as instructed on the product label
Duration:	Minimum of three months and up to six months
Complementary supplements:	600 mg n-Acetyl cysteine once or twice daily; 1,000 mg vitamins C with 250–500 mg bioflavonoids daily; 5,000 IU of vitamin D daily
Complementary essential oils:	Inhale or diffuse rosemary, eucalyptus, myrtle, and peppermint essential oil

Cognitive Function

Recommended mushrooms:	Chaga, lion's mane, stout camphor, turkey tail, white jelly
Form/Dosage:	Mushroom complex containing at least two of the above recommended mushrooms as instructed on the product label; 1,000 mg lion's mane supplement three times daily; 1,500 mg turkey tail twice daily; 200–400 mg of white jelly three times daily
Duration:	Minimum of eight weeks; indefinitely to maintain cognition throughout life or to improve cognitive dysfunction
Complementary supplements:	400–450 mg of bacopa daily; 1,500 mg Panax ginseng, three times daily; 200 mcg of huperzine A daily
Complementary essential oils:	Take 1 drop of Spanish sage in a capsule daily

Cold

See Viral Infection

Colitis, Ulcerative

Recommended mushrooms:	Chaga, Cordyceps militaris, lion's mane, reishi
Form/Dosage:	1,800 mg reishi three times daily; mushroom complex with the above as instructed on the product label
Duration:	Until symptoms significantly improve plus two additional months

Complementary supplements:	500 mg of bromelain before each meal; multistrain probiotic as instructed on the product label
Complementary essential oils:	Take a capsule filled with 1 drop each of spearmint, rosemary, copaiba, fennel, peppermint, and ginger, twice daily

Dementia

See Cognitive Function

Depression

Recommended mushrooms:	Lion's mane, psilocybin
Form/Dosage:	1–2.5 mg of psilocybin every three to four days, titrated up to 5 mg if necessary, for four to eight weeks, followed by a two-week rest, or 25 mg under the guidance of a health-care professional as instructed; 1,000 mg lion's mane supplement, three times daily
Duration:	As instructed by a health-care professional
Complementary supplements:	St. John's wort extract (Perika) as instructed on the product label; heal the gut with the strategies in *Heal the Gut, Heal the Immune System*
Complementary essential oils:	Add 5 drops of frankincense, 5 drops of sweet orange, and 1 drop of ylang ylang to a 10 mL roller bottle, and fill the rest with carrier oil, apply over the heart area of the chest a few times daily

Detoxification

Recommended mushrooms:	Oyster, king oyster, turkey tail, reishi, shiitake, Cordyceps sinensis
Form/Dosage:	Start with a colon cleanse and then support liver function with 1,000 mg three times daily of oyster, king oyster, or turkey tail followed by reishi or shiitake; then use 1,000 mg of Cordyceps sinensis to aid kidney function
Duration:	Use liver and kidney supportive mushrooms for 30 to 60 days each
Complementary supplements:	See *Heal the Gut, Heal the Immune System* for a complete cleansing and detoxification protocol
Complementary essential oils:	Add a few drops of citrus essential oils to your water daily

Diabetes

Recommended mushrooms: Almond, chaga, Cordyceps sinensis, king oyster, maitake, oyster, pink oyster, poria, reishi

Form/Dosage: Mushroom complex as instructed on the supplement label or by an informed health-care professional; 1,000 mg oyster supplement, three times daily

Duration: At least three months and until glucose is well managed

Complementary supplements: 250–500 mg of mulberry leaf extract (providing a minimum of 7.5 mg of DNJ) before your largest meal of the day; 500 mg of berberine HCl twice daily

Complementary essential oils: Take a capsule filled with 1 drop each of cinnamon bark, fennel, lemongrass, and geranium essential oil morning and evening with a meal

Dysbiosis

Recommended mushrooms: Chaga, Cordyceps sinensis, Cordyceps militaris, enoki, king oyster, lion's mane, maitake, poria, reishi, turkey tail, white jelly, wood ear

Form/Dosage: 1,000 mg lion's mane supplement, three times daily; 1,200 mg of turkey tail supplement three times daily on an empty stomach; mushroom complex as instructed on the product label

Duration: 60 to 120 days

Complementary supplements: High-potency multistrain probiotic daily with a meal

Complementary essential oils: Add a few drops of citrus essential oils to your water daily

Eczema

Recommended mushrooms: Oyster

Form/Dosage: Topical Imunoglukan P4H cream or cream containing oyster mushroom extract

Duration: Until symptoms completely resolve

Complementary supplements: Heal the gut using the strategies in *Heal the Gut, Heal the Immune System*

Complementary essential oils: Homeopathic cardiospermum cream instead

Endometriosis

Recommended mushrooms: Chaga

Form/Dosage: 1,000 mg Chaga daily

Duration: Until symptoms resolve plus an additional month

Complementary supplements: Molecular progesterone complex as instructed on the product label; 600 mg of n-Acetyl cysteine with 500 mg of turmeric and 250–500 mg of quercetin three times daily

Complementary essential oils: Take a capsule filled with 4 drops of copaiba and 1 drop each of geranium and clary sage essential oils one to three times daily

Fatigue

Recommended mushrooms: Chaga, Cordyceps sinensis, Cordyceps militaris, reishi

Form/Dosage: Mushroom complex with the above mushrooms as instructed on the supplement label; 1,000 mg of reishi three times daily

Duration: Minimum of four weeks or until fatigue is corrected

Complementary supplements: 1,000 mg of Panax ginseng twice daily; 2,000 mg of D-ribose one to three times daily; 400–600 mg of ashwagandha, twice daily

Complementary essential oils: Add 1 drop of peppermint essential oil to 16 ounces of water and consume; inhale peppermint essential oil as needed

Fatty Liver, Alcoholic

Recommended mushrooms: Stout camphor

Form/Dosage: 300 mg stout camphor one to two times daily

Duration: Minimum of twelve weeks

Complementary supplements: High-potency multistrain probiotic as instructed on the product label; 200–300 mg of milk thistle (standardized to silymarin content) daily; 500 mg of berberine HCl twice daily

Complementary essential oils: Take a capsule filled with 1 drop each of ginger, lemon, lime, and tangerine, three times daily

Fertility, Female

Recommended mushrooms: Maitake

Form/Dosage: 250 mg maitake plus 18 mg of SX-fraction, three times daily between meals beginning at the first day of menses

Duration: At least three menstrual cycles and up to seven or until conception

Complementary supplements: 1,500 mg of evening primrose oil once or twice daily; molecular progesterone complex as instructed on the product label

Complementary essential oils: Dilute to 5%–10% and apply 2 to 4 drops of clary sage to the lower abdomen and mons pubis 2 times daily. Apply 1 drop of diluted clary sage to the inside and outside of the right ankle; take a capsule filled with 1 drop each of ylang ylang, frankincense, fennel, clary sage, and geranium, 2 times daily.

Fibromyalgia

Recommended mushrooms: Psylocibin, reishi

Form/Dosage: 1–2.5 mg of psilocybin every three to four days, titrated up to 5 mg if necessary, for four to eight weeks, followed by a two-week rest, or 25 mg under the guidance of a health-care professional; 3,000 mg of reishi twice daily

Duration: As determined by health-care professional

Complementary supplements: 500 mg of acetyl L-carnitine three times daily; Fish oil providing 1,000 mg of EPA and 500 mg of DHA two to four times daily; 5,000 IU of vitamin D daily; 200–400 mg magnesium citrate daily (alternatively, spray or rub magnesium on the legs and arms twice daily); 100 mg of 5-HTP three times daily

Complementary essential oils: Take a capsule filled with 2 drops of frankincense and 1 drop each of lemongrass, basil, myrrh, and German chamomile, 2 times daily.

Flu (Influenza)

See Viral Infection

Gastritis

Recommended mushrooms:	Lion's mane
Form/Dosage:	1,000 mg lion's mane three times daily
Duration:	Minimum of two weeks and up to six months
Complementary supplements:	760 mg of DGL (deglycyrrhizinated licorice) tablets prior to each meal; multistrain probiotic as instructed on the product label; 1,100 mg of ginger two to three times daily; zinc L-carnosine as instructed on the product label
Complementary essential oils:	Take a capsule filled with 1 drop each of copaiba, peppermint, fennel, ginger, and lemongrass, one to three times daily.

Gout

Recommended mushrooms:	Chaga, Cordyceps militaris, honey, reishi
Form/Dosage:	Mushroom complex as instructed on the product label
Duration:	Until symptoms resolve plus an additional month
Complementary supplements:	30 mL of unsweetened tart cherry juice once or twice daily
Complementary essential oils:	Dilute to 25%, and gently apply 1 drop each of frankincense, peppermint, and cypress to affected joints, several times daily.

Graves' Disease

Recommended mushrooms:	Cordyceps sinensis
Form/Dosage:	2,000 mg of fermented powder (Corbin) three times daily
Duration:	As determined by disease remission markers
Complementary supplements:	See *Beating Autoimmune Thyroid Disorders Naturally* for a complete program
Complementary essential oils:	Create a roller bottle with 5 drops frankincense, 3 drops each of myrtle, myrrh, and German chamomile, filling the rest of the bottle with carrier oil, and apply over the thyroid area of the neck two to three times daily

Hashimoto's Disease

Recommended mushrooms: Cordyceps sinensis

Form/Dosage: 2,000 mg of fermented powder (Corbin) three times daily

Duration: As determined by disease remission markers

Complementary supplements: See *Beating Autoimmune Thyroid Disorders Naturally* for a complete program

Complementary essential oils: Create a roller bottle with 5 drops frankincense, 3 drops each of myrtle, myrrh, and German chamomile, filling the rest of the bottle with carrier oil, and apply over the thyroid area of the neck two to three times daily

Headache, Cluster

Recommended mushrooms: Psilocybin

Form/Dosage: 1–2.5 mg of psilocybin every three to four days, titrated up to 5 mg if necessary, for four to eight weeks, followed by a two-week rest, or 10 mg under the guidance of a health-care professional as instructed

Duration: Work closely with a health-care professional to determine

Complementary supplements: 400–800 mg of white willow bark daily; 200–400 mg of magnesium citrate daily

Complementary essential oils: Create a roller bottle with 10 drops peppermint, 7 drops each of rosemary, hinoki, and lavender, 6 drops copaiba, and 3 drops German chamomile or blue tansy essential oils, fill the rest of the bottle with carrier oil, and roll onto the temples, back of the neck, and forehead as needed.

Healthy Aging (Reduce Risk of Oxidative Stress-Related Conditions)

Recommended mushrooms: Chaga, Cordyceps sinensis, pink oyster, reishi

Form/Dosage: 225 mg reishi daily after a meal; mushroom complex as instructed on the product label

Duration: Six months

Complementary supplements: 100–300 mg of S-Acetyl L-glutathione daily

Complementary essential oils: Take 1 drop each of clove, frankincense, and sweet orange essential oil once or twice daily

Hepatitis B or C

Recommended mushrooms:	Cordyceps sinensis, reishi, shiitake
Form/Dosage:	1,800 mg reishi three times daily; 1,000 mg shiitake three times daily
Duration:	Minimum of twelve weeks
Complementary supplements:	450–500 mg of black cumin seed oil (minimum 1.5% thymoquinone) three times daily; 200–300 mg of milk thistle (standardized to silymarin content) two to three times daily
Complementary essential oils:	Take a capsule filled with 2 drops each of sweet orange, helichrysum, and German chamomile, two to four times daily.

Herpes Simplex Virus Type 1

Recommended mushrooms:	Oyster
Form/Dosage:	300 mg oyster pleuran (Imunoglukan P4H ACUTE!) each morning on an empty stomach for 10 days, followed by 100 mg for 120 days
Duration:	Three to six months
Complementary supplements:	1,000 mg of monolaurin three times daily during outbreaks, 500–1,000 mg six days per week as a preventive; 1,000 mg of lysine three times daily on an empty stomach
Complementary essential oils:	Take a capsule filled with 1 drop each of melissa, thyme, peppermint, and sandalwood essential oil once or twice daily.

Human Papillomavirus (HPV) Infection

Recommended mushrooms:	Turkey tail, reishi, shiitake, cordyceps
Form/Dosage:	Papilocare or Palomacare vaginal gel as instructed on the product label; 1,000 mg of shiitake or cordyceps three times daily; or 400 mg of a combination of turkey tail and reishi daily; 3,000 mg shiitake supplement on an empty stomach daily
Duration:	Minimum of two months and up to twelve months
Complementary supplements:	220 mg zinc sulfate twice daily for three moths
Complementary essential oils:	Myrtle vaginal suppositories (0.5% essential oil, 10% aqueous extract)

Hypercholesterolemia (High Cholesterol)

Recommended mushrooms: King oyster, maitake, oyster

Form/Dosage: 1,000 mg oyster supplement, three times daily; mushroom complex as instructed on the product label

Duration: Minimum six weeks and up to 26 weeks

Complementary supplements: 1,200 mg of Armolipid Plus red yeast rice extract daily; 300–500 mg of berberine HCl two to three times daily

Complementary essential oils: Take a capsule filled with 2 drops each of lemongrass, lime, clove, and lemon, morning and evening.

Insomnia

Recommended mushrooms: Honey, lion's mane, poria, shiitake

Form/Dosage: 1,000 mg lion's mane supplement, three times daily; 1,000 mg shiitake supplement, three times daily before a meal; 500 mg poria up to three times daily; honey mushroom as part of a mushroom complex

Duration: Until sleep cycle regulates

Complementary supplements: 530–600 mg of valerian root twice daily; homeopathic Neurexan as directed on the product label

Complementary essential oils: Apply a combination of lavender, Virginia cedarwood, sandalwood, vetiver, marjoram, and valerian essential oils diluted to 5%–10% to the chest area

Kidney Disease

Recommended mushrooms: Cordyceps sinensis

Form/Dosage: 600–2,000 mg Cordyceps sinensis three times daily

Duration: As determined by a health-care professional

Complementary supplements: 600 mg of n-Acetyl cysteine three times daily

Complementary essential oils: Take a capsule filled with 2 drops of lemongrass essential oil twice daily.

Kidney Stones

Recommended mushrooms: Poria

Form/Dosage: 500 mg poria three times daily

Duration: Until stones are passed plus one week

Complementary supplements: 400–500 mg of Chanca Piedra three times daily thirty minutes prior to a meal

Complementary essential oils: Take 1 capsule filled with 4 drops each of lemon and orange, and 1 drop of juniper berry two to three times, daily.

Kidney Transplant Support

Recommended mushrooms: Cordyceps sinensis

Form/Dosage: 1,000–2,000 mg Cordyceps sinensis three times daily

Duration: As instructed by your health-care professional

Complementary supplements: n/a

Complementary essential oils: n/a

Leaky Gut

Recommended mushrooms: Poria, reishi

Form/Dosage: Mushroom complex as instructed on the product label; 500 mg poria up to three times daily; 1,000 mg reishi up to three times daily

Duration: 60 to 120 days

Complementary supplements: 5,000 mg of powdered L-glutamine on an empty stomach, once or twice daily; see *Heal the Gut, Heal the Immune System* for additional recommendations

Complementary essential oils: Take a capsule with 1 drop each of oregano, sweet orange, and ginger twice daily

Lupus (Systemic Lupus Erythematosus)

Recommended mushrooms: Cordyceps sinensis, psylocibin

Form/Dosage: 1–2.5 mg of psilocybin every three to four days, titrated up to 5 mg if necessary, for four to eight weeks, followed by a two-week rest, or 25 mg under the guidance of a health-care professional; 1,000–1,500 mg Cordyceps sinensis three times daily

Duration:	Until symptoms are regulated well and for an additional two months after
Complementary supplements:	600 mg of n-Acetyl cysteine three times daily; fish oil supplying 1,125 mg each of DHA and EPA twice daily; 100 mg of S-acetyl L-glutathione twice daily; 600 mg of white peony root (standardized to paeoniflorin) two to three times daily
Complementary essential oils:	Massage most of your body with 3 drops each of lemongrass, copaiba, marjoram, and frankincense mixed with 5 teaspoons of carrier oil, 3 times per week.

Metabolic Syndrome

Recommended mushrooms:	Chaga, king oyster, reishi
Form/Dosage:	Mushroom complex as instructed by the product label; 1,000 mg Chaga daily; 1,000 mg king oyster up to three times daily; 720–1,000 mg reishi two to three times daily
Duration:	Until metabolic markers are improved significantly
Complementary supplements:	500 mg berberine HCl two to three times daily; 1,000–1,500 mg bitter melon twice daily
Complementary essential oils:	Two drops of cumin essential oil in a capsule three times daily

Migraine

Recommended mushrooms:	Psilocybin
Form/Dosage:	1–2.5 mg of psilocybin every three to four days, titrated up to 5 mg if necessary, for four to eight weeks, followed by a two-week rest, or 10 mg under the guidance of a health-care professional as instructed
Duration:	Work closely with a health-care professional to determine
Complementary supplements:	380 mg feverfew extract daily; 75 mg butterbur (standardized to 15% petasins) twice daily
Complementary essential oils:	Create a roller bottle with 10 drops peppermint, 7 drops each of rosemary, hinoki, and lavender, 6

drops copaiba, and 3 drops German chamomile or blue tansy essential oils, fill the rest of the bottle with carrier oil, and roll onto the temples, back of the neck, and forehead as needed.

Neuropathic Pain (Neuropathy)

Recommended mushrooms: Psilocybin

Form/Dosage: 1–2.5 mg of psilocybin every three to four days, titrated up to 5 mg if necessary, for four to eight weeks, followed by a two-week rest, or a low dose as determined by an informed health-care professional

Duration: As determined by health-care professional

Complementary supplements: 100 mg stabilized R-Alpha lipoic acid two to three times daily; 1,000 mg acetyl-L-carnitine two to three times daily

Complementary essential oils: Dilute to 15%–25% and apply 1 to 2 drops each of frankincense, spruce, peppermint, vetiver, helichrysum, lavender, and eucalyptus to affected area, three to five times daily

Nonalcoholic Fatty Liver Disease

Recommended mushrooms: Cordyceps militaris, poria, stout camphor

Form/Dosage: 300 mg stout camphor one to two times daily; mushroom complex with the above as instructed on the product label

Duration: Minimum of 12 weeks

Complementary supplements: High-potency multistrain probiotic as instructed on the product label; 200–300 mg of milk thistle (standardized to silymarin content) daily; 500 mg of berberine HCl twice daily

Complementary essential oils: Take a capsule filled with 1 drop each of ginger, lemon, lime, and tangerine, three times daily

Obesity

Recommended mushrooms: Cordyceps militaris, maitake, psilocybin

Form/Dosage: 1–2.5 mg of psilocybin every three to four days, titrated up to 5 mg if necessary, for four to eight weeks, followed by a two-week rest, or 1.75–20

mg weekly under the guidance of a health-care professional; mushroom complex rich in beta-glucans as instructed on the product label

Duration: Until desired weight is reached

Complementary supplements: 5,000 mg calcium pyruvate powder twice daily; 1,000 mg L-carnitine twice daily

Complementary essential oils: Take a capsule filled with 3 drops of grapefruit, and 1 drop each of orange and lemongrass, two to three times daily.

Obsessive-Compulsive Disorder

Recommended mushrooms: Psilocybin

Form/Dosage: 1–2.5 mg of psilocybin every three to four days, titrated up to 5 mg if necessary, for four to eight weeks, followed by a two-week rest, or 1.75–20 mg weekly under the guidance of a health-care professional

Duration: As determined by symptoms

Complementary supplements: 600 mg n-Acetyl cysteine three times daily (titrated up to five times daily over six weeks to reach the most effective dose of 3,000 mg/day); 1,000 mg sarcosine one to two times daily

Complementary essential oils: Dilute to 25% and apply 1 drop of lavender on each big toe and the bottoms of the feet, two to four times daily, particularly before going to bed.

Osteoarthritis

Recommended mushrooms: Mesima

Form/Dosage: 750 mg mesima twice daily

Duration: Minimum of eight weeks and for as long as symptoms persist

Complementary supplements: Combination of glucosamine, chondroitin, MSM supplement as instructed on the product label; Boswellia extract as instructed on the product label; 6 mg calcium fructoborate daily

Complementary essential oils: Dilute to 5%–10% and apply 1 to 2 drops each of balsam fir, peppermint, cypress, and wintergreen on affected area, two to three times daily.

Parkinson's Disease

Recommended mushrooms: Almond, lion's mane, reishi

Form/Dosage: Mushroom complex containing the above as instructed on the product label

Duration: As long as needed to manage symptoms and disease progression

Complementary supplements: Mucuna pruriens as directed on the supplement label (a clinical study used doses supplying 500 or 1,000 mg L-DOPA once weekly; but this is not recommended unless doing so under the care of health professional); 20 mg PQQ daily

Complementary essential oils: Take a capsule with two drops each of geranium and black pepper, and one drop of clove twice daily

Physical Performance or Endurance

Recommended mushrooms: Cordyceps militaris, reishi

Form/Dosage: 3,000 mg reishi dissolved in warm water twice daily; 1,000 mg reishi three times daily; 1,300 mg cordyceps three times daily

Duration: Six to twelve weeks

Complementary supplements: 3,000 mg L-arginine daily; 500 mg rhodiola three times daily; beet root supplement at least two hours prior to physical exertion

Complementary essential oils: Add 1 drop of peppermint essential oil to 16 ounces of water and consume; apply a 5% dilution of spearmint and peppermint essential oil to the chest prior to physical exertion

Postprandial (After-Meal) Blood Sugar Control

Recommended mushrooms: Oyster

Form/Dosage: 1,000 mg oyster supplement before each meal

Duration: Until blood glucose regulates

Complementary supplements: 250–500 mg of mulberry leaf extract (providing a minimum of 7.5 mg of DNJ) before your two largest meals of the day; 500 mg of berberine HCl twice daily

Complementary essential oils: 1 drop of cinnamon bark essential oil in a capsule before a meal

Posttraumatic Stress Disorder (PTSD)

Recommended mushrooms: Psylocibin,

Form/Dosage: 1–2.5 mg of psilocybin every three to four days, titrated up to 5 mg if necessary, for four to eight weeks, followed by a two-week rest, or up to three 10–25 mg doses weeks to months apart under the guidance of a health-care professional as instructed

Duration: Until stabilized

Complementary supplements: 500 mg rhodiola (standardized to 5% rosavins) with breakfast; 200–300 mg phosphatidylserine at bedtime; high-quality multistrain probiotic with evening meal

Complementary essential oils: Inhale sweet orange essential oil as needed throughout the day

Recurrent Respiratory Tract Infections (Children Aged 1 to 12)

Recommended mushrooms: Oyster

Form/Dosage: 1 mL/5 kg body weight of Imunoglukan P4HW syrup each morning on an empty stomach

Duration: Up to six months

Complementary supplements: 1,000–2,000 IU vitamin D daily; elderberry (Sambucol) as instructed on the product label

Complementary essential oils: Diffuse lemon and frankincense essential oil while sleeping

Rheumatoid Arthritis

Recommended mushrooms: Mesima, reishi

Form/Dosage: Mushroom complex as instructed on the product label; 500–1,100 mg mesima up to three times daily; 1,000 mg reishi up to three times daily

Duration: While symptoms persists and for one to two months after resolution of symptoms

Complementary supplements: 500 mg turmeric two to four times daily; Boswellia extract as instructed on the product label; 1,000 mg cat's claw two to three times daily

Complementary essential oils: Oral—Take 1 capsule filled with 3 drops each of frankincense, balsam fir, and copaiba essential oil two times daily.

Sleep Disturbance

See Insomnia

Traumatic Brain Injury (TBI)

Recommended mushrooms:	Cordyceps militaris, Cordyceps sinensis, psylocibin
Form/Dosage:	Mushroom complex as instructed on the product label;
Duration:	Works best immediately following injury and for the next four to six weeks; take mushrooms daily for long-term TBI
Complementary supplements:	2,000 mg n-Acetyl cysteine immediately following injury, 2,000 mg 4 hours later, then 1,000 mg daily; 1,000 mg taurine one to two times daily; 800 mg of wild green oat extract daily for 2 weeks
Complementary essential oils:	Take a capsule filled with 1 drop each of Spanish sage, turmeric, rosemary, and lavender, three times daily

Viral Infection

Recommended mushrooms:	Enoki, king oyster, mesima, reishi, shiitake, turkey tail
Form/Dosage:	Mushroom complex rich in beta-glucans as instructed on the product label; 200–350 mg reishi beta-glucans daily before breakfast; 500 mg mesima twice daily; 1,000 mg shiitake or turkey tail three times daily
Duration:	While symptoms persist and for three to five days after resolution of symptoms
Complementary supplements:	30 mg chelated zinc three times daily; 1,000 mg of vitamin C plus 100–250 mg bioflavonoids and 100–250 mg of quercetin three to five times daily; 600 mg n-Acetyl cysteine two to three times daily
Complementary essential oils:	Take a capsule filled with 1 drop each of oregano, lemon, clove, geranium, cinnamon, and lemongrass two to three times daily

Wound Healing

Recommended mushrooms: Enoki, white jelly

Form/Dosage: Topically as part of a cream, gel, or poultice

Duration: Until wound heals, plus three to five days after

Complementary supplements: n/a

Complementary essential oils: Dilute to 5% and apply helichrysum, frankincense, lavender, tea tree to the wound two to three times daily

Mushroom foraging is not only a hobby but a means to collect valuable natural remedies. That being said, it is crucial to learn which mushrooms are safe to eat because the downside to mushroom foraging is that if it goes wrong, it could be deadly. The following is meant to provide tips to help you as you search for wild mushrooms.

Leverage apps, books, communities, and videos. Some apps, like Mushroom Identificator and Picture Mushroom – Mushrooms ID, allow you to snap a photo of the mushroom to help identify the species. Other apps require you to enter features and characteristics to identify the mushroom. If apps aren't your thing, purchase a book on mushroom foraging and take it with you. A key way to expand your mushroom knowledge is to connect with experts in a community. Look for local, regional, or national groups on social media to build your mushroom foraging community. Lastly, you can find mushroom identification videos on video services like YouTube.

Know your local laws. Each park and forest has different laws regarding foraging. May American parks advise visitors to limit the collection of edibles, like mushrooms and berries, to what you will consume during your visit.

Forage after heavy rain. As fungi, mushrooms thrive in moist, damp, and humid conditions. The best time to find these conditions in the woods is after heavy rain, which triggers rapid mushroom growth.

Learn the best places to find mushrooms. Forests and wooded areas are vast, making finding mushrooms difficult. Look under downed logs or around tree stumps. Check around tree roots. Burned areas of forests or fields are frequent habitats of mushrooms. Some mushrooms prefer loamy soil—a mixture of sand, clay, and organic matter. Examine areas along streams or creeks, which provide a moist environment for mushrooms to grow.

Become familiar with dangerous and poisonous mushrooms. Learn how to identify inedible, poisonous, and toxic mushrooms. Some of the most common poisonous mushrooms found in the wild are: 1) death caps (*Amanita phalloides*), which have a round cap that ranges from green to yellow and is held up by a thin, white stalk; 2) fly agaric (*Amanita muscaria*), identifiable by their striking white-spotted, usually red cap; 3) destroying angel (*Amanita bisporigera*), which have a narrow stem and sold white cap that somewhat resembles an egg with gills under the cap; and 4) false parasol

(*Chlorophyllum molybdites*), characterized by a large, whitish to light brown, funnel-shaped cap and coarse brownish scales.

Cut, don't pull up. Pulling up mushroom roots stops them from regrowing. Instead, cut the mushrooms so they can grow back in the future.

Take only what you need. The sustainability of mushrooms for future generations to enjoy requires constraint. Only harvest what you are going to eat or use medicinally and avoid overharvesting.

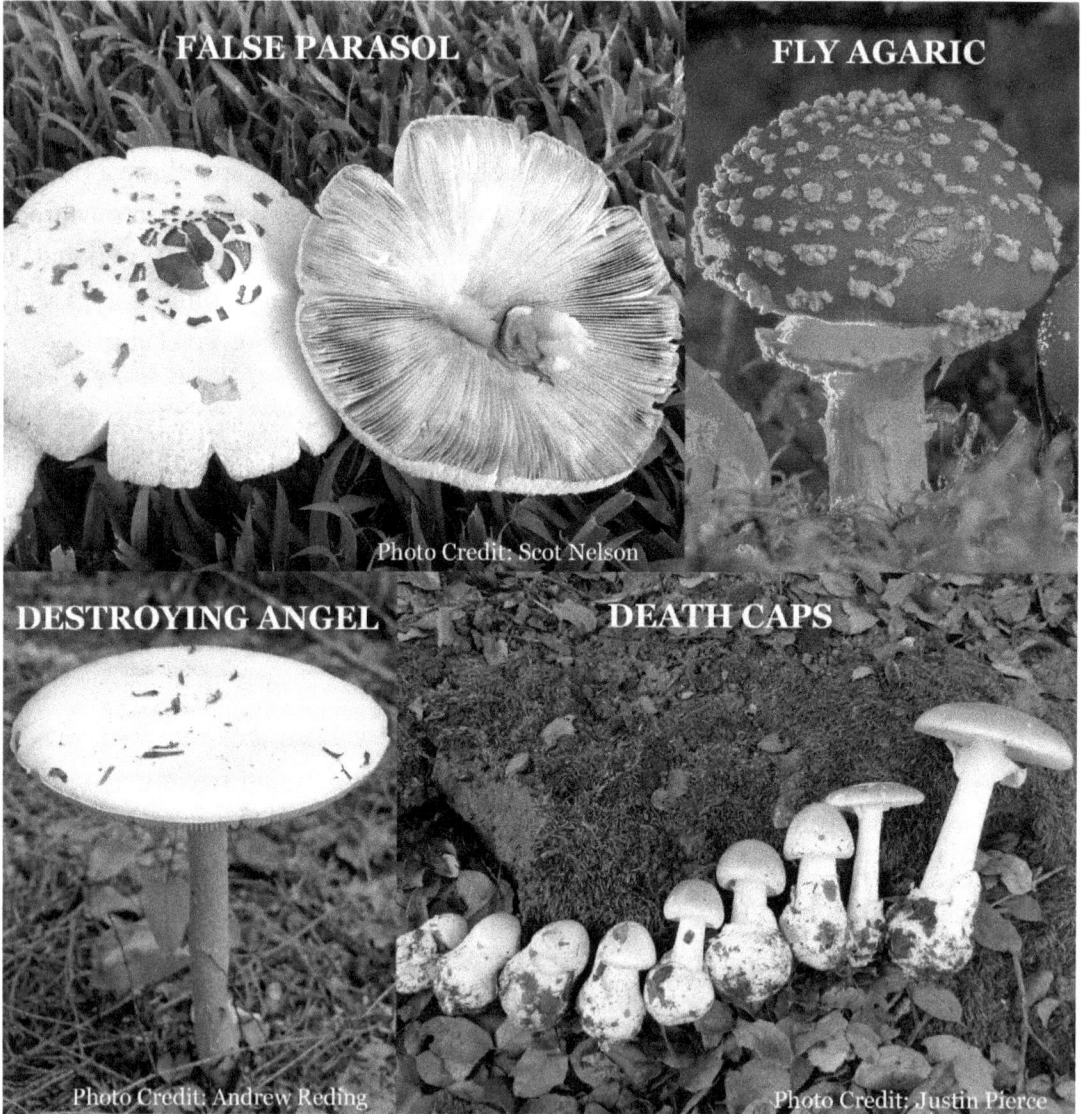
FALSE PARASOL
FLY AGARIC
Photo Credit: Scot Nelson
DESTROYING ANGEL
DEATH CAPS
Photo Credit: Andrew Reding
Photo Credit: Justin Pierce

Identification of the medicinal mushrooms in this book:

Agarikon. Agarikon mushrooms can be very large and hang like a fruit on a tree trunk where branches connect to the trunks. They are typically found growing high in trees.

The exterior resembles a beehive with chunky pale white flesh. The mushroom is soft and has a chalky consistency.

Almond. Growing in rich, humusy soil and compost, the almond mushroom starts out bell shaped. They are brownish to reddish-brown and occasionally buff or tan (especially when young). The top of the cap is covered in very fine silk-like fibers. The cap flattens out as they age with the edges rolling under a little bit. The cap top also shifts to a scaly appearance with brownish fiber tufts arranged in an outward radiating concentric pattern as it ages. Some people say it looks like snakeskin. The cap averages two to seven inches wide and is stained yellowish-brown with age. The gills start out white, then turn pinkish, followed finally by dark black-brown. They are covered in a white scaly fibrous veil when young that splits during aging to produce a cottony material. The stem is whitish or buff colored, smooth and thick with a bulbous base and averages from two to six inches long. The spore print is dark purplish-brown.

Chaga. Chaga mushrooms grow larger and develop a hardened, black outer layer that feels rough as they age. The outside is characterized by deep crevices and ridges and may appear cracked. When cut open, chaga mushrooms have a yellow-golden color and resemble a mass of fibrous tissue. Remarkably, these mushrooms are from five to twenty years old when ready to be harvested for medicinal purposes. A sign of a chaga that has lost its medicinal value because it is overly aged is brittleness and gray or white masses.

Cordyceps. The rarest and most expensive cordyceps species is *Cordyceps sinensis*, which grow between one and a half to four inches tall and has a yellowish-orange color—most are tan, brown, or black—that changes to brown or black when dry. They are long and slender and have a club-like appearance at the end instead of a cap. It should be noted that since these mushrooms grow on and take over a host's body, they can be more unique and reminiscent of their host. *Cordyceps militaris* mushrooms grow from just under an inch to over three inches and are also long and slender with a club-shaped end (the top is wider than the base). The upper portion is orange and pimply, while the lower portion is smooth and orange to pale orange.

Enoki. Enoki mushrooms have convex caps ranging from about half inch to nearly three inches wide. They are sticky and moist when fresh. The color varies from dark orange-brown to yellowish-brown that tends to fade during age. The gills are whitish to pale yellow and broadly or narrowly attached to the stem. The stem is about three-quarters of an inch to just over four inches and roughly one to four inches wide. The spore print is white.

Honey. Honey mushrooms have a cap that varies in color, often approximating the color of honey, hence their name. The cap measures from one to six inches in diameter, frequently appearing slimy when moist. The stem is normally two to six inches long with a distinctive white ring or skirt near the top. The white to pale yellow gills are attached to the stem.

King oyster. The largest of the Pleurotus species, king oyster mushrooms have a convex cap that is from one to five inches that flattens out as it ages. At full maturity, the cap margins roll inwards giving it a characteristic oyster look. The stem is white and thick, measuring from one to four inches. The gills are thin and distant from each other.

Lion's mane. Distinguished by their icicle-like clumps of teeth—spine-like structures that can be up to two inches long—hanging from a central stalk, lion's mane mushrooms are easily identifiable. This distinctive feature looks like a shaggy, white lion's mane, hence their name. They are roughly the size of a dinner plate. Another distinguishing feature is their unmistakable mild seafood aroma.

Maitake. Maitake mushrooms grow in densely clustered rosettes that spring from a single stem. The entire mushroom is normally six to twelve inches across and four to twelve inches high. The caps (fronds) are pale gray to brown with concentric zones of coloring. Aged mushrooms turn more yellowish and unattractive. The frond tops are frequently finely velvety with tiny hairs, but can also be bald and smooth. Each individual frond is normally one to six inches wide and shaped like a fan with wavy edges. The pores are light gray, turning to white, and smooth. Maitake mushrooms have no gills. The interior flesh is white and firm. The spore print is white.

Mesima. Mesima mushrooms have a hoof-shaped, asymmetrical, usually dark brown cap that turns black as it dries. The pore surface is pale reddish- or yellowish-brown when fresh and brown when dried. The body of the mushroom grows on a tree trunk in a shelf-like manner.

Oyster. The cap of the oyster mushroom is light brown to brownish. Measuring about two to ten inches across, the cap usually contains overlapping clusters that give it an oyster-like appearance. The gills running down the stem are whitish to gray unless they are older, which makes them yellowish or brown. The stem is very short, maybe even absent, whitish and fuzzy or hairy. Oyster mushrooms have white, yellowish, or lilac spore print.

Pink oyster. Pink oyster mushrooms have a unique vibrant pinkish-orange colored caps that makes them easily identifiable. The caps are fan/oyster-shaped that are arranged in overlapping layers. The most intense pink color is found at the cap folds that meet the underside. Wild pink oyster mushrooms tend to be paler than cultivated varieties that may appear beige more than pink. Each cap is attached to a short, thick central stem that varies in color from white to brownish. The underside contains closely spaced pale pink gills that extend from the stem to the edge of the cap and are typically thin and wavy in shape. Pink oyster mushroom spores are small and elliptical, ranging in color from beige to light brown.

Poria. Colored from pale red to white to light brown, the sclerotium of poria mushrooms is up to twelve inches long. These mushrooms can weigh over two pounds, grow underground, and somewhat resemble a large potato in shape.

Psilocybe. Given the dozens of species of psilocybe mushrooms, it is best to rely on a field guide or app to identify them. However, they can often be recognized by their color, shape, and stem bruising, which is bluish in color.

Reishi. Reishi mushrooms have kidney or fan-shaped caps that appear reddish when wet. Their shiny, lacquered red-brown appearance is one of their primary identifying features. Young reishi mushrooms haven't developed their fan-shaped appearance and instead have knobs or ladles with long handles. Their shape at maturity is largely dependent on where they grow. Reishi growing on the side of a tree grows outward horizontally; whereas those fruiting on logs frequently develop stems that arch so they can grow horizontally. Reishi caps can be larger than a foot across and an inch or two thick. Their spore print is brown.

Shiitake. Shiitake mushrooms have a cap that measures from two to six inches and is usually convex (though sometimes it presents as flat) and light to dark brown, gradually darkening toward the center. The cap's edge rolls down and inward. The gills are whitish to cream-colored. Younger mushrooms have smooth caps that start to crack with age, exposing white flesh. The stem is relatively thin and ranges from one to three inches in height. It is white or cream at first, but turns brown as it ages. Shiitake mushrooms bruise brown when damaged.

Stout camphor. Growing exclusively on decaying wood, stout camphor mushrooms have a distinctive orange-red exterior. It appears as a fuzzy, irregular shaped fungus.

Turkey tail. Turkey tail mushrooms have distinct, starkly contrasting concentric color zones on the cap that resemble the feathers of a turkey's tail. One of the distinguishing features of turkey tail mushrooms are the pores on its underside that are very small. This feature helps differentiate it from false turkey tail mushrooms (*Stereum ostrea*, *Stereum hirstum*, and *Trichaptum abietinum*), which have a smooth underside. The surface of turkey tail mushrooms should feel velvety or fuzzy. They are also thin and flexible until they age, where they become hard and rigid.

White jelly. A parasitic yeast, white jelly mushrooms start growing as a jelly blob until it merges with a specific wood-decomposing fungus, most commonly *Annulohypoxylon archeri.* This merger allows the jelly to turn into a translucent whitish-yellowish jellyfish-like mushroom. As the mushroom transforms, it forms ear-shaped leaflets that are frilly looking,

Wood ear. Without an official cap, wood ear mushroom fruiting bodies are thin, irregular, ear-shaped lobes that are rubbery and gelatinous. They are reddish-brown in color with one side—generally the upper—being smooth and the other side covered in very fine hairs that appear whitish but are actually grayish to brown. The individual lobes grow low to the wood, reaching widths of one to four inches across. They can also appear translucent, depending on maturity. These mushrooms have no gills or stem, so the fruiting body is attached to the substrate directly. Wood ear spore prints are white.

Foraging for mushrooms is challenging but rewarding. With practice and consistency, you'll get the hang of it, and with some luck, you may score the medicinal mushroom you need for your health. Be on the lookout for look-alike mushrooms, especially those that could be harmful. Ultimately, you reconnect with nature as you search for edible and medicinal mushrooms that could potentially benefit your health further.

REFERENCES

[1] Stamets P. Can mushrooms help save the world? Interview by Bonnie J. Horrigan. *Explore (NY)*. 2006 Mar;2(2):152-61.

[2] Altannavch N, Zhou X, Khan MA, et al. Anti-oxidant and Anticancerous Effect of Fomitopsis officinalis (Vill. ex Fr. Bond. et Sing) Mushroom on Hepatocellular Carcinoma Cells In Vitro through NF-kB Pathway. *Anticancer Agents Med Chem.* 2022;22(8):1561-1570.

[3] Vedenicheva NP, Al-Maali GA, Bisko NA, et al. Effect of Cytokinin-Containing Extracts from Some Medicinal Mushroom Mycelia on HepG2 Cells In Vitro. *Int J Med Mushrooms*. 2021;23(3):15-28.

[4] Wu HT, Lu FH, Su YC, et al. In vivo and in vitro anti-tumor effects of fungal extracts. *Molecules*. 2014 Feb 21;19(2):2546-56.

[5] Fijałkowska A, Muszyńska B, Sułkowska-Ziaja K, et al. Medicinal potential of mycelium and fruiting bodies of an arboreal mushroom Fomitopsis officinalis in therapy of lifestyle diseases. *Sci Rep*. 2020 Nov 18;10(1):20081.

[6] Wu HT, Lu FH, Su YC, et al. In vivo and in vitro anti-tumor effects of fungal extracts. *Molecules*. 2014 Feb 21;19(2):2546-56.

[7] Wu HT, Lu FH, Su YC, et al. In vivo and in vitro anti-tumor effects of fungal extracts. *Molecules*. 2014 Feb 21;19(2):2546-56.

[8] Garmanchuk LV, Vedenicheva NP, Al-Maali GA, et al. ANTIPROLIFERATIVE ACTIVITIES Of EXTRACTS FROM MYCELIAL BIOMASS OF SOME MEDICINAL BASIDIOMYCETES IN HUMAN COLON CANCER CELLS COLO 205. *Exp Oncol*. 2022 Nov;44(3):213-216.

[9] Wu HT, Lu FH, Su YC, et al. In vivo and in vitro anti-tumor effects of fungal extracts. *Molecules*. 2014 Feb 21;19(2):2546-56.

[10] Golovchenko VV, Naranmandakh S, Ganbaatar J, et al. Structural investigation and comparative cytotoxic activity of water-soluble polysaccharides from fruit bodies of the medicinal fungus quinine conk. *Phytochemistry*. 2020 Jul;175:112313.

[11] Shi ZT, Bao HY, Feng S. [Antitumor activity and structure-activity relationship of seven lanostane-type triterpenes from Fomitopsis pinicola and F. officinalis]. *Zhongguo Zhong Yao Za Zhi*. 2017 Mar;42(5):915-922.

[12] Wu HT, Lu FH, Su YC, et al. In vivo and in vitro anti-tumor effects of fungal extracts. *Molecules*. 2014 Feb 21;19(2):2546-56.

[13] Vazirian M, Faridfar S, Eftekhari M. "Gharikon"/"Agharikon" a Valuable Medicinal Mushroom in Iranian Traditional Medicine. *Iran J Med Sci*. 2016 May;41(3 Suppl):S34.

[14] Muszyńska B, Fijałkowska A, Sułkowska-Ziaja K, et al. Fomitopsis officinalis: a Species of Arboreal Mushroom with Promising Biological and Medicinal Properties. *Chem Biodivers*. 2020 Jun;17(6):e2000213.

[15] Vazirian M, Faridfar S, Eftekhari M. "Gharikon"/"Agharikon" a Valuable Medicinal Mushroom in Iranian Traditional Medicine. *Iran J Med Sci*. 2016 May;41(3 Suppl):S34.

[16] Teplyakova TV, Psurtseva NV, Kosogova TA, et al. Antiviral activity of polyporoid mushrooms (higher Basidiomycetes) from Altai Mountains (Russia). *Int J Med Mushrooms*. 2012;14(1):37-45.

[17] Vazirian M, Faridfar S, Eftekhari M. "Gharikon"/"Agharikon" a Valuable Medicinal Mushroom in Iranian Traditional Medicine. *Iran J Med Sci*. 2016 May;41(3 Suppl):S34.

[18] Girometta C. Antimicrobial properties of Fomitopsis officinalis in the light of its bioactive metabolites: a review. *Mycology*. 2018 Oct 25;10(1):32-39.

[19] Flores GA, Cusumano G, Ianni F, et al. Fomitopsis officinalis: Spatial (Pileus and Hymenophore) Metabolomic Variations Affect Functional Components and Biological Activities. *Antibiotics (Basel)*. 2023 Apr 16;12(4):766.

[20] Sidorenko ML, Buzoleva LS. [Search for new types of raw materials for antibacterial drugs]. *Antibiot Khimioter*. 2012;57(5-6):7-10.

[21] Vazirian M, Faridfar S, Eftekhari M. "Gharikon"/"Agharikon" a Valuable Medicinal Mushroom in Iranian Traditional Medicine. *Iran J Med Sci*. 2016 May;41(3 Suppl):S34.

[22] Vazirian M, Faridfar S, Eftekhari M. "Gharikon"/"Agharikon" a Valuable Medicinal Mushroom in Iranian Traditional Medicine. *Iran J Med Sci*. 2016 May;41(3 Suppl):S34.

[23] Hwang CH, Jaki BU, Klein LL, et al. Chlorinated coumarins from the polypore mushroom Fomitopsis officinalis and their activity against Mycobacterium tuberculosis. *J Nat Prod*. 2013 Oct 25;76(10):1916-22.

[24] Vazirian M, Faridfar S, Eftekhari M. "Gharikon"/"Agharikon" a Valuable Medicinal Mushroom in Iranian Traditional Medicine. *Iran J Med Sci*. 2016 May;41(3 Suppl):S34.

[25] Naranmandakh S, Murata T, Odonbayar B, et al. Lanostane triterpenoids from Fomitopsis officinalis and their trypanocidal activity. *J Nat Med*. 2018 Mar;72(2):523-529.

[26] Altannavch N, Zhou X, Khan MA, et al. Anti-oxidant and Anticancerous Effect of Fomitopsis officinalis (Vill. ex Fr. Bond. et Sing) Mushroom on Hepatocellular Carcinoma Cells In Vitro through NF-kB Pathway. *Anticancer Agents Med Chem.* 2022;22(8):1561-1570.

[27] Fijałkowska A, Muszyńska B, Sułkowska-Ziaja K, et al. Medicinal potential of mycelium and fruiting bodies of an arboreal mushroom Fomitopsis officinalis in therapy of lifestyle diseases. *Sci Rep*. 2020 Nov 18;10(1):20081.

[28] Bertéli MB, Lopes AD, Colla IM, et al. Agaricus subrufescens: substratum nitrogen concentration and mycelial extraction method on antitumor activity. *An Acad Bras Cienc*. 2016 Oct-Dec;88(4):2239-2246.

[29] Wen C, Geervliet M, de Vries H, et al. Agaricus subrufescens fermented rye affects the development of intestinal microbiota, local intestinal and innate immunity in suckling-to-nursery pigs. *Anim Microbiome*. 2023 Apr 11;5(1):24.

[30] Wen C, Geervliet M, de Vries H, et al. Agaricus subrufescens fermented rye affects the development of intestinal microbiota, local intestinal and innate immunity in suckling-to-nursery pigs. *Anim Microbiome*. 2023 Apr 11;5(1):24.

[31] de Groot N, Fariñas F, Fabà L, et al. Fermented rye with Agaricus subrufescens and mannan-rich hydrolysate based feed additive to modulate post-weaning piglet immune response. *Porcine Health Manag*. 2021 Dec 9;7(1):60.

[32] da Costa MC, Regina M, et al. Photoprotective and Antimutagenic Activity of Agaricus subrufescens Basidiocarp Extracts. *Curr Microbiol*. 2015 Oct;71(4):476-82.

[33] da Costa MC, Regina M, et al. Photoprotective and Antimutagenic Activity of Agaricus subrufescens Basidiocarp Extracts. *Curr Microbiol*. 2015 Oct;71(4):476-82.

[34] Sousa FTG, Biering SB, Patel TS, et al. Sulfated β-glucan from Agaricus subrufescens inhibits flavivirus infection and nonstructural protein 1-mediated pathogenesis. *Antiviral Res*. 2022 Jul;203:105330.

[35] Merel D, Savoie JM, Mata G, et al. Methanolic Extracts from Cultivated Mushrooms Affect the Production of Fumonisins B and Fusaric Acid by Fusarium verticillioides. *Toxins (Basel)*. 2020 Jun 2;12(6):366.

[36] Sun Y, Cheng M, Dong L, et al. Agaricus blazei extract (FA-2-b-β) induces apoptosis in chronic myeloid leukemia cells. *Oncol Lett*. 2020 Nov;20(5):270.

[37] Kim MO, Moon DO, Jung JM, et al. Agaricus blazei Extract Induces Apoptosis through ROS-Dependent JNK Activation Involving the Mitochondrial Pathway and Suppression of Constitutive NF-κB in THP-1 Cells. *Evid Based Complement Alternat Med*. 2011;2011:838172.

[38] Ogasawara A, Doi H, Matsui T, et al. Agaritine derived from Agaricus blazei Murrill induces apoptosis via mitochondrial membrane depolarization in hematological tumor cell lines. *Fujita Med J*. 2023 May;9(2):147-153.

[39] Kim CF, Jiang JJ, Leung KN, et al. Inhibitory effects of Agaricus blazei extracts on human myeloid leukemia cells. *J Ethnopharmacol*. 2009 Mar 18;122(2):320-6.

[40] Akiyama H, Endo M, Matsui T, et al. Agaritine from Agaricus blazei Murrill induces apoptosis in the leukemic cell line U937. *Biochim Biophys Acta*. 2011 May;1810(5):519-25.

[41] Endo M, Beppu H, Akiyama H, et al. Agaritine purified from Agaricus blazei Murrill exerts anti-tumor activity against leukemic cells. *Biochim Biophys Acta*. 2010 Jul;1800(7):669-73.

[42] Cheng MX, Yu SR, Wang ZD, et al. [Inhibitory Effects of Agaricus Blazei Murrill (FA-2-b-β) on Proliferation of Chronic Myeloid Leukemia Cells in vivo and Its Mechanism]. *Zhongguo Shi Yan Xue Ye Xue Za Zhi*. 2020 Dec;28(6):1885-1891.

[43] Feng WW, Bai Y, Wang DP, et al. [Study on the Mechanism of Multi-Drug Resistance of Agaricus Blazei Extract FA-2-b-β Mediated Wnt Signaling Pathway to Reverse Acute T Lymphoblastic Leukemia]. *Zhongguo Shi Yan Xue Ye Xue Za Zhi*. 2023 Jun;31(3):621-627.

[44] Li X, Zhao X, Wang H, et al. A polysaccharide from the fruiting bodies of Agaricus blazei Murill induces caspase-dependent apoptosis in human leukemia HL-60 cells. *Tumour Biol*. 2014 Sep;35(9):8963-8.

[45] Jin CY, Moon DO, Choi YH, et al. Bcl-2 and caspase-3 are major regulators in Agaricus blazei-induced human leukemic U937 cell apoptosis through dephoshorylation of Akt. *Biol Pharm Bull*. 2007 Aug;30(8):1432-7.

[46] Gao L, Sun Y, Chen C, et al. Primary mechanism of apoptosis induction in a leukemia cell line by fraction FA-2-b-ss prepared from the mushroom Agaricus blazei Murill. *Braz J Med Biol Res*. 2007 Nov;40(11):1545-55.

[47] Tangen JM, Holien T, Mirlashari MR, et al. Cytotoxic Effect on Human Myeloma Cells and Leukemic Cells by the Agaricus blazei Murill Based Mushroom Extract, Andosan™. *Biomed Res Int*. 2017;2017:2059825.

[48] Yu CH, Kan SF, Shu CH, et al. Inhibitory mechanisms of Agaricus blazei Murill on the growth of prostate cancer in vitro and in vivo. *J Nutr Biochem*. 2009 Oct;20(10):753-64.

[49] Matsushita Y, Furutani Y, Matsuoka R, et al. Hot water extract of Agaricus blazei Murrill specifically inhibits growth and induces apoptosis in human pancreatic cancer cells. *BMC Complement Altern Med*. 2018 Dec 4;18(1):319.

[50] Tung YC, Su ZY, Kuo ML, et al. Ethanolic Extract of Agaricus blazei Fermentation Product Inhibits the Growth and Invasion of Human Hepatoma HA22T/VGH and SK-Hep-1 Cells. *J Tradit Complement Med*. 2012 Apr;2(2):145-53.

[51] Su ZY, Tung YC, Hwang LS, et al. Blazeispirol A from Agaricus blazei fermentation product induces cell death in human hepatoma Hep 3B cells through caspase-dependent and caspase-independent pathways. *J Agric Food Chem*. 2011 May 11;59(9):5109-16.

[52] Yeh MY, Shang HS, Lu HF, et al. Chitosan oligosaccharides in combination with Agaricus blazei Murill extract reduces hepatoma formation in mice with severe combined immunodeficiency. *Mol Med Rep*. 2015 Jul;12(1):133-40.

[53] Niu YC, Liu JC, Zhao XM, et al. A low molecular weight polysaccharide isolated from Agaricus blazei Murill (LMPAB) exhibits its anti-metastatic effect by down-regulating metalloproteinase-9 and up-regulating Nm23-H1. *Am J Chin Med*. 2009;37(5):909-21.

[54] Wu MF, Lu HF, Hsu YM, et al. Possible reduction of hepatoma formation by Smmu 7721 cells in SCID mice and metastasis formation by B16F10 melanoma cells in C57BL/6 mice by Agaricus blazei murill extract. *In Vivo*. 2011 May-Jun;25(3):399-404.

[55] da Silva AF, Sartori D, Macedo FC Jr, et al. Effects of β-glucan extracted from Agaricus blazei on the expression of ERCC5, CASP9, and CYP1A1 genes and metabolic profile in HepG2 cells. *Hum Exp Toxicol*. 2013 Jun;32(6):647-54.

[56] Pinheiro F, Faria RR, de Camargo JL, et al. Chemoprevention of preneoplastic liver foci development by dietary mushroom Agaricus blazei Murrill in the rat. *Food Chem Toxicol*. 2003 Nov;41(11):1543-50.

[57] Wu B, Cui J, Zhang C, Li Z. A polysaccharide from Agaricus blazei inhibits proliferation and promotes apoptosis of osteosarcoma cells. *Int J Biol Macromol*. 2012 May 1;50(4):1116-20.

[58] Kobayashi H, Yoshida R, Kanada Y, et al. Suppressing effects of daily oral supplementation of beta-glucan extracted from Agaricus blazei Murill on spontaneous and peritoneal disseminated metastasis in mouse model. *J Cancer Res Clin Oncol*. 2005 Aug;131(8):527-38.

[59] Shimizu T, Kawai J, Ouchi K, et al. Agarol, an ergosterol derivative from Agaricus blazei, induces caspase-independent apoptosis in human cancer cells. *Int J Oncol*. 2016 Apr;48(4):1670-8.

[60] Itoh H, Ito H, Hibasami H. Blazein of a new steroid isolated from Agaricus blazei Murrill (himematsutake) induces cell death and morphological change indicative of apoptotic chromatin condensation in human lung cancer LU99 and stomach cancer KATO III cells. *Oncol Rep*. 2008 Dec;20(6):1359-61.

[61] Kimura Y, Kido T, Takaku T, et al. Isolation of an anti-angiogenic substance from Agaricus blazei Murill: its antitumor and antimetastatic actions. *Cancer Sci*. 2004 Sep;95(9):758-64.

[62] Wu MF, Chen YL, Lee MH, et al. Effect of Agaricus blazei Murrill extract on HT-29 human colon cancer cells in SCID mice in vivo. *In Vivo*. 2011 Jul-Aug;25(4):673-7.

[63] Shimizu T, Kawai J, Ouchi K, et al. Agarol, an ergosterol derivative from Agaricus blazei, induces caspase-independent apoptosis in human cancer cells. *Int J Oncol*. 2016 Apr;48(4):1670-8.

194

[64] Jin CY, Choi YH, Moon DO, et al. Induction of G2/M arrest and apoptosis in human gastric epithelial AGS cells by aqueous extract of Agaricus blazei. *Oncol Rep*. 2006 Dec;16(6):1349-55.

[65] Hetland G, Eide DM, Tangen JM, et al. The Agaricus blazei-Based Mushroom Extract, Andosan™, Protects against Intestinal Tumorigenesis in the A/J Min/+ Mouse. *PLoS One*. 2016 Dec 21;11(12):e0167754.

[66] Ishii PL, Prado CK, Mauro Mde O, et al. Evaluation of Agaricus blazei in vivo for antigenotoxic, anticarcinogenic, phagocytic and immunomodulatory activities. *Regul Toxicol Pharmacol*. 2011 Apr;59(3):412-22.

[67] Ziliotto L, Pinheiro F, Barbisan LF, et al. Screening for in vitro and in vivo antitumor activities of the mushroom Agaricus blazei. *Nutr Cancer*. 2009;61(2):245-50.

[68] Ziliotto L, Barbisan LF, Rodrigues MA. Lack of chemoprevention of dietary Agaricus blazei against rat colonic aberrant crypt foci. *Hum Exp Toxicol*. 2008 Jun;27(6):505-11.

[69] Lee JS, Hong EK. Agaricus blazei Murill enhances doxorubicin-induced apoptosis in human hepatocellular carcinoma cells by NFκB-mediated increase of intracellular doxorubicin accumulation. *Int J Oncol*. 2011 Feb;38(2):401-8

[70] Delmanto RD, de Lima PL, Sugui MM, et al. Antimutagenic effect of Agaricus blazei Murrill mushroom on the genotoxicity induced by cyclophosphamide. *Mutat Res*. 2001 Sep 20;496(1-2):15-21.

[71] Bertéli MB, Umeo SH, Bertéli A, et al. Mycelial antineoplastic activity of Agaricus blazei. *World J Microbiol Biotechnol*. 2014 Aug;30(8):2307-13.

[72] Kobayashi H, Masumoto J. Endotoxin contamination of Agaricus blazei Murrill extract enhances murine immunologic responses and inhibits the growth of sarcoma 180 implants in vivo. *J Environ Pathol Toxicol Oncol*. 2010;29(2):159-68.

[73] Mizuno M, Minato K, Ito H, et al. Anti-tumor polysaccharide from the mycelium of liquid-cultured Agaricus blazei mill. *Biochem Mol Biol Int*. 1999 Apr;47(4):707-14.

[74] Lee YL, Kim HJ, Lee MS, et al. Oral administration of Agaricus blazei (H1 strain) inhibited tumor growth in a sarcoma 180 inoculation model. *Exp Anim*. 2003 Oct;52(5):371-5.

[75] Niu YC, Liu JC, Zhao XM, et al. A low molecular weight polysaccharide isolated from Agaricus blazei suppresses tumor growth and angiogenesis in vivo. *Oncol Rep*. 2009 Jan;21(1):145-52.

[76] Takaku T, Kimura Y, Okuda H. et al. Isolation of an antitumor compound from Agaricus blazei Murill and its mechanism of action. *J Nutr*. 2001 May;131(5):1409-13.

[77] Ohno N, Furukawa M, Miura NN, et al. Antitumor beta glucan from the cultured fruit body of Agaricus blazei. *Biol Pharm Bull*. 2001 Jul;24(7):820-8.

[78] Gonzaga ML, Bezerra DP, Alves AP, et al. In vivo growth-inhibition of Sarcoma 180 by an alpha-(1-->4)-glucan-beta-(1-->6)-glucan-protein complex polysaccharide obtained from Agaricus blazei Murill. *J Nat Med*. 2009 Jan;63(1):32-40.

[79] Niu YC, Liu JC, Zhao XM, et al. Immunostimulatory activities of a low molecular weight antitumoral polysaccharide isolated from Agaricus blazei Murill (LMPAB) in Sarcoma 180 ascitic tumor-bearing mice. *Pharmazie*. 2009 Jul;64(7):472-6.

[80] Ito H, Shimura K, Itoh H, et al. Antitumor effects of a new polysaccharide-protein complex (ATOM) prepared from Agaricus blazei (Iwade strain 101) "Himematsutake" and its mechanisms in tumor-bearing mice. *Anticancer Res*. 1997 Jan-Feb;17(1A):277-84.

[81] Fernandes MB, Habu S, de Lima MA, et al. Influence of drying methods over in vitro antitumoral effects of exopolysaccharides produced by Agaricus blazei LPB 03 on submerged fermentation. *Bioprocess Biosyst Eng*. 2011 Mar;34(3):253-61.

[82] Kaneno R, Fontanari LM, Santos SA, et al. Effects of extracts from Brazilian sun-mushroom (Agaricus blazei) on the NK activity and lymphoproliferative responsiveness of Ehrlich tumor-bearing mice. *Food Chem Toxicol*. 2004 Jun;42(6):909-16.

[83] Itoh H, Ito H, Amano H, et al. Inhibitory action of a (1-->6)-beta-D-glucan-protein complex (F III-2-b) isolated from Agaricus blazei Murill ("himematsutake") on Meth A fibrosarcoma-bearing mice and its antitumor mechanism. *Jpn J Pharmacol*. 1994 Oct;66(2):265-71.

[84] Fujimiya Y, Suzuki Y, Katakura R, et al. Tumor-specific cytocidal and immunopotentiating effects of relatively low molecular weight products derived from the basidiomycete, Agaricus blazei Murill. *Anticancer Res*. 1999 Jan-Feb;19(1A):113-8.

[85] Wu MF, Lu HF, Hsu YM, et al. Possible reduction of hepatoma formation by Smmu 7721 cells in SCID mice and metastasis formation by B16F10 melanoma cells in C57BL/6 mice by Agaricus blazei murill extract. *In Vivo*. 2011 May-Jun;25(3):399-404.

[86] Ali MM, Baig MT, Huma A, et al. Effect of Agaricus blazei Murill on exploratory behavior of mice-model. *Braz J Biol*. 2021 Dec 20;84:e252575.

[87] de Santi-Rampazzo AP, Schoffen JP, Cirilo CP, et al. Aqueous Extract of Agaricus blazei Murill Prevents Age-Related Changes in the Myenteric Plexus of the Jejunum in Rats. *Evid Based Complement Alternat Med*. 2015;2015:287153.

[88] de Sá-Nakanishi AB, Soares AA, et al. Effects of treating old rats with an aqueous Agaricus blazei extract on oxidative and functional parameters of the brain tissue and brain mitochondria. *Oxid Med Cell Longev*. 2014;2014:563179.

[89] Venkatesh Gobi V, Rajasankar S, Ramkumar M, et al. Agaricus blazei extract abrogates rotenone-induced dopamine depletion and motor deficits by its anti-oxidative and anti-inflammatory properties in Parkinsonic mice. *Nutr Neurosci*. 2018 Nov;21(9):657-666.

[90] Venkatesh Gobi V, Rajasankar S, Ramkumar M, et al. Agaricus blazei extract attenuates rotenone-induced apoptosis through its mitochondrial protective and antioxidant properties in SH-SY5Y neuroblastoma cells. *Nutr Neurosci*. 2018 Feb;21(2):97-107.

[91] Venkatesh Gobi V, Rajasankar S, Swaminathan Johnson WM, et al. Antiapoptotic role of Agaricus blazei extract in rodent model of Parkinson's disease. *Front Biosci (Elite Ed)*. 2019 Jan 1;11(1):12-19.

[92] Yasuma T, Toda M, Kobori H, et al. Subcritical Water Extracts from Agaricus blazei Murrill's Mycelium Inhibit the Expression of Immune Checkpoint Molecules and Axl Receptor. *J Fungi (Basel)*. 2021 Jul 23;7(8):590.

[93] Jiang L, Yu Z, Lin Y, et al. Low-molecular-weight polysaccharides from Agaricus blazei Murrill modulate the Th1 response in cancer immunity. *Oncol Lett*. 2018 Mar;15(3):3429-3436.

[94] Zou XG, Chi Y, Cao YQ, et al. Preparation Process Optimization of Peptides from Agaricus blazei Murrill, and Comparison of Their Antioxidant and Immune-Enhancing Activities Separated by Ultrafiltration Membrane Technology. *Foods*. 2023 Jan 5;12(2):251.

[95] Yuminamochi E, Koike T, Takeda K, et al. Interleukin-12- and interferon-gamma-mediated natural killer cell activation by Agaricus blazei Murill. *Immunology*. 2007 Jun;121(2):197-206.

[96] Mizuno M, Morimoto M, Minato K, et al. Polysaccharides from Agaricus blazei stimulate lymphocyte T-cell subsets in mice. *Biosci Biotechnol Biochem*. 1998 Mar;62(3):434-7.

[97] Cui L, Sun Y, Xu H, et al. A polysaccharide isolated from Agaricus blazei Murill (ABP-AW1) as a potential Th1 immunity-stimulating adjuvant. *Oncol Lett*. 2013 Oct;6(4):1039-1044.

[98] Shimizu S, Kitada H, Yokota H, et al. Activation of the alternative complement pathway by Agaricus blazei Murill. *Phytomedicine*. 2002 Sep;9(6):536-45.

[99] Tang NY, Yang JS, Lin JP, et al. Effects of Agaricus blazei Murill extract on immune responses in normal BALB/c mice. *In Vivo*. 2009 Sep-Oct;23(5):761-6.

[100] Ni WY, Wu MF, Liao NC, et al. Extract of medicinal mushroom Agaricus blazei Murill enhances the non-specific and adaptive immune activities in BALB/c mice. *In Vivo*. 2013 Nov-Dec;27(6):779-86.

[101] Kasai H, He LM, Kawamura M, et al. IL-12 Production Induced by Agaricus blazei Fraction H (ABH) Involves Toll-like Receptor (TLR). *Evid Based Complement Alternat Med*. 2004 Dec;1(3):259-267.

[102] Chan Y, Chang T, Chan CH, et al. Immunomodulatory effects of Agaricus blazei Murill in Balb/cByJ mice. *J Microbiol Immunol Infect*. 2007 Jun;40(3):201-8.

[103] Kimura N, Fujino E, Urabe S, et al. Effect of supplementation of Agaricus mushroom meal extracts on enzyme activities in peripheral leukocytes of calves. *Res Vet Sci*. 2007 Feb;82(1):7-10.

[104] Nakajima A, Ishida T, Koga M, et al. Effect of hot water extract from Agaricus blazei Murill on antibody-producing cells in mice. *Int Immunopharmacol*. 2002 Jul;2(8):1205-11.

[105] Førland DT, Johnson E, Tryggestad AM, et al. An extract based on the medicinal mushroom Agaricus blazei Murill stimulates monocyte-derived dendritic cells to cytokine and chemokine production in vitro. *Cytokine*. 2010 Mar;49(3):245-50.

[106] Bernardshaw S, Lyberg T, Hetland G, et al. Effect of an extract of the mushroom Agaricus blazei Murill on expression of adhesion molecules and production of reactive oxygen species in monocytes and granulocytes in human whole blood ex vivo. *APMIS*. 2007 Jun;115(6):719-25.

[107] Bernardshaw S, Hetland G, Ellertsen LK, et al. An extract of the medicinal mushroom Agaricus blazei Murill differentially stimulates production of pro-inflammatory cytokines in human monocytes and human vein endothelial cells in vitro. *Inflammation*. 2005 Dec;29(4-6):147-53.

[108] Sorimachi K, Akimoto K, Ikehara Y, et al. Secretion of TNF-alpha, IL-8 and nitric oxide by macrophages activated with Agaricus blazei Murill fractions in vitro. *Cell Struct Funct*. 2001 Apr;26(2):103-8.

[109] Kim GY, Lee MY, Lee HJ, et al. Effect of water-soluble proteoglycan isolated from Agaricus blazei on the maturation of murine bone marrow-derived dendritic cells. *Int Immunopharmacol*. 2005 Sep;5(10):1523-32.

[110] Shu CH, Wen BJ, Lin KJ. Monitoring the polysaccharide quality of Agaricus blazei in submerged culture by examining molecular weight distribution and TNF-alpha release capability of macrophage cell line RAW 264.7. *Biotechnol Lett*. 2004 Feb;26(4):2061-4.

[111] Zhong M, Tai A, Yamamoto I. In vitro augmentation of natural killer activity and interferon-gamma production in murine spleen cells with Agaricus blazei fruiting body fractions. *Biosci Biotechnol Biochem*. 2005 Dec;69(12):2466-9.

[112] Liu Y, Zhang L, Zhu X, et al. Polysaccharide Agaricus blazei Murill stimulates myeloid derived suppressor cell differentiation from M2 to M1 type, which mediates inhibition of tumour immune-evasion via the Toll-like receptor 2 pathway. *Immunology*. 2015 Nov;146(3):379-91.

[113] Lin JG, Fan MJ, Tang NY, et al. An extract of Agaricus blazei Murill administered orally promotes immune responses in murine leukemia BALB/c mice in vivo. *Integr Cancer Ther*. 2012 Mar;11(1):29-36.

[114] Huang TT, Ojcius DM, Young JD, et al. The anti-tumorigenic mushroom Agaricus blazei Murill enhances IL-1β production and activates the NLRP3 inflammasome in human macrophages. *PLoS One*. 2012;7(7):e41383.

[115] Cheng F, Yan X, Zhang M, et al. Regulation of RAW 264.7 cell-mediated immunity by polysaccharides from Agaricus blazei Murill via the MAPK signal transduction pathway. *Food Funct*. 2017 Apr 19;8(4):1475-1480.

[116] Berven L, Karppinen P, Hetland G, et al. The polar high molecular weight fraction of the Agaricus blazei Murill extract, AndoSan™, reduces the activity of the tumor-associated protease, legumain, in RAW 264.7 cells. *J Med Food*. 2015 Apr;18(4):429-38.

[117] Gu Y, Fujimiya Y, Itokawa Y, et al. Tumoricidal effects of beta-glucans: mechanisms include both antioxidant activity plus enhanced systemic and topical immunity. *Nutr Cancer*. 2008;60(5):685-91.

[118] Ellertsen LK, Hetland G, Johnson E, et al. Effect of a medicinal extract from Agaricus blazei Murill on gene expression in a human monocyte cell line as examined by microarrays and immuno assays. *Int Immunopharmacol*. 2006 Feb;6(2):133-43.

[119] Tsai WJ, Yang SC, Huang YL, et al. 4-Hydroxy-17-methylincisterol from Agaricus blazei Decreased Cytokine Production and Cell Proliferation in Human Peripheral Blood Mononuclear Cells via Inhibition of NF-AT and NF-κB Activation. *Evid Based Complement Alternat Med*. 2013;2013:435916.

[120] Kawamura M, Kasai H, He L, et al. Antithetical effects of hemicellulase-treated Agaricus blazei on the maturation of murine bone-marrow-derived dendritic cells. *Immunology*. 2005 Mar;114(3):397-409.

[121] Yamanaka D, Motoi M, Ishibashi K, et al. Effect of Agaricus brasiliensis-derived cold water extract on Toll-like receptor 2-dependent cytokine production in vitro. *Immunopharmacol Immunotoxicol*. 2012 Aug;34(4):561-70.

[122] Kuo YC, Huang YL, Chen CC, et al. Cell cycle progression and cytokine gene expression of human peripheral blood mononuclear cells modulated by Agaricus blazei. *J Lab Clin Med*. 2002 Sep;140(3):176-87.

[123] Takimoto H, Kato H, Kaneko M, et al. Amelioration of skewed Th1/Th2 balance in tumor-bearing and asthma-induced mice by oral administration of Agaricus blazei extracts. *Immunopharmacol Immunotoxicol*. 2008;30(4):747-60.

[124] Xie W, Lv A, Li R, et al. Agaricus blazei Murill Polysaccharides Protect Against Cadmium-Induced Oxidative Stress and Inflammatory Damage in Chicken Spleens. *Biol Trace Elem Res*. 2018 Jul;184(1):247-258.

[125] Liu W, Ge M, Hu X, et al. The Effects of Agaricus blazei Murill Polysaccharides on Cadmium-Induced Apoptosis and the TLR4 Signaling Pathway of Peripheral Blood Lymphocytes in Chicken. *Biol Trace Elem Res*. 2017 Nov;180(1):153-163.

[126] Song HH, Chae HS, Oh SR, et al. Anti-inflammatory and anti-allergic effect of Agaricus blazei extract in bone marrow-derived mast cells. *Am J Chin Med*. 2012;40(5):1073-84.

[127] Padilha MM, Avila AA, Sousa PJ, et al. Anti-inflammatory activity of aqueous and alkaline extracts from mushrooms (Agaricus blazei Murill). *J Med Food.* 2009 Apr;12(2):359-64.

[128] Johnson E, Førland DT, Hetland G, et al. Effect of AndoSan™ on expression of adhesion molecules and production of reactive oxygen species in human monocytes and granulocytes in vivo. *Scand J Gastroenterol.* 2012 Sep;47(8-9):984-92.

[129] Wang P, Li XT, Sun L, et al. Anti-Inflammatory Activity of Water-Soluble Polysaccharide of Agaricus blazei Murill on Ovariectomized Osteopenic Rats. *Evid Based Complement Alternat Med.* 2013;2013:164817.

[130] Hetland G, Johnson E, Lyberg T, et al. The Mushroom Agaricus blazei Murill Elicits Medicinal Effects on Tumor, Infection, Allergy, and Inflammation through Its Modulation of Innate Immunity and Amelioration of Th1/Th2 Imbalance and Inflammation. *Adv Pharmacol Sci.* 2011;2011:157015.

[131] Song HH, Chae HS, Oh SR, et al. Anti-inflammatory and anti-allergic effect of Agaricus blazei extract in bone marrow-derived mast cells. *Am J Chin Med.* 2012;40(5):1073-84.

[132] Ellertsen LK, Hetland G. An extract of the medicinal mushroom Agaricus blazei Murill can protect against allergy.

[133] Choi YH, Yan GH, Chai OH, et al. Inhibitory effects of Agaricus blazei on mast cell-mediated anaphylaxis-like reactions. *Biol Pharm Bull.* 2006 Jul;29(7):1366-71. *Clin Mol Allergy.* 2009 May 5;7:6.

[134] Li Y, Lu X, Li X, et al. Effects of Agaricus blazei Murrill polysaccharides on hyperlipidemic rats by regulation of intestinal microflora. *Food Sci Nutr.* 2020 Apr 19;8(6):2758-2772.

[135] Vincent M, Philippe E, Everard A, et al. Dietary supplementation with Agaricus blazei murill extract prevents diet-induced obesity and insulin resistance in rats. *Obesity (Silver Spring).* 2013 Mar;21(3):553-61.

[136] Wei Q, Zhan Y, Chen B, et al. Assessment of antioxidant and antidiabetic properties of Agaricus blazei Murill extracts. *Food Sci Nutr.* 2019 Dec 5;8(1):332-339.

[137] Niwa A, Tajiri T, Higashino H. Ipomoea batatas and Agarics blazei ameliorate diabetic disorders with therapeutic antioxidant potential in streptozotocin-induced diabetic rats. *J Clin Biochem Nutr.* 2011 May;48(3):194-202.

[138] Wei Q, Li J, Zhan Y, Zhong Q, et al. Enhancement of glucose homeostasis through the PI3K/Akt signaling pathway by dietary with Agaricus blazei Murrill in STZ-induced diabetic rats. *Food Sci Nutr.* 2020 Jan 13;8(2):1104-1114.

[139] Vincent M, Philippe E, Everard A, et al. Dietary supplementation with Agaricus blazei murill extract prevents diet-induced obesity and insulin resistance in rats. *Obesity (Silver Spring).* 2013 Mar;21(3):553-61.

[140] Kim YW, Kim KH, Choi HJ, et al. Anti-diabetic activity of beta-glucans and their enzymatically hydrolyzed oligosaccharides from Agaricus blazei. *Biotechnol Lett.* 2005 Apr;27(7):483-7.

[141] Oh TW, Kim YA, Jang WJ, et al. Semipurified fractions from the submerged-culture broth of Agaricus blazei Murill reduce blood glucose levels in streptozotocin-induced diabetic rats. *J Agric Food Chem.* 2010 Apr 14;58(7):4113-9.

[142] Jonathan SG, Adeoyo OR. Evaluation of ten wild nigerian mushrooms for amylase and cellulase activities. *Mycobiology.* 2011 Jun;39(2):103-8.

[143] Wei Q, Huang L, Li J, et al. The beneficial effects of Agaricus blazei Murrill on hepatic antioxidant enzymes and the pancreatic tissue recovery in streptozotocin-induced diabetic rats. *J Food Biochem.* 2020 May;44(5):e13170.

[144] Di Naso FC, de Mello RN, Bona S, et al. Effect of Agaricus blazei Murill on the pulmonary tissue of animals with streptozotocin-induced diabetes. *Exp Diabetes Res.* 2010;2010:543926.

[145] Soares AA, de Oliveira AL, Sá-Nakanishi AB, et al. Effects of an Agaricus blazei aqueous extract pretreatment on paracetamol-induced brain and liver injury in rats. *Biomed Res Int.* 2013;2013:469180.

[146] Al-Dbass AM, Al-Daihan SK, Bhat RS. Agaricus blazei Murill as an efficient hepatoprotective and antioxidant agent against CCl4-induced liver injury in rats. *Saudi J Biol Sci.* 2012 Jul;19(3):303-9.

[147] Wu MF, Hsu YM, Tang MC, et al. Agaricus blazei Murill extract abrogates CCl4-induced liver injury in rats. *In Vivo.* 2011 Jan-Feb;25(1):35-40.

[148] Hu X, Zhang R, Xie Y, et al. The Protective Effects of Polysaccharides from Agaricus blazei Murill Against Cadmium-Induced Oxidant Stress and Inflammatory Damage in Chicken Livers. *Biol Trace Elem Res.* 2017 Jul;178(1):117-126.

[149] Wang H, Li G, Zhang W, et al. The protective effect of Agaricus blazei Murrill, submerged culture using the optimized medium composition, on alcohol-induced liver injury. *Biomed Res Int.* 2014;2014:573978.

[150] Chang JB, Wu MF, Yang YY, et al. Carbon tetrachloride-induced hepatotoxicity and its amelioration by Agaricus blazei Murrill extract in a mouse model. *In Vivo.* 2011 Nov-Dec;25(6):971-6.

[151] Barbisan LF, Miyamoto M, Scolastici C, et al. Influence of aqueous extract of Agaricus blazei on rat liver toxicity induced by different doses of diethylnitrosamine. *J Ethnopharmacol.* 2002 Nov;83(1-2):25-32.

[152] Barbisan LF, Scolastici C, Miyamoto M, et al. Effects of crude extracts of Agaricus blazei on DNA damage and on rat liver carcinogenesis induced by diethylnitrosamine. *Genet Mol Res.* 2003 Sep 30;2(3):295-308.

[153] Bernardshaw S, Hetland G, Grinde B, et al. An extract of the mushroom Agaricus blazei Murill protects against lethal septicemia in a mouse model of fecal peritonitis. *Shock.* 2006 Apr;25(4):420-5.

[154] Tontowiputro DK, Sargowo D, Tjokroprawiro A, et al. The significance of Agaricus blazei as an immunomodulator of the level of IL-17 in Balb/C mice with atherosclerosis. *Cent Eur J Immunol.* 2020;45(1):1-8.

[155] Dong S, Furutani Y, Suto Y, et al. Estrogen-like activity and dual roles in cell signaling of an Agaricus blazei Murrill mycelia-dikaryon extract. *Microbiol Res.* 2012 Apr 20;167(4):231-7.

[156] Gonçalves JL, Roma EH, Gomes-Santos AC, et al. Pro-inflammatory effects of the mushroom Agaricus blazei and its consequences on atherosclerosis development. *Eur J Nutr.* 2012 Dec;51(8):927-37.

[157] Tsubone H, Makimura Y, Hanafusa M, et al. Agaricus brasiliensis KA21 improves circulatory functions in spontaneously hypertensive rats. *J Med Food.* 2014 Mar;17(3):295-301.

[158] Li Y, Lu X, Li X, et al. Effects of Agaricus blazei Murrill polysaccharides on hyperlipidemic rats by regulation of intestinal microflora. *Food Sci Nutr.* 2020 Apr 19;8(6):2758-2772.

[159] Li Y, Sheng Y, Lu X, et al. Isolation and purification of acidic polysaccharides from Agaricus blazei Murill and evaluation of their lipid-lowering mechanism. *Int J Biol Macromol.* 2020 Aug 15;157:276-287.

[160] de Miranda AM, Ribeiro GM, Cunha AC, et al. Hypolipidemic effect of the edible mushroom Agaricus blazei in rats subjected to a hypercholesterolemic diet. *J Physiol Biochem.* 2014 Mar;70(1):215-24.

[161] Câmara Neto JF, Campelo MDS, Cerqueira GS, et al. Gastroprotective effect of hydroalcoholic extract from Agaricus blazei Murill against ethanol-induced gastric ulcer in mice. *J Ethnopharmacol*. 2022 Jun 28;292:115191.

[162] Song Y, Zhang R, Wang H, et al. Protective Effect of Agaricus blazei Polysaccharide Against Cadmium-Induced Damage on the Testis of Chicken. *Biol Trace Elem Res*. 2018 Aug;184(2):491-500.

[163] Živković L, Borozan S, Čabarkapa A, et al. Antigenotoxic Properties of Agaricus blazei against Hydrogen Peroxide in Human Peripheral Blood Cells. *Oxid Med Cell Longev*. 2017;2017:8759764.

[164] Bellini MF, Angeli JP, Matuo R, et al. Antigenotoxicity of Agaricus blazei mushroom organic and aqueous extracts in chromosomal aberration and cytokinesis block micronucleus assays in CHO-k1 and HTC cells. *Toxicol In Vitro*. 2006 Apr;20(3):355-60.

[165] Angeli JP, Ribeiro LR, Bellini MF, et al. Beta-glucan extracted from the medicinal mushroom Agaricus blazei prevents the genotoxic effects of benzo[a]pyrene in the human hepatoma cell line HepG2. *Arch Toxicol*. 2009 Jan;83(1):81-6.

[166] Guterrez ZR, Mantovani MS, Eira AF, et al. Variation of the antimutagenicity effects of water extracts of Agaricus blazei Murrill in vitro. *Toxicol In Vitro*. 2004 Jun;18(3):301-9.

[167] Machado MP, Filho ER, Terezan AP, et al. Cytotoxicity, genotoxicity and antimutagenicity of hexane extracts of Agaricus blazei determined in vitro by the comet assay and CHO/HGPRT gene mutation assay. *Toxicol In Vitro*. 2005 Jun;19(4):533-9.

[168] Martins de Oliveira J, Jordão BQ, et al. Anti-genotoxic effect of aqueous extracts of sun mushroom (Agaricus blazei Murill lineage 99/26) in mammalian cells in vitro. *Food Chem Toxicol*. 2002 Dec;40(12):1775-80.

[169] Osaki Y, Kato T, Yamamoto K, Okubo J, et al. [Antimutagenic and bactericidal substances in the fruit body of a Basidiomycete Agaricus blazei, Jun-17]. *Yakugaku Zasshi*. 1994 May;114(5):342-50.

[170] Menoli RC, Mantovani MS, Ribeiro LR, et al. Antimutagenic effects of the mushroom Agaricus blazei Murrill extracts on V79 cells. *Mutat Res*. 2001 Sep 20;496(1-2):5-13.

[171] Matuo R, Oliveira RJ, Silva AF, et al. Anticlastogenic Activity of Aqueous Extract of Agaricus blazei in Drug-Metabolizing Cells (HTCs) During Cell Cycle. *Toxicol Mech Methods*. 2007;17(3):147-52.

[172] Angeli JP, Ribeiro LR, Gonzaga ML, et al. Protective effects of beta-glucan extracted from Agaricus brasiliensis against chemically induced DNA damage in human lymphocytes. *Cell Biol Toxicol*. 2006 Jul;22(4):285-91.

[173] Bellini MF, Giacomini NL, Eira AF, et al. Anticlastogenic effect of aqueous extracts of Agaricus blazei on CHO-k1 cells, studying different developmental phases of the mushroom. *Toxicol In Vitro*. 2003 Aug;17(4):465-9.

[174] Luiz RC, Jordão BQ, da Eira AF, et al. Mechanism of anticlastogenicity of Agaricus blazei Murill mushroom organic extracts in wild type CHO (K(1)) and repair deficient (xrs5) cells by chromosome aberration and sister chromatid exchange assays. *Mutat Res*. 2003 Jul 25;528(1-2):75-9.

[175] Xie W, Lv A, Li R, et al. Agaricus blazei Murill Polysaccharides Protect Against Cadmium-Induced Oxidative Stress and Inflammatory Damage in Chicken Spleens. *Biol Trace Elem Res*. 2018 Jul;184(1):247-258.

[176] Lv A, Ge M, Hu X, et al. Effects of Agaricus blazei Murill Polysaccharide on Cadmium Poisoning on the MDA5 Signaling Pathway and Antioxidant Function of Chicken Peripheral Blood Lymphocytes. *Biol Trace Elem Res*. 2018 Jan;181(1):122-132.

[177] Oliveira OM, Vellosa JC, Fernandes AS, et al. Antioxidant activity of Agaricus blazei. *Fitoterapia*. 2007 Apr;78(3):263-4.

[178] Zou XG, Chi Y, Cao YQ, et al. Preparation Process Optimization of Peptides from Agaricus blazei Murrill, and Comparison of Their Antioxidant and Immune-Enhancing Activities Separated by Ultrafiltration Membrane Technology. *Foods*. 2023 Jan 5;12(2):251.

[179] Wu S, Li F, Jia S, et al. Drying effects on the antioxidant properties of polysaccharides obtained from Agaricus blazei Murrill. *Carbohydr Polym*. 2014 Mar 15;103:414-7.

[180] Hakime-Silva RA, Vellosa JC, Khalil NM, et al. Chemical, enzymatic and cellular antioxidant activity studies of Agaricus blazei Murrill. *An Acad Bras Cienc*. 2013 Sep;85(3):1073-81.

[181] Jia S, Li F, Liu Y, Ren H, et al. Effects of extraction methods on the antioxidant activities of polysaccharides from Agaricus blazei Murrill. *Int J Biol Macromol*. 2013 Nov;62:66-9.

[182] Ker YB, Chen KC, Chyau CC, et al. Antioxidant capability of polysaccharides fractionated from submerge-cultured Agaricus blazei mycelia. *J Agric Food Chem*. 2005 Sep 7;53(18):7052-8.

[183] Izawa S, Inoue Y. A screening system for antioxidants using thioredoxin-deficient yeast: discovery of thermostable antioxidant activity from Agaricus blazei Murill. *Appl Microbiol Biotechnol*. 2004 May;64(4):537-42.

[184] Dong S, Furutani Y, Kimura S, et al. Brefeldin A is an estrogenic, Erk1/2-activating component in the extract of Agaricus blazei mycelia. *J Agric Food Chem*. 2013 Jan 9;61(1):128-36.

[185] Dong S, Furutani Y, Suto Y, et al. Estrogen-like activity and dual roles in cell signaling of an Agaricus blazei Murrill mycelia-dikaryon extract. *Microbiol Res*. 2012 Apr 20;167(4):231-7.

[186] Zhao Y, Tian N, Wang H, et al. Chemically Sulfated Polysaccharides from Agaricus blazei Murill: Synthesis, Characterization and Anti-HIV Activity. *Chem Biodivers*. 2021 Sep;18(9):e2100338.

[187] Val CH, Brant F, Miranda AS, et al. Effect of mushroom Agaricus blazei on immune response and development of experimental cerebral malaria. *Malar J*. 2015 Aug 11;14:311.

[188] Sorimachi K, Ikehara Y, Maezato G, et al. Inhibition by Agaricus blazei Murill fractions of cytopathic effect induced by western equine encephalitis (WEE) virus on VERO cells in vitro. *Biosci Biotechnol Biochem*. 2001 Jul;65(7):1645-7.

[189] Soković M, Ćirić A, Glamočlija J, et al. Agaricus blazei hot water extract shows anti quorum sensing activity in the nosocomial human pathogen Pseudomonas aeruginosa. *Molecules*. 2014 Apr 3;19(4):4189-99.

[190] Bernardshaw S, Johnson E, Hetland G. An extract of the mushroom Agaricus blazei Murill administered orally protects against systemic Streptococcus pneumoniae infection in mice. *Scand J Immunol*. 2005 Oct;62(4):393-8.

[191] Osaki Y, Kato T, Yamamoto K, Okubo J, et al. [Antimutagenic and bactericidal substances in the fruit body of a Basidiomycete Agaricus blazei, Jun-17]. *Yakugaku Zasshi*. 1994 May;114(5):342-50.

[192] Valadares DG, Duarte MC, Oliveira JS, et al. Leishmanicidal activity of the Agaricus blazei Murill in different Leishmania species. *Parasitol Int*. 2011 Dec;60(4):357-63.

[193] Valadares DG, Duarte MC, Ramírez L, et al. Prophylactic or therapeutic administration of Agaricus blazei Murill is effective in treatment of murine visceral leishmaniasis. *Exp Parasitol*. 2012 Oct;132(2):228-36.

[194] de Jesus Pereira NC, Régis WC, Costa LE, et al. Evaluation of adjuvant activity of fractions derived from Agaricus blazei, when in association with the recombinant LiHyp1 protein, to protect against visceral leishmaniasis. *Exp Parasitol*. 2015 Jun;153:180-90.

[195] Valadares DG, Duarte MC, Ramírez L, et al. Therapeutic efficacy induced by the oral administration of Agaricus blazei Murill against Leishmania amazonensis. *Parasitol Res*. 2012 Oct;111(4):1807-16.

[196] Feng Q, Li Y, Lu X, et al. Agaricus blazei polypeptide exerts a protective effect on D-galactose-induced aging mice via the Keap1/Nrf2/ARE and P53/Trim32 signaling pathways. *J Food Biochem*. 2021 Jan;45(1):e13555.

[197] Yuan W, Huang M, Wu Y, et al. Agaricus blazei Murrill Polysaccharide Attenuates Periodontitis via H2 S/NRF2 Axis-Boosted Appropriate Level of Autophagy in PDLCs. *Mol Nutr Food Res*. 2023 Sep 29:e2300112.

[198] Saraiva MM, Campelo MDS, Câmara Neto JF, et al. Agaricus blazei Murill polysaccharides/alginate/poly(vinyl alcohol) blend as dressings for wound healing. *Int J Biol Macromol*. 2023 Jul 31;244:125278.

[199] Campelo MDS, Mota LB, Câmara Neto JF, et al. Agaricus blazei Murill extract-loaded in alginate/poly(vinyl alcohol) films prepared by Ca2+ cross-linking for wound healing applications. *J Biomed Mater Res B Appl Biomater*. 2023 May;111(5):1035-1047.

[200] Sui Z, Yang R, Liu B, et al. Chemical analysis of Agaricus blazei polysaccharides and effect of the polysaccharides on IL-1beta mRNA expression in skin of burn wound-treated rats. *Int J Biol Macromol*. 2010 Aug 1;47(2):155-7.

[201] Mahmood F, Hetland G, Nentwich I, et al. Agaricus blazei-Based Mushroom Extract Supplementation to Birch Allergic Blood Donors: A Randomized Clinical Trial. *Nutrients*. 2019 Oct 2;11(10):2339.

[202] Hsu CH, Hwang KC, Chiang YH, et al. The mushroom Agaricus blazei Murill extract normalizes liver function in patients with chronic hepatitis B. *J Altern Complement Med*. 2008 Apr;14(3):299-301.

[203] Grinde B, Hetland G, Johnson E. Effects on gene expression and viral load of a medicinal extract from Agaricus blazei in patients with chronic hepatitis C infection. *Int Immunopharmacol*. 2006 Aug;6(8):1311-4.

[204] Hsu CH, Liao YL, Lin SC, et al. The mushroom Agaricus Blazei Murill in combination with metformin and gliclazide improves insulin resistance in type 2 diabetes: a randomized, double-blinded, and placebo-controlled clinical trial. *J Altern Complement Med*. 2007 Jan-Feb;13(1):97-102.

[205] Therkelsen SP, Hetland G, Lyberg T, et al. Effect of a Medicinal Agaricus blazei Murill-Based Mushroom Extract, AndoSan™, on Symptoms, Fatigue and Quality of Life in Patients with Ulcerative Colitis in a Randomized Single-Blinded Placebo Controlled Study. *PLoS One*. 2016 Mar 2;11(3):e0150191.

[206] Førland DT, Johnson E, Saetre L, et al. Effect of an extract based on the medicinal mushroom Agaricus blazei Murill on expression of cytokines and calprotectin in patients *with ulcerative colitis and Crohn's disease. Scand J Immunol*. 2011 Jan;73(1):66-75.

[207] Therkelsen SP, Hetland G, Lyberg T, et al. Effect of the Medicinal Agaricus blazei Murill-Based Mushroom Extract, AndoSanTM, on Symptoms, Fatigue and Quality of Life in Patients with Crohn's Disease in a Randomized Single-Blinded Placebo Controlled Study. *PLoS One*. 2016 Jul 14;11(7):e0159288.

[208] Therkelsen SP, Hetland G, Lyberg T, et al. Cytokine Levels After Consumption of a Medicinal Agaricus blazei Murill-Based Mushroom Extract, AndoSan™ , in Patients with Crohn's Disease and Ulcerative Colitis in a Randomized Single-Blinded Placebo-Controlled Study. *Scand J Immunol*. 2016 Dec;84(6):323-331.

[209] Johnson E, Forland DT, Saetre L, et al. Effect of an extract based on the medicinal mushroom Agaricus blazei murill on release of cytokines, chemokines and leukocyte growth factors in human blood ex vivo and in vivo. *Scand J Immunol*. 2009 Mar;69(3):242-50.

[210] Ohno S, Sumiyoshi Y, Hashine K, et al. Quality of life improvements among cancer patients in remission following the consumption of Agaricus blazei Murill mushroom extract. *Complement Ther Med*. 2013 Oct;21(5):460-7.

[211] Ahn WS, Kim DJ, Chae GT, et al. Natural killer cell activity and quality of life were improved by consumption of a mushroom extract, Agaricus blazei Murill Kyowa, in gynecological cancer patients undergoing chemotherapy. *Int J Gynecol Cancer*. 2004 Jul-Aug;14(4):589-94.

[212] Tangen JM, Tierens A, Caers J, et al. Immunomodulatory effects of the Agaricus blazei Murrill-based mushroom extract AndoSan in patients with multiple myeloma undergoing high dose chemotherapy and autologous stem cell transplantation: a randomized, double blinded clinical study. *Biomed Res Int*. 2015;2015:718539.

[213] Lima CU, Souza VC, Morita MC, et al. Agaricus blazei Murrill and inflammatory mediators in elderly women: a randomized clinical trial. *Scand J Immunol*. 2012 Mar;75(3):336-41.

[214] Fan MJ, Lin YC, Shih HD, et al. Crude extracts of Agaricus brasiliensis induce apoptosis in human oral cancer CAL 27 cells through a mitochondria-dependent pathway. *In Vivo*. 2011 May-Jun;25(3):355-66.

[215] Baranoski A, Tempesta Oliveira M, Semprebon SC, et al. Effects of sulfated and non-sulfated β-glucan extracted from Agaricus brasiliensis in breast adenocarcinoma cells - MCF-7. *Toxicol Mech Methods*. 2015;25(9):672-9.

[216] Tajima K, Amano H, Motoi A, et al. Outdoor-Cultivated Royal Sun Medicinal Mushroom Agaricus brasiliensis KA21 (Agaricomycetes) Reduces Anticancer Medicine Side Effects. *Int J Med Mushrooms*. 2020;22(1):31-43.

[217] Jumes FM, Lugarini D, Pereira AL, et al. Effects of Agaricus brasiliensis mushroom in Walker-256 tumor-bearing rats. *Can J Physiol Pharmacol*. 2010 Jan;88(1):21-7.

[218] Mourão F, Linde GA, Messa V, et al. Antineoplasic activity of Agaricus brasiliensis basidiocarps on different maturation phases. *Braz J Microbiol*. 2009 Oct;40(4):901-5.

[219] Sovrani V, da Rosa J, Drewinski MP, et al. In Vitro and In Vivo Antitumoral Activity of Exobiopolymers from the Royal Sun Culinary-Medicinal Mushroom Agaricus brasiliensis (Agaricomycetes). *Int J Med Mushrooms*. 2017;19(9):767-775.

[220] Pinto AV, Martins PR, Romagnoli GG, et al. Polysaccharide fraction of Agaricus brasiliensis avoids tumor-induced IL-10 production and changes the microenvironment of subcutaneous Ehrlich adenocarcinoma. *Cell Immunol*. 2009;256(1-2):27-38.

[221] Xin Y, Zhang Y, Zhang X. Antidepressant Effect of Water Extract of Royal Sun Medicinal Mushroom, Agaricus brasiliensis (Agaricomycetes), in Mice Exposed to Chronic Unpredictable Mild Stress. *Int J Med Mushrooms*. 2022;24(4):63-73.

[222] Zhang C, Gao X, Sun Y, et al. Anxiolytic Effects of Royal Sun Medicinal Mushroom, Agaricus brasiliensis (Higher Basidiomycetes) on Ischemia-Induced Anxiety in Rats. *Int J Med Mushrooms*. 2015;17(1):1-10.

[223] Yamanaka D, Tada R, Adachi Y, et al. Agaricus brasiliensis-derived β-glucans exert immunoenhancing effects via a dectin-1-dependent pathway. *Int Immunopharmacol.* 2012 Nov;14(3):311-9.

[224] Smiderle FR, Ruthes AC, van Arkel J, et al. Polysaccharides from Agaricus bisporus and Agaricus brasiliensis show similarities in their structures and their immunomodulatory effects on human monocytic THP-1 cells. *BMC Complement Altern Med.* 2011 Jul 25;11:58.

[225] Martins PR, de Campos Soares ÂMV, da Silva Pinto Domeneghini AV, et al. Agaricus brasiliensis polysaccharides stimulate human monocytes to capture Candida albicans, express toll-like receptors 2 and 4, and produce pro-inflammatory cytokines. *J Venom Anim Toxins Incl Trop Dis.* 2017 Mar 23;23:17.

[226] Smiderle FR, Alquini G, Tadra-Sfeir MZ, et al. Agaricus bisporus and Agaricus brasiliensis (1→6)-β-D-glucans show immunostimulatory activity on human THP-1 derived macrophages. *Carbohydr Polym.* 2013 Apr 15;94(1):91-9.

[227] Zhang Y, Liu D, Fang L, et al. A galactomannoglucan derived from Agaricus brasiliensis: Purification, characterization and macrophage activation via MAPK and IκB/NFκB pathways. *Food Chem.* 2018 Jan 15;239:603-611.

[228] Yamanaka D, Motoi M, Ishibashi K, et al. Effect of Agaricus brasiliensis-derived cold water extract on Toll-like receptor 2-dependent cytokine production in vitro. *Immunopharmacol Immunotoxicol.* 2012 Aug;34(4):561-70.

[229] Fang L, Zhang Y, Xie J, et al. Royal Sun Medicinal Mushroom, Agaricus brasiliensis (Agaricomycetidae), Derived Polysaccharides Exert Immunomodulatory Activities In Vitro and In Vivo. *Int J Med Mushrooms.* 2016;18(2):123-32.

[230] Martins PR, Gameiro MC, Castoldi L, et al. Polysaccharide-rich fraction of Agaricus brasiliensis enhances the candidacidal activity of murine macrophages. *Mem Inst Oswaldo Cruz.* 2008 May;103(3):244-50.

[231] Mizuno M, Nishitani Y. Macrophage activation-mediated hydrogen peroxide generation by the royal sun medicinal mushroom Agaricus brasiliensis (Higher Basidiomycetes). *Int J Med Mushrooms.* 2013;15(4):365-71.

[232] Berven L, Karppinen P, Hetland G, et al. The polar high molecular weight fraction of the Agaricus blazei Murill extract, AndoSan™, reduces the activity of the tumor-associated protease, legumain, in RAW 264.7 cells. *J Med Food.* 2015 Apr;18(4):429-38.

[233] Komura DL, Carbonero ER, Gracher AH, et al. Structure of Agaricus spp. fucogalactans and their anti-inflammatory and antinociceptive properties. *Bioresour Technol.* 2010 Aug;101(15):6192-9

[234] Saiki P, Kawano Y, Van Griensven LJLD, et al. The anti-inflammatory effect of Agaricus brasiliensis is partly due to its linoleic acid content. *Food Funct.* 2017 Nov 15;8(11):4150-4158.

[235] Komura DL, Carbonero ER, Gracher AH, et al. Structure of Agaricus spp. fucogalactans and their anti-inflammatory and antinociceptive properties. *Bioresour Technol.* 2010 Aug;101(15):6192-9

[236] de Souza ACDS, Goncalves GA, Soares AA, et al. Antioxidant Action of an Aqueous Extract of Royal Sun Medicinal Mushroom, Agaricus brasiliensis (Agaricomycetes), in Rats with Adjuvant-Induced Arthritis. *Int J Med Mushrooms.* 2018;20(2):101-117.

[237] Croccia C, Lopes AJ, Pinto LF, et al. Royal sun medicinal mushroom Agaricus brasiliensis (higher Basidiomycetes) and the attenuation of pulmonary inflammation induced by 4-(methylnitrosamino)-1-(3-pyridyl)-1-butanone (NNK). *Int J Med Mushrooms.* 2013;15(4):345-55.

[238] Yu H, Han C, Sun Y, et al. The agaricoglyceride of royal sun medicinal mushroom, Agaricus brasiliensis (higher basidiomycetes) is anti-inflammatory and reverses diabetic glycemia in the liver of mice. *Int J Med Mushrooms.* 2013;15(4):357-64.

[239] Ji W, Huang H, Chao J, et al. Protective Effect of Agaricus brasiliensis on STZ-Induced Diabetic Neuropathic Pain in Rats. *Evid Based Complement Alternat Med.* 2014;2014:679259.

[240] Caetano ELA, Viroel FJM, Laurino LF, et al. Royal Sun Culinary-Medicinal Mushroom Agaricus brasiliensis (Agaricomycetes) as a Functional Food in Gestational Diabetes Mellitus Before and After Fetus Implantation. *Int J Med Mushrooms.* 2021;23(9):15-27.

[241] Zhang L, Yuan B, Wang H, et al. Therapeutic effect of Agaricus brasiliensis on phenylhydrazine-induced neonatal jaundice in rats. *Biomed Res Int.* 2015;2015:651218.

[242] Zhang S, He B, Ge J, et al. Characterization of chemical composition of Agaricus brasiliensis polysaccharides and its effect on myocardial SOD activity, MDA and caspase-3 level in ischemia-reperfusion rats. *Int J Biol Macromol.* 2010 Apr 1;46(3):363-6.

[243] Tsubone H, Makimura Y, Hanafusa M, et al. Agaricus brasiliensis KA21 improves circulatory functions in spontaneously hypertensive rats. *J Med Food.* 2014 Mar;17(3):295-301. *Foods.* 2019 Nov 4;8(11):546.

[244] de Miranda AM, Rossoni Júnior JV, Souza E Silva L, et al. Agaricus brasiliensis (sun mushroom) affects the expression of genes related to cholesterol homeostasis. *Eur J Nutr.* 2017 Jun;56(4):1707-1717.

[245] Akahane K, Satoh K, Ohta M, et al. Hot Water Extracts of the Royal Sun Mushroom, Agaricus brasiliensis (Higher Basidiomycetes), Inhibit Platelet Activation via the P2Y1 Receptor. *Int J Med Mushrooms.* 2015;17(8):763-70.

[246] de Oliveira AL, Eler GJ, Bracht A, et al. Purinergic effects of a hydroalcoholic Agaricus brasiliensis (A. blazei) extract on liver functions. *J Agric Food Chem.* 2010 Jun 23;58(12):7202-10.

[247] Yamanaka D, Motoi M, Motoi A, et al. Differences in antioxidant activities of outdoor- and indoor-cultivated Agaricus brasiliensis, and protective effects against carbon tetrachloride-induced acute hepatic injury in mice. *BMC Complement Altern Med.* 2014 Nov 24;14:454.

[248] Zhang C, Han C, Zhao B, et al. The protective effects of aqueous extracts of wild-growing and fermented Royal Sun mushroom, Agaricus brasiliensis S. Wasser et al. (higher basidiomycetes), in CCl4-induced oxidative damage in rats. *Int J Med Mushrooms.* 2012;14(6):557-61.

[249] Nakamura A, Zhu Q, Yokoyama Y, et al. Agaricus brasiliensis KA21 May Prevent Diet-Induced Nash Through Its Antioxidant, Anti-Inflammatory, and Anti-Fibrotic Activities in the Liver. *Biocontrol Sci.* 2017;22(3):171-174.

[250] Uyanoglu M, Canbek M, van Griensven LJ, et al. Effects of polysaccharide from fruiting bodies of Agaricus bisporus, Agaricus brasiliensis, and Phellinus linteus on alcoholic liver injury. *Int J Food Sci Nutr.* 2014 Jun;65(4):482-8.

[251] Câmara Neto JF, Campelo MDS, Cerqueira GS, et al. Gastroprotective effect of hydroalcoholic extract from Agaricus blazei Murill against ethanol-induced gastric ulcer in mice. *J Ethnopharmacol.* 2022 Jun 28;292:115191.

[252] Navegantes-Lima KC, Monteiro VVS, de França Gaspar SL, et al. Agaricus brasiliensis Mushroom Protects Against Sepsis by Alleviating Oxidative and Inflammatory Response. *Front Immunol.* 2020 Jul 1;11:1238.

[253] Gameiro PH, Nascimento JS, Rocha BH, et al. Antimutagenic effect of aqueous extract from Agaricus brasiliensis on culture of human lymphocytes. *J Med Food.* 2013 Feb;16(2):180-3.

[254] Angeli JP, Ribeiro LR, Gonzaga ML, et al. Protective effects of beta-glucan extracted from Agaricus brasiliensis against chemically induced DNA damage in human lymphocytes. *Cell Biol Toxicol.* 2006 Jul;22(4):285-91.

[255] Stojković D, Reis FS, Glamočlija J, et al. Cultivated strains of Agaricus bisporus and A. brasiliensis: chemical characterization and evaluation of antioxidant and antimicrobial properties for the final healthy product--natural preservatives in yoghurt. *Food Funct.* 2014 Jul 25;5(7):1602-12.

[256] Mourão F, Harue Umco S, Seiko Takemura O, et al. Antioxidant Activity of Agaricus brasiliensis Basidiocarps on Different Maturation Phases. *Braz J Microbiol.* 2011 Jan;42(1):197-202.

[257] Yurkiv B, Wasser SP, Nevo E, et al. Antioxidant Effects of Medicinal Mushrooms Agaricus brasiliensis and Ganoderma lucidum (Higher Basidiomycetes): Evidence from Animal Studies. *Int J Med Mushrooms.* 2015;17(10):943-55.

[258] Cardozo FT, Camelini CM, Cordeiro MN, et al. Characterization and cytotoxic activity of sulfated derivatives of polysaccharides from Agaricus brasiliensis. *Int J Biol Macromol.* 2013 Jun;57:265-72.

[259] Zhang J, Gao Z, Li S, et al. Purification, Characterization, Antioxidation, and Antiaging Properties of Exopolysaccharides and Endopolysaccharides of the Royal Sun Medicinal Mushroom, Agaricus brasiliensis (Agaricomycetes). *Int J Med Mushrooms.* 2016;18(12):1071-1081.

[260] Faccin LC, Benati F, Rincão VP, et al. Antiviral activity of aqueous and ethanol extracts and of an isolated polysaccharide from Agaricus brasiliensis against poliovirus type 1. *Lett Appl Microbiol.* 2007 Jul;45(1):24-8.

[261] Eguchi N, Fujino K, Thanasut K, et al. In vitro Anti-Influenza Virus Activity of Agaricus brasiliensis KA21.

[262] Yamamoto KA, Galhardi LC, Rincão VP, et al. Antiherpetic activity of an Agaricus brasiliensis polysaccharide, its sulfated derivative and fractions. *Int J Biol Macromol.* 2013 Jan;52:9-13.

[263] Cardozo FT, Camelini CM, Mascarello A, et al. Immunomodulatory and Antitumoral Properties of Ganoderma lucidum and Agaricus brasiliensis (Agaricomycetes) Medicinal Mushrooms. *Int J Med Mushrooms.* 2018;20(4):393-403.

[264] Minari MC, Rincão VP, Soares SA, et al. Antiviral properties of polysaccharides from Agaricus brasiliensis in the replication of bovine herpesvirus 1. *Acta Virol.* 2011;55(3):255-9.

[265] Cardozo FT, Camelini CM, Leal PC, et al. Antiherpetic mechanism of a sulfated derivative of Agaricus brasiliensis fruiting bodies polysaccharide. *Intervirology.* 2014;57(6):375-83.

[266] Cardozo FT, Larsen IV, Carballo EV, et al. In vivo anti-herpes simplex virus activity of a sulfated derivative of Agaricus brasiliensis mycelial polysaccharide. *Antimicrob Agents Chemother.* 2013 Jun;57(6):2541-9.

[267] Stojković D, Reis FS, Glamočlija J, et al. Cultivated strains of Agaricus bisporus and A. brasiliensis: chemical characterization and evaluation of antioxidant and antimicrobial properties for the final healthy product--natural preservatives in yoghurt. *Food Funct.* 2014 Jul 25;5(7):1602-12.

[268] Saraiva MM, Campelo MDS, Câmara Neto JF, et al. Agaricus blazei Murill polysaccharides/alginate/poly(vinyl alcohol) blend as dressings for wound healing. *Int J Biol Macromol.* 2023 Jul 31;244:125278.

[269] Campelo MDS, Mota LB, Câmara Neto JF, et al. Agaricus blazei Murill extract-loaded in alginate/poly(vinyl alcohol) films prepared by Ca2+ cross-linking for wound healing applications. *Biomed Mater Res B Appl Biomater.* 2023 May;111(5):1035-1047.

[270] Silva FF, de Oliveira GAC, Martins Costa HC, et al. Royal Sun Culinary-Medicinal Mushroom, Agaricus brasiliensis (Agaricomycetes), Supplement in Training Capacity Improvement Parameters. *Int J Med Mushrooms.* 2017;19(9):759-766.

[271] Yamanaka D, Shoda M, Matsubara T, et al. Open-Label Study of the Influence of Food Containing the Royal Sun Mushroom, Agaricus brasiliensis KA21 (Agaricomycetes), on β-Glucan-Specific Antibody Production in Healthy Human Volunteers. *Int J Med Mushrooms.* 2021;23(2):13-28.

[272] Liu Y, Fukuwatari Y, Okumura K, et al. Immunomodulating Activity of Agaricus brasiliensis KA21 in Mice and in Human Volunteers. *Evid Based Complement Alternat Med.* 2008 Jun;5(2):205-19.

[273] Motoi M, Motoi A, Yamanaka D, et al. Open-Label Study of the Influence of Food Containing the Royal Sun Mushroom, Agaricus brasiliensis KA21 (Higher Basidiomycetes), on the Quality of Life of Healthy Human Volunteers. *Int J Med Mushrooms.* 2015;17(9):799-817.

[274] Szychowski KA, Skora B, Pomianek T, et al. Inonotus obliquus – from folk medicine to clinical use. *J Tradit Complement Med.* 2021 Jul;11(4):293-302.

[275] Xin X, Qu J, Veeraraghavan VP, et al. Assessment of the Gastroprotective Effect of the Chaga Medicinal Mushroom, Inonotus obliquus (Agaricomycetes), Against the Gastric Mucosal Ulceration Induced by Ethanol in Experimental Rats. *Int J Med Mushrooms.* 2019;21(8):805-816.

[276] Chen YF, Zheng JJ, Qu C, et al. Inonotus obliquus polysaccharide ameliorates dextran sulphate sodium induced colitis involving modulation of Th1/Th2 and Th17/Treg balance. *Artif Cells Nanomed Biotechnol.* 2019 Dec;47(1):757-766.

[277] Choi SY, Hur SJ, An CS, et al. Anti-inflammatory effects of Inonotus obliquus in colitis induced by dextran sodium sulfate. *J Biomed Biotechnol.* 2010;2010:943516.

[278] Zhang J, Cheng S, Liang J, et al. Polysaccharide from fermented mycelium of Inonotus obliquus attenuates the ulcerative colitis and adjusts the gut microbiota in mice. *Microb Pathog.* 2023 Apr;177:105990.

[279] Sun R, Jin D, Fei F, et al. Mushroom polysaccharides from Grifola frondosa (Dicks.) Gray and Inonotus obliquus (Fr.) Pilat ameliorated dextran sulfate sodium-induced colitis in mice by global modulation of systemic metabolism and the gut microbiota. *Front Pharmacol.* 2023 Jun 7;14:1172963.

[280] Mishra SK, Kang JH, Kim DK, et al. Orally administered aqueous extract of Inonotus obliquus ameliorates acute inflammation in dextran sulfate sodium (DSS)-induced colitis in mice. *J Ethnopharmacol.* 2012 Sep 28;143(2):524-32.

[281] Li J, Qu C, Li F, et al. Inonotus obliquus Polysaccharide Ameliorates Azoxymethane/Dextran Sulfate Sodium-Induced Colitis-Associated Cancer in Mice via Activation of the NLRP3 Inflammasome. *Front Pharmacol.* 2021 Feb 2;11:621835.

[282] Ji Y, Tao T, Zhang J, et al. Comparison of effects on colitis-associated tumorigenesis and gut microbiota in mice between Ophiocordyceps sinensis and Cordyceps militaris. *Phytomedicine*. 2021 Sep;90:153653.

[283] Zhao Y, Zheng W. Deciphering the antitumoral potential of the bioactive metabolites from medicinal mushroom Inonotus obliquus. *J Ethnopharmacol*. 2021 Jan 30;265:113321.

[284] Gery A, Dubreule C, Andre V, et al. Chaga (Inonotus obliquus), a Future Potential Medicinal Fungus in Oncology? A Chemical Study and a Comparison of the Cytotoxicity Against Human Lung Adenocarcinoma Cells (A549) and Human Bronchial Epithelial Cells (BEAS-2B). *Integr Cancer Ther*. 2018 Sep;17(3):832-843.

[285] Jiang S, Shi F, Lin H, et al. Inonotus obliquus polysaccharides induces apoptosis of lung cancer cells and alters energy metabolism via the LKB1/AMPK axis. *Int J Biol Macromol*. 2020 May 15;151:1277-1286.

[286] Zhao F, Mai Q, Ma J, et al. Triterpenoids from Inonotus obliquus and their antitumor activities. *Fitoterapia*. 2015 Mar;101:34-40.

[287] Liu C, Zhao C, Pan HH, et al. Chemical constituents from Inonotus obliquus and their biological activities. *J Nat Prod*. 2014 Jan 24;77(1):35-41.

[288] Lee KR, Lee JS, Song JE, et al. Inonotus obliquus-derived polysaccharide inhibits the migration and invasion of human non-small cell lung carcinoma cells via suppression of MMP-2 and MMP-9. *Int J Oncol*. 2014 Dec;45(6):2533-40.

[289] Wang Q, Mu H, Zhang L, et al. Characterization of two water-soluble lignin metabolites with antiproliferative activities from Inonotus obliquus. *Int J Biol Macromol*. 2015 Mar;74:507-14.

[290] Mazurkiewicz W, Rydel K, Pogocki D, et al. Separation of an aqueous extract Inonotus obliquus (Chaga). A novel look at the efficiency of its influence on proliferation of A549 human lung carcinoma cells. *Acta Pol Pharm*. 2010 Jul-Aug;67(4):397-406.

[291] Zhong XH, Wang LB, Sun DZ. Effects of inotodiol extracts from inonotus obliquus on proliferation cycle and apoptotic gene of human lung adenocarcinoma cell line A549. *Chin J Integr Med*. 2011 Mar;17(3):218-23.

[292] Baek J, Roh HS, Baek KH, et al. Bioactivity-based analysis and chemical characterization of cytotoxic constituents from Chaga mushroom (Inonotus obliquus) that induce apoptosis in human lung adenocarcinoma cells. *J Ethnopharmacol*. 2018 Oct 5;224:63-75.

[293] Alzand Kim Unal S, Boufaris MSM. Lanostane-Type Triterpenes and Abietane-Type Diterpene from the Sclerotia of Chaga Medicinal Mushroom, Inonotus obliquus (Agaricomycetes), and Their Biological Activities. *Int J Med Mushrooms*. 2018;20(6):507-516.

[294] Chung MJ, Chung CK, Jeong Y, et al. Anticancer activity of subfractions containing pure compounds of Chaga mushroom (Inonotus obliquus) extract in human cancer cells and in Balbc/c mice bearing Sarcoma-180 cells. *Nutr Res Pract*. 2010 Jun;4(3):177-82.

[295] Nakajima Y, Nishida H, Matsugo S, et al. Cancer cell cytotoxicity of extracts and small phenolic compounds from Chaga [Inonotus obliquus (persoon) Pilat]. *J Med Food*. 2009 Jun;12(3):501-7.

[296] Sun Y, Yin T, Chen XH, et al. In vitro antitumor activity and structure characterization of ethanol extracts from wild and cultivated Chaga medicinal mushroom, Inonotus obliquus (Pers.:Fr.) Pilát (Aphyllophoromycetideae). *Int J Med Mushrooms*. 2011;13(2):121-30.

[297] Lemieszek MK, Langner E, Kaczor J, et al. Anticancer effects of fraction isolated from fruiting bodies of Chaga medicinal mushroom, Inonotus obliquus (Pers.:Fr.) Pilát (Aphyllophoromycetideae): in vitro studies. *Int J Med Mushrooms*. 2011;13(2):131-43.

[298] Arata S, Watanabe J, Maeda M, et al. Continuous intake of the Chaga mushroom (Inonotus obliquus) aqueous extract suppresses cancer progression and maintains body temperature in mice. *Heliyon*. 2016 May 12;2(5):e00111.

[299] Tsai CC, Li YS, Lin PP. Inonotus obliquus extract induces apoptosis in the human colorectal carcinoma's HCT-116 cell line. *Biomed Pharmacother*. 2017 Dec;96:1119-1126.

[300] Zhao F, Mai Q, Ma J, et al. Triterpenoids from Inonotus obliquus and their antitumor activities. *Fitoterapia*. 2015 Mar;101:34-40.

[301] Kang JH, Jang JE, Mishra SK, et al. Ergosterol peroxide from Chaga mushroom (Inonotus obliquus) exhibits anti-cancer activity by down-regulation of the β-catenin pathway in colorectal cancer. *J Ethnopharmacol*. 2015 Sep 15;173:303-12.

[302] Lee SH, Hwang HS, Yun JW. Antitumor activity of water extract of a mushroom, Inonotus obliquus, against HT-29 human colon cancer cells. *Phytother Res*. 2009 Dec;23(12):1784-9.

[303] Lee HS, Kim EJ, Kim SH. Ethanol extract of Innotus obliquus (Chaga mushroom) induces G1 cell cycle arrest in HT-29 human colon cancer cells. *Nutr Res Pract*. 2015 Apr;9(2):111-6.

[304] Kuriyama I, Nakajima Y, Nishida H, et al. Inhibitory effects of low molecular weight polyphenolics from Inonotus obliquus on human DNA topoisomerase activity and cancer cell proliferation. *Mol Med Rep*. 2013 Aug;8(2):535-42.

[305] Hu H, Zhang Z, Lei Z, et al. Comparative study of antioxidant activity and antiproliferative effect of hot water and ethanol extracts from the mushroom Inonotus obliquus. *J Biosci Bioeng*. 2009 Jan;107(1):42-8.

[306] Kim J, Yang SC, Hwang AY, et al. Composition of Triterpenoids in Inonotus obliquus and Their Anti-Proliferative Activity on Cancer Cell Lines. *Molecules*. 2020 Sep 6;25(18):4066.

[307] Zhou F, Zia G, Chen L, et al. Chemical constituents from Inonotus obliquus and their antitumor activities. *J Nat Med*. 2016 Oct;70(4):721-30.

[308] Shan P, Wang C, Chen H, et al. Inonotsutriol E from Inonotus obliquus exhibits promising anti breast cancer activity via regulating the JAK2/STAT3 signaling pathway. *Bioorg Chem*. 2023 Oct;139:106741.

[309] Lee MG, Kwon YS, Nam KS, et al. Chaga mushroom extract induces autophagy via the AMPK-mTOR signaling pathway in breast cancer cells. *J Ethnopharmacol*. 2021 Jun 28;274:114081.

[310] Ma L, Chen H, Dong P, et al. Anti-inflammatory and anticancer activities of extracts and compounds from the mushroom Inonotus obliquus. *Food Chem*. 2013 Aug 15;139(1-4):503-8.

[311] Chung MJ, Chung CK, Jeong Y, et al. Anticancer activity of subfractions containing pure compounds of Chaga mushroom (Inonotus obliquus) extract in human cancer cells and in Balbc/c mice bearing Sarcoma-180 cells. *Nutr Res Pract*. 2010 Jun;4(3):177-82.

[312] Kim J, Yang SC, Hwang AY, et al. Composition of Triterpenoids in Inonotus obliquus and Their Anti-Proliferative Activity on Cancer Cell Lines. *Molecules.* 2020 Sep 6;25(18):4066.

[313] Ma L, Chen H, Dong P, et al. Anti-inflammatory and anticancer activities of extracts and compounds from the mushroom Inonotus obliquus. *Food Chem.* 2013 Aug 15;139(1-4):503-8.

[314] Kim J, Yang SC, Hwang AY, et al. Composition of Triterpenoids in Inonotus obliquus and Their Anti-Proliferative Activity on Cancer Cell Lines. *Molecules.* 2020 Sep 6;25(18):4066.

[315] Fan L, Ding S, Ai L, et al. Antitumor and immunomodulatory activity of water-soluble polysaccharide from Inonotus obliquus. *Carbohydr Polym.* 2012 Oct 1;90(2):870-4.

[316] Chung MJ, Chung CK, Jeong Y, et al. Anticancer activity of subfractions containing pure compounds of Chaga mushroom (Inonotus obliquus) extract in human cancer cells and in Balbc/c mice bearing Sarcoma-180 cells. *Nutr Res Pract.* 2010 Jun;4(3):177-82.

[317] Su B, Yan X, Li Y, et al. Effects of Inonotus obliquus Polysaccharides on Proliferation, Invasion, Migration, and Apoptosis of Osteosarcoma Cells. *Anal Cell Pathol (Amst).* 2020 Nov 17;2020:4282036.

[318] Zhao F, Mai Q, Ma J, et al. Triterpenoids from Inonotus obliquus and their antitumor activities. *Fitoterapia.* 2015 Mar;101:34-40.

[319] Rzymowska J. The effect of aqueous extracts from Inonotus obliquus on the mitotic index and enzyme activities. *Boll Chim Farm.* 1998 Jan;137(1):13-5.

[320] Chung MJ, Chung CK, Jeong Y, et al. Anticancer activity of subfractions containing pure compounds of Chaga mushroom (Inonotus obliquus) extract in human cancer cells and in Balbc/c mice bearing Sarcoma-180 cells. *Nutr Res Pract.* 2010 Jun;4(3):177-82.

[321] Jarosz A, Skórska M, Rzymowska J, et al. Effect of the extracts from fungus Inonotus obliquus on catalase level in HeLa and nocardia cells. *Acta Biochim Pol.* 1990;37(1):149-51.

[322] Zhang SD, Yu L, Wang P, et al. Inotodiol inhibits cells migration and invasion and induces apoptosis via p53-dependent pathway in HeLa cells. *Phytomedicine.* 2019 Jul;60:152957.

[323] Kuriyama I, Nakajima Y, Nishida H, et al. Inhibitory effects of low molecular weight polyphenolics from Inonotus obliquus on human DNA topoisomerase activity and cancer cell proliferation. *Mol Med Rep.* 2013 Aug;8(2):535-42.

[324] Burczyk J, Gawron A, Slotwinska M, et al. Antimitotic activity of aqueous extracts of Inonotus obliquus. *Boll Chim Farm.* 1996 May;135(5):306-9.

[325] Youn MJ, Kim JK, Park SY, et al. Potential anticancer properties of the water extract of Inonotus [corrected] obliquus by induction of apoptosis in melanoma B16-F10 cells. *J Ethnopharmacol.* 2009 Jan 21;121(2):221-8.

[326] Song Y, Hui J, Kou W, et al. Identification of Inonotus obliquus and analysis of antioxidation and antitumor activities of polysaccharides. *Curr Microbiol.* 2008 Nov;57(5):454-62.

[327] Youn MJ, Kim JK, Park SY, et al. Chaga mushroom (Inonotus obliquus) induces G0/G1 arrest and apoptosis in human hepatoma HepG2 cells. *World J Gastroenterol.* 2008 Jan 28;14(4):511-7.

[328] Alzand Kim Unal S, Boufaris MSM. Lanostane-Type Triterpenes and Abietane-Type Diterpene from the Sclerotia of Chaga Medicinal Mushroom, Inonotus obliquus (Agaricomycetes), and Their Biological Activities. *Int J Med Mushrooms.* 2018;20(6):507-516.

[329] Park JR, Park JS, Jo EH, et al. Reversal of the TPA-induced inhibition of gap junctional intercellular communication by Chaga mushroom (Inonotus obliquus) extracts: effects on MAP kinases. *Biofactors.* 2006;27(1-4):147-55.

[330] Ryu K, Nakamura S, Nakashima S, et al. Triterpenes with Anti-invasive Activity from Sclerotia of Inonotus obliquus. *Nat Prod Commun.* 2017 Feb;12(2):225-228.

[331] Ning X, Luo Q, Li C, et al. Inhibitory effects of a polysaccharide extract from the Chaga medicinal mushroom, Inonotus obliquus (higher Basidiomycetes), on the proliferation of human neurogliocytoma cells. *Int J Med Mushrooms.* 2014;16(1):29-36.

[332] Chen Y, Gu X, Huang SQ, et al. Optimization of ultrasonic/microwave assisted extraction (UMAE) of polysaccharides from Inonotus obliquus and evaluation of its anti-tumor activities. *Int J Biol Macromol.* 2010 May 1;46(4):429-35.

[333] Kuriyama I, Nakajima Y, Nishida H, et al. Inhibitory effects of low molecular weight polyphenolics from Inonotus obliquus on human DNA topoisomerase activity and cancer cell proliferation. *Mol Med Rep.* 2013 Aug;8(2):535-42.

[334] Abugomaa A, Elbadawy M, Ishihara Y, et al. Anti-cancer activity of Chaga mushroom (Inonotus obliquus) against dog bladder cancer organoids. *Front Pharmacol.* 2023 Apr 19;14:1159516.

[335] Lee KR, Lee JS, Kim YR, et al. Polysaccharide from Inonotus obliquus inhibits migration and invasion in B16-F10 cells by suppressing MMP-2 and MMP-9 via downregulation of NF-κB signaling pathway. *Oncol Rep.* 2014 May;31(5):2447-53.

[336] Lee KR, Lee JS, Lee S, et al. Polysaccharide isolated from the liquid culture broth of Inonotus obliquus suppresses invasion of B16-F10 melanoma cells via AKT/NF-κB signaling pathway. *Mol Med Rep.* 2016 Nov;14(5):4429-4435.

[337] Taji S, Yamada T, Wada S, et al. Lanostane-type triterpenoids from the sclerotia of Inonotus obliquus possessing anti-tumor promoting activity. *Eur J Med Chem.* 2008 Nov;43(11):2373-9.

[338] Nakata T, Yamada T, Taji S, et al. Structure determination of inonotsuoxides A and B and in vivo anti-tumor promoting activity of inotodiol from the sclerotia of Inonotus obliquus. *Bioorg Med Chem.* 2007 Jan 1;15(1):257-64.

[339] Fang J, Gao S, Islam R, et al. Extracts of Phellinus linteus, Bamboo (Sasa senanensis) Leaf and Chaga Mushroom (Inonotus obliquus) Exhibit Antitumor Activity through Activating Innate Immunity. *Nutrients.* 2020 Jul 29;12(8):2279.

[340] Nomura M, Takahashi T, Uesugi A, et al. Inotodiol, a lanostane triterpenoid, from Inonotus obliquus inhibits cell proliferation through caspase-3-dependent apoptosis. *Anticancer Res.* 2008 Sep-Oct;28(5A):2691-6.

[341] Zhao Y, Zheng W. Deciphering the antitumoral potential of the bioactive metabolites from medicinal mushroom Inonotus obliquus. *J Ethnopharmacol.* 2021 Jan 30;265:113321.

[342] Javed S, Mitchell K, Sidsworth D, et al. Inonotus obliquus attenuates histamine-induced microvascular inflammation. *PLoS One.* 2019 Aug 22;14(8):e0220776.

[343] Sun Y, Deng X, Li Z, et al. Polysaccharide derived from Inonotus obliquus inhibits lipopolysaccharide-induced acute endometritis in mice. *Am J Transl Res.* 2022 Nov 15;14(11):8332-8342.

344 Hu B, Dong Y, Zhou W, et al. Effect of Inonotus obliquus polysaccharide on composition of the intestinal flora in mice with acute endometritis. *PLoS One*. 2021 Nov 5;16(11):e0259570.

345 Luo LS, Wang Y, Dai LJ, et al. Triterpenoid acids from medicinal mushroom Inonotus obliquus (Chaga) alleviate hyperuricemia and inflammation in hyperuricemic mice: Possible inhibitory effects on xanthine oxidase activity. *J Food Biochem*. 2022 Mar;46(3):e13932.

346 Yong T, Chen S, Liang D, et al. Actions of Inonotus obliquus against Hyperuricemia through XOD and Bioactives Screened by Molecular Modeling. *Int J Mol Sci*. 2018 Oct 18;19(10):3222.

347 Song J, Chen M, Meng F, et al. Studies on the interaction mechanism between xanthine oxidase and osmundacetone: Molecular docking, multi-spectroscopy and dynamical simulation. *Spectrochim Acta A Mol Biomol Spectrosc*. 2023 Oct 15;299:122861.

348 Kim HG, Yoon DH, Kim CH, et al. Ethanol extract of Inonotus obliquus inhibits lipopolysaccharide-induced inflammation in RAW 264.7 macrophage cells. *J Med Food*. 2007 Mar;10(1):80-9.

349 Ma L, Chen H, Dong P, et al. Anti-inflammatory and anticancer activities of extracts and compounds from the mushroom Inonotus obliquus. *Food Chem*. 2013 Aug 15;139(1-4):503-8.

350 Debnath T, Park SR, Kim DH, et al. Anti-oxidant and anti-inflammatory activities of Inonotus obliquus and germinated brown rice extracts. *Molecules*. 2013 Aug 2;18(8):9293-304.

351 Van Q, Nayak BN, Reimer M, et al. Anti-inflammatory effect of Inonotus obliquus, Polygala senega L., and Viburnum trilobum in a cell screening assay. *J Ethnopharmacol*. 2009 Sep 25;125(3):487-93.

352 Alhallaf W, Perkins LB. The Anti-Inflammatory Properties of Chaga Extracts Obtained by Different Extraction Methods against LPS-Induced RAW 264.7. *Molecules*. 2022 Jun 30;27(13):4207.

353 Park YM, Won JH, Kim YH, et al. In vivo and in vitro anti-inflammatory and anti-nociceptive effects of the methanol extract of Inonotus obliquus. *J Ethnopharmacol*. 2005 Oct 3;101(1-3):120-8.

354 Sun R, Jin D, Fei F, et al. Mushroom polysaccharides from Grifola frondosa (Dicks.) Gray and Inonotus obliquus (Fr.) Pilat ameliorated dextran sulfate sodium-induced colitis in mice by global modulation of systemic metabolism and the gut microbiota. *Front Pharmacol*. 2023 Jun 7;14:1172963.

355 Xu T, Li G, Wang X, et al. Inonotus obliquus polysaccharide ameliorates serum profiling in STZ-induced diabetic mice model. *BMC Chem*. 2021 Dec 17;15(1):64.

356 Chen SD, Yong TQ, Xiao C, et al. Inhibitory effect of triterpenoids from the mushroom Inonotus obliquus against α-glucosidase and their interaction: Inhibition kinetics and molecular stimulations. *Bioorg Chem*. 2021 Oct;115:105276.

357 Liu P, Xue J, Tong S, et al. Structure Characterization and Hypoglycaemic Activities of Two Polysaccharides from Inonotus obliquus. *Molecules*. 2018 Aug 4;23(8):1948.

358 Wang J, Wang C, Li S, et al. Anti-diabetic effects of Inonotus obliquus polysaccharides in streptozotocin-induced type 2 diabetic mice and potential mechanism via PI3K-Akt signal pathway. *Biomed Pharmacother*. 2017 Nov;95:1669-1677.

359 Ying YM, Zhang LY, Zhang X, et al. Terpenoids with alpha-glucosidase inhibitory activity from the submerged culture of Inonotus obliquus. *Phytochemistry*. 2014 Dec;108:171-6.

360 Xue J, Tong S, Wang Z, et al. Chemical Characterization and Hypoglycaemic Activities In Vitro of Two Polysaccharides from Inonotus obliquus by Submerged Culture. *Molecules*. 2018 Dec 10;23(12):3261.

361 Wang C, Gao X, Santhanam RK, et al. Effects of polysaccharides from Inonotus obliquus and its chromium (III) complex on advanced glycation end-products formation, α-amylase, α-glucosidase activity and H2O2-induced oxidative damage in hepatic L02 cells. *Food Chem Toxicol*. 2018 Jun;116(Pt B):335-345.

362 Joo JI, Kim DH, Yun JW. Extract of Chaga mushroom (Inonotus obliquus) stimulates 3T3-L1 adipocyte differentiation. *Phytother Res*. 2010 Nov;24(11):1592-9.

363 Zhang Y, Zhao Y, Cui H, et al. Comparison of hypoglycemic activity of fermented mushroom of Inonotus obliquus rich in vanadium and wild-growing I. obliquus. *Biol Trace Elem Res*. 2011 Dec;144(1-3):1351-7.

364 Wang C, Chen Z, Pan Y, et al. Anti-diabetic effects of Inonotus obliquus polysaccharides-chromium (III) complex in type 2 diabetic mice and its sub-acute toxicity evaluation in normal mice. *Food Chem Toxicol*. 2017 Oct;108(Pt B):498-509.

365 Diao BZ, Jin WR, Yu XJ. Protective Effect of Polysaccharides from Inonotus obliquus on Streptozotocin-Induced Diabetic Symptoms and Their Potential Mechanisms in Rats. *Evid Based Complement Alternat Med*. 2014;2014:841496.

366 Wang M, Zhao Z, Zhou X, et al. Simultaneous Use of Stimulatory Agents to Enhance the Production and Hypoglycaemic Activity of Polysaccharides from Inonotus obliquus by Submerged Fermentation. *Molecules*. 2019 Dec 2;24(23):4400.

367 Wang J, Hu W, Li L, et al. Antidiabetic activities of polysaccharides separated from Inonotus obliquus via the modulation of oxidative stress in mice with streptozotocin-induced diabetes. *PLoS One*. 2017 Jun 29;12(6):e0180476.

368 Lu X, Chen H, Dong P, et al. Phytochemical characteristics and hypoglycaemic activity of fraction from mushroom Inonotus obliquus. *J Sci Food Agric*. 2010 Jan 30;90(2):276-80.

369 Wang C, Li W, Chen Z, et al. Effects of simulated gastrointestinal digestion in vitro on the chemical properties, antioxidant activity, α-amylase and α-glucosidase inhibitory activity of polysaccharides from Inonotus obliquus. *Food Res Int*. 2018 Jan;103:280-288.

370 Lu X, Zhao Y, Wang C, et al. Necessity of Different Lignocellulose on Exopolysaccharide Synthesis and Its Hypoglycemic Activity In Vitro of Inonotus obliquus. *Appl Biochem Biotechnol*. 2023 Sep 2. Online ahead of print.

371 Gao X, Santhanam RK, Xue Z, et al. Antioxidant, α-amylase and α-glucosidase activity of various solvent fractions of I. obliquus and the preventive role of active fraction against H2 O2 induced damage in hepatic L02 cells as fungisome. *J Food Sci*. 2020 Apr;85(4):1060-1069.

372 Zhang Z, Liang X, Tong L, et al. Effect of Inonotus obliquus (Fr.) Pilat extract on the regulation of glycolipid metabolism via PI3K/Akt and AMPK/ACC pathways in mice. *J Ethnopharmacol*. 2021 Jun 12;273:113963.

373 Lee JH, Hyun CK. Insulin-sensitizing and beneficial lipid-metabolic effects of the water-soluble melanin complex extracted from Inonotus obliquus. *Phytother Res*. 2014 Sep;28(9):1320-8.

374 Sun JE, Ao ZH, Lu ZM, et al. Antihyperglycemic and antilipidperoxidative effects of dry matter of culture broth of Inonotus obliquus in submerged culture on normal and alloxan-diabetes mice. *J Ethnopharmacol*. 2008 Jun 19;118(1):7-13.

375 Sim YC, Lee JS, Lee S, et al. Effects of polysaccharides isolated from Inonotus obliquus against hydrogen peroxide-induced oxidative damage in RINm5F pancreatic β-cells. *Mol Med Rep*. 2016 Nov;14(5):4263-4270.

376 Xu HY, Sun JE, Lu ZM, et al. Beneficial effects of the ethanol extract from the dry matter of a culture broth of Inonotus obliquus in submerged culture on the antioxidant defence system and regeneration of pancreatic beta-cells in experimental diabetes in mice. *Nat Prod Res*. 2010 Apr;24(6):542-53.

377 Ye X, Wu K, Xu L, et al. Methanol extract of Inonotus obliquus improves type 2 diabetes mellitus through modifying intestinal flora. *Front Endocrinol (Lausanne)*. 2023 Jan 6;13:1103972.

378 Chen S, Ma Y, Li H, et al. Anti-diabetic effects of Inonotus obliquus extract in high fat diet combined streptozotocin-induced type 2 diabetic mice. *Nutr Hosp*. 2022 Dec 20;39(6):1256-1263.

379 Yang M, Hu D, Cui Z, et al. Lipid-Lowering Effects of Inonotus obliquus Polysaccharide In Vivo and In Vitro. *Foods*. 2021 Dec 12;10(12):3085.

380 Lin F, Li X, Guo X, et al. Study on the hypolipidemic effect of Inonotus obliquus polysaccharide in hyperlipidemia rats based on the regulation of intestinal flora. *Food Sci Nutr*. 2022 Sep 25;11(1):191-203.

381 Joo JI, Kim DH, Yun JW. Extract of Chaga mushroom (Inonotus obliquus) stimulates 3T3-L1 adipocyte differentiation. *Phytother Res*. 2010 Nov;24(11):1592-9.

382 Hu Y, Sheng Y, Yu M, et al. Antioxidant activity of Inonotus obliquus polysaccharide and its amelioration for chronic pancreatitis in mice. *Int J Biol Macromol*. 2016 Jun;87:348-56.

383 Hu B, Dong Y, Zhou W, et al. Effect of Inonotus obliquus polysaccharide on composition of the intestinal flora in mice with acute endometritis. *PLoS One*. 2021 Nov 5;16(11):e0259570.

384 Hu Y, Teng C, Yu S, et al. Inonotus obliquus polysaccharide regulates gut microbiota of chronic pancreatitis in mice. *AMB Express*. 2017 Dec;7(1):39.

385 Yu J, Xiang H, Xie Q. The difference of regulatory effect of two Inonotus obliquus extracts on high-fat diet mice in relation to the fatty acid elongation function of gut microbiota. *Food Sci Nutr*. 2020 Nov 24;9(1):449-458.

386 Hu B, He X, Tan J, et al. Gender-related differences in the effects of Inonotus obliquus polysaccharide on intestinal microorganisms in SD rats model. *Front Vet Sci*. 2022 Sep 20;9:957053.

387 Lin F, Li X, Guo X, et al. Study on the hypolipidemic effect of Inonotus obliquus polysaccharide in hyperlipidemia rats based on the regulation of intestinal flora. *Food Sci Nutr*. 2022 Sep 25;11(1):191-203.

388 Sun R, Jin D, Fei F, et al. Mushroom polysaccharides from Grifola frondosa (Dicks.) Gray and Inonotus obliquus (Fr.) Pilat ameliorated dextran sulfate sodium-induced colitis in mice by global modulation of systemic metabolism and the gut microbiota. *Front Pharmacol*. 2023 Jun 7;14:1172963.

389 Burmasova MA, Utenaeva AA, Sysoeva EV, et al. Melanins of Inonotus Obliquus: Bifidogenic and Antioxidant Properties. *Biomolecules*. 2019 Jun 24;9(6):248.

390 Ji Y, Tao T, Zhang J, et al. Comparison of effects on colitis-associated tumorigenesis and gut microbiota in mice between Ophiocordyceps sinensis and Cordyceps militaris. *Phytomedicine*. 2021 Sep;90:153653.

391 Su L, Xin C, Yang J, et al. A polysaccharide from Inonotus obliquus ameliorates intestinal barrier dysfunction in mice with type 2 diabetes mellitus. *Int J Biol Macromol*. 2022 Aug 1;214:312-323.

392 Maza PAMA, Lee JH, Kim YS, et al. Inotodiol From Inonotus obliquus Chaga Mushroom Induces Atypical Maturation in Dendritic Cells. *Front Immunol*. 2021 Mar 12;12:650841.

393 Shen D, Feng Y, Zhang X, et al. In Vitro Immunomodulatory Effects of Inonotus obliquus Extracts on Resting M0 Macrophages and LPS-Induced M1 Macrophages. *Evid Based Complement Alternat Med*. 2022 Apr 21;2022:8251344.

394 Ko SK, Jin M, Pyo MY. Inonotus obliquus extracts suppress antigen-specific IgE production through the modulation of Th1/Th2 cytokines in ovalbumin-sensitized mice. *J Ethnopharmacol*. 2011 Oct 11;137(3):1077-82.

395 Harikrishnan R, Balasundaram C, Heo MS. Inonotus obliquus containing diet enhances the innate immune mechanism and disease resistance in olive flounder Paralichythys olivaceus against Uronema marinum. *Fish Shellfish Immunol*. 2012 Jun;32(6):1148-54.

396 Niu H, Song D, Mu H, et al. Investigation of three lignin complexes with antioxidant and immunological capacities from Inonotus obliquus. *Int J Biol Macromol*. 2016 May;86:587-93.

397 Xu X, Li J, Hu Y. Polysaccharides from Inonotus obliquus sclerotia and cultured mycelia stimulate cytokine production of human peripheral blood mononuclear cells in vitro and their chemical characterization. *Int Immunopharmacol*. 2014 Aug;21(2):269-78.

398 Fan L, Ding S, Ai L, et al. Antitumor and immunomodulatory activity of water-soluble polysaccharide from Inonotus obliquus. *Carbohydr Polym*. 2012 Oct 1;90(2):870-4.

399 Kim YR. Immunomodulatory Activity of the Water Extract from Medicinal Mushroom Inonotus obliquus. *Mycobiology*. 2005 Sep;33(3):158-62.

400 Won DP, Lee JS, Kwon DS, et al. Immunostimulating activity by polysaccharides isolated from fruiting body of Inonotus obliquus. *Mol Cells*. 2011 Feb;31(2):165-73.

401 Kim YO, Han SB, Lee HW, et al. Immuno-stimulating effect of the endo-polysaccharide produced by submerged culture of Inonotus obliquus. *Life Sci*. 2005 Sep 23;77(19):2438-56.

402 Sang R, Sun F, Zhou H, et al. Immunomodulatory effects of Inonotus obliquus polysaccharide on splenic lymphocytes infected with Toxoplasma gondii via NF-κB and MAPKs pathways. *Immunopharmacol Immunotoxicol*. 2022 Feb;44(1):129-138.

403 Xu L, Yu Y, Sang R, et al. Inonotus obliquus polysaccharide protects against adverse pregnancy caused by Toxoplasma gondii infection through regulating Th17/Treg balance via TLR4/NF-κB pathway. *Int J Biol Macromol*. 2020 Mar 1;146:832-840.

404 Ding X, Ge B, Wang M, et al. Inonotus obliquus polysaccharide ameliorates impaired reproductive function caused by Toxoplasma gondii infection in male mice via regulating Nrf2-PI3K/AKT pathway. *Int J Biol Macromol*. 2020 May 15;151:449-458.

405 Yan K, Zhou H, Wang M, et al. Inhibitory Effects of Inonotus obliquus Polysaccharide on Inflammatory Response in Toxoplasma gondii-Infected RAW264.7 Macrophages. *Evid Based Complement Alternat Med*. 2021 Dec 29;2021:2245496.

[406] Xu L, Sang R, Yu Y, et al. The polysaccharide from Inonotus obliquus protects mice from Toxoplasma gondii-induced liver injury. *Int J Biol Macromol*. 2019 Mar 15;125:1-8.

[407] Yu J, Xiang H, Xie Q. The difference of regulatory effect of two Inonotus obliquus extracts on high-fat diet mice in relation to the fatty acid elongation function of gut microbiota. *Food Sci Nutr*. 2020 Nov 24;9(1):449-458.

[408] Wu T, Shu Q, Yang K, et al. Ameliorating effects of Inonotus obliquus on high fat diet-induced obese rats. *Acta Biochim Biophys Sin (Shanghai)*. 2015 Sep;47(9):755-7.

[409] Yu J, Xiang JY, Xiang H, et al. Cecal Butyrate (Not Propionate) Was Connected with Metabolism-Related Chemicals of Mice, Based on the Different Effects of the Two Inonotus obliquus Extracts on Obesity and Their Mechanisms. *ACS Omega*. 2020 Jun 30;5(27):16690-16700.

[410] Yun JS, Pahk JW, Lee JS, et al. Inonotus obliquus protects against oxidative stress-induced apoptosis and premature senescence. *Mol Cells*. 2011 May;31(5):423-9.

[411] Wei YM, yang L, Mei WL, et al. Phenolic compounds from the sclerotia of Inonotus obliquus. *Nat Prod Res*. 2022 May;36(9):2413-2417.

[412] Zou CX, Dong SH, Hou ZL, et al. Modified lanostane-type triterpenoids with neuroprotective effects from the fungus Inonotus obliquus. *Bioorg Chem*. 2020 Dec;105:104438.

[413] Zou CX, Wang XB, Lv TM, et al. Flavan derivative enantiomers and drimane sesquiterpene lactones from the Inonotus obliquus with neuroprotective effects. *Bioorg Chem*. 2020 Mar;96:103588.

[414] Xin Y, Zhang Y, Zhang X. Protective Effects of Chaga Medicinal Mushroom, Inonotus obliquus (Agaricomycetes), Extract on β-Amyloid-Induced Neurotoxicity in PC12 Cells and Aging Rats: In Vitro and In Vivo Studies. *Int J Med Mushrooms*. 2021;23(9):55-62.

[415] Giridharan VV, Thandavarayan RA, Konishi T. Amelioration of scopolamine induced cognitive dysfunction and oxidative stress by Inonotus obliquus - a medicinal mushroom. *Food Funct*. 2011 Jun;2(6):320-7.

[416] Kou RW, Xia B, Han R, et al. Neuroprotective effects of a new triterpenoid from edible mushroom on oxidative stress and apoptosis through the BDNF/TrkB/ERK/CREB and Nrf2 signaling pathway in vitro and in vivo. *Food Funct*. 2022 Nov 28;13(23):12121-12134.

[417] Yang W, Chen C, Chen J, et al. PrPSc Inhibition and Cellular Protection of DBL on a Prion-Infected Cultured Cell via Multiple Pathways. *Mol Neurobiol*. 2022 May;59(5):3310-3321.

[418] Han Y, Nan S, Fan J, et al. Inonotus obliquus polysaccharides protect against Alzheimer's disease by regulating Nrf2 signaling and exerting antioxidative and antiapoptotic effects. *Int J Biol Macromol*. 2019 Jun 15;131:769-778.

[419] Wei YM, Yang L, Wang H, et al. Triterpenoids as bivalent and dual inhibitors of acetylcholinesterase/ butyrylcholinesterase from the fruiting bodies of Inonotus obliquus. *Phytochemistry*. 2022 Aug;200:113182.

[420] Kou RW, Han R, Gao YQ, et al. Anti-neuroinflammatory polyoxygenated lanostanoids from Chaga mushroom Inonotus obliquus. *Phytochemistry*. 2021 Apr;184:112647.

[421] Ishfaq PM, Mishra S, Mishra A, et al. Inonotus obliquus aqueous extract prevents histopathological alterations in liver induced by environmental toxicant Microcystin. *Curr Res Pharmacol Drug Discov*. 2022 Jul 8;3:100118.

[422] Li Z, Mei J, Jiang L, Geng C, et al. Chaga Medicinal Mushroom, Inonotus obliquus (Agaricomycetes) Polysaccharides Suppress Tacrine-induced Apoptosis by ROS-scavenging and Mitochondrial Pathway in HepG2 Cells. *Int J Med Mushrooms*. 2019;21(6):583-593.

[423] Alzand Kim Unal S, Boufaris MSM. Lanostane-Type Triterpenes and Abietane-Type Diterpene from the Sclerotia of Chaga Medicinal Mushroom, Inonotus obliquus (Agaricomycetes), and Their Biological Activities. *Int J Med Mushrooms*. 2018;20(6):507-516.

[424] Hong KB, Noh DO, Park Y, et al. Hepatoprotective Activity of Water Extracts from Chaga Medicinal Mushroom, Inonotus obliquus (Higher Basidiomycetes) Against Tert-Butyl Hydroperoxide-Induced Oxidative Liver Injury in Primary Cultured Rat Hepatocytes. *Int J Med Mushrooms*. 2015;17(11):1069-76.

[425] Peng A, Liu Sm Fang L, et al. Inonotus obliquus and its bioactive compounds alleviate non-alcoholic fatty liver disease via regulating FXR/SHP/SREBP-1c axis. *Eur J Pharmacol*. 2022 Apr 15;921:174841.

[426] Wu Y, Cui H, Zhang Y, et al. Inonotus obliquus extract alleviates myocardial ischemia/reperfusion injury by suppressing endoplasmic reticulum stress. *Mol Med Rep*. 2021 Jan;23(1):77.

[427] Chiang KH, Chiu YC, Yar N, et al. Ethanol-Ethyl Acetate Extract on Combined Streptozotocin and Unilateral Nephrectomy-Induced Diabetic Nephropathy in Mice. *Int J Mol Sci*. 2023 Feb 23;24(5):4443.

[428] Zhang Y, Liao H, Shen D, et al. Renal Protective Effects of Inonotus obliquus on High-Fat Diet/Streptozotocin-Induced Diabetic Kidney Disease Rats: Biochemical, Color Doppler Ultrasound and Histopathological Evidence. *Front Pharmacol*. 2022 Jan 17;12:743931.

[429] Li Y, Zhou Y, Wu J, et al. Phelligridin D from Inonotus obliquus attenuates oxidative stress and accumulation of ECM in mesangial cells under high glucose via activating Nrf2. *J Nat Med*. 2021 Sep;75(4):1021-1029.

[430] Chou YJ, Kan WC, Chang CM, et al. Renal Protective Effects of Low Molecular Weight of Inonotus obliquus Polysaccharide (LIOP) on HFD/STZ-Induced Nephropathy in Mice. *Int J Mol Sci*. 2016 Sep 13;17(9):1535.

[431] Duan Q, Tian L, Feng J, et al. Trametenolic Acid Ameliorates the Progression of Diabetic Nephropathy in db/db Mice via Nrf2/HO-1 and NF-κB-Mediated Pathways. *J Immunol Res*. 2022 Aug 30;2022:6151847.

[432] Yoon TJ, Lee SJ, Kim EY, et al. Inhibitory effect of chaga mushroom extract on compound 48/80-induced anaphylactic shock and IgE production in mice. *Int Immunopharmacol*. 2013 Apr;15(4):666-70.

[433] Nguyet TMN, Lomunova M, Le BV, et al. The mast cell stabilizing activity of Chaga mushroom critical for its therapeutic effect on food allergy is derived from inotodiol. *Int Immunopharmacol*. 2018 Jan;54:286-295.

[434] Nguyen TMN, Le HS, Le BV, et al. Anti-allergic effect of inotodiol, a lanostane triterpenoid from Chaga mushroom, via selective inhibition of mast cell function. *Int Immunopharmacol*. 2020 Apr;81:106244

[435] Yan G, Jin G, Li L, et al. [Protective effects and mechanism of Inonotus obliquus on asthmatic mice]. *Zhongguo Zhong Yao Za Zhi*. 2011 Apr;36(8):1067-70.

[436] Chen YM, Chiu WC, Chiu YS. Effect of Inonotus obliquus Extract Supplementation on Endurance Exercise and Energy-Consuming Processes through Lipid Transport in Mice. *Nutrients*. 2022 Nov 25;14(23):5007.

[437] Zhang CJ, Guo JY, Cheng H, et al. Spatial structure and anti-fatigue of polysaccharide from Inonotus obliquus. *Int J Biol Macromol*. 2020 May 15;151:855-860.

[438] Yue Z, Xiuhong Z, Shuyan Y, et al. Effect of Inonotus Obliquus Polysaccharides on physical fatigue in mice. *J Tradit Chin Med*. 2015 Aug;35(4):468-72.

[439] Basal WT, Elfiky A, Eid J. Chaga Medicinal Mushroom Inonotus obliquus (Agaricomycetes) Terpenoids May Interfere with SARS-CoV-2 Spike Protein Recognition of the Host Cell: A Molecular Docking Study. *Int J Med Mushrooms*. 2021;23(3):1-14.

[440] Teplyakova TV, Pyankov OV, Safatov AS, et al. Water Extract of the Chaga Medicinal Mushroom, Inonotus obliquus (Agaricomycetes), Inhibits SARS-CoV-2 Replication in Vero E6 and Vero Cell Culture Experiments. *Int J Med Mushrooms*. 2022;24(2):23-30.

[441] Shipovalov AV, Kudrov GA, Kartashov MY, et al. [Antiviral activity of basidial fungus Inonotus obliquus aqueous extract against SARS-CoV-2 virus (Coronaviridae: Betacoronavirus: Sarbecovirus) in vivo in BALB/c mice model]. *Vopr Virusol*. 2023 May 18;68(2):152-160.

[442] Eid JI, Das B, Al-Tuwaijri MM, et al. Targeting SARS-CoV-2 with Chaga mushroom: An in silico study toward developing a natural antiviral compound. *Food Sci Nutr*. 2021 Oct 20;9(12):6513-6523.

[443] Elshemey WM, Elfiky AA, Ibrahim IM, et al. Interference of Chaga mushroom terpenoids with the attachment of SARS-CoV-2; in silico perspective. *Comput Biol Med*. 2022 Jun;145:105478.

[444] Shibnev VA, Garaev TM, Finogenova MP, et al. [Antiviral activity of aqueous extracts of the birch fungus Inonotus obliquus on the human immunodeficiency virus]. *Vopr Virusol*. 2015;60(2):35-8.

[445] Teplyakova TV, Ilyicheva TN, Kosogova TA, et al. Medicinal Mushrooms against Influenza Viruses. *Int J Med Mushrooms*. 2021;23(2):1-11.

[446] Shibnev VA, Mishin DV, Garaev TM, et al. Antiviral activity of Inonotus obliquus fungus extract towards infection caused by hepatitis C virus in cell cultures. *Bull Exp Biol Med*. 2011 Sep;151(5):612-4.

[447] Pan HH, Yu XT, Li T, et al. Aqueous extract from a Chaga medicinal mushroom, Inonotus obliquus (higher Basidiomycetes), prevents herpes simplex virus entry through inhibition of viral-induced membrane fusion. *Int J Med Mushrooms*. 2013;15(1):29-38.

[448] Polkovnikova MV, Nosik NN, Garaev TM, et al. [A study of the antiherpetic activity of the chaga mushroom (Inonotus obliquus) extracts in the Vero cells infected with the herpes simplex virus]. *Vopr Virusol*. 2014 Mar-Apr;59(2):45-8.

[449] Tian J, Hu X, Liu D, et al. Identification of Inonotus obliquus polysaccharide with broad-spectrum antiviral activity against multi-feline viruses. *Int J Biol Macromol*. 2017 Feb;95:160-167.

[450] Seetaha S, Ratanabunyong S, Tabtimmai L, et al. Anti-feline immunodeficiency virus reverse transcriptase properties of some medicinal and edible mushrooms. *Vet World*. 2020 Sep;13(9):1798-1806.

[451] Seo DJ, Choi C. Inhibition of Murine Norovirus and Feline Calicivirus by Edible Herbal Extracts. *Food Environ Virol*. 2017 Mar;9(1):35-44.

[452] Glamočlija J, Ćirić A, Nikolić M, et al. Chemical characterization and biological activity of Chaga (Inonotus obliquus), a medicinal "mushroom". *J Ethnopharmacol*. 2015 Mar 13;162:323-32.

[453] Liao H, Jia D, Zhao X, et al. Effects of Chaga Medicinal Mushroom Inonotus obliquus (Agaricomycetes) Extracts on NOS-cGMP-PDE5 Pathway in Rat Penile Smooth Muscle Cells. *Int J Med Mushrooms*. 2020;22(10):979-990.

[454] Sagayama K, Tanaka N, Fukumoto T, et al. Lanostane-type triterpenes from the sclerotium of Inonotus obliquus (Chaga mushrooms) as proproliferative agents on human follicle dermal papilla cells. *J Nat Med*. 2019 Jun;73(3):597-601.

[455] Yan ZF, Yang Y, Tian FH, et al. Inhibitory and Acceleratory Effects of Inonotus obliquus on Tyrosinase Activity and Melanin Formation in B16 Melanoma Cells. *Evid Based Complement Alternat Med*. 2014;2014:259836.

[456] Eid JI, Al-Tuwaijri MM, Mohanty S, et al. Chaga mushroom (Inonotus obliquus) polysaccharides exhibit genoprotective effects in UVB-exposed embryonic zebrafish (Danio rerio) through coordinated expression of DNA repair genes. *Heliyon*. 2021 Feb 4;7(2):e06003.

[457] Ham SS, Kim SH, Moon SY, et al. Antimutagenic effects of subfractions of Chaga mushroom (Inonotus obliquus) extract. *Mutat Res*. 2009 Jan;672(1):55-9.

[458] Burmasova MA, Utenaeva AA, Sysoeva EV, et al. Melanins of Inonotus Obliquus: Bifidogenic and Antioxidant Properties. *Biomolecules*. 2019 Jun 24;9(6):248.

[459] Wang Y, Ouyang F, Teng C, et al. Optimization for the extraction of polyphenols from Inonotus obliquus and its antioxidation activity. *Prep Biochem Biotechnol*. 2021;51(9):852-859.

[460] Cui Y, Kim DS, Park KC. Antioxidant effect of Inonotus obliquus. *J Ethnopharmacol*. 2005 Jan 4;96(1-2):79-85.

[461] Mu H, Zhang A, Zhang W, et al. Antioxidative properties of crude polysaccharides from Inonotus obliquus. *Int J Mol Sci*. 2012;13(7):9194-9206.

[462] Hwang BS, Lee IK, Yun BS. Phenolic compounds from the fungus Inonotus obliquus and their antioxidant properties. *J Antibiot (Tokyo)*. 2016 Feb;69(2):108-10.

[463] Zhao W, Huang P, Zhu Z, et al. Production of phenolic compounds and antioxidant activity via bioconversion of wheat straw by Inonotus obliquus under submerged fermentation with the aid of a surfactant. *J Sci Food Agric*. 2021 Feb;101(3):1021-1029.

[464] Huang SQ, Ding S, Fan L. Antioxidant activities of five polysaccharides from Inonotus obliquus. *Int J Biol Macromol*. 2012 Jun 1;50(5):1183-7.

[465] Song Y, Hui J, Kou W, et al. Identification of Inonotus obliquus and analysis of antioxidation and antitumor activities of polysaccharides. *Curr Microbiol*. 2008 Nov;57(5):454-62.

[466] Zhang N, Chen H, Ma L, et al. Physical modifications of polysaccharide from Inonotus obliquus and the antioxidant properties. *Int J Biol Macromol*. 2013 Mar;54:209-15.

[467] Du X, Mu H, Zhou S, et al. Chemical analysis and antioxidant activity of polysaccharides extracted from Inonotus obliquus sclerotia. *Int J Biol Macromol*. 2013 Nov;62:691-6.

468 Xu X, Quan L, Shen M. Effect of chemicals on production, composition and antioxidant activity of polysaccharides of Inonotus obliquus. *Int J Biol Macromol*. 2015;77:143-50.

469 Debnath T, Park SR, Kim DH, et al. Anti-oxidant and anti-inflammatory activities of Inonotus obliquus and germinated brown rice extracts. *Molecules*. 2013 Aug 2;18(8):9293-304.

470 Ma L, Chen H, Zhang Y, et al. Chemical modification and antioxidant activities of polysaccharide from mushroom Inonotus obliquus. *Carbohydr Polym*. 2012 Jun 20;89(2):371-8.

471 Liang L, Zhang Z, Wang H. Antioxidant activities of extracts and subfractions from Inonotus Obliquus. *Int J Food Sci Nutr*. 2009;60 Suppl 2:175-84.

472 Xu X, Hu Y, Quan L. Production of bioactive polysaccharides by Inonotus obliquus under submerged fermentation supplemented with lignocellulosic biomass and their antioxidant activity. *Bioprocess Biosyst Eng*. 2014 Dec;37(12):2483-92.

473 Eid JI, Das B. Molecular insights and cell cycle assessment upon exposure to Chaga (Inonotus obliquus) mushroom polysaccharides in zebrafish (Danio rerio). *Sci Rep*. 2020 May 4;10(1):7406.

474 Lee IK, Kim YS, Jang YW, et al. New antioxidant polyphenols from the medicinal mushroom Inonotus obliquus. *Bioorg Med Chem Lett*. 2007 Dec 15;17(24):6678-81.

475 Nakajima Y, Sato Y, Konishi T. Antioxidant small phenolic ingredients in Inonotus obliquus (persoon) Pilat (Chaga). *Chem Pharm Bull (Tokyo)*. 2007 Aug;55(8):1222-6.

476 Lin SY, Yeh CC, Liang CH, et al. Preparation of Chaga medicinal mushroom, Inonotus obliquus-fermented rice using solid-state fermentation and its taste quality and antioxidant property. *Int J Med Mushrooms*. 2012;14(6):581-92.

477 Wang C, Li W, Chen Z, et al. Effects of simulated gastrointestinal digestion in vitro on the chemical properties, antioxidant activity, α-amylase and α-glucosidase inhibitory activity of polysaccharides from Inonotus obliquus. *Food Res Int*. 2018 Jan;103:280-288.

478 Chen H, Yan M, Zhu J, et al. Enhancement of exo-polysaccharide production and antioxidant activity in submerged cultures of Inonotus obliquus by lignocellulose decomposition. *J Ind Microbiol Biotechnol*. 2011 Feb;38(2):291-8.

479 Fu L, Chen H, Dong P, et al. Effects of ultrasonic treatment on the physicochemical properties and DPPH radical scavenging activity of polysaccharides from mushroom Inonotus obliquus. *J Food Sci*. 2010 May;75(4):C322-7.

480 Xu X, Shen M, Quan L. Stimulatory Agents Simultaneously Improving the Production and Antioxidant Activity of Polyphenols from Inonotus obliquus by Submerged Fermentation. *Appl Biochem Biotechnol*. 2015 Jul;176(5):1237-50.

481 Zheng W, Zhang M, Zhao Y, et al. Analysis of antioxidant metabolites by solvent extraction from sclerotia of Inonotus obliquus (Chaga). *Phytochem Anal*. 2011 Mar-Apr;22(2):95-102.

482 Xiang Y, Xu X, Li J. Chemical properties and antioxidant activity of exopolysaccharides fractions from mycelial culture of Inonotus obliquus in a ground corn stover medium. *Food Chem*. 2012 Oct 15;134(4):1899-905.

483 Zheng W, Zhang M, Zhao Y, et al. NMR-based metabonomic analysis on effect of light on production of antioxidant phenolic compounds in submerged cultures of Inonotus obliquus. *Bioresour Technol*. 2009 Oct;100(19):4481-7.

484 Hu H, Zhang Z, Lei Z, et al. Comparative study of antioxidant activity and antiproliferative effect of hot water and ethanol extracts from the mushroom Inonotus obliquus. *J Biosci Bioeng*. 2009 Jan;107(1):42-8.

485 Gao X, Santhanam RK, Xue Z, et al. Antioxidant, α-amylase and α-glucosidase activity of various solvent fractions of I. obliquus and the preventive role of active fraction against H2 O2 induced damage in hepatic L02 cells as fungisome. *J Food Sci*. 2020 Apr;85(4):1060-1069.

486 Chen H, Xu X, Zhu Y. Optimization of hydroxyl radical scavenging activity of exo-polysaccharides from Inonotus obliquus in submerged fermentation using response surface methodology. *J Microbiol Biotechnol*. 2010 Apr;20(4):835-43.

487 Hu Y, Sheng Y, Yu M, et al. Antioxidant activity of Inonotus obliquus polysaccharide and its amelioration for chronic pancreatitis in mice. *Int J Biol Macromol*. 2016 Jun;87:348-56.

488 Zhao FQ, Yan L, Cui XH, et al. [Triterpenoids from Inonotus obliquus protect mice against oxidative damage induced by CCl4]. *Yao Xue Xue Bao*. 2012 May;47(5):680-4.

489 Nakajima Y, Nishida H, Nakamura Y, et al. Prevention of hydrogen peroxide-induced oxidative stress in PC12 cells by 3,4-dihydroxybenzalacetone isolated from Chaga (Inonotus obliquus (persoon) Pilat). *Free Radic Biol Med*. 2009 Oct 15;47(8):1154-61.

490 Ikemoto MJ, Aihara Y, Ishii N, et al. 3,4-Dihydroxybenzalacetone Inhibits the Propagation of Hydrogen Peroxide-Induced Oxidative Effect via Secretory Components from SH-SY5Y Cells. *Biol Pharm Bull*. 2023;46(4):599-607.

491 Park YK, Lee HB, Jeon EJ, et al. Chaga mushroom extract inhibits oxidative DNA damage in human lymphocytes as assessed by comet assay. *Biofactors*. 2004;21(1-4):109-12.

492 Han SH, Ahn Y, Lee HJ, et al. Antioxidant and Immunostimulatory Activities of a Submerged Culture of Cordyceps sinensis Using Spent Coffee. *Foods*. 2021 Jul 22;10(8):1697.

493 Li J, Cai H, Sun H, et al. Extracts of Cordyceps sinensis inhibit breast cancer growth through promoting M1 macrophage polarization via NF-κB pathway activation. *J Ethnopharmacol*. 2020 Oct 5;260:112969.

494 Cai H, Li J, Gu B, et al. Extracts of Cordyceps sinensis inhibit breast cancer cell metastasis via down-regulation of metastasis-related cytokines expression. *J Ethnopharmacol*. 2018 Mar 25;214:106-112.

495 Lee EJ, Jang KH, Im SY, et al. Physico-chemical properties and cytotoxic potential of Cordyceps sinensis metabolites. *Nat Prod Res*. 2015;29(5):455-9.

496 Sang Q, Pan Y, Jiang Z, et al. HPLC determination of massoia lactone in fermented Cordyceps sinensis mycelium Cs-4 and its anticancer activity in vitro. *J Food Biochem*. 2020 Sep;44(9):e13336.

497 Wu JY, Zhang QX, Leung PH. Inhibitory effects of ethyl acetate extract of Cordyceps sinensis mycelium on various cancer cells in culture and B16 melanoma in C57BL/6 mice. *Phytomedicine*. 2007 Jan;14(1):43-9.

498 Wang D, Zhang Y, Lu J, et al. Cordycepin, a Natural Antineoplastic Agent, Induces Apoptosis of Breast Cancer Cells via Caspase-dependent Pathways. *Nat Prod Commun*. 2016 Jan;11(1):63-8.

499 Ko BS, Lu YJ, Yao WL, et al. Cordycepin regulates GSK-3β/β-catenin signaling in human leukemia cells. *PLoS One*. 2013 Sep 26;8(9):e76320.

[500] Qi W, Zhou X, Wang J, et al. Cordyceps sinensis polysaccharide inhibits colon cancer cells growth by inducing apoptosis and autophagy flux blockage via mTOR signaling. *Carbohydr Polym*. 2020 Jun 1;237:116113.

[501] Sang Q, Pan Y, Jiang Z, et al. HPLC determination of massoia lactone in fermented Cordyceps sinensis mycelium Cs-4 and its anticancer activity in vitro. *J Food Biochem*. 2020 Sep;44(9):e13336.

[502] Wang BJ, Won SJ, Yu ZR, et al. Free radical scavenging and apoptotic effects of Cordyceps sinensis fractionated by supercritical carbon dioxide. *Food Chem Toxicol*. 2005 Apr;43(4):543-52.

[503] Zhang X, Xiao Y, Huang Q. The cellular uptake of Cordyceps sinensis exopolysaccharide-selenium nanoparticles and their induced apoptosis of HepG2 cells via mitochondria- and death receptor-mediated pathways. *Int J Biol Macromol*. 2023 Aug 30;247:125747.

[504] Lee EJ, Jang KH, Im SY, et al. Physico-chemical properties and cytotoxic potential of Cordyceps sinensis metabolites. *Nat Prod Res*. 2015;29(5):455-9.

[505] Sang Q, Pan Y, Jiang Z, et al. HPLC determination of massoia lactone in fermented Cordyceps sinensis mycelium Cs-4 and its anticancer activity in vitro. *J Food Biochem*. 2020 Sep;44(9):e13336.

[506] Tan L, Liu S, Li X, et al. The Large Molecular Weight Polysaccharide from Wild Cordyceps and Its Antitumor Activity on H22 Tumor-Bearing Mice. *Molecules*. 2023 Apr 10;28(8):3351.

[507] Wu JY, Zhang QX, Leung PH. Inhibitory effects of ethyl acetate extract of Cordyceps sinensis mycelium on various cancer cells in culture and B16 melanoma in C57BL/6 mice. *Phytomedicine*. 2007 Jan;14(1):43-9.

[508] Wang BJ, Won SJ, Yu ZR, et al. Free radical scavenging and apoptotic effects of Cordyceps sinensis fractionated by supercritical carbon dioxide. *Food Chem Toxicol*. 2005 Apr;43(4):543-52.

[509] Shao LW, Huang LH, Yan S, et al. Cordycepin induces apoptosis in human liver cancer HepG2 cells through extrinsic and intrinsic signaling pathways. *Oncol Lett*. 2016 Aug;12(2):995-1000.

[510] Ko BS, Lu YJ, Yao WL, et al. Cordycepin regulates GSK-3β/β-catenin signaling in human leukemia cells. *PLoS One*. 2013 Sep 26;8(9):e76320.

[511] Lee EJ, Jang KH, Im SY, et al. Physico-chemical properties and cytotoxic potential of Cordyceps sinensis metabolites. *Nat Prod Res*. 2015;29(5):455-9.

[512] Nakamura K, Konoha K, Yamaguchi Y, et al. Combined effects of Cordyceps sinensis and methotrexate on hematogenic lung metastasis in mice. *Recept Channels*. 2003;9(5):329-34.

[513] Thakur A, Hui R, Hongyan Z, et al. Pro-apoptotic effects of Paecilomyces hepiali, a Cordyceps sinensis extract on human lung adenocarcinoma A549 cells in vitro. *J Cancer Res Ther*. 2011 Oct-Dec;7(4):421-6.

[514] Zhang SL. [Lewis lung cancer of mice treated with Cordyceps sinensis and its artificial cultured mycelia]. *Zhong Yao Tong Bao*. 1987 Feb;12(2):53-4.

[515] Ko BS, Lu YJ, Yao WL, et al. Cordycepin regulates GSK-3β/β-catenin signaling in human leukemia cells. *PLoS One*. 2013 Sep 26;8(9):e76320.

[516] Wang Z, Wu X, Liang YN, et al. Cordycepin Induces Apoptosis and Inhibits Proliferation of Human Lung Cancer Cell Line H1975 via Inhibiting the Phosphorylation of EGFR. *Molecules*. 2016 Sep 27;21(10):1267.

[517] Ji NF, Yao LS, Li Y, et al. Polysaccharide of Cordyceps sinensis enhances cisplatin cytotoxicity in non-small cell lung cancer H157 cell line. *Integr Cancer Ther*. 2011 Dec;10(4):359-67.

[518] Wei C, Yao X, Jiang Z, et al. Cordycepin Inhibits Drug-resistance Non-Small Cell Lung Cancer Progression by Activating AMPK Signaling Pathway. *Pharmacol Res*. 2019 Jun;144:79-89.

[519] Sang Q, Pan Y, Jiang Z, et al. HPLC determination of massoia lactone in fermented Cordyceps sinensis mycelium Cs-4 and its anticancer activity in vitro. *J Food Biochem*. 2020 Sep;44(9):e13336.

[520] Hahne JC, Meyer SR, Dietl J, et al. The effect of Cordyceps extract and a mixture of Ganoderma lucidum/Agaricus Blazi Murill extract on human endometrial cancer cell lines in vitro. *Int J Oncol*. 2014 Jul;45(1):373-82.

[521] Chang MM, Hong SY, Yang SH, et al. Anti-Cancer Effect of Cordycepin on FGF9-Induced Testicular Tumorigenesis. *Int J Mol Sci*. 2020 Nov 6;21(21):8336.

[522] Lee YP, Huang WR, Wu WS, et al. Cordycepin enhances radiosensitivity to induce apoptosis through cell cycle arrest, caspase pathway and ER stress in MA-10 rodent Leydig tumor cells. *Am J Cancer Res*. 2022 Aug 15;12(8):3601-3624.

[523] Sang Q, Pan Y, Jiang Z, et al. HPLC determination of massoia lactone in fermented Cordyceps sinensis mycelium Cs-4 and its anticancer activity in vitro. *J Food Biochem*. 2020 Sep;44(9):e13336.

[524] Zhang Y, Zhang XX, Yuan RY, et al. Cordycepin induces apoptosis in human pancreatic cancer cells via the mitochondrial-mediated intrinsic pathway and suppresses tumor growth in vivo. *Onco Targets Ther*. 2018 Aug 1;11:4479-4490.

[525] Dos Santos LF, Rubel R, Ribeiro Bonatto SJ, et al. Effects of Cordyceps sinensis on macrophage function in high-fat diet fed rats and its anti-proliferative effects on IMR-32 human neuroblastoma cells. *Pak J Pharm Sci*. 2018 Jan;31(1):1-8.

[526] Chen Y, Yang SH, Hueng DY, et al. Cordycepin induces apoptosis of C6 glioma cells through the adenosine 2A receptor-p53-caspase-7-PARP pathway. *Chem Biol Interact*. 2014 Jun 5;216:17-25.

[527] Sang Q, Pan Y, Jiang Z, et al. HPLC determination of massoia lactone in fermented Cordyceps sinensis mycelium Cs-4 and its anticancer activity in vitro. *J Food Biochem*. 2020 Sep;44(9):e13336.

[528] Chen YJ, Shiao MS, Lee SS, et al. Effect of Cordyceps sinensis on the proliferation and differentiation of human leukemic U937 cells. *Life Sci*. 1997;60(25):2349-59.

[529] Bok JW, Lermer L, Chilton J, et al. Antitumor sterols from the mycelia of Cordyceps sinensis. *Phytochemistry*. 1999 Aug;51(7):891-8.

[530] Matsuda H, Akaki J, Nakamura S, et al. Apoptosis-inducing effects of sterols from the dried powder of cultured mycelium of Cordyceps sinensis. *Chem Pharm Bull (Tokyo)*. 2009 Apr;57(4):411-4.

[531] Wu JY, Zhang QX, Leung PH. Inhibitory effects of ethyl acetate extract of Cordyceps sinensis mycelium on various cancer cells in culture and B16 melanoma in C57BL/6 mice. *Phytomedicine*. 2007 Jan;14(1):43-9.

[532] Zhang Q, Wu J, Hu Z, et al. Induction of HL-60 apoptosis by ethyl acetate extract of Cordyceps sinensis fungal mycelium. *Life Sci*. 2004 Oct 29;75(24):2911-9.

[533] Zhang QX, Wu JY. Cordyceps sinensis mycelium extract induces human premyelocytic leukemia cell apoptosis through mitochondrion pathway. *Exp Biol Med (Maywood)*. 2007 Jan;232(1):52-7.

[534] Bai XL, Yang SX, Shan Y, et al. [Effects of cultivated Cordyceps sinensis on proliferation and apoptosis of human leukemia K562 cells]. *Zhongguo Zhong Yao Za Zhi*. 2018 May;43(10):2134-2139.

[535] Kuo YC, Lin CY, Tsai WJ, et al. Growth inhibitors against tumor cells in Cordyceps sinensis other than cordycepin and polysaccharides. *Cancer Invest*. 1994;12(6):611-5.

[536] Liu C, Lu S, Ji MR. [Effects of Cordyceps sinensis (CS) on in vitro natural killer cells]. *Zhongguo Zhong Xi Yi Jie He Za Zhi*. 1992 May;12(5):267-9, 259.

[537] Ko BS, Lu YJ, Yao WL, et al. Cordycepin regulates GSK-3β/β-catenin signaling in human leukemia cells. *PLoS One*. 2013 Sep 26;8(9):e76320.

[538] Shen YD, Shao XT, Ni YD, et al. [Cordyceps sinensis polysaccharide enhances apoptosis of HL-60 cells induced by triptolide]. *Zhejiang Da Xue Xue Bao Yi Xue Ban*. 2009 Mar;38(2):158-62.

[539] Sang Q, Pan Y, Jiang Z, et al. HPLC determination of massoia lactone in fermented Cordyceps sinensis mycelium Cs-4 and its anticancer activity in vitro. *J Food Biochem*. 2020 Sep;44(9):e13336.

[540] Yamaguchi N, Yoshida J, Ren LJ, et al. Augmentation of various immune reactivities of tumor-bearing hosts with an extract of Cordyceps sinensis. *Biotherapy*. 1990;2(3):199-205.

[541] Ko BS, Lu YJ, Yao WL, et al. Cordycepin regulates GSK-3β/β-catenin signaling in human leukemia cells. *PLoS One*. 2013 Sep 26;8(9):e76320.

[542] Sang Q, Pan Y, Jiang Z, et al. HPLC determination of massoia lactone in fermented Cordyceps sinensis mycelium Cs-4 and its anticancer activity in vitro. *J Food Biochem*. 2020 Sep;44(9):e13336.

[543] Chen Y, Chen YC, Lin YT, et al. Cordycepin induces apoptosis of CGTH W-2 thyroid carcinoma cells through the calcium-calpain-caspase 7-PARP pathway. *J Agric Food Chem*. 2010 Nov 24;58(22):11645-52.

[544] Ko BS, Lu YJ, Yao WL, et al. Cordycepin regulates GSK-3β/β-catenin signaling in human leukemia cells. *PLoS One*. 2013 Sep 26;8(9):e76320.

[545] Wang CY, Tsai SW, Chien HH, et al. Cordycepin Inhibits Human Gestational Choriocarcinoma Cell Growth by Disrupting Centrosome Homeostasis. *Drug Des Devel Ther*. 2020 Jul 27;14:2987-3000.

[546] Xu JC, Zhou XP, Wang XA, et al. Cordycepin Induces Apoptosis and G2/M Phase Arrest through the ERK Pathways in Esophageal Cancer Cells. *J Cancer*. 2019 May 26;10(11):2415-2424.

[547] Wu WC, Hsiao JR, Lian YY, et al. The apoptotic effect of cordycepin on human OEC-M1 oral cancer cell line. *Cancer Chemother Pharmacol*. 2007 Jun;60(1):103-11.

[548] Su NW, Wu SH, Chi CW, et al. Cordycepin, isolated from medicinal fungus Cordyceps sinensis, enhances radiosensitivity of oral cancer associated with modulation of DNA damage repair. *Food Chem Toxicol*. 2019 Feb;124:400-410.

[549] Chen YH, Wang JY, Pan BS, et al. Cordycepin enhances cisplatin apoptotic effect through caspase/MAPK pathways in human head and neck tumor cells. *Onco Targets Ther*. 2013 Jul 25;6:983-98.

[550] Chiu JH, Ju CH, Wu LH, et al. Cordyceps sinensis increases the expression of major histocompatibility complex class II antigens on human hepatoma cell line HA22T/VGH cells. *Am J Chin Med*. 1998;26(2):159-70.

[551] Kubo E, Yoshikawa N, Kunitomo M, et al. Inhibitory effect of Cordyceps sinensis on experimental hepatic metastasis of melanoma by suppressing tumor cell invasion. *Anticancer Res*. 2010 Sep;30(9):3429-33.

[552] Nakamura K, Yamaguchi Y, Kagota S, et al. Inhibitory effect of Cordyceps sinensis on spontaneous liver metastasis of Lewis lung carcinoma and B16 melanoma cells in syngeneic mice. *Jpn J Pharmacol*. 1999 Mar;79(3):335-41.

[553] Nakamura K, Yamaguchi Y, Kagota S, et al. Activation of in vivo Kupffer cell function by oral administration of Cordyceps sinensis in rats. *Jpn J Pharmacol*. 1999 Apr;79(4):505-8.

[554] Yoshikawa N, Kunitomo M, Kagota S, et al. Inhibitory effect of cordycepin on hematogenic metastasis of B16-F1 rodent melanoma cells accelerated by adenosine-5'-diphosphate. *Anticancer Res*. 2009 Oct;29(10):3857-60.

[555] Jordan JL, Nowak A, Lee TD. Activation of innate immunity to reduce lung metastases in breast cancer. *Cancer Immunol Immunother*. 2010 May;59(5):789-97.

[556] Sato A, Yoshikawa N, Kubo E, et al. Inhibitory effect of cordycepin on experimental hepatic metastasis of B16-F0 rodent melanoma cells. *In Vivo*. 2013 Nov-Dec;27(6):729-32.

[557] Mei YX, Yang W, Zhu PX, et al. Isolation, characterization, and antitumor activity of a novel heteroglycan from cultured mycelia of Cordyceps sinensis. *Planta Med*. 2014 Aug;80(13):1107-12.

[558] Yoshida J, Takamura S, Yamaguchi N, et al. Antitumor activity of an extract of Cordyceps sinensis (Berk.) Sacc. against murine tumor cell lines. *Jpn J Exp Med*. 1989 Aug;59(4):157-61.

[559] Chen J, Zhang W, Lu T, et al. Morphological and genetic characterization of a cultivated Cordyceps sinensis fungus and its polysaccharide component possessing antioxidant property in H22 tumor-bearing mice. *Life Sci*. 2006 May 1;78(23):2742-8.

[560] Zhang W, Li J, Qiu S, et al. Effects of the exopolysaccharide fraction (EPSF) from a cultivated Cordyceps sinensis on immunocytes of H22 tumor bearing mice. *Fitoterapia*. 2008 Apr;79(3):168-73.

[561] Wu JY, Zhang QX, Leung PH. Inhibitory effects of ethyl acetate extract of Cordyceps sinensis mycelium on various cancer cells in culture and B16 melanoma in C57BL/6 mice. *Phytomedicine*. 2007 Jan;14(1):43-9.

[562] Jayakumar T, Chiu CC, Wang SH, et al. Anti-cancer effects of CME-1, a novel polysaccharide, purified from the mycelia of Cordyceps sinensis against B16-F10 melanoma cells. *J Cancer Res Ther*. 2014 Jan-Mar;10(1):43-9.

[563] Zhang W, Yang J, Chen J, et al. Immunomodulatory and antitumour effects of an exopolysaccharide fraction from cultivated Cordyceps sinensis (Chinese caterpillar fungus) on tumour-bearing mice. *Biotechnol Appl Biochem*. 2005 Aug;42(Pt 1):9-15.

[564] Yang J, Zhang W, Shi P, et al. Effects of exopolysaccharide fraction (EPSF) from a cultivated Cordyceps sinensis fungus on c-Myc, c-Fos, and VEGF expression in B16 melanoma-bearing mice. *Pathol Res Pract*. 2005;201(11):745-50.

[565] Xu RH, Peng XE, Chen GZ, et al. Effects of cordyceps sinensis on natural killer activity and colony formation of B16 melanoma. *Chin Med J (Engl)*. 1992 Feb;105(2):97-101.

[566] Yoshikawa N, Nakamura K, Yamaguchi Y, et al. Antitumour activity of cordycepin in mice. *Clin Exp Pharmacol Physiol*. 2004 Dec;31 Suppl 2:S51-3.

567 Yoshikawa N, Yamada S, Takeuchi C, et al. Cordycepin (3'-deoxyadenosine) inhibits the growth of B16-BL6 rodent melanoma cells through the stimulation of adenosine A3 receptor followed by glycogen synthase kinase-3beta activation and cyclin D1 suppression. *Naunyn Schmiedebergs Arch Pharmacol*. 2008 Jun;377(4-6):591-5.

568 Yoshikawa N, Nakamura K, Yamaguchi Y, et al. Reinforcement of antitumor effect of Cordyceps sinensis by 2'-deoxycoformycin, an adenosine deaminase inhibitor. *In Vivo*. 2007 Mar-Apr;21(2):291-5.

569 Yoshida J, Takamura S, Yamaguchi N, et al. Antitumor activity of an extract of Cordyceps sinensis (Berk.) Sacc. against murine tumor cell lines. *Jpn J Exp Med*. 1989 Aug;59(4):157-61.

570 Liu WC, Chuang WL, Tsai ML, et al. Cordyceps sinensis health supplement enhances recovery from taxol-induced leukopenia. *Exp Biol Med (Maywood)*. 2008 Apr;233(4):447-55.

571 Ying M, Yu Q, Zheng B, et al. Cultured Cordyceps sinensis polysaccharides modulate intestinal mucosal immunity and gut microbiota in cyclophosphamide-treated mice. *Carbohydr Polym*. 2020 May 1;235:115957.

572 Chen S , Wang J , Fang Q, et al. A polysaccharide from natural Cordyceps sinensis regulates the intestinal immunity and gut microbiota in mice with cyclophosphamide-induced intestinal injury. *Food Funct*. 2021 Jul 21;12(14):6271-6282.

573 Wu GD, Pan A, Zhang X, et al. Cordyceps Improves Obesity and its Related Inflammation via Modulation of Enterococcus cecorum Abundance and Bile Acid Metabolism. *Am J Chin Med*. 2022;50(3):817-838.

574 Mao YH, Song AX, Li LQ, et al. Effects of exopolysaccharide fractions with different molecular weights and compositions on fecal microflora during in vitro fermentation. *Int J Biol Macromol*. 2020 Feb 1;144:76-84.

575 Mao YH, Song AX, Wang ZM, et al. Protection of Bifidobacterial cells against antibiotics by a high molecular weight exopolysaccharide of a medicinal fungus Cs-HK1 through physical interactions. *Int J Biol Macromol*. 2018 Nov;119:312-319.

576 Ying M, Yu Q, Zheng B, et al. Cultured Cordyceps sinensis polysaccharides modulate intestinal mucosal immunity and gut microbiota in cyclophosphamide-treated mice. *Carbohydr Polym*. 2020 May 1;235:115957.

577 Chen S , Wang J , Fang Q, et al. A polysaccharide from natural Cordyceps sinensis regulates the intestinal immunity and gut microbiota in mice with cyclophosphamide-induced intestinal injury. *Food Funct*. 2021 Jul 21;12(14):6271-6282.

578 Gu GS, Ren JA, Li GW, et al. Cordyceps sinensis preserves intestinal mucosal barrier and may be an adjunct therapy in endotoxin-induced sepsis rat model: a pilot study. *Int J Clin Exp Med*. 2015 May 15;8(5):7333-41.

579 Zhang X, Wang M, Qiao Y, et al. Exploring the mechanisms of action of Cordyceps sinensis for the treatment of depression using network pharmacology and molecular docking. *Ann Transl Med*. 2022 Mar;10(6):282.

580 Yang X, Chen L, Zhao L, et al. Cordyceps sinensis-derived fungus Isaria felina ameliorates experimental autoimmune thyroiditis in mice. *Biomed Pharmacother*. 2021 Aug;140:111733.

581 Cheng C, Zhu X. Cordycepin mitigates MPTP-induced Parkinson's disease through inhibiting TLR/NF-κB signaling pathway. *Life Sci*. 2019 Apr 15;223:120-127.

582 Xiang F, Lin L, Hu M, et al. Therapeutic efficacy of a polysaccharide isolated from Cordyceps sinensis on hypertensive rats. *Int J Biol Macromol*. 2016 Jan;82:308-14.

583 Chiou WF, Chang PC, Chou CJ, et al. Protein constituent contributes to the hypotensive and vasorelaxant activities of Cordyceps sinensis. *Life Sci*. 2000 Feb 25;66(14):1369-76.

584 Feng MG, Zhou QG, Feng GH. [Vasodilating effect of cultured Cordyceps sinensis (Berk) Sacc. mycelia in anesthetized dogs]. *Zhong Yao Tong Bao*. 1987 Dec;12(12):41-5, 60.

585 Luitel H, Novoyatleva T, Sydykov A, et al. Yarsagumba is a Promising Therapeutic Option for Treatment of Pulmonary Hypertension due to the Potent Anti-Proliferative and Vasorelaxant Properties. *Medicina (Kaunas)*. 2020 Mar 16;56(3):131.

586 Yang L, Jiao X, Wu J, et al. Cordyceps sinensis inhibits airway remodeling in rats with chronic obstructive pulmonary disease. *Exp Ther Med*. 2018 Mar;15(3):2731-2738.

587 Sun X, Feng X, Zheng D, et al. Ergosterol attenuates cigarette smoke extract-induced COPD by modulating inflammation, oxidative stress and apoptosis in vitro and in vivo. *Clin Sci (Lond)*. 2019 Jul 15;133(13):1523-1536.

588 Chen J, Chan WM, Leung HY, et al. Anti-Inflammatory Effects of a Cordyceps sinensis Mycelium Culture Extract (Cs-4) on Rodent Models of Allergic Rhinitis and Asthma. *Molecules*. 2020 Sep 4;25(18):4051.

589 Lin XX, Xie QM, Shen WH, et al. [Effects of fermented Cordyceps powder on pulmonary function in sensitized guinea pigs and airway inflammation in sensitized rats]. *Zhongguo Zhong Yao Za Zhi*. 2001 Sep;26(9):622-5.

590 Wang RL, Liu SH, Shen SH, et al. Protective Mechanism of Cordyceps sinensis Treatment on Acute Kidney Injury-Induced Acute Lung Injury through AMPK/mTOR Signaling Pathway. *Chin J Integr Med*. 2023 Feb 27. Online ahead of print.

591 Fu S, Lu W, Yu W, et al. Protective effect of Cordyceps sinensis extract on lipopolysaccharide-induced acute lung injury in mice. *Biosci Rep*. 2019 Jun 25;39(6):BSR20190789.

592 Chen M, Cheung FW, Chan MH, et al. Protective roles of Cordyceps on lung fibrosis in cellular and rat models. *J Ethnopharmacol*. 2012 Sep 28;143(2):448-54.

593 Chiou YL, Lin CY. The extract of Cordyceps sinensis inhibited airway inflammation by blocking NF-κB activity. *Inflammation*. 2012 Jun;35(3):985-93.

594 Yue GG, Lau CB, Fung KP, et al. Effects of Cordyceps sinensis, Cordyceps militaris and their isolated compounds on ion transport in Calu-3 human airway epithelial cells. *J Ethnopharmacol*. 2008 Apr 17;117(1):92-101.

595 Kuo YC, Tsai WJ, Wang JY, et al. Regulation of bronchoalveolar lavage fluids cell function by the immunomodulatory agents from Cordyceps sinensis. *Life Sci*. 2001 Jan 19;68(9):1067-82.

596 Liu A, Wu J, Li A, et al. The inhibitory mechanism of Cordyceps sinensis on cigarette smoke extract-induced senescence in human bronchial epithelial cells. *Int J Chron Obstruct Pulmon Dis*. 2016 Jul 28;11:1721-31.

597 Liu Q, Zhang W, Cui H, et al. [Study on effect of cordyceps sinensis on early-stage silicotic pulmonary fibrosis in rabbits]. *Zhonghua Lao Dong Wei Sheng Zhi Ye Bing Za Zhi*. 2014 Jul;32(7):530-2.

598 Xu H, Li S, Lin Y, et al. [Effectiveness of cultured Cordyceps sinensis combined with glucocorticosteroid on pulmonary fibrosis induced by bleomycin in rats]. *Zhongguo Zhong Yao Za Zhi*. 2011 Aug;36(16):2265-70.

599 Singh M, Tulsawani R, Koganti P, et al. Cordyceps sinensis increases hypoxia tolerance by inducing heme oxygenase-1 and metallothionein via Nrf2 activation in human lung epithelial cells. *Biomed Res Int*. 2013;2013:569206.

[600] Mishra J, Khan W, Ahmad S, et al. Supercritical Carbon Dioxide Extracts of Cordyceps sinensis: Chromatography-based Metabolite Profiling and Protective Efficacy Against Hypobaric Hypoxia. *Front Pharmacol*. 2021 Aug 26;12:628924.

[601] Gao BA, Yang J, Huang J, et al. Cordyceps sinensis extract suppresses hypoxia-induced proliferation of rat pulmonary artery smooth muscle cells. *Saudi Med J*. 2010 Sep;31(9):974-9.

[602] Li DG, Ren ZX. Cordyceps sinensis promotes immune regulation and enhances bacteriostatic activity of PA-824 via IL-10 in Mycobacterium tuberculosis disease. *Braz J Med Biol Res*. 2017 Aug 7;50(9):e6188.

[603] Liu H, Cao D, Liu H, et al. The Herbal Medicine Cordyceps sinensis Protects Pancreatic Beta Cells from Streptozotocin-Induced Endoplasmic Reticulum Stress. *Can J Diabetes*. 2016 Aug;40(4):329-35.

[604] Lo HC, Hsu TH, Tu ST, et al. Anti-hyperglycemic activity of natural and fermented Cordyceps sinensis in rats with diabetes induced by nicotinamide and streptozotocin. *Am J Chin Med*. 2006;34(5):819-32.

[605] Zhang G, Huang Y, Bian Y, et al. Hypoglycemic activity of the fungi Cordyceps militaris, Cordyceps sinensis, Tricholoma mongolicum, and Omphalia lapidescens in streptozotocin-induced diabetic rats. *Appl Microbiol Biotechnol*. 2006 Oct;72(6):1152-6.

[606] Kan WC, Wang HY, Chien CC, et al. Effects of Extract from Solid-State Fermented Cordyceps sinensis on Type 2 Diabetes Mellitus. *Evid Based Complement Alternat Med*. 2012;2012:743107.

[607] Kiho T, Yamane A, Hui J, et al. Polysaccharides in fungi. XXXVI. Hypoglycemic activity of a polysaccharide (CS-F30) from the cultural mycelium of Cordyceps sinensis and its effect on glucose metabolism in rodent liver. *Biol Pharm Bull*. 1996 Feb;19(2):294-6.

[608] Kiho T, Ookubo K, Usui S, et al. Structural features and hypoglycemic activity of a polysaccharide (CS-F10) from the cultured mycelium of Cordyceps sinensis. *Biol Pharm Bull*. 1999 Sep;22(9):966-70.

[609] Kiho T, Hui J, Yamane A, et al. Polysaccharides in fungi. XXXII. Hypoglycemic activity and chemical properties of a polysaccharide from the cultural mycelium of Cordyceps sinensis. *Biol Pharm Bull*. 1993 Dec;16(12):1291-3.

[610] Li SP, Zhang GH, Zeng Q, et al. Hypoglycemic activity of polysaccharide, with antioxidation, isolated from cultured Cordyceps mycelia. *Phytomedicine*. 2006 Jun;13(6):428-33.

[611] Zhang X, Zhang H, Qiang W, et al. Oral administration of human FGF21 expressed by mycelium of Cordyceps militaris improves blood glucose and lipid in type II diabetes mellitus. *Cell Mol Biol (Noisy-le-grand)*. 2022 Sep 30;68(10):54-62.

[612] El Zahraa Z El Ashry F, Mahmoud MF, et al. Effect of Cordyceps sinensis and taurine either alone or in combination on streptozotocin induced diabetes. *Food Chem Toxicol*. 2012 Mar;50(3-4):1159-65.

[613] Balon TW, Jasman AP, Zhu JS. A fermentation product of Cordyceps sinensis increases whole-body insulin sensitivity in rats. *J Altern Complement Med*. 2002 Jun;8(3):315-23.

[614] Zhao CS, Yin WT, Wang JY, et al. CordyMax Cs-4 improves glucose metabolism and increases insulin sensitivity in normal rats. *J Altern Complement Med*. 2002 Jun;8(3):309-14.

[615] Shi B, Wang Z, Jin H, et al. Immunoregulatory Cordyceps sinensis increases regulatory T cells to Th17 cell ratio and delays diabetes in NOD mice. *Int Immunopharmacol*. 2009 May;9(5):582-6.

[616] Wang MF, Zhu QH, He YG. Treatment with Cordyceps sinensis enriches Treg population in peripheral lymph nodes and delays type I diabetes development in NOD mice. *Pharmazie*. 2013 Sep;68(9):768-71.

[617] Singh KP, Meena HS, Negi PS. Enhancement of Neuromuscular Activity by Natural Specimens and Cultured Mycelia of Cordyceps sinensis in Mice. *Indian J Pharm Sci*. 2014 Sep;76(5):458-61.

[618] Nishizawa K, Torii K, Kawasaki A, et al. Antidepressant-like effect of Cordyceps sinensis in the rodent tail suspension test. *Biol Pharm Bull*. 2007 Sep;30(9):1758-62.

[619] Chen S, Wang J, Dong N, et al. Polysaccharides from natural Cordyceps sinensis attenuated dextran sodium sulfate-induced colitis in C57BL/6J mice. *Food Funct*. 2023 Jan 23;14(2):720-733.

[620] Marchbank T, Ojobo E, Playford CJ, et al. Reparative properties of the traditional Chinese medicine Cordyceps sinensis (Chinese caterpillar mushroom) using HT29 cell culture and rat gastric damage models of injury. *Br J Nutr*. 2011 May;105(9):1303-10.

[621] Liu WC, Wang SC, Tsai ML, et al. Protection against radiation-induced bone marrow and intestinal injuries by Cordyceps sinensis, a Chinese herbal medicine. *Radiat Res*. 2006 Dec;166(6):900-7.

[622] Yang ML, Kuo PC, Hwang TL, et al. Anti-inflammatory principles from Cordyceps sinensis. *J Nat Prod*. 2011 Sep 23;74(9):1996-2000.

[623] Wang Y, Wang Y, Liu D, et al. Cordyceps sinensis polysaccharide inhibits PDGF-BB-induced inflammation and ROS production in human mesangial cells. *Carbohydr Polym*. 2015 Jul 10;125:135-45.

[624] Li LQ, Song AX, Yin JY, et al. Anti-inflammation activity of exopolysaccharides produced by a medicinal fungus Cordyceps sinensis Cs-HK1 in cell and animal models. *Int J Biol Macromol*. 2020 Apr 15;149:1042-1050.

[625] Qian GM, Pan GF, Guo JY. Anti-inflammatory and antinociceptive effects of cordymin, a peptide purified from the medicinal mushroom Cordyceps sinensis. *Nat Prod Res*. 2012;26(24):2358-62.

[626] Rao YK, Fang SH, Tzeng YM. Evaluation of the anti-inflammatory and anti-proliferation tumoral cells activities of Antrodia camphorata, Cordyceps sinensis, and Cinnamomum osmophloeum bark extracts. *J Ethnopharmacol*. 2007 Oct 8;114(1):78-85.

[627] Qian GM, Pan GF, Guo JY. Anti-inflammatory and antinociceptive effects of cordymin, a peptide purified from the medicinal mushroom Cordyceps sinensis. *Nat Prod Res*. 2012;26(24):2358-62.

[628] Qi W, Yan YB, Lei W, et al. Prevention of disuse osteoporosis in rats by Cordyceps sinensis extract. *Osteoporos Int*. 2012 Sep;23(9):2347-57.

[629] Mizuha Y, Yamamoto H, Sato T, et al. Water extract of Cordyceps sinensis (WECS) inhibits the RANKL-induced osteoclast differentiation. *Biofactors*. 2007;30(2):105-16.

[630] Zhang DW, Wang ZL, Qi W, et al. The effects of Cordyceps sinensis phytoestrogen on estrogen deficiency-induced osteoporosis in ovariectomized rats. *BMC Complement Altern Med*. 2014 Dec 13;14:484.

[631] Qi W, Wang PJ, Guo WJ, et al. The mechanism of Cordyceps sinensis and strontium in prevention of osteoporosis in rats. *Biol Trace Elem Res*. 2011 Oct;143(1):302-9.

[632] Qi W, Yan YB, Wang PJ, et al. The co-effect of Cordyceps sinensis and strontium on osteoporosis in ovariectomized osteopenic rats. *Biol Trace Elem Res*. 2011 Jun;141(1-3):216-23.

[633] Qi W, Zhang Y, Yan YB, et al. The Protective Effect of Cordymin, a Peptide Purified from the Medicinal Mushroom Cordyceps sinensis, on Diabetic Osteopenia in Alloxan-Induced Diabetic Rats. *Evid Based Complement Alternat Med*. 2013;2013:985636.

[634] Chen JL, Chen YC, Yang SH, et al. Immunological alterations in lupus-prone autoimmune (NZB/NZW) F1 mice by mycelia Chinese medicinal fungus Cordyceps sinensis-induced redistributions of peripheral mononuclear T lymphocytes. *Clin Exp Med*. 2009 Dec;9(4):277-84.

[635] Fu T, Lin J. [Effect of Cordyceps sinensis on inhibiting systemic lupus erythematosus in MRL 1pr/1pr mice (correction of rats)]. *Zhong Yao Cai*. 2001 Sep;24(9):658-9.

[636] Chen JR, Yen JH, Lin CC, et al. The effects of Chinese herbs on improving survival and inhibiting anti-ds DNA antibody production in lupus mice. *Am J Chin Med*. 1993;21(3-4):257-62.

[637] Kuo YC, Tsai WJ, Shiao MS, et al. Cordyceps sinensis as an immunomodulatory agent. *Am J Chin Med*. 1996;24(2):111-25.

[638] Wu R, Jia Q, Li X, et al. Preparation of the sphingolipid fraction from mycelia of Cordyceps sinensis and its immunosuppressive activity. *J Ethnopharmacol*. 2022 Jun 12;291:115126.

[639] Zhou X, Luo L, Dressel W, et al. Cordycepin is an immunoregulatory active ingredient of Cordyceps sinensis. *Am J Chin Med*. 2008;36(5):967-80.

[640] Zhang Z, Xia SS. Cordyceps Sinensis-I as an immunosuppressant in heterotopic heart allograft model in rats. *J Tongji Med Univ*. 1990;10(2):100-3.

[641] Xiao G, Miyazato A, Abe Y, et al. Activation of myeloid dendritic cells by deoxynucleic acids from Cordyceps sinensis via a Toll-like receptor 9-dependent pathway. *Cell Immunol*. 2010;263(2):241-50.

[642] Li CY, Chiang CS, Tsai ML, et al. Two-sided effect of Cordyceps sinensis on dendritic cells in different physiological stages. *J Leukoc Biol*. 2009 Jun;85(6):987-95.

[643] Park DK, Choi WS, Park PJ, et al. Immunoglobulin and cytokine production from mesenteric lymph node lymphocytes is regulated by extracts of Cordyceps sinensis in C57Bl/6N mice. *J Med Food*. 2008 Dec;11(4):784-8.

[644] Yang LY, Chen A, Kuo YC, et al. Efficacy of a pure compound H1-A extracted from Cordyceps sinensis on autoimmune disease of MRL lpr/lpr mice. *J Lab Clin Med*. 1999 Nov;134(5):492-500.

[645] Ding C, Tian P, Jia L, et al. The synergistic effects of C. Sinensis with CsA in preventing allograft rejection. *Front Biosci (Landmark Ed)*. 2009 Jan 1;14(10):3864-71.

[646] Zhu XY, Yu HY. [Immunosuppressive effect of cultured Cordyceps sinensis on cellular immune response]. *Zhong Xi Yi Jie He Za Zhi*. 1990 Aug;10(8):485-7, 454.

[647] Ka Wai Lee S, Kwok Wong C, Kai Kong S, et al. Immunomodulatory activities of HERBSnSENSES Cordyceps -- in vitro and in vivo studies. *Immunopharmacol Immunotoxicol*. 2006;28(2):341-60.

[648] Yap ACS, Li X, Yap YHY, et al. Immunomodulatory Properties of Water-Soluble Polysaccharides Extracted from the Fruiting Body of Chinese Caterpillar Mushroom, Ophiocordyceps sinensis Cultivar OCS02® (Ascomycetes). *Int J Med Mushrooms*. 2020;22(10):967-977.

[649] Jordan JL, Hirsch GM, Lee TD. C. sinensis ablates allograft vasculopathy when used as an adjuvant therapy with cyclosporin A. *Transpl Immunol*. 2008 Jul;19(3-4):159-66.

[650] Yang LY, Huang WJ, Hsieh HG, et al. H1-A extracted from Cordyceps sinensis suppresses the proliferation of human mesangial cells and promotes apoptosis, probably by inhibiting the tyrosine phosphorylation of Bcl-2 and Bcl-XL. *J Lab Clin Med*. 2003 Jan;141(1):74-83.

[651] Wei S, Peng W, Zhang C, et al. Cordyceps sinensis aqueous extract regulates the adaptive immunity of mice subjected to 60 Co γ irradiation. *Phytother Res*. 2021 Sep;35(9):5163-5177.

[652] Zhang Y, Liu J, Wang Y, et al. Nucleosides and amino acids, isolated from Cordyceps sinensis, protected against cyclophosphamide-induced myelosuppression in mice. *Nat Prod Res*. 2022 Dec;36(23):6056-6059.

[653] Hu T, Jiang C, Huang Q, et al. A comb-like branched β-D-glucan produced by a Cordyceps sinensis fungus and its protective effect against cyclophosphamide-induced immunosuppression in mice. *Carbohydr Polym*. 2016 May 20;142:259-67.

[654] Zhang J, Yu Y, Zhang Z, et al. Effect of polysaccharide from cultured Cordyceps sinensis on immune function and anti-oxidation activity of mice exposed to 60Co. *Int Immunopharmacol*. 2011 Dec;11(12):2251-7.

[655] Han SH, Ahn Y, Lee HJ, et al. Antioxidant and Immunostimulatory Activities of a Submerged Culture of Cordyceps sinensis Using Spent Coffee. *Foods*. 2021 Jul 22;10(8):1697.

[656] Meng LZ, Lin BQ, Wang B, et al. Mycelia extracts of fungal strains isolated from Cordyceps sinensis differently enhance the function of RAW 264.7 macrophages. *J Ethnopharmacol*. 2013 Jul 30;148(3):818-25.

[657] Sheng L, Chen J, Li J, Zhang W. An exopolysaccharide from cultivated Cordyceps sinensis and its effects on cytokine expressions of immunocytes. *Appl Biochem Biotechnol*. 2011 Mar;163(5):669-78.

[658] Wu DT, Meng LZ, Wang LY, et al. Chain conformation and immunomodulatory activity of a hyperbranched polysaccharide from Cordyceps sinensis. *Carbohydr Polym*. 2014 Sep 22;110:405-14.

[659] Hao T, Li JJ, Du ZY, et al. [Cordyceps sinensis enhances lymphocyte proliferation and CD markers expression in simulated microgravity environment]. *Zhongguo Shi Yan Xue Ye Xue Za Zhi*. 2012 Oct;20(5):1212-5.

[660] Jordan JL, Sullivan AM, Lee TD. Immune activation by a sterile aqueous extract of Cordyceps sinensis: mechanism of action. *Immunopharmacol Immunotoxicol*. 2008;30(1):53-70.

[661] Yoon TJ, Yu KW, Shin KS, et al. Innate immune stimulation of exo-polymers prepared from Cordyceps sinensis by submerged culture. *Appl Microbiol Biotechnol*. 2008 Oct;80(6):1087-93.

[662] Chen W, Zhang W, Shen W, et al. Effects of the acid polysaccharide fraction isolated from a cultivated Cordyceps sinensis on macrophages in vitro. *Cell Immunol*. 2010;262(1):69-74.

[663] Kuo MC, Chang CY, Cheng TL, et al. Immunomodulatory effect of exo-polysaccharides from submerged cultured Cordyceps sinensis: enhancement of cytokine synthesis, CD11b expression, and phagocytosis. *Appl Microbiol Biotechnol*. 2007 Jun;75(4):769-75.

664 Chen W, Yuan F, Wang K, et al. Modulatory effects of the acid polysaccharide fraction from one of anamorph of Cordyceps sinensis on Ana-1 cells. *J Ethnopharmacol*. 2012 Aug 1;142(3):739-45.

665 Wu Y, Sun H, Qin F, et al. Effect of various extracts and a polysaccharide from the edible mycelia of Cordyceps sinensis on cellular and humoral immune response against ovalbumin in mice. *Phytother Res*. 2006 Aug;20(8):646-52.

666 Koh JH, Yu KW, Suh HJ, et al. Activation of macrophages and the intestinal immune system by an orally administered decoction from cultured mycelia of Cordyceps sinensis. *Biosci Biotechnol Biochem*. 2002 Feb,66(2).407-11.

667 Chen GZ, Chen GL, Sun T, et al. Effects of Cordyceps sinensis on murine T lymphocyte subsets. *Chin Med J (Engl)*. 1991 Jan;104(1):4-8.

668 Cheung JK, Li J, Cheung AW, et al. Cordysinocan, a polysaccharide isolated from cultured Cordyceps, activates immune responses in cultured T-lymphocytes and macrophages: signaling cascade and induction of cytokines. *J Ethnopharmacol*. 2009 Jul 6;124(1):61-8.

669 Liu P, Zhu J, Huang Y, et al. [Influence of Cordyceps sinensis (Berk.) Sacc. and rat serum containing same medicine on IL-1, IFN and TNF produced by rat Kupffer cells]. *Zhongguo Zhong Yao Za Zhi*. 1996 Jun;21(6):367-9, 384.

670 Zhang SL. [Activation of murine peritoneal macrophages by natural Cordyceps sinensis and its cultured mycelia]. *Zhong Xi Yi Jie He Za Zhi*. 1985 Jan;5(1):45-7, 5.

671 Song D, Lin J, Yuan F, et al. Ex vivo stimulation of murine dendritic cells by an exopolysaccharide from one of the anamorph of Cordyceps sinensis. *Cell Biochem Funct*. 2011 Oct;29(7):555-61.

672 Ma LL, Yang XY, Gao JZ. [Experimental study on effect of Bailing Cpsule on dendritic cells in mice]. *Zhongguo Zhong Xi Yi Jie He Za Zhi*. 2007 Oct;27(10):905-8.

673 Zhu ZY, Meng M, Sun H, et al. Structural analysis and immunostimulatory activity of glycopeptides from Paecilomyces sinensis. *Food Funct*. 2016 Mar;7(3):1593-600.

674 Hsu TL, Cheng SC, Yang WB, et al. Profiling carbohydrate-receptor interaction with recombinant innate immunity receptor-Fc fusion proteins. *J Biol Chem*. 2009 Dec 11;284(50):34479-89.

675 Zhu ZY, Chen J, Si CL, et al. Immunomodulatory effect of polysaccharides from submerged cultured Cordyceps gunnii. *Pharm Biol*. 2012 Sep;50(9):1103-10.

676 Cheng Q. [Effect of cordyceps sinensis on cellular immunity in rats with chronic renal insufficiency]. *Zhonghua Yi Xue Za Zhi*. 1992 Jan;72(1):27-9, 63.

677 Zhong SS, Xiang YJ, Liu PJ, et al. Effect of Cordyceps sinensis on the Treatment of Experimental Autoimmune Encephalomyelitis: A Pilot Study on Mice Model. *Chin Med J (Engl)*. 2017 Oct 5;130(19):2296-2301.

678 Kuo CF, Chen CC, et al. Cordyceps sinensis mycelium protects mice from group A streptococcal infection. *J Med Microbiol*. 2005 Aug;54(Pt 8):795-802.

679 Zhu Y, Ma L, Hu Q, et al. [In Vitro Anti-HIV-1 Activity of Cordyceps sinensis Extracts]. *Bing Du Xue Bao*. 2016 Jul;32(4):417-22.

680 Kuo CF, Chen CC, Lin CF, et al. Abrogation of streptococcal pyrogenic exotoxin B-mediated suppression of phagocytosis in U937 cells by Cordyceps sinensis mycelium via production of cytokines. *Food Chem Toxicol*. 2007 Feb;45(2):278-85.

681 Li X, Wu M, Chen L, et al. A Sphingosine-1-Phosphate Modulator Ameliorates Polycystic Kidney Disease in Han:SPRD Rats. *Am J Nephrol*. 2020;51(1):1-10.

682 He P, Lei J, Miao JN, et al. Cordyceps sinensis attenuates HBx-induced cell apoptosis in HK-2 cells through suppressing the PI3K/Akt pathway. *Int J Mol Med*. 2020 Apr;45(4):1261-1269.

683 Zhang Q, Xiao X, Li M, et al. Bailing capsule (Cordyceps sinensis) ameliorates renal triglyceride accumulation through the PPARα pathway in diabetic rats. *Front Pharmacol*. 2022 Aug 25;13:915592.

684 Zhao K, Gao Q, Zong C, et al. Cordyceps sinensis prevents contrast-induced nephropathy in diabetic rats: its underlying mechanism. *Int J Clin Exp Pathol*. 2018 Dec 1;11(12):5571-5580.

685 Zhang Y, Xu L, Lu Y, et al. Protective effect of Cordyceps sinensis against diabetic kidney disease through promoting proliferation and inhibiting apoptosis of renal proximal tubular cells. *BMC Complement Med Ther*. 2023 Apr 6;23(1):109.

686 Li Y, Wang L, Xu B, et al. Based on Network Pharmacology Tools to Investigate the Molecular Mechanism of Cordyceps sinensis on the Treatment of Diabetic Nephropathy. *J Diabetes Res*. 2021 Feb 5;2021:8891093.

687 Hao L, Pan MS, Zheng Y, et al. Effect of Cordyceps sinensis and Tripterygium wilfordii polyglycosidium on podocytes in rats with diabetic nephropathy. *Exp Ther Med*. 2014 Jun;7(6):1465-1470.

688 Dong Z, Sun Y, Wei G, et al. A Nucleoside/Nucleobase-Rich Extract from Cordyceps Sinensis Inhibits the Epithelial-Mesenchymal Transition and Protects against Renal Fibrosis in Diabetic Nephropathy. *Molecules*. 2019 Nov 14;24(22):4119.

689 Yuan M, Tang R, Zhou Q, et al. [Effect of Cordyceps sinensis on expressions of HIF-1α and VEGF in the kidney of rats with diabetic nephropathy]. *Zhong Nan Da Xue Xue Bao Yi Xue Ban*. 2013 May;38(5):448-57.

690 Xu J, Yuan Q, Wu K, et al. Effects of Bailing capsule on diabetic nephropathy based on UPLC-MS urine metabolomics. *RSC Adv*. 2019 Nov 5;9(62):35969-35975.

691 Xiao ZH, Zhou JH, Wu HS. [Effect of myriocin on the expression of cyclinD1 in high glucose-induced hypertrophy mesangial cells]. *Zhongguo Dang Dai Er Ke Za Zhi*. 2011 Aug;13(8):677-9.

692 Du F, Li S, Wang T, et al. Cordyceps sinensis attenuates renal fibrosis and suppresses BAG3 induction in obstructed rat kidney. *Am J Transl Res*. 2015 May 15;7(5):932-40.

693 Xiao C, Xiao P, Li X, et al. Cordyceps sinensis may inhibit Th22 cell chemotaxis to improve kidney function in IgA nephropathy. *Am J Transl Res*. 2018 Mar 15;10(3):857-865.

694 Wang HP, Liu CW, Chang HW, et al. Cordyceps sinensis protects against renal ischemia/reperfusion injury in rats. *Mol Biol Rep*. 2013 Mar;40(3):2347-55.

695 Wang Y, Liu D, Zhao H, et al. Cordyceps sinensis polysaccharide CPS-2 protects human mesangial cells from PDGF-BB-induced proliferation through the PDGF/ERK and TGF-β1/Smad pathways. *Mol Cell Endocrinol*. 2014 Feb 15;382(2):979-88.

696 Zhao-Long W, Xiao-Xia W, et al. Inhibitory effect of Cordyceps sinensis and Cordyceps militaris on human glomerular mesangial cell proliferation induced by native LDL. *Cell Biochem Funct*. 2000 Jun;18(2):93-7.

[697] Yu H, Zhou Q, Huang R, et al. [Effect of Cordyceps sinensis on the expression of HIF-1α and NGAL in rats with renal ischemia-reperfusion injury]. *Zhong Nan Da Xue Xue Bao Yi Xue Ban*. 2012 Jan;37(1):57-66.

[698] Wang Y, Yin H, Lv X, et al. Protection of chronic renal failure by a polysaccharide from Cordyceps sinensis. *Fitoterapia*. 2010 Jul;81(5):397-402.

[699] Pan MM, Zhang MH, Ni HF, et al. Inhibition of TGF-β1/Smad signal pathway is involved in the effect of Cordyceps sinensis against renal fibrosis in 5/6 nephrectomy rats. *Food Chem Toxicol*. 2013 Aug;58:487-94.

[700] Liu BH, He WM, Wan YG, et al. [Molecular mechanisms of mycelium of Cordyceps sinensis ameliorating renal tubular epithelial cells aging induced by D-galactose via inhibiting autophagy-related AMPK/ULK1 signaling activation]. *Zhongguo Zhong Yao Za Zhi*. 2019 Mar;44(6):1258-1265.

[701] Tu S, Zhou Q, Tang R, et al. [Proapoptotic effect of angiotensin II on renal tubular epithelial cells and protective effect of Cordyceps sinensis]. *Zhong Nan Da Xue Xue Bao Yi Xue Ban*. 2012 Jan;37(1):67-72.

[702] Shahed AR, Kim SI, Shoskes DA. Down-regulation of apoptotic and inflammatory genes by Cordyceps sinensis extract in rat kidney following ischemia/reperfusion. *Transplant Proc*. 2001 Sep;33(6):2986-7.

[703] Zhong F, Liu X, Zhou Q, et al. 1H NMR spectroscopy analysis of metabolites in the kidneys provides new insight into pathophysiological mechanisms: applications for treatment with Cordyceps sinensis. *Nephrol Dial Transplant*. 2012 Feb;27(2):556-65.

[704] Hao L, Pan MS, Zheng Y. [Effects of Cordyceps Sinensis and Tiptervgium wilfordii Polyglycosidium on the podocytes in rats with diabetic nephropathy]. *Zhongguo Zhong Xi Yi Jie He Za Zhi*. 2012 Feb;32(2):261-5.

[705] Han F, Dou M, Wang Y, et al. Cordycepin protects renal ischemia/reperfusion injury through regulating inflammation, apoptosis, and oxidative stress. *Acta Biochim Biophys Sin (Shanghai)*. 2020 Feb 3;52(2):125-132.

[706] Li LS, Zheng F, Liu ZH. [Experimental study on effect of Cordyceps sinensis in ameliorating aminoglycoside induced nephrotoxicity]. *Zhongguo Zhong Xi Yi Jie He Za Zhi*. 1996 Dec;16(12):733-7.

[707] Zhen F, Tian J, Li LS. [Mechanisms and therapeutic effect of Cordyceps sinensis (CS) on aminoglycoside induced acute renal failure (ARF) in rats]. *Zhongguo Zhong Xi Yi Jie He Za Zhi*. 1992 May;12(5):288-91, 262.

[708] Hong T, Cui LK, Wen J, et al. [Cordycepin protects podocytes from injury mediated by complements complex C5b-9]. *Sichuan Da Xue Xue Bao Yi Xue Ban*. 2015 Mar;46(2):173-8, 227.

[709] Zhang Y, Ao X, Li H, et al. [Cordyceps sinensis protects HK2 cells from ischemia-reperfusion injury through Sirt1 pathway]. *Zhong Nan Da Xue Xue Bao Yi Xue Ban*. 2017 Nov 28;42(11):1263-1269.

[710] Lin CY, Ku FM, Kuo YC, et al. Inhibition of activated human mesangial cell proliferation by the natural product of Cordyceps sinensis (H1-A): an implication for treatment of IgA mesangial nephropathy. *J Lab Clin Med*. 1999 Jan;133(1):55-63.

[711] Tang R, Zhou Q, Shu J, et al. [Effect of cordyceps sinensis extract on Klotho expression and apoptosis in renal tubular epithelial cells induced by angiotensin II]. *Zhong Nan Da Xue Xue Bao Yi Xue Ban*. 2009 Apr;34(4):300-7.

[712] Zhang MH, Pan MM, Ni HF, et al. [Effect of Cordyceps sinensis powder on renal oxidative stress and mitochondria functions in 5/6 nephrectomized rats]. Zhongguo Zhong Xi Yi Jie He Za Zhi. 2015 Apr;35(4):443-9.

[713] Tian J, Chen XM, Li LS. [Effects of Cordyceps sinensis, rhubarb and serum renotropin on tubular epithelial cell growth]. *Zhong Xi Yi Jie He Za Zhi*. 1991 Sep;11(9):547-9, 518.

[714] Cheng YJ, Cheng SM, Teng YH, et al. Cordyceps sinensis prevents apoptosis in rodent liver with D-galactosamine/lipopolysaccharide-induced fulminant hepatic failure. *Am J Chin Med*. 2014;42(2):427-41.

[715] Freire Dos Santos L, Rubel R, Bonatto SJ, et al. Cordyceps sinensis biomass produced by submerged fermentation in high-fat diet feed rats normalizes the blood lipid and the low testosterone induced by diet. *EXCLI J*. 2012 Dec 3;11:767-775.

[716] Liu X, Zhong F, Tang XL, et al. Cordyceps sinensis protects against liver and heart injuries in a rat model of chronic kidney disease: a metabolomic analysis. *Acta Pharmacol Sin*. 2014 May;35(5):697-706.

[717] Peng J, Li X, Feng Q, et al. Anti-fibrotic effect of Cordyceps sinensis polysaccharide: Inhibiting HSC activation, TGF-β1/Smad signalling, MMPs and TIMPs. *Exp Biol Med (Maywood)*. 2013 Jun;238(6):668-77.

[718] Zhao X, Li L. [Cordyceps sinensis in protection of the kidney from cyclosporine A nephrotoxicity]. *Zhonghua Yi Xue Za Zhi*. 1993 Jul;73(7):410-2, 447.

[719] Ahmed AF, El-Maraghy NN, Abdel Ghaney RH, et al. Therapeutic effect of captopril, pentoxifylline, and cordyceps sinensis in pre-hepatic portal hypertensive rats. *Saudi J Gastroenterol*. 2012 May-Jun;18(3):182-7.

[720] Peng Y, Tao Y, Wang Q, et al. Ergosterol Is the Active Compound of Cultured Mycelium Cordyceps sinensis on Antiliver Fibrosis. *Evid Based Complement Alternat Med*. 2014;2014:537234.

[721] Liu YK, Shen W. Inhibitive effect of cordyceps sinensis on experimental hepatic fibrosis and its possible mechanism. *World J Gastroenterol*. 2003 Mar;9(3):529-33.

[722] Tang H, Wei W, Wang W, et al. Effects of cultured Cordyceps mycelia polysaccharide A on tumor neurosis factor-α induced hepatocyte injury with mitochondrial abnormality. *Carbohydr Polym*. 2017 May 1;163:43-53.

[723] Li FH, Liu P, Xiong WG, et al. [Effects of Cordyceps sinensis on dimethylnitrosamine-induced liver fibrosis in rats]. *Zhong Xi Yi Jie He Xue Bao*. 2006 Sep;4(5):514-7.

[724] Peng Y, Huang K, Shen L, et al. Cultured Mycelium Cordyceps sinensis allevi¬ates CCl4-induced liver inflammation and fibrosis in mice by activating hepatic natural killer cells. *Acta Pharmacol Sin*. 2016 Feb;37(2):204-16.

[725] Peng Y, Chen Q, Yang T, et al. Cultured mycelium Cordyceps sinensis protects liver sinusoidal endothelial cells in acute liver injured mice. *Mol Biol Rep*. 2014 Mar;41(3):1815-27.

[726] Zhang X, Liu YK, Shen W, et al. Dynamical influence of Cordyceps sinensis on the activity of hepatic insulinase of experimental liver cirrhosis. *Hepatobiliary Pancreat Dis Int*. 2004 Feb;3(1):99-101.

[727] Cheng YJ, Shyu WC, Teng YH, et al. Antagonistic interaction between cordyceps sinensis and exercise on protection in fulminant hepatic failure. *Am J Chin Med*. 2014;42(5):1199-213.

[728] Zhang X, Liu YK, Zheng Q, et al. [Influence of Cordyceps sinensis on pancreatic islet beta cells in rats with experimental liver fibrogenesis]. *Zhonghua Gan Zang Bing Za Zhi*. 2003 Feb;11(2):93-4.

[729] Liu WC, Wang SC, Tsai ML, et al. Protection against radiation-induced bone marrow and intestinal injuries by Cordyceps sinensis, a Chinese herbal medicine. *Radiat Res.* 2006 Dec;166(6):900-7.

[730] Li Y, Chen GZ, Jiang DZ. Effect of Cordyceps sinensis on erythropoiesis in rodent bone marrow. *Chin Med J (Engl).* 1993 Apr;106(4):313-6.

[731] Liu X, Zhong F, Tang XL, et al. Cordyceps sinensis protects against liver and heart injuries in a rat model of chronic kidney disease: a metabolomic analysis. *Acta Pharmacol Sin.* 2014 May;35(5):697-706.

[732] Gu YY, Wang H, Wang S, et al. Effects of Cordyceps sinensis on the Expressions of NF-κB and TGF-β1 in Myocardium of Diabetic Rats. *Evid Based Complement Alternat Med.* 2015;2015:369631.

[733] Yan XF, Zhang ZM, Yao HY, et al. Cardiovascular protection and antioxidant activity of the extracts from the mycelia of Cordyceps sinensis act partially via adenosine receptors. *Phytother Res.* 2013 Nov;27(11):1597-604.

[734] Ku CW, Ho TJ, Huang CY, et al. Cordycepin Attenuates Palmitic Acid-Induced Inflammation and Apoptosis of Vascular Endothelial Cells through Mediating PI3K/Akt/eNOS Signaling Pathway. *Am J Chin Med.* 2021;49(7):1703-1722.

[735] Wu R, Yao PA, Wang HL, et al. Effect of fermented Cordyceps sinensis on doxorubicin-induced cardiotoxicity in rats. *Mol Med Rep.* 2018 Sep;18(3):3229-3241.

[736] Chang Y, Hsu WH, Lu WJ, et al. Inhibitory mechanisms of CME-1, a novel polysaccharide from the mycelia of Cordyceps sinensis, in platelet activation. *Curr Pharm Biotechnol.* 2015;16(5):451-61.

[737] Lu WJ, Chang NC, Jayakumar T, et al. Ex vivo and in vivo studies of CME-1, a novel polysaccharide purified from the mycelia of Cordyceps sinensis that inhibits human platelet activation by activating adenylate cyclase/cyclic AMP. *Thromb Res.* 2014 Dec;134(6):1301-10.

[738] Chang YI, Hsu WH, Lu WJ, et al. Inhibitory Mechanisms of CME-1, a Novel Polysaccharide from the Mycelia of Cordyceps sinensis, in Platelet Activation. *Curr Pharm Biotechnol.* 2015 Mar 3.

[739] Mao YH, Song FL, Xu YX, et al. Extraction, Characterization, and Platelet Inhibitory Effects of Two Polysaccharides from the Cs-4 Fungus. *Int J Mol Sci.* 2022 Oct 20;23(20):12608.

[740] Mei QB, Tao JY, Gao SB, et al. [Antiarrhythmic effects of Cordyceps sinensis (Berk.) Sacc]. *Zhongguo Zhong Yao Za Zhi.* 1989 Oct;14(10):616-8, 640.

[741] Zhao Y. [Inhibitory effects of alcoholic extract of Cordyceps sinensis on abdominal aortic thrombus formation in rabbits]. *Zhonghua Yi Xue Za Zhi.* 1991 Nov;71(11):612-5, 42.

[742] Li F, Gao XY, Rao BF, et al. [Effects of cordyceps sinensis alcohol extractive on serum interferon-gamma level and splenic T lymphocyte subset in mice with viral myocarditis]. *Xi Bao Yu Fen Zi Mian Yi Xue Za Zhi.* 2006 May;22(3):321-3.

[743] Bai X, Tan TY, Li YX, et al. The protective effect of cordyceps sinensis extract on cerebral ischemic injury via modulating the mitochondrial respiratory chain and inhibiting the mitochondrial apoptotic pathway. *Biomed Pharmacother.* 2020 Apr;124:109834.

[744] Zou YX, Liu YX, Ruan MH, et al. Cordyceps sinensis Oral Liquid Inhibits Damage Induced by Oxygen and Glucose Deprivation in SH-SY5Y Cells. *Altern Ther Health Med.* 2016 Mar-Apr;22(2):37-42.

[745] Liu Z, Li P, Zhao D, et al. Protective effect of extract of Cordyceps sinensis in middle cerebral artery occlusion-induced focal cerebral ischemia in rats. *Behav Brain Funct.* 2010 Oct 19;6:61.

[746] Liu Z, Li P, Zhao D, et al. Anti-inflammation effects of Cordyceps sinensis mycelium in focal cerebral ischemic injury rats. *Inflammation.* 2011 Dec;34(6):639-44.

[747] Li SP, Zhao KJ, Ji ZN, et al. A polysaccharide isolated from Cordyceps sinensis, a traditional Chinese medicine, protects PC12 cells against hydrogen peroxide-induced injury. *Life Sci.* 2003 Sep 26;73(19):2503-13.

[748] Wang J, Liu YM, Cao W, et al. Anti-inflammation and antioxidant effect of Cordymin, a peptide purified from the medicinal mushroom Cordyceps sinensis, in middle cerebral artery occlusion-induced focal cerebral ischemia in rats. *Metab Brain Dis.* 2012 Jun;27(2):159-65.

[749] Pal M, Bhardwaj A, Manickam M, et al. Protective Efficacy of the Caterpillar Mushroom, Ophiocordyceps sinensis (Ascomycetes), from India in Neuronal Hippocampal Cells against Hypoxia. *Int J Med Mushrooms.* 2015;17(9):829-40.

[750] Zhou Q, Hu S. [Effect of Cordyceps Cinensis extractant on apoptosis and expression of Toll-like receptor 4 mRNA in the ischemia-reperfusion injured NRK-52E cells]. *Zhong Nan Da Xue Xue Bao Yi Xue Ban.* 2010 Jan;35(1):77-84.

[751] Zhu XY, Ma TT, Li Y, et al. Fingolimod protects against neurovascular unit injury in a rat model of focal cerebral ischemia/reperfusion injury. *Neural Regen Res.* 2023 Apr;18(4):869-874.

[752] Chen Y, Fu L, Han M, et al. The Prophylactic and Therapeutic Effects of Fermented Cordyceps sinensis Powder, Cs-C-Q80, on Subcortical Ischemic Vascular Dementia in Mice. *Evid Based Complement Alternat Med.* 2018 Dec 18;2018:4362715.

[753] Gong MF, Xu JP, et al. [Effect of Cordyceps sinensis sporocarp on learning-memory in mice]. *Zhong Yao Cai.* 2011 Sep;34(9):1403-5.

[754] Zhang Y, Yang M, Gong S, et al. Cordyceps sinensis extracts attenuate aortic transplant arteriosclerosis in rats. *J Surg Res.* 2012 Jun 1;175(1):123-30.

[755] Ji DB, Ye J, Li CL, et al. Antiaging effect of Cordyceps sinensis extract. *Phytother Res.* 2009 Jan;23(1):116-22.

[756] Zou Y, Liu Y, Ruan M, et al. Cordyceps sinensis oral liquid prolongs the lifespan of the fruit fly, Drosophila melanogaster, by inhibiting oxidative stress. *Int J Mol Med.* 2015 Oct;36(4):939-46.

[757] Chen YY, Chen CH, Lin WC, et al. The Role of Autophagy in Anti-Cancer and Health Promoting Effects of Cordycepin. *Molecules.* 2021 Aug 16;26(16):4954.

[758] Freire Dos Santos L, Rubel R, Bonatto SJ, et al. Cordyceps sinensis biomass produced by submerged fermentation in high-fat diet feed rats normalizes the blood lipid and the low testosterone induced by diet. *EXCLI J.* 2012 Dec 3;11:767-775.

[759] Tiamyom K, Sirichaiwetchakoon K, Hengpratom T, et al. The Effects of Cordyceps sinensis (Berk.) Sacc. and Gymnema inodorum (Lour.) Decne. Extracts on Adipogenesis and Lipase Activity In Vitro. *Evid Based Complement Alternat Med.* 2019 Apr 1;2019:5370473.

[760] Koh JH, Kim JM, Chang UJ, et al. Hypocholesterolemic effect of hot-water extract from mycelia of Cordyceps sinensis. *Biol Pharm Bull.* 2003 Jan;26(1):84-7.

[761] Yamaguchi Y, Kagota S, Nakamura K, et al. Inhibitory effects of water extracts from fruiting bodies of cultured Cordyceps sinensis on raised serum lipid peroxide levels and aortic cholesterol deposition in atherosclerotic mice. *Phytother Res.* 2000 Dec;14(8):650-2.

[762] Tiamyom K, Sirichaiwetchakoon K, Hengpratom T, et al. The Effects of Cordyceps sinensis (Berk.) Sacc. and Gymnema inodorum (Lour.) Decne. Extracts on Adipogenesis and Lipase Activity In Vitro. *Evid Based Complement Alternat Med.* 2019 Apr 1;2019:5370473.

[763] Wu GD, Pan A, Zhang X, et al. Cordyceps Improves Obesity and its Related Inflammation via Modulation of Enterococcus cecorum Abundance and Bile Acid Metabolism. *Am J Chin Med.* 2022;50(3):817-838.

[764] Hu Z, Lee CI, Shah VK, et al. Cordycepin Increases Nonrapid Eye Movement Sleep via Adenosine Receptors in Rats. *Evid Based Complement Alternat Med.* 2013;2013:840134.

[765] Ma MW, Gao XS, Yu HL, et al. Cordyceps sinensis Promotes the Growth of Prostate Cancer Cells. *Nutr Cancer.* 2018 Oct;70(7):1166-1172.

[766] Freire Dos Santos L, Rubel R, Bonatto SJ, et al. Cordyceps sinensis biomass produced by submerged fermentation in high-fat diet feed rats normalizes the blood lipid and the low testosterone induced by diet. *EXCLI J.* 2012 Dec 3;11:767-775.

[767] Huang BM, Hsu CC, Tsai SJ, et al. Effects of Cordyceps sinensis on testosterone production in normal rodent Leydig cells. *Life Sci.* 2001 Oct 19;69(22):2593-602.

[768] Hsu CC, Huang YL, Tsai SJ, et al. In vivo and in vitro stimulatory effects of Cordyceps sinensis on testosterone production in rodent Leydig cells. *Life Sci.* 2003 Sep 5;73(16):2127-36.

[769] Huang BM, Chuang YM, Chen CF, et al. Effects of extracted Cordyceps sinensis on steroidogenesis in MA-10 rodent Leydig tumor cells. *Biol Pharm Bull.* 2000 Dec;23(12):1532-5.

[770] Huang BM, Hsiao KY, Chuang PC, et al. Upregulation of steroidogenic enzymes and ovarian 17beta-estradiol in human granulosa-lutein cells by Cordyceps sinensis mycelium. *Biol Reprod.* 2004 May;70(5):1358-64.

[771] Chen YC, Huang BM. Regulatory mechanisms of Cordyceps sinensis on steroidogenesis in MA-10 rodent Leydig tumor cells. *Biosci Biotechnol Biochem.* 2010;74(9):1855-9.

[772] Huang BM, Ju SY, Wu CS, et al. Cordyceps sinensis and its fractions stimulate MA-10 rodent Leydig tumor cell steroidogenesis. *J Androl.* 2001 Sep-Oct;22(5):831-7.

[773] Chen YC, Huang YL, Huang BM. Cordyceps sinensis mycelium activates PKA and PKC signal pathways to stimulate steroidogenesis in MA-10 rodent Leydig tumor cells. *Int J Biochem Cell Biol.* 2005 Jan;37(1):214-23.

[774] Hsu CC, Tsai SJ, Huang YL, et al. Regulatory mechanism of Cordyceps sinensis mycelium on rodent Leydig cell steroidogenesis. *FEBS Lett.* 2003 May 22;543(1-3):140-3.

[775] Wong KL, So EC, Chen CC, et al. Regulation of steroidogenesis by Cordyceps sinensis mycelium extracted fractions with (hCG) treatment in rodent Leydig cells. *Arch Androl.* 2007 Mar-Apr;53(2):75-7.

[776] Huang YL, Leu SF, Liu BC, et al. In vivo stimulatory effect of Cordyceps sinensis mycelium and its fractions on reproductive functions in male rodent. *Life Sci.* 2004 Jul 16;75(9):1051-62.

[777] Pan BS, Lin CY, Huang BM. The Effect of Cordycepin on Steroidogenesis and Apoptosis in MA-10 Rodent Leydig Tumor Cells. *Evid Based Complement Alternat Med.* 2011;2011:750468.

[778] Leu SF, Poon SL, Pao HY, et al. The in vivo and in vitro stimulatory effects of cordycepin on rodent leydig cell steroidogenesis. *Biosci Biotechnol Biochem.* 2011;75(4):723-31.

[779] Pao HY, Pan BS, Leu SF, et al. Cordycepin stimulated steroidogenesis in MA-10 rodent Leydig tumor cells through the protein kinase C Pathway. *J Agric Food Chem.* 2012 May 16;60(19):4905-13.

[780] Leu SF, Chien CH, Tseng CY, et al. The in vivo effect of Cordyceps sinensis mycelium on plasma corticosterone level in male rodent. *Biol Pharm Bull.* 2005 Sep;28(9):1722-5.

[781] Wang SM, Lee LJ, Lin WW, et al. Effects of a water-soluble extract of Cordyceps sinensis on steroidogenesis and capsular morphology of lipid droplets in cultured rat adrenocortical cells. *Cell Biochem.* 1998 Jun 15;69(4):483-9.

[782] Kumar R, Negi PS, Singh B, et al. Cordyceps sinensis promotes exercise endurance capacity of rats by activating skeletal muscle metabolic regulators. *J Ethnopharmacol.* 2011 Jun 14;136(1):260-6.

[783] Yan F, Wang B, Zhang Y. Polysaccharides from Cordyceps sinensis mycelium ameliorate exhaustive swimming exercise-induced oxidative stress. *Pharm Biol.* 2014 Feb;52(2):157-61.

[784] Singh KP, Meena HS, Negi PS. Enhancement of Neuromuscular Activity by Natural Specimens and Cultured Mycelia of Cordyceps sinensis in Mice. *Indian J Pharm Sci.* 2014 Sep;76(5):458-61.

[785] Koh JH, Kim KM, et al. Antifatigue and antistress effect of the hot-water fraction from mycelia of Cordyceps sinensis. *Biol Pharm Bull.* 2003 May;26(5):691-4.

[786] Dai G, Bao T, Xu C, et al. CordyMax Cs-4 improves steady-state bioenergy status in rodent liver. *J Altern Complement Med.* 2001 Jun;7(3):231-40.

[787] Manabe N, Sugimoto M, Azuma Y, et al. Effects of the mycelial extract of cultured Cordyceps sinensis on in vivo hepatic energy metabolism in the rodent. *Jpn J Pharmacol.* 1996 Jan;70(1):85-8.

[788] Manabe N, Azuma Y, Sugimoto M, et al. Effects of the mycelial extract of cultured Cordyceps sinensis on in vivo hepatic energy metabolism and blood flow in dietary hypoferric anaemic mice. *Br J Nutr.* 2000 Feb;83(2):197-204.

[789] Ma H, Wang G, Guo X, et al. Network Pharmacology and Molecular Docking Analysis Explores the Mechanisms of Cordyceps sinensis in the Treatment of Oral Lichen Planus. *J Oncol.* 2022 Aug 29;2022:3156785.

[790] Cheng WY, Wei XQ, Siu KC, et al. Cosmetic and Skincare Benefits of Cultivated Mycelia from the Chinese Caterpillar Mushroom, Ophiocordyceps sinensis (Ascomycetes). *Int J Med Mushrooms.* 2018;20(7):623-636.

[791] Wong WC, Wu JY, Benzie IF. Photoprotective potential of Cordyceps polysaccharides against ultraviolet B radiation-induced DNA damage to human skin cells. *Br J Dermatol.* 2011 May;164(5):980-6.

[792] Zhou L, Yang W, Xu Y, et al. [Short-term curative effect of cultured Cordyceps sinensis (Berk.) Sacc. Mycelia in chronic hepatitis B]. *Zhongguo Zhong Yao Za Zhi.* 1990 Jan;15(1):53-5, 65.

[793] Seetaha S, Ratanabunyong S, Tabtimmai L, et al. Anti-feline immunodeficiency virus reverse transcriptase properties of some medicinal and edible mushrooms. *Vet World.* 2020 Sep;13(9):1798-1806.

[794] Mamta, Mehrotra S, Amitabh, et al. Phytochemical and antimicrobial activities of Himalayan Cordyceps sinensis (Berk.) Sacc. *Indian J Exp Biol*. 2015 Jan;53(1):36-43.

[795] Mishra J, Rajput R, Singh K, et al. Antioxidant-Rich Peptide Fractions Derived from High-Altitude Chinese Caterpillar Medicinal Mushroom Ophiocordyceps sinensis (Ascomycetes) Inhibit Bacterial Pathogens. *Int J Med Mushrooms*. 2019;21(2):155-168.

[796] Siu KM, Mak DH, Chiu PY, et al. Pharmacological basis of 'Yin-nourishing' and 'Yang-invigorating' actions of Cordyceps, a Chinese tonifying herb. *Life Sci*. 2004 Dec 10;76(4):385-95.

[797] Wang Y, Wang Y, Liu D, et al. Cordyceps sinensis polysaccharide inhibits PDGF-BB-induced inflammation and ROS production in human mesangial cells. *Carbohydr Polym*. 2015 Jul 10;125:135-45.

[798] Li SP, Li P, Dong TT, et al. Anti-oxidation activity of different types of natural Cordyceps sinensis and cultured Cordyceps mycelia. *Phytomedicine*. 2001 May;8(3):207-12.

[799] Han SH, Ahn Y, Lee HJ, et al. Antioxidant and Immunostimulatory Activities of a Submerged Culture of Cordyceps sinensis Using Spent Coffee. *Foods*. 2021 Jul 22;10(8):1697.

[800] Wang J, Nie S, Kan L, et al. Comparison of structural features and antioxidant activity of polysaccharides from natural and cultured Cordyceps sinensis. *Food Sci Biotechnol*. 2017 Feb 28;26(1):55-62.

[801] Yamaguchi Y, Kagota S, Nakamura K, et al. Antioxidant activity of the extracts from fruiting bodies of cultured Cordyceps sinensis. *Phytother Res*. 2000 Dec;14(8):647-9.

[802] Yan JK, Wang WQ, Ma HL, et al. Sulfation and enhanced antioxidant capacity of an exopolysaccharide produced by the medicinal fungus Cordyceps sinensis. *Molecules*. 2012 Dec 24;18(1):167-77.

[803] Li SP, Su ZR, Dong TT, et al. The fruiting body and its caterpillar host of Cordyceps sinensis show close resemblance in main constituents and anti-oxidation activity. *Phytomedicine*. 2002 May;9(4):319-24.

[804] Dong CH, Yao YJ. In vitro evaluation of antioxidant activities of aqueous extracts from natural and cultured mycelia of Cordyceps sinensis. *Lebensm Wiss Technol*. 2008 May;41(4):669-677.

[805] Wang BJ, Won SJ, Yu ZR, et al. Free radical scavenging and apoptotic effects of Cordyceps sinensis fractionated by supercritical carbon dioxide. *Food Chem Toxicol*. 2005 Apr;43(4):543-52.

[806] Mamta, Mehrotra S, Amitabh, et al. Phytochemical and antimicrobial activities of Himalayan Cordyceps sinensis (Berk.) Sacc. *Indian J Exp Biol*. 2015 Jan;53(1):36-43.

[807] Chen X, Ding ZY, Wang WQ, et al. An antioxidative galactomannan-protein complex isolated from fermentation broth of a medicinal fungus Cs-HK1. *Carbohydr Polym*. 2014 Nov 4;112:469-74.

[808] Gu YX, Song YW, Fan LQ, et al. [Antioxidant activity of natural and cultured Cordyceps sp]. *Zhongguo Zhong Yao Za Zhi*. 2007 Jun;32(11):1028-31.

[809] Chen S, Siu KC, Wang WQ, et al. Structure and antioxidant activity of a novel poly-N-acetylhexosamine produced by a medicinal fungus. *Carbohydr Polym*. 2013 Apr 15;94(1):332-8.

[810] Wang Y, Wang M, Ling Y, et al. Structural determination and antioxidant activity of a polysaccharide from the fruiting bodies of cultured Cordyceps sinensis. *Am J Chin Med*. 2009;37(5):977-89.

[811] Chen J, Zhang W, Lu T, et al. Morphological and genetic characterization of a cultivated Cordyceps sinensis fungus and its polysaccharide component possessing antioxidant property in H22 tumor-bearing mice. *Life Sci*. 2006 May 1;78(23):2742-8.

[812] Xiao Y, Zhang X, Huang Q. Protective effects of Cordyceps sinensis exopolysaccharide-selenium nanoparticles on H2O2-induced oxidative stress in HepG2 cells. *Int J Biol Macromol*. 2022 Jul 31;213:339-351.

[813] Zou Y, Liu Y, Ruan M, et al. Cordyceps sinensis oral liquid prolongs the lifespan of the fruit fly, Drosophila melanogaster, by inhibiting oxidative stress. *Int J Mol Med*. 2015 Oct;36(4):939-46.

[814] Yan F, Wang B, Zhang Y. Polysaccharides from Cordyceps sinensis mycelium ameliorate exhaustive swimming exercise-induced oxidative stress. *Pharm Biol*. 2014 Feb;52(2):157-61.

[815] Vasiljevic JD, Zivkovic LP, Cabarkapa AM, et al. Cordyceps sinensis: Genotoxic Potential in Human Peripheral Blood Cells and Antigenotoxic Properties Against Hydrogen Peroxide by Comet Assay. *Altern Ther Health Med*. 2016 Jun;22 Suppl 2:24-31.

[816] Wu R, Gao JP, Wang HL, et al. Effects of fermented Cordyceps sinensis on oxidative stress in doxorubicin treated rats. *Pharmacogn Mag*. 2015 Oct-Dec;11(44):724-31.

[817] Yu HM, Wang BS, Huang SC, et al. Comparison of protective effects between cultured Cordyceps militaris and natural Cordyceps sinensis against oxidative damage. *J Agric Food Chem*. 2006 Apr 19;54(8):3132-8.

[818] Chu HL, Chien JC, Duh PD. Protective effect of Cordyceps militaris against high glucose-induced oxidative stress in human umbilical vein endothelial cells. *Food Chem*. 2011 Dec 1;129(3):871-6.

[819] Wang SH, Yang WB, Liu YC, et al. A potent sphingomyelinase inhibitor from Cordyceps mycelia contributes its cytoprotective effect against oxidative stress in macrophages. *J Lipid Res*. 2011 Mar;52(3):471-9.

[820] Shen W, Song D, Wu J, et al. Protective effect of a polysaccharide isolated from a cultivated Cordyceps mycelia on hydrogen peroxide-induced oxidative damage in PC12 cells. *Phytother Res*. 2011 May;25(5):675-80.

[821] Ong BY, Aziz Z. Efficacy of Cordyceps sinensis as an adjunctive treatment in kidney transplant patients: A systematic-review and meta-analysis. *Complement Ther Med*. 2017 Feb;30:84-92.

[822] Hong T, Zhang M, Fan J. Cordyceps sinensis (a traditional Chinese medicine) for kidney transplant recipients (Review). *Cochrane Database Syst Rev*. 2015;(10):CD009698.

[823] Ding C, Tian PX, Xue W, et al. Efficacy of Cordyceps sinensis in long term treatment of renal transplant patients. *Front Biosci (Elite Ed)*. 2011 Jan 1;3(1):301-7.

[824] Zhang Z, Wang X, Zhang Y, et al. Effect of Cordyceps sinensis on renal function of patients with chronic allograft nephropathy. *Urol Int*. 2011;86(3):298-301.

[825] Li Y, Xue WJ, Tian PX, et al. Clinical application of Cordyceps sinensis on immunosuppressive therapy in renal transplantation. *Transplant Proc*. 2009 Jun;41(5):1565-9.

[826] He XL, Chen JH, Wang YM. [Clinical observation on treatment of chronic allograft nephropathy with bailing capsule]. *Zhongguo Zhong Xi Yi Jie He Za Zhi*. 2006 Feb;26(2):102-5.

[827] Sun M, Yang YR, Lu YP, et al. [Clinical study on application of bailing capsule after renal transplantation]. *Zhongguo Zhong Xi Yi Jie He Za Zhi*. 2004 Sep;24(9):808-10.

[828] Wang W, Zhang XN, Yin H, et al. Effects of Bailing capsules for renal transplant recipients: a retrospective clinical study. *Chin Med J (Engl)*. 2013;126(10):1895-9.

[829] He T, Zhao R, Lu Y, et al. Dual-Directional Immunomodulatory Effects of Corbrin Capsule on Autoimmune Thyroid Diseases. *Evid Based Complement Alternat Med*. 2016;2016:1360386.

[830] Yu X, Mao Y, Shergis JL, et al. Effectiveness and Safety of Oral Cordyceps sinensis on Stable COPD of GOLD Stages 2-3: Systematic Review and Meta-Analysis. *Evid Based Complement Alternat Med*. 2019 Apr 3;2019:4903671.

[831] Wang N, Li J, Huang X, Chen W, et al. Herbal Medicine Cordyceps sinensis Improves Health-Related Quality of Life in Moderate-to-Severe Asthma. *Evid Based Complement Alternat Med*. 2016;2016:6134593.

[832] Zhang HW, Lin ZX, Tung YS, et al. Cordyceps sinensis (a traditional Chinese medicine) for treating chronic kidney disease (Review). *Cochrane Database Syst Rev*. 2014;(12):CD008353.

[833] Bao ZD, Wu ZG, Zheng F. [Amelioration of aminoglycoside nephrotoxicity by Cordyceps sinensis in old patients]. *Zhongguo Zhong Xi Yi Jie He Za Zhi*. 1994 May;14(5):271-3, 259.

[834] Bee Yean O, Zoriah A. Efficacy of Cordyceps sinensis as an adjunctive treatment in hemodialysis patients: a systematic review and Meta-analysis. *J Tradit Chin Med*. 2019 Feb;39(1):1-14.

[835] Luo Y, Yang SK, Zhou X, et al. Use of Ophiocordyceps sinensis (syn. Cordyceps sinensis) combined with angiotensin-converting enzyme inhibitors (ACEI)/angiotensin receptor blockers (ARB) versus ACEI/ARB alone in the treatment of diabetic kidney disease: a meta-analysis. *Ren Fail*. 2015 May;37(4):614-34.

[836] Zhao K, Lin Y, Li YJ, et al. Efficacy of short-term cordyceps sinensis for prevention of contrast-induced nephropathy in patients with acute coronary syndrome undergoing elective percutaneous coronary intervention. *Int J Clin Exp Med*. 2014 Dec 15;7(12):5758-64.

[837] Gong HY, Wang KQ, Tang SG. [Effects of cordyceps sinensis on T lymphocyte subsets and hepatofibrosis in patients with chronic hepatitis B]. *Hunan Yi Ke Da Xue Xue Bao*. 2000 Jun 28;25(3):248-50.

[838] Wang XB, Jiang YY, Zhao CY. [Clinical research of xinganbao capsule on the treatment of chronic hepatitis B liver fibrosis]. *Zhongguo Zhong Xi Yi Jie He Za Zhi*. 2012 Mar;32(3):325-8.

[839] Gao Q, Wu G, He D. [Effect of Cordyceps sinensis on the Th1/Th2 cytokines in patients with Condyloma Acuminatum]. *Zhong Yao Cai*. 2000 Jul;23(7):402-4.

[840] Chen S, Li Z, Krochmal R, Abrazado M, et al. Effect of Cs-4 (Cordyceps sinensis) on exercise performance in healthy older subjects: a double-blind, placebo-controlled trial. *J Altern Complement Med*. 2010 May;16(5):585-90.

[841] Parcell AC, Smith JM, Schulthies SS, et al. Cordyceps Sinensis (CordyMax Cs-4) supplementation does not improve endurance exercise performance. *Int J Sport Nutr Exerc Metab*. 2004 Apr;14(2):236-42.

[842] Jo E, Jang HJ, Shen L, et al. Cordyceps militaris Exerts Anticancer Effect on Non-Small Cell Lung Cancer by Inhibiting Hedgehog Signaling via Suppression of TCTN3. *Integr Cancer Ther*. 2020 Jan-Dec;19:1534735420923756.

[843] Bizarro A, Ferreira IC, Soković M, et al. Cordyceps militaris (L.) Link Fruiting Body Reduces the Growth of a Non-Small Cell Lung Cancer Cell Line by Increasing Cellular Levels of p53 and p21. *Molecules*. 2015 Jul 31;20(8):13927-40.

[844] Jeong MK, Yoo HS, Kang IC. The Extract of Cordyceps Militaris Inhibited the Proliferation of Cisplatin-Resistant A549 Lung Cancer Cells by Downregulation of H-Ras. *J Med Food*. 2019 Aug;22(8):823-832.

[845] Park SE, Kim J, Lee YW, et al. Antitumor activity of water extracts from Cordyceps militaris in NCI-H460 cell xenografted nude mice. *J Acupunct Meridian Stud*. 2009 Dec;2(4):294-300.

[846] Reis FS, Barros L, Calhelha RC, et al. The methanolic extract of Cordyceps militaris (L.) Link fruiting body shows antioxidant, antibacterial, antifungal and antihuman tumor cell lines properties. *Food Chem Toxicol*. 2013 Dec;62:91-8.

[847] Liu XC, Zhu ZY, Liu YL, et al. Comparisons of the anti-tumor activity of polysaccharides from fermented mycelia and cultivated fruiting bodies of Cordyceps militaris in vitro. *Int J Biol Macromol*. 2019 Jun 1;130:307-314.

[848] Dong CH, Yang T, Lian T. A comparative study of the antimicrobial, antioxidant, and cytotoxic activities of methanol extracts from fruit bodies and fermented mycelia of caterpillar medicinal mushroom Cordyceps militaris (Ascomycetes). *Int J Med Mushrooms*. 2014;16(5):485-95.

[849] Park SE, Yoo HS, Jin CY, et al. Induction of apoptosis and inhibition of telomerase activity in human lung carcinoma cells by the water extract of Cordyceps militaris. *Food Chem Toxicol*. 2009 Jul;47(7):1667-75.

[850] Jo E, Jang HJ, Shen L, et al. Cordyceps militaris Exerts Anticancer Effect on Non-Small Cell Lung Cancer by Inhibiting Hedgehog Signaling via Suppression of TCTN3. *Integr Cancer Ther*. 2020 Jan-Dec;19:1534735420923756.

[851] Lu YY, Huang X, Luo ZC, et al. [Mechanism of Cordyceps militaris against non-small cell lung cancer: based on serum metabolomics]. *Zhongguo Zhong Yao Za Zhi*. 2022 Sep;47(18):5032-5039.

[852] Luo L, Ran R, Yao J, et al. Se-Enriched Cordyceps militaris Inhibits Cell Proliferation, Induces Cell Apoptosis, And Causes G2/M Phase Arrest In Human Non-Small Cell Lung Cancer Cells. *Onco Targets Ther*. 2019 Oct 23;12:8751-8763.

[853] Zhou Q, Zhang Z, Song L, et al. Cordyceps militaris fraction inhibits the invasion and metastasis of lung cancer cells through the protein kinase B/glycogen synthase kinase 3β/β-catenin signaling pathway. *Oncol Lett*. 2018 Dec;16(6):6930-6939.

[854] Hu Z, Lai Y, Ma C, et al. Cordyceps militaris extract induces apoptosis and pyroptosis via caspase-3/PARP/GSDME pathways in A549 cell line. *Food Sci Nutr*. 2021 Oct 30;10(1):21-38.

[855] Aramwit P, Porasuphatana S, Srichana T, et al. Toxicity evaluation of cordycepin and its delivery system for sustained in vitro anti-lung cancer activity. *Nanoscale Res Lett*. 2015 Mar 27;10:152.

[856] Wang Z, Wu X, Liang YN, et al. Cordycepin Induces Apoptosis and Inhibits Proliferation of Human Lung Cancer Cell Line H1975 via Inhibiting the Phosphorylation of EGFR. *Molecules*. 2016 Sep 27;21(10):1267.

[857] Yu X, Ling J, Liu X, et al. Cordycepin induces autophagy-mediated c-FLIPL degradation and leads to apoptosis in human non-small cell lung cancer cells. *Oncotarget*. 2017 Jan 24;8(4):6691-6699.

[858] Jo E, Jang HJ, Yang KE, et al. Cordyceps militaris induces apoptosis in ovarian cancer cells through TNF-α/TNFR1-mediated inhibition of NF-κB phosphorylation. *BMC Complement Med Ther*. 2020 Jan 13;20(1):1.

[859] Yoon SY, Lindroth AM, Kwon S, et al. Adenosine derivatives from Cordyceps exert antitumor effects against ovarian cancer cells through ENT1-mediated transport, induction of AMPK signaling, and consequent autophagic cell death. *Biomed Pharmacother*. 2022 Sep;153:113491.

[860] Jang HJ, Yang KE, Hwang IH, et al. Cordycepin inhibits human ovarian cancer by inducing autophagy and apoptosis through Dickkopf-related protein 1/β-catenin signaling. *Am J Transl Res*. 2019 Nov 15;11(11):6890-6906.

[861] Reis FS, Barros L, Calhelha RC, et al. The methanolic extract of Cordyceps militaris (L.) Link fruiting body shows antioxidant, antibacterial, antifungal and antihuman tumor cell lines properties. *Food Chem Toxicol*. 2013 Dec;62:91-8.

[862] Jing Y, Cui X, Chen Z, et al. Elucidation and biological activities of a new polysaccharide from cultured Cordyceps militaris. *Carbohydr Polym*. 2014 Feb 15;102:288-96.

[863] Seo H, Song J, Kim M, et al. Cordyceps militaris Grown on Germinated Soybean Suppresses KRAS-Driven Colorectal Cancer by Inhibiting the RAS/ERK Pathway. *Nutrients*. 2018 Dec 21;11(1):20.

[864] Lee HH, Lee S, Lee K, et al. Anti-cancer effect of Cordyceps militaris in human colorectal carcinoma RKO cells via cell cycle arrest and mitochondrial apoptosis. *Daru*. 2015 Jul 4;23(1):35.

[865] Rao YK, Fang SH, Wu WS, et al. Constituents isolated from Cordyceps militaris suppress enhanced inflammatory mediator's production and human cancer cell proliferation. *J Ethnopharmacol*. 2010 Sep 15;131(2):363-7.

[866] Chantawannakul J, Chatpattanasiri P, Wattayagorn V, et al. Virtual Screening for Biomimetic Anti-Cancer Peptides from Cordyceps militaris Putative Pepsinized Peptidome and Validation on Colon Cancer Cell Line. *Molecules*. 2021 Sep 23;26(19):5767.

[867] Reis FS, Barros L, Calhelha RC, et al. The methanolic extract of Cordyceps militaris (L.) Link fruiting body shows antioxidant, antibacterial, antifungal and antihuman tumor cell lines properties. *Food Chem Toxicol*. 2013 Dec;62:91-8.

[868] Jing Y, Cui X, Chen Z, et al. Elucidation and biological activities of a new polysaccharide from cultured Cordyceps militaris. *Carbohydr Polym*. 2014 Feb 15;102:288-96.

[869] Mollah ML, Park DK, Park HJ. Cordyceps militaris Grown on Germinated Soybean Induces G2/M Cell Cycle Arrest through Downregulation of Cyclin B1 and Cdc25c in Human Colon Cancer HT-29 Cells. *Evid Based Complement Alternat Med*. 2012;2012:249217.

[870] Xu J, Shen X, Sun D, et al. Cordycepin Suppresses The Malignant Phenotypes of Colon Cancer Cells through The GSK3ß/ß-catenin/cyclin D1 Signaling Pathway. *Cell J*. 2022 May;24(5):255-260.

[871] Deng Q, Li X, Fang C, et al. Cordycepin enhances anti-tumor immunity in colon cancer by inhibiting phagocytosis immune checkpoint CD47 expression. *Int Immunopharmacol*. 2022 Jun;107:108695.

[872] Zhang Z, Li K, Zheng Z, et al. Cordycepin inhibits colon cancer proliferation by suppressing MYC expression. *BMC Pharmacol Toxicol*. 2022 Feb 4;23(1):12.

[873] Li SZ, Ren JW, Fei J, et al. Cordycepin induces Bax-dependent apoptosis in colorectal cancer cells. *Mol Med Rep*. 2019 Feb;19(2):901-908.

[874] Song J, Wang Y, Teng M, et al. Cordyceps militaris induces tumor cell death via the caspase-dependent mitochondrial pathway in HepG2 and MCF-7 cells. *Mol Med Rep*. 2016 Jun;13(6):5132-40.

[875] Ji Y, Cao Y, Song Y. Green synthesis of gold nanoparticles using a Cordyceps militaris extract and their antiproliferative effect in liver cancer cells (HepG2). *Artif Cells Nanomed Biotechnol*. 2019 Dec;47(1):2737-2745.

[876] Shi P, Huang Z, Tan X, et al. Proteomic detection of changes in protein expression induced by cordycepin in human hepatocellular carcinoma BEL-7402 cells. *Methods Find Exp Clin Pharmacol*. 2008 Jun;30(5):347-53.

[877] Guo Z, Chen W, Dai G, et al. Cordycepin suppresses the migration and invasion of human liver cancer cells by downregulating the expression of CXCR4. *Int J Mol Med*. 2020 Jan;45(1):141-150.

[878] Lee HH, Jeong JW, Lee JH, et al. Cordycepin increases sensitivity of Hep3B human hepatocellular carcinoma cells to TRAIL-mediated apoptosis by inactivating the JNK signaling pathway. *Oncol Rep*. 2013 Sep;30(3):1257-64.

[879] Yamamoto K, Shichiri H, Uda A, et al. Apoptotic Effects of the Extracts of Cordyceps militaris via Erk Phosphorylation in a Renal Cell Carcinoma Cell Line. *Phytother Res*. 2015 May;29(5):707-13.

[880] Yang C, Zhao L, Yuan W, et al. Cordycepin induces apoptotic cell death and inhibits cell migration in renal cell carcinoma via regulation of microRNA-21 and PTEN phosphatase. *Biomed Res*. 2017;38(5):313-320.

[881] Song J, Wang Y, Teng M, et al. Cordyceps militaris induces tumor cell death via the caspase-dependent mitochondrial pathway in HepG2 and MCF-7 cells. *Mol Med Rep*. 2016 Jun;13(6):5132-40.

[882] Jeong MH, Lee CM, Lee SW, et al. Cordycepin-enriched Cordyceps militaris induces immunomodulation and tumor growth delay in mouse-derived breast cancer. *Oncol Rep*. 2013 Oct;30(4):1996-2002.

[883] Reis FS, Barros L, Calhelha RC, et al. The methanolic extract of Cordyceps militaris (L.) Link fruiting body shows antioxidant, antibacterial, antifungal and antihuman tumor cell lines properties. *Food Chem Toxicol*. 2013 Dec;62:91-8.

[884] Wu HC, Chen ST, Chang JC, et al. Radical Scavenging and Antiproliferative Effects of Cordycepin-Rich Ethanol Extract from Brown Rice-Cultivated Cordyceps militaris (Ascomycetes) Mycelium on Breast Cancer Cell Lines. *Int J Med Mushrooms*. 2019;21(7):657-669.

[885] Lee D, Lee WY, Jung K, et al. The Inhibitory Effect of Cordycepin on the Proliferation of MCF-7 Breast Cancer Cells, and its Mechanism: An Investigation Using Network Pharmacology-Based Analysis. *Biomolecules*. 2019 Aug 23;9(9):407.

[886] Jin CY, Kim GY, Choi YH. Induction of apoptosis by aqueous extract of Cordyceps militaris through activation of caspases and inactivation of Akt in human breast cancer MDA-MB-231 Cells. *J Microbiol Biotechnol*. 2008 Dec;18(12):1997-2003.

[887] Park BT, Na KH, Jung EC, et al. Antifungal and Anticancer Activities of a Protein from the Mushroom Cordyceps militaris. *Korean J Physiol Pharmacol*. 2009 Feb;13(1):49-54.

[888] Lee D, Lee WY, Jung K, et al. The Inhibitory Effect of Cordycepin on the Proliferation of MCF-7 Breast Cancer Cells, and its Mechanism: An Investigation Using Network Pharmacology-Based Analysis. *Biomolecules*. 2019 Aug 26;9(9):414.

[889] Suksiriworapong J, Pongprasert N, Bunsupa S, et al. CD44-Targeted Lipid Polymer Hybrid Nanoparticles Enhance Anti-Breast Cancer Effect of Cordyceps militaris Extracts. *Pharmaceutics*. 2023 Jun 20;15(6):1771.

[890] Wen Z, Du X, Meng N, et al. Tussah silkmoth pupae improve anti-tumor properties of Cordyceps militaris (L.) Link by increasing the levels of major metabolite cordycepin. *RSC Adv*. 2019 Feb 13;9(10):5480-5491.

[891] Quan X, Kwak BS, Lee JY, et al. Cordyceps militaris Induces Immunogenic Cell Death and Enhances Antitumor Immunogenic Response in Breast Cancer. *Evid Based Complement Alternat Med.* 2020 Sep 3;2020:9053274.

[892] Wu W, Li X, Qi M, et al. Cordycepin Inhibits Growth and Metastasis Formation of MDA-MB-231 Xenografts in Nude Mice by Modulating the Hedgehog Pathway. *Int J Mol Sci.* 2022 Sep 8;23(18):10362.

[893] Marslin G, Khandelwal V, Franklin G. Cordycepin Nanoencapsulated in Poly(Lactic-Co-Glycolic Acid) Exhibits Better Cytotoxicity and Lower Hemotoxicity Than Free Drug. *Nanotechnol Sci Appl.* 2020 Jun 12;13:37-45.

[894] Rao YK, Fang SH, Wu WS, et al. Constituents isolated from Cordyceps militaris suppress enhanced inflammatory mediator's production and human cancer cell proliferation. *J Ethnopharmacol.* 2010 Sep 15;131(2):363-7.

[895] Lee HH, Park C, Jeong JW, et al. Apoptosis induction of human prostate carcinoma cells by cordycepin through reactive oxygen species-mediated mitochondrial death pathway. *Int J Oncol.* 2013 Mar;42(3):1036-44.

[896] Jeong JW, Jin CY, Park C, et al. Inhibition of migration and invasion of LNCaP human prostate carcinoma cells by cordycepin through inactivation of Akt. *Int J Oncol.* 2012 May;40(5):1697-704.

[897] Cao HL, Liu ZJ, Chang Z. Cordycepin induces apoptosis in human bladder cancer cells via activation of A3 adenosine receptors. *Tumour Biol.* 2017 Jul;39(7):1010428317706915.

[898] Park BT, Na KH, Jung EC, et al. Antifungal and Anticancer Activities of a Protein from the Mushroom Cordyceps militaris. *Korean J Physiol Pharmacol.* 2009 Feb;13(1):49-54.

[899] Lee EJ, Kim WJ, Moon SK. Cordycepin suppresses TNF-alpha-induced invasion, migration and matrix metalloproteinase-9 expression in human bladder cancer cells. *Phytother Res.* 2010 Dec;24(12):1755-61.

[900] Lee SJ, Kim SK, Choi WS, et al. Cordycepin causes p21WAF1-mediated G2/M cell-cycle arrest by regulating c-Jun N-terminal kinase activation in human bladder cancer cells. *Arch Biochem Biophys.* 2009 Oct 15;490(2):103-9.

[901] Li XY, Tao H, Jin C, et al. Cordycepin inhibits pancreatic cancer cell growth in vitro and in vivo via targeting FGFR2 and blocking ERK signaling. *Chin J Nat Med.* 2020 May;18(5):345-355.

[902] Nasser MI, Masood M, Wei W, et al. Cordycepin induces apoptosis in SGC-7901 cells through mitochondrial extrinsic phosphorylation of PI3K/Akt by generating ROS. *Int J Oncol.* 2017 Mar;50(3):911-919.

[903] Yang CH, Kao YH, Huang KS, et al. Cordyceps militaris and mycelial fermentation induced apoptosis and autophagy of human glioblastoma cells. *Cell Death Dis.* 2012 Nov 29;3(11):e431.

[904] Hueng DY, Hsieh CH, Cheng YC, et al. Cordycepin inhibits migration of human glioblastoma cells by affecting lysosomal degradation and protein phosphatase activation. *J Nutr Biochem.* 2017 Mar;41:109-116.

[905] Baik JS, Kwon HY, Kim KS, et al. Cordycepin induces apoptosis in human neuroblastoma SK-N-BE(2)-C and melanoma SK-MEL-2 cells. *Indian J Biochem Biophys.* 2012 Apr;49(2):86-91.

[906] Baik JS, Kwon HY, Kim KS, et al. Cordycepin induces apoptosis in human neuroblastoma SK-N-BE(2)-C and melanoma SK-MEL-2 cells. *Indian J Biochem Biophys.* 2012 Apr;49(2):86-91.

[907] Ruma IM, Putranto EW, Kondo E, et al. Extract of Cordyceps militaris inhibits angiogenesis and suppresses tumor growth of human malignant melanoma cells. *Int J Oncol.* 2014 Jul;45(1):209-18.

[908] Wada T, Sumardika IW, Saito S, et al. Identification of a novel component leading to anti-tumor activity besides the major ingredient cordycepin in Cordyceps militaris extract. *J Chromatogr B Analyt Technol Biomed Life Sci.* 2017 Sep 1;1061-1062:209-219.

[909] Lan YH, Lu YS, Wu JY, et al. Cordyceps militaris Reduces Oxidative Stress and Regulates Immune T Cells to Inhibit Metastatic Melanoma Invasion. *Antioxidants (Basel).* 2022 Jul 30;11(8):1502.

[910] Zheng Q, Shao Y, Zheng W, et al. [Cordycepin, a metabolite of Cordyceps militaris, inhibits xenograft tumor growth of tongue squamous cell carcinoma in nude mice]. *Nan Fang Yi Ke Da Xue Xue Bao.* 2023 Jun 20;43(6):873-878.

[911] Lee S, Lee HH, Kim J, et al. Anti-tumor effect of Cordyceps militaris in HCV-infected human hepatocarcinoma 7.5 cells. *J Microbiol.* 2015 Jul;53(7):468-74.

[912] Oh J, Choi E, Yoon DH, et al. 1H-NMR-Based Metabolic Profiling of Cordyceps militaris to Correlate the Development Process and Anti-Cancer Effect. *J Microbiol Biotechnol.* 2019 Aug 28;29(8):1212-1220.

[913] Jing Y, Cui X, Chen Z, et al. Elucidation and biological activities of a new polysaccharide from cultured Cordyceps militaris. *Carbohydr Polym.* 2014 Feb 15;102:288-96.

[914] Chou SM, Lai WJ, Hong TW, et al. Synergistic property of cordycepin in cultivated Cordyceps militaris-mediated apoptosis in human leukemia cells. *Phytomedicine.* 2014 Oct 15;21(12):1516-24.

[915] Chou SM, Lai WJ, Hong T, et al. Involvement of p38 MAPK in the Anticancer Activity of Cultivated Cordyceps militaris. *Am J Chin Med.* 2015;43(5):1043-57.

[916] Lee H, Kim YJ, Kim HW, et al. Induction of apoptosis by Cordyceps militaris through activation of caspase-3 in leukemia HL-60 cells. *Biol Pharm Bull.* 2006 Apr;29(4):670-4.

[917] Park C, Hong SH, Lee JY, et al. Growth inhibition of U937 leukemia cells by aqueous extract of Cordyceps militaris through induction of apoptosis. *Oncol Rep.* 2005 Jun;13(6):1211-6.

[918] Gao YL, Wang YJ, Chung HH, et al. Molecular networking as a dereplication strategy for monitoring metabolites of natural product treated cancer cells. *Rapid Commun Mass Spectrom.* 2020 Apr;34 Suppl 1:e8549.

[919] Jeong JW, Jin CY, Park C, et al. Induction of apoptosis by cordycepin via reactive oxygen species generation in human leukemia cells. *Toxicol In Vitro.* 2011 Jun;25(4):817-24.

[920] Tima S, Tapingkae T, To-Anun C, et al. Antileukaemic Cell Proliferation and Cytotoxic Activity of Edible Golden Cordyceps (Cordyceps militaris) Extracts. *Evid Based Complement Alternat Med.* 2022 Apr 22;2022:5347718.

[921] Jang KJ, Kwon GS, Jeong JW, et al. Cordyceptin induces apoptosis through repressing hTERT expression and inducing extranuclear export of hTERT. *J Biosci Bioeng.* 2015 Mar;119(3):351-7.

[922] Liao Y, Ling J, Zhang G, et al. Cordycepin induces cell cycle arrest and apoptosis by inducing DNA damage and up-regulation of p53 in Leukemia cells. *Cell Cycle.* 2015;14(5):761-71.

[923] Jing Y, Cui X, Chen Z, et al. Elucidation and biological activities of a new polysaccharide from cultured Cordyceps militaris. *Carbohydr Polym.* 2014 Feb 15;102:288-96.

924 Tian T, Song L, Zheng Q, et al. Induction of apoptosis by Cordyceps militaris fraction in human chronic myeloid leukemia K562 cells involved with mitochondrial dysfunction. *Pharmacogn Mag*. 2014 Jul;10(39):325-31.

925 Tima S, Tapingkae T, To-Anun C, et al. Antileukaemic Cell Proliferation and Cytotoxic Activity of Edible Golden Cordyceps (Cordyceps militaris) Extracts. *Evid Based Complement Alternat Med*. 2022 Apr 22;2022:5347718.

926 Tima S, Tapingkae T, To-Anun C, et al. Antileukaemic Cell Proliferation and Cytotoxic Activity of Edible Golden Cordyceps (Cordyceps militaris) Extracts. *Evid Based Complement Alternat Med*. 2022 Apr 22;2022:5347718.

927 Park JG, Son YJ, Lee TH, et al. Anticancer Efficacy of Cordyceps militaris Ethanol Extract in a Xenografted Leukemia Model. *Evid Based Complement Alternat Med*. 2017;2017:8474703.

928 Lin LT, Lai YJ, Wu SC, et al. Optimal conditions for cordycepin production in surface liquid-cultured Cordyceps militaris treated with porcine liver extracts for suppression of oral cancer. *J Food Drug Anal*. 2018 Jan;26(1):135-144.

929 Xie W, Zhang Z, Song L, et al. Cordyceps militaris Fraction induces apoptosis and G2/M Arrest via c-Jun N-Terminal kinase signaling pathway in oral squamous carcinoma KB Cells. *Pharmacogn Mag*. 2018 Jan-Mar;14(53):116-123.

930 Nurmamat E, Xiao H, Zhang Y, et al. Effects of Different Temperatures on the Chemical Structure and Antitumor Activities of Polysaccharides from Cordyceps militaris. *Polymers (Basel)*. 2018 Apr 12;10(4):430.

931 Bi S, Huang W, Chen S, et al. Cordyceps militaris polysaccharide converts immunosuppressive macrophages into M1-like phenotype and activates T lymphocytes by inhibiting the PD-L1/PD-1 axis between TAMs and T lymphocytes. *Int J Biol Macromol*. 2020 May 1;150:261-280.

932 Lee MJ, Lee JC, Hsieh JH, et al. Cordycepin inhibits the proliferation of malignant peripheral nerve sheath tumor cells through the p53/Sp1/tubulin pathway. *Am J Cancer Res*. 2021 Apr 15;11(4):1247-1266.

933 Yoo HS, Shin JW, Cho JH, et al. Effects of Cordyceps militaris extract on angiogenesis and tumor growth. *Acta Pharmacol Sin*. 2004 May;25(5):657-65.

934 Avtonomova AV, Krasnopolskaya LM, Shuktueva MI, et al. [Assessment of Antitumor Effect of Submerged Culture of Ophiocordyceps sinensis and Cordyceps militaris]. *Antibiot Khimioter*. 2015;60(7-8):14-7.

935 Bai KC, Sheu F. A novel protein from edible fungi Cordyceps militaris that induces apoptosis. *J Food Drug Anal*. 2018 Jan;26(1):21-30.

936 Chen Y, Wu Y, Li S, et al. Large-scale isolation and antitumor mechanism evaluation of compounds from the traditional Chinese medicine Cordyceps Militaris. *Eur J Med Chem*. 2021 Feb 15;212:113142.

937 Yang Q, Yin Y, Yu G, et al. A novel protein with anti-metastasis activity on 4T1 carcinoma from medicinal fungus Cordyceps militaris. *Int J Biol Macromol*. 2015 Sep;80:385-91.

938 Yoo HS, Shin JW, Cho JH, et al. Effects of Cordyceps militaris extract on angiogenesis and tumor growth. *Acta Pharmacol Sin*. 2004 May;25(5):657-65.

939 Kim YS, Kim EK, Hwang JW, et al. Fermented Asterina pectinifera with Cordyceps militaris Mycelia Induced Apoptosis in B16F10 Melanoma Cells. *Adv Exp Med Biol*. 2017;975 Pt 2:1141-1152.

940 Hsu PY, Lin YH, Yeh EL, et al. Cordycepin and a preparation from Cordyceps militaris inhibit malignant transformation and proliferation by decreasing EGFR and IL-17RA signaling in a murine oral cancer model. *Oncotarget*. 2017 Oct 4;8(55):93712-93728.

941 Liu J, Yang S, Yang X, et al. [Anticarcinogenic effect and hormonal effect of Cordyceps militaris Link]. *Zhongguo Zhong Yao Za Zhi*. 1997 Feb;22(2):111-3, inside back cover.

942 Lin RK, Choong CY, Hsu WH, et al. Polysaccharides obtained from mycelia of Cordyceps militaris attenuated doxorubicin-induced cytotoxic effects in chemotherapy. *Afr Health Sci*. 2019 Jun;19(2):2156-2163.

943 Raghu SV, Kudva AK, Rao S, et al. Dietary agents in mitigating chemotherapy-related cognitive impairment (chemobrain or chemofog): first review addressing the benefits, gaps, challenges and ways forward. *Food Funct*. 2021 Nov 15;12(22):11132-11153.

944 Jeong MH, Park YS, Jeong DH, et al. In vitro evaluation of Cordyceps militaris as a potential radioprotective agent. *Int J Mol Med*. 2014 Nov;34(5):1349-57.

945 Oh J, Choi E, Kim J, et al. Efficacy of Ethyl Acetate Fraction of Cordyceps militaris for Cancer-Related Fatigue in Blood Biochemical and 1H-Nuclear Magnetic Resonance Metabolomic Analyses. *Integr Cancer Ther*. 2020 Jan-Dec;19:1534735420932635.

946 Omak G, Yilmaz-Ersan L. Effect of Cordyceps militaris on formation of short-chain fatty acids as postbiotic metabolites. *Prep Biochem Biotechnol*. 2022;52(10):1142-1150.

947 Zhao H, Li M, Liu L, et al. Cordyceps militaris polysaccharide alleviates diabetic symptoms by regulating gut microbiota against TLR4/NF-κB pathway. *Int J Biol Macromol*. 2023 Mar 1;230:123241.

948 Huang S, Zou Y, Tang H, et al. Cordyceps militaris polysaccharides modulate gut microbiota and improve metabolic disorders in mice with diet-induced obesity. *J Sci Food Agric*. 2023 Mar 15;103(4):1885-1894.

949 Huang R, Zhu Z, Wu S, et al. Polysaccharides from Cordyceps militaris prevent obesity in association with modulating gut microbiota and metabolites in high-fat diet-fed mice. *Food Res Int*. 2022 Jul;157:111197.

950 Chen J, Zou Y, Zheng T, et al. The in Vitro Fermentation of Cordyceps militaris Polysaccharides Changed the Simulated Gut Condition and Influenced Gut Bacterial Motility and Translocation. *J Agric Food Chem*. 2022 Nov 9;70(44):14193-14204.

951 Wu S, Wu Q, Wang J, et al. Novel Selenium Peptides Obtained from Selenium-Enriched Cordyceps militaris Alleviate Neuroinflammation and Gut Microbiota Dysbacteriosis in LPS-Injured Mice. *J Agric Food Chem*. 2022 Mar 16;70(10):3194-3206.

952 Yu WQ, Wang XL, Ji HH, et al. CM3-SII polysaccharide obtained from Cordyceps militaris ameliorates hyperlipidemia in heterozygous LDLR-deficient hamsters by modulating gut microbiota and NPC1L1 and PPARα levels. *Int J Biol Macromol*. 2023 Jun 1;239:124293.

953 Zheng H, Cao H, Zhang D, et al. Cordyceps militaris Modulates Intestinal Barrier Function and Gut Microbiota in a Pig Model. *Front Microbiol*. 2022 Mar 17;13:810230.

954 Zhao H, Li M, Liu L, et al. Cordyceps militaris polysaccharide alleviates diabetic symptoms by regulating gut microbiota against TLR4/NF-κB pathway. *Int J Biol Macromol*. 2023 Mar 1;230:123241.

955 Zheng H, Cao H, Zhang D, et al. Cordyceps militaris Modulates Intestinal Barrier Function and Gut Microbiota in a Pig Model. *Front Microbiol*. 2022 Mar 17;13:810230.

956 Han ES, Oh JY, Park HJ. Cordyceps militaris extract suppresses dextran sodium sulfate-induced acute colitis in mice and production of inflammatory mediators from macrophages and mast cells. *J Ethnopharmacol*. 2011 Apr 12;134(3):703-10.

957 Park DK, Park HJ. Ethanol extract of Cordyceps militaris grown on germinated soybeans attenuates dextran-sodium-sulfate-(DSS-) induced colitis by suppressing the expression of matrix metalloproteinases and inflammatory mediators. *Biomed Res Int*. 2013;2013:102918.

958 Park DK, Park HJ. Ethanol extract of Cordyceps militaris grown on germinated soybeans attenuates dextran-sodium-sulfate-(DSS-) induced colitis by suppressing the expression of matrix metalloproteinases and inflammatory mediators. *Biomed Res Int*. 2013;2013:102918.

959 Sun J, Xu J, Wang S, et al. A new cerebroside from cordyceps militaris with anti-PTP1B activity. *Fitoterapia*. 2019 Oct;138:104342.

960 Sun H, Yu X, Li T, et al. Structure and hypoglycemic activity of a novel exopolysaccharide of Cordyceps militaris. *Int J Biol Macromol*. 2021 Jan 1;166:496-508.

961 Ren YY, Sun PP, Ji YP, et al. Carboxymethylation and acetylation of the polysaccharide from Cordyceps militaris and their α-glucosidase inhibitory activities. *Nat Prod Res*. 2020 Feb;34(3):369-377.

962 Wu L, Sun H, Hao Y, et al. Chemical structure and inhibition on α-glucosidase of the polysaccharides from Cordyceps militaris with different developmental stages. *Int J Biol Macromol*. 2020 Apr 1;148:722-736.

963 Dong Y, Jing T, Meng Q, et al. Studies on the antidiabetic activities of Cordyceps militaris extract in diet-streptozotocin-induced diabetic Sprague-Dawley rats. *Biomed Res Int*. 2014;2014:160980.

964 Shang XL, Pan LC, Tang Y, et al. 1H NMR-based metabonomics of the hypoglycemic effect of polysaccharides from Cordyceps militaris on streptozotocin-induced diabetes in mice. *Nat Prod Res*. 2020 May;34(10):1366-1372.

965 Zhang G, Huang Y, Bian Y, et al. Hypoglycemic activity of the fungi Cordyceps militaris, Cordyceps sinensis, Tricholoma mongolicum, and Omphalia lapidescens in streptozotocin-induced diabetic rats. *Appl Microbiol Biotechnol*. 2006 Oct;72(6):1152-6.

966 Zhu ZY, Guo MZ, Liu F, et al. Preparation and inhibition on α-d-glucosidase of low molecular weight polysaccharide from Cordyceps militaris. *Int J Biol Macromol*. 2016 Dec;93(Pt A):27-33.

967 Zhao H, Lai Q, Zhang J, et al. Antioxidant and Hypoglycemic Effects of Acidic-Extractable Polysaccharides from Cordyceps militaris on Type 2 Diabetes Mice. *Oxid Med Cell Longev*. 2018 Nov 25;2018:9150807.

968 Liu C, Song J, Teng M, et al. Antidiabetic and Antinephritic Activities of Aqueous Extract of Cordyceps militaris Fruit Body in Diet-Streptozotocin-Induced Diabetic Sprague Dawley Rats. *Oxid Med Cell Longev*. 2016;2016:9685257.

969 Cheng YW, Chen YI, Tzeng CY, et al. Aqueous extracts of Cordyceps militaris (Ascomycetes) lower the levels of plasma glucose by activating the cholinergic nerve in streptozotocin-induced diabetic rats. *Int J Med Mushrooms*. 2013;15(3):277-86.

970 Ma L, Zhang S, Du M. Cordycepin from Cordyceps militaris prevents hyperglycemia in alloxan-induced diabetic mice. *Nutr Res*. 2015 May;35(5):431-9.

971 Han X, Liu LH, Fang XY, et al. Cordythiazole A, the first member of thiazole alkaloids from Chinese cordyceps, with α-glucosidase inhibitory activity. *J Nat Med*. 2023 Sep;77(4):986-991.

972 Lee BH, Chen CH, Hsu YY, et al. Polysaccharides Obtained from Cordyceps militaris Alleviate Hyperglycemia by Regulating Gut Microbiota in Mice Fed a High-Fat/Sucrose Diet. *Foods*. 2021 Aug 12;10(8):1870.

973 Yu SH, Chen SY, Li WS, et al. Hypoglycemic Activity through a Novel Combination of Fruiting Body and Mycelia of Cordyceps militaris in High-Fat Diet-Induced Type 2 Diabetes Mellitus Mice. *J Diabetes Res*. 2015;2015:723190.

974 Liu X, Dun M, Jian T, et al. Cordyceps militaris extracts and cordycepin ameliorate type 2 diabetes mellitus by modulating the gut microbiota and metabolites. *Front Pharmacol*. 2023 Mar 9;14:1134429.

975 Yan B, Gong Y, Meng W, et al. Cordycepin protects islet β-cells against glucotoxicity and lipotoxicity via modulating related proteins of ROS/JNK signaling pathway. *Biomed Pharmacother*. 2023 Jul;163:114776.

976 Huang T, Zhou Y, Lu X, et al. Cordycepin, a major bioactive component of Cordyceps militaris, ameliorates diabetes-induced testicular damage through the Sirt1/Foxo3a pathway. *Andrologia*. 2022 Feb;54(1):e14294.

977 Xue B, Li L, Gu XD, et al. Protective Effect of Cordycepin on Impairment of Endothelial Function in Type 2 Diabetes Mellitus. *Int J Med Mushrooms*. 2022;24(3):65-75.

978 Liu C, Song J, Teng M, et al. Antidiabetic and Antinephritic Activities of Aqueous Extract of Cordyceps militaris Fruit Body in Diet-Streptozotocin-Induced Diabetic Sprague Dawley Rats. *Oxid Med Cell Longev*. 2016;2016:9685257.

979 Chen DD , Xu R , Zhou JY et al. Cordyceps militaris polysaccharides exerted protective effects on diabetic nephropathy in mice via regulation of autophagy. *Food Funct*. 2019 Aug 1;10(8):5102-5114.

980 Yu SH, Dubey NK, Li WS, et al. Cordyceps militaris Treatment Preserves Renal Function in Type 2 Diabetic Nephropathy Mice. *PLoS One*. 2016 Nov 10;11(11):e0166342.

981 Zhao H, Li M, Liu L, et al. Cordyceps militaris polysaccharide alleviates diabetic symptoms by regulating gut microbiota against TLR4/NF-κB pathway. *Int J Biol Macromol*. 2023 Mar 1;230:123241.

982 Huang S, Zou Y, Tang H, et al. Cordyceps militaris polysaccharides modulate gut microbiota and improve metabolic disorders in mice with diet-induced obesity. *J Sci Food Agric*. 2023 Mar 15;103(4):1885-1894.

983 Yu WQ, Wang XL, Ji HH, et al. CM3-SII polysaccharide obtained from Cordyceps militaris ameliorates hyperlipidemia in heterozygous LDLR-deficient hamsters by modulating gut microbiota and NPC1L1 and PPARα levels. *Int J Biol Macromol*. 2023 Jun 1;239:124293.

984 Cheng YW, Chen YI, Tzeng CY, et al. Extracts of Cordyceps militaris lower blood glucose via the stimulation of cholinergic activation and insulin secretion in normal rats. *Phytother Res*. 2012 Aug;26(8):1173-7.

985 Choi SB, Park CH, Choi MK, et al. Improvement of insulin resistance and insulin secretion by water extracts of Cordyceps militaris, Phellinus linteus, and Paecilomyces tenuipes in 90% pancreatectomized rats. *Biosci Biotechnol Biochem*. 2004 Nov;68(11):2257-64.

[986] Cheng YW, Chen YI, Tzeng CY, et al. Extracts of Cordyceps militaris lower blood glucose via the stimulation of cholinergic activation and insulin secretion in normal rats. *Phytother Res.* 2012 Aug;26(8):1173-7.

[987] Niu YJ, Tao RY, Liu Q, et al. Improvement on lipid metabolic disorder by 3'-deoxyadenosine in high-fat-diet-induced fatty mice. *Am J Chin Med.* 2010;38(6):1065-75.

[988] Kim DJ, Kang YH, Kim KK, et al. Increased glucose metabolism and alpha-glucosidase inhibition in Cordyceps militaris water extract-treated HepG2 cells. *Nutr Res Pract.* 2017 Jun;11(3):180-189.

[989] Sun H, Zhang A, Gong Y, et al. Improving effect of cordycepin on insulin synthesis and secretion in normal and oxidative-damaged INS-1 cells. *Eur J Pharmacol.* 2022 Apr 5;920:174843.

[990] Nguyen TV, Chumnanpuen P, Parunyakul K, et al. A study of the aphrodisiac properties of Cordyceps militaris in streptozotocin-induced diabetic male rats. *Vet World.* 2021 Feb;14(2):537-544.

[991] Wang J, Wang Y, Yang X, et al. Purification, structural characterization, and PCSK9 secretion inhibitory effect of the novel alkali-extracted polysaccharide from Cordyceps militaris. *Int J Biol Macromol.* 2021 May 15;179:407-417.

[992] Kim SB, Ahn B, Kim M, et al. Effect of Cordyceps militaris extract and active constituents on metabolic parameters of obesity induced by high-fat diet in C58BL/6J mice. *J Ethnopharmacol.* 2014;151(1):478-84.

[993] Yu WQ, Yin F, Shen N, et al. Polysaccharide CM1 from Cordyceps militaris hinders adipocyte differentiation and alleviates hyperlipidemia in LDLR(+/-) hamsters. *Lipids Health Dis.* 2021 Dec 13;20(1):178.

[994] Wang L, Xu N, Zhang J, et al. Antihyperlipidemic and hepatoprotective activities of residue polysaccharide from Cordyceps militaris SU-12. *Carbohydr Polym.* 2015 Oct 20;131:355-62.

[995] Gao J, Lian ZQ, Zhu P, et al. Lipid-lowering effect of cordycepin (3'-deoxyadenosine) from Cordyceps militaris on hyperlipidemic hamsters and rats. *Yao Xue Xue Bao.* 2011 Jun;46(6):669-76.

[996] Guo P, Kai Q, Gao J, et al. Cordycepin prevents hyperlipidemia in hamsters fed a high-fat diet via activation of AMP-activated protein kinase. *J Pharmacol Sci.* 2010;113(4):395-403.

[997] Li Y, Miao M, Yin F, et al. The polysaccharide-peptide complex from mushroom Cordyceps militaris ameliorates atherosclerosis by modulating the lncRNA-miRNA-mRNA axis. *Food Funct.* 2022 Mar 21;13(6):3185-3197.

[998] Yang X, Lin P, Wang J, et al. Purification, characterization and anti-atherosclerotic effects of the polysaccharides from the fruiting body of Cordyceps militaris. *Int J Biol Macromol.* 2021 Jun 30;181:890-904.

[999] Jung SM, Park SS, Kim WJ, et al. Ras/ERK1 pathway regulation of p27KIP1-mediated G1-phase cell-cycle arrest in cordycepin-induced inhibition of the proliferation of vascular smooth muscle cells. *Eur J Pharmacol.* 2012 Apr 15;681(1-3):15-22.

[1000] Won KJ, Lee SC, Lee CK, et al. Cordycepin attenuates neointimal formation by inhibiting reactive oxygen species-mediated responses in vascular smooth muscle cells in rats. *J Pharmacol Sci.* 2009 Mar;109(3):403-12.

[1001] Yin F, Lin P, Yu WQ, et al. The Cordyceps militaris-Derived Polysaccharide CM1 Alleviates Atherosclerosis in LDLR(-/-) Mice by Improving Hyperlipidemia. *Front Mol Biosci.* 2021 Dec 13;8:783807.

[1002] Wang Y, Huang C, Lu F, et al. In-situ and real-time monitoring of two-stage enzymatic preparation of ACE inhibitory peptides from Cordyceps militaris medium residues by ultrasonic-assisted pretreatment. *Food Chem.* 2023 Aug 30;418:135886.

[1003] Wang Y, Yang Z, Bao D, et al. Improving Hypoxia Adaption Causes Distinct Effects on Growth and Bioactive Compounds Synthesis in an Entomopathogenic Fungus Cordyceps militaris. *Front Microbiol.* 2021 Jun 22;12:698436.

[1004] Valdez-Solana MA, Corral-Guerrero IA, et al. Cordyceps militaris Inhibited Angiotensin-Converting Enzyme through Molecular Interaction between Cordycepin and ACE C-Domain. *Life (Basel).* 2022 Sep 19;12(9):1450.

[1005] Kwon HW, Shin JH, Lim DH, et al. Antiplatelet and antithrombotic effects of cordycepin-enriched WIB-801CE from Cordyceps militaris ex vivo, in vivo, and in vitro. *BMC Complement Altern Med.* 2016 Dec 7;16(1):508.

[1006] Cho HJ, Cho JY, Rhee MH, et al. Inhibitory effects of cordycepin (3'-deoxyadenosine), a component of Cordyceps militaris, on human platelet aggregation induced by thapsigargin. *J Microbiol Biotechnol.* 2007 Jul;17(7):1134-8.

[1007] Lee DH, Kwon HW, Kim HH, et al. Cordycepin-enriched WIB801C from Cordyceps militaris inhibits ADP-induced [Ca(2+)]i mobilization and fibrinogen binding via phosphorylation of IP 3R and VASP. *Arch Pharm Res.* 2015 Jan;38(1):81-97.

[1008] Lee DH, Kim HH, Lim DH, et al. Effect of Cordycepin-Enriched WIB801C from Cordyceps militaris Suppressing Fibrinogen Binding to Glycoprotein IIb/IIIa. *Biomol Ther (Seoul).* 2015 Jan;23(1):60-70.

[1009] Lee DH, Kim HH, Cho HJ, et al. Cordycepin-Enriched WIB801C From Cordyceps militaris Inhibits Collagen-Induced [Ca(2+)]i Mobilization via cAMP-Dependent Phosphorylation of Inositol 1, 4, 5-Trisphosphate Receptor in Human Platelets. *Biomol Ther (Seoul).* 2014 May;22(3):223-31.

[1010] Cho HJ, Cho JY, Rhee MH, et al. Cordycepin (3'-deoxyadenosine) inhibits human platelet aggregation induced by U46619, a TXA2 analogue. *J Pharm Pharmacol.* 2006 Dec;58(12):1677-82.

[1011] Cho HJ, Cho JY, Rhee MH, et al. Cordycepin (3'-deoxyadenosine) inhibits human platelet aggregation in a cyclic AMP- and cyclic GMP-dependent manner. *Eur J Pharmacol.* 2007 Mar 8;558(1-3):43-51.

[1012] Takakura K, Ito S, Sonoda J, et al. Cordyceps militaris improves the survival of Dahl salt-sensitive hypertensive rats possibly via influences of mitochondria and autophagy functions. *Heliyon.* 2017 Nov 24;3(11):e00462.

[1013] Zhou M, Zha Z, Zheng Z, et al. Cordycepin suppresses vascular inflammation, apoptosis and oxidative stress of arterial smooth muscle cell in thoracic aortic aneurysm with VEGF inhibition. *Int Immunopharmacol.* 2023 Mar;116:109759.

[1014] Park ES, Kang DH, Yang MK, et al. Cordycepin, 3'-deoxyadenosine, prevents rat hearts from ischemia/reperfusion injury via activation of Akt/GSK-3β/p70S6K signaling pathway and HO-1 expression. *Cardiovasc Toxicol.* 2014 Mar;14(1):1-9.

[1015] Wang HB, Duan MX, Xu M, et al. Cordycepin ameliorates cardiac hypertrophy via activating the AMPKα pathway. *J Cell Mol Med.* 2019 Aug;23(8):5715-5727.

[1016] Huang S, Zou Y, Tang H, et al. Cordyceps militaris polysaccharides modulate gut microbiota and improve metabolic disorders in mice with diet-induced obesity. *J Sci Food Agric.* 2023 Mar 15;103(4):1885-1894.

[1017] Huang R, Zhu Z, Wu S, et al. Polysaccharides from Cordyceps militaris prevent obesity in association with modulating gut microbiota and metabolites in high-fat diet-fed mice. *Food Res Int.* 2022 Jul;157:111197.

[1018] Yu WQ, Yin F, Shen N, et al. Polysaccharide CM1 from Cordyceps militaris hinders adipocyte differentiation and alleviates hyperlipidemia in LDLR(+/-) hamsters. *Lipids Health Dis.* 2021 Dec 13;20(1):178.

[1019] Jang D, Lee E, Lee S, et al. System-level investigation of anti-obesity effects and the potential pathways of Cordyceps militaris in ovariectomized rats. *BMC Complement Med Ther.* 2022 May 12;22(1):132.

[1020] Shimada T, Hiramatsu N, Kasai A, et al. Suppression of adipocyte differentiation by Cordyceps militaris through activation of the aryl hydrocarbon receptor. *Am J Physiol Endocrinol Metab.* 2008 Oct;295(4):E859-67.

[1021] Liu Q, Hong IP, Ahn MJ, et al. Anti-adipogenic activity of Cordyceps militaris in 3T3-L1 cells. *Nat Prod Commun.* 2011 Dec;6(12):1839-41.

[1022] Li Y, Li Y, Wang X, et al. Cordycepin Modulates Body Weight by Reducing Prolactin Via an Adenosine A1 Receptor. *Curr Pharm Des.* 2018;24(27):3240-3249.

[1023] Takahashi S, Tamai M, Nakajima S, et al. Blockade of adipocyte differentiation by cordycepin. *Br J Pharmacol.* 2012 Oct;167(3):561-75.

[1024] Tian JY, Chen L, Zhang XL, et al. [Investigation of a compound, compatibility of Rhodiola crenulata, Cordyceps militaris, and Rheum palmatum, on metabolic syndrome treatment II - improving obesity]. *Zhongguo Zhong Yao Za Zhi.* 2013 May;38(9):1411-5.

[1025] Yang CH, Kuo WS, Wang JS, et al. Improvement in the Blood Urea Nitrogen and Serum Creatinine Using New Cultivation of Cordyceps militaris. *Evid Based Complement Alternat Med.* 2022 Mar 23;2022:4321298.

[1026] Tsai CH, Yen YH, Yang JP. Finding of polysaccharide-peptide complexes in Cordyceps militaris and evaluation of its acetylcholinesterase inhibition activity. *J Food Drug Anal.* 2015 Mar;23(1):63-70.

[1027] Phan CW, David P, Naidu M, et al. Neurite outgrowth stimulatory effects of culinary-medicinal mushrooms and their toxicity assessment using differentiating Neuro-2a and embryonic fibroblast BALB/3T3. *BMC Complement Altern Med.* 2013 Oct 11;13:261.

[1028] Cai ZL, Wang CY, Jiang ZJ, et al. Effects of cordycepin on Y-maze learning task in mice. *Eur J Pharmacol.* 2013 Aug 15;714(1-3):249-53.

[1029] Bai L, Tan C, Ren J, et al. Cordyceps militaris acidic polysaccharides improve learning and memory impairment in mice with exercise fatigue through the PI3K/NRF2/HO-1 signalling pathway. *Int J Biol Macromol.* 2023 Feb 1;227:158-172.

[1030] Li Z, Zhang Z, Zhang J, et al. Cordyceps militaris extract attenuates D-galactose-induced memory impairment in mice. *J Med Food.* 2012 Dec;15(12):1057-63.

[1031] Cai ZL, Wang CY, Jiang ZJ, et al. Effects of cordycepin on Y-maze learning task in mice. *Eur J Pharmacol.* 2013 Aug 15;714(1-3):249-53.

[1032] Yuan G, An L, Sun Y, et al. Improvement of Learning and Memory Induced by Cordyceps Polypeptide Treatment and the Underlying Mechanism. *Evid Based Complement Alternat Med.* 2018 Mar 15;2018:9419264.

[1033] Wang J, Gong Y, Tan H, et al. Cordycepin suppresses glutamatergic and GABAergic synaptic transmission through activation of A1 adenosine receptor in rat hippocampal CA1 pyramidal neurons. *Biomed Pharmacother.* 2022 Jan;145:112446.

[1034] He MT, Lee AY, Kim JH, et al. Protective role of Cordyceps militaris in Aβ1-42-induced Alzheimer's disease in vivo. *Food Sci Biotechnol.* 2018 Dec 4;28(3):865-872.

[1035] Thai NM, Dat TTH, Hai NTT, et al. Identification of potential inhibitors against Alzheimer-related proteins in Cordyceps militaris ethanol extract: experimental evidence and computational analyses. *3 Biotech.* 2023 Sep;13(9):292.

[1036] Jiao L, Yu Z, Zhong X, et al. Cordycepin improved neuronal synaptic plasticity through CREB-induced NGF upregulation driven by MG-M2 polarization: a microglia-neuron symphony in AD. *Biomed Pharmacother.* 2023 Jan;157:114054.

[1037] He MT, Park CH, Shin YS, et al. Caterpillar Medicinal Mushroom, Cordyceps militaris (Ascomycetes), Protects Aβ1-42-Induced Neurologic Damage in C6 Glial Cells. *Int J Med Mushrooms.* 2020;22(12):1203-1213.

[1038] He MT, Park CH, Cho EJ. Caterpillar Medicinal Mushroom, Cordyceps militaris (Ascomycota), Attenuates Aβ1-42-Induced Amyloidogenesis and Inflammatory Response by Suppressing Amyloid Precursor Protein Progression and p38 MAPK/JNK Activation. *Int J Med Mushrooms.* 2021;23(11):71-83.

[1039] Hwang IK, Lim SS, Yoo KY, et al. A Phytochemically characterized extract of Cordyceps militaris and cordycepin protect hippocampal neurons from ischemic injury in gerbils. *Planta Med.* 2008 Feb;74(2):114-9.

[1040] Hwang S, Cho GS, Ryu S, et al. Post-ischemic treatment of WIB801C, standardized Cordyceps extract, reduces cerebral ischemic injury via inhibition of inflammatory cell migration. *J Ethnopharmacol.* 2016 Jun 20;186:169-180.

[1041] Kim YO, Kim HJ, Abu-Taweel GM, et al. Neuroprotective and therapeutic effect of Cordyceps militaris on ischemia-induced neuronal death and cognitive impairments. *Saudi J Biol Sci.* 2019 Nov;26(7):1352-1357.

[1042] Yin L, Zhang Y, Wang L, et al. Neuroprotective potency of a soy whey fermented by Cordyceps militaris SN-18 against hydrogen peroxide-induced oxidative injury in PC12 cells. *Eur J Nutr.* 2022 Mar;61(2):779-792.

[1043] Hwang S, Cho GS, Ryu S, et al. Post-ischemic treatment of WIB801C, standardized Cordyceps extract, reduces cerebral ischemic injury via inhibition of inflammatory cell migration. *J Ethnopharmacol.* 2016 Jun 20;186:169-180.

[1044] Jiang X, Tang P-C, Chen Q, et al. Cordycepin Exerts Neuroprotective Effects via an Anti-Apoptotic Mechanism based on the Mitochondrial Pathway in a Rotenone-Induced Parkinsonism Rat Model. *CNS Neurol Disord Drug Targets.* 2019;18(8):609-620.

[1045] Cheng Z, He W, Zhou X, et al. Cordycepin protects against cerebral ischemia/reperfusion injury in vivo and in vitro. *Eur J Pharmacol.* 2011 Aug 16;664(1-3):20-8.

[1046] Zhang XL, Huang WM, Tang PC, et al. Anti-inflammatory and neuroprotective effects of natural cordycepin in rotenone-induced PD models through inhibiting Drp1-mediated mitochondrial fission. *Neurotoxicology.* 2021 May;84:1-13.

[1047] Wei P, Wang K, Luo C, et al. Cordycepin confers long-term neuroprotection via inhibiting neutrophil infiltration and neuroinflammation after traumatic brain injury. *J Neuroinflammation.* 2021 Jun 15;18(1):137.

[1048] Wu S, Wu Q, Wang J, et al. Novel Selenium Peptides Obtained from Selenium-Enriched Cordyceps militaris Alleviate Neuroinflammation and Gut Microbiota Dysbacteriosis in LPS-Injured Mice. *J Agric Food Chem.* 2022 Mar 16;70(10):3194-3206.

[1049] Nallathamby N, Malek SNA, Vidyadaran S, et al. Lipids in an Ethyl Acetate Fraction of Caterpillar Medicinal Mushroom, Cordyceps militaris (Ascomycetes), Reduce Nitric Oxide Production in BV2 Cells via NRF2 and NF-κB Pathways. *Int J Med Mushrooms.* 2020;22(12):1215-1223.

[1050] Nallathamby N, Guan-Serm L, Vidyadaran S, et al. Ergosterol of Cordyceps militaris Attenuates LPS Induced Inflammation in BV2 Microglia Cells. *Nat Prod Commun.* 2015 Jun;10(6):885-6.

[1051] Govindula A, Pai A, Baghel S, et al. Molecular mechanisms of cordycepin emphasizing its potential against neuroinflammation: An update. *Eur J Pharmacol*. 2021 Oct 5;908:174364.

[1052] Zhang XL, Huang WM, Tang PC, et al. Anti-inflammatory and neuroprotective effects of natural cordycepin in rotenone-induced PD models through inhibiting Drp1-mediated mitochondrial fission. *Neurotoxicology*. 2021 May;84:1-13.

[1053] Lee JY, Choi HY, Baik HH, et al. Cordycepin-enriched WIB-801C from Cordyceps militaris improves functional recovery by attenuating blood-spinal cord barrier disruption after spinal cord injury. *J Ethnopharmacol*. 2017 May 5;203:90-100.

[1054] Lin YE, Chen YC, Lu KH, et al. Antidepressant-like effects of water extract of Cordyceps militaris (Linn.) Link by modulation of ROCK2/PTEN/Akt signaling in an unpredictable chronic mild stress-induced animal model. *J Ethnopharmacol*. 2021 Aug 10;276:114194.

[1055] Tianzhu Z, Shihai Y, Juan D. Antidepressant-like effects of cordycepin in a mice model of chronic unpredictable mild stress. *Evid Based Complement Alternat Med*. 2014;2014:438506.

[1056] Dong Y, Hu S, Liu C, et al. Purification of polysaccharides from Cordyceps militaris and their anti-hypoxic effect. *Mol Med Rep*. 2015 Feb;11(2):1312-7.

[1057] Xu YF. Effect of Polysaccharide from Cordyceps militaris (Ascomycetes) on Physical Fatigue Induced by Forced Swimming. *Int J Med Mushrooms*. 2016;18(12):1083-1092.

[1058] Zhong L, Zhao L, Yang F, et al. Evaluation of anti-fatigue property of the extruded product of cereal grains mixed with Cordyceps militaris on mice. *J Int Soc Sports Nutr*. 2017 Jun 2;14:15.

[1059] Song J, Wang Y, Teng M, et al. Studies on the Antifatigue Activities of Cordyceps militaris Fruit Body Extract in Mouse Model. *Evid Based Complement Alternat Med*. 2015;2015:174616.

[1060] Chai X, Pan M, Wang J, et al. Cordycepin exhibits anti-fatigue effect via activating TIGAR/SIRT1/PGC-1α signaling pathway. *Biochem Biophys Res Commun*. 2022 Dec 31;637:127-135.

[1061] Choi E, Oh J, Sung GH. Beneficial Effect of Cordyceps militaris on Exercise Performance via Promoting Cellular Energy Production. *Mycobiology*. 2020 Nov 9;48(6):512-517.

[1062] Jung K, Kim IH, Han D. Effect of medicinal plant extracts on forced swimming capacity in mice. *J Ethnopharmacol*. 2004 Jul;93(1):75-81.

[1063] Song J, Wang Y, Liu C, et al. Cordyceps militaris fruit body extract ameliorates membranous glomerulonephritis by attenuating oxidative stress and renal inflammation via the NF-κB pathway. *Food Funct*. 2016 Apr;7(4):2006-15.

[1064] Song Q, Zhu Z. Using Cordyceps militaris extracellular polysaccharides to prevent Pb2+-induced liver and kidney toxicity by activating Nrf2 signals and modulating gut microbiota. *Food Funct*. 2020 Oct 21;11(10):9226-9239.

[1065] Gu LB, Bian RW, Tu Y, et al. [Mechanisms of cordycepin on improving renal interstitial fibrosis via regulating eIF2α/TGF-β/Smad signaling pathway]. *Zhongguo Zhong Yao Za Zhi*. 2014 Nov;39(21):4096-101.

[1066] Sun T, Dong W, Jiang G, et al. Cordyceps militaris Improves Chronic Kidney Disease by Affecting TLR4/NF-κB Redox Signaling Pathway. *Oxid Med Cell Longev*. 2019 Mar 31;2019:7850863.

[1067] Wang L, Xu N, Zhang J, et al. Antihyperlipidemic and hepatoprotective activities of residue polysaccharide from Cordyceps militaris SU-12. *Carbohydr Polym*. 2015 Oct 20;131:355-62.

[1068] Song Q, Zhu Z. Using Cordyceps militaris extracellular polysaccharides to prevent Pb2+-induced liver and kidney toxicity by activating Nrf2 signals and modulating gut microbiota. *Food Funct*. 2020 Oct 21;11(10):9226-9239.

[1069] Li J, Zhong L, Zhu H, et al. The Protective Effect of Cordycepin on D-Galactosamine/Lipopolysaccharide-Induced Acute Liver Injury. *Mediators Inflamm*. 2017;2017:3946706.

[1070] Hung YP, Lee CL. Higher Anti-Liver Fibrosis Effect of Cordyceps militaris-Fermented Product Cultured with Deep Ocean Water via Inhibiting Proinflammatory Factors and Fibrosis-Related Factors Expressions. *Mar Drugs*. 2017 Jun 8;15(6):168.

[1071] Hung YP, Lee CL. Higher Anti-Liver Fibrosis Effect of Cordyceps militaris-Fermented Product Cultured with Deep Ocean Water via Inhibiting Proinflammatory Factors and Fibrosis-Related Factors Expressions. *Mar Drugs*. 2017 Jun 8;15(6):168.

[1072] Nan JX, Park EJ, Yang BK, et al. Antifibrotic effect of extracellular biopolymer from submerged mycelial cultures of Cordyceps militaris on liver fibrosis induced by bile duct ligation and scission in rats. *Arch Pharm Res*. 2001 Aug;24(4):327-32.

[1073] Cha JY, Ahn HY, Cho YS, et al. Protective effect of cordycepin-enriched Cordyceps militaris on alcoholic hepatotoxicity in Sprague-Dawley rats. *Food Chem Toxicol*. 2013 Oct;60:52-7.

[1074] Yang J, Zhou Y, Shi J. Cordycepin protects against acute pancreatitis by modulating NF-κB and NLRP3 inflammasome activation via AMPK. *Life Sci*. 2020 Jun 15;251:117645.

[1075] Wang J, Chen C, Jiang Z, et al. Protective effect of Cordyceps militaris extract against bisphenol A induced reproductive damage. *Syst Biol Reprod Med*. 2016 Aug;62(4):249-57.

[1076] Lee HS, Kim MK, Kim YK, et al. Stimulation of osteoblastic differentiation and mineralization in MC3T3-E1 cells by antler and fermented antler using Cordyceps militaris. *J Ethnopharmacol*. 2011 Jan 27;133(2):710-7.

[1077] Shang X, Tan Q, Liu R, et al. In vitro anti-Helicobacter pylori effects of medicinal mushroom extracts, with special emphasis on the Lion's Mane mushroom, Hericium erinaceus (higher Basidiomycetes). *Int J Med Mushrooms*. 2013;15(2):165-74.

[1078] Yang J, Cao Y, Lv Z, et al. Cordycepin protected against the TNF-α-induced inhibition of osteogenic differentiation of human adipose-derived mesenchymal stem cells. *Int J Immunopathol Pharmacol*. 2015 Sep;28(3):296-307.

[1079] Kim J, Lee H, Kang KS, et al. Cordyceps militaris mushroom and cordycepin inhibit RANKL-induced osteoclast differentiation. *J Med Food*. 2015 Apr;18(4):446-52.

[1080] Wang F, Yin P, Lu Y, et al. Cordycepin prevents oxidative stress-induced inhibition of osteogenesis. *Oncotarget*. 2015 Nov 3;6(34):35496-508.

[1081] Lee KT, Su CH, Liu SC, et al. Cordycerebroside A inhibits ICAM-1-dependent M1 monocyte adhesion to osteoarthritis synovial fibroblasts. *J Food Biochem*. 2022 Jul;46(7):e14108.

[1082] Noh EM, Kim JS, Hur H, et al. Cordycepin inhibits IL-1beta-induced MMP-1 and MMP-3 expression in rheumatoid arthritis synovial fibroblasts. *Rheumatology (Oxford)*. 2009 Jan;48(1):45-8.

[1083] Tran NKS, Kim GT, Lee DY, et al. Fermented Cordyceps militaris Extract Ameliorates Hepatosteatosis via Activation of Fatty Acid Oxidation. *J Med Food*. 2019 Apr;22(4):325-336.

226

[1084] Tran NKS, Kim GT, Park SH et al. Fermented Cordyceps militaris Extract Prevents Hepatosteatosis and Adipocyte Hypertrophy in High Fat Diet-Fed Mice. *Nutrients*. 2019 May 6;11(5):1015.

[1085] Choi HN, Jang YH, Kim MJ, et al. Cordyceps militaris alleviates non-alcoholic fatty liver disease in ob/ob mice. *Nutr Res Pract*. 2014 Apr;8(2):172-6.

[1086] Li T, Wen L, Cheng B. Cordycepin alleviates hepatic lipid accumulation by inducing protective autophagy via PKA/mTOR pathway. *Biochem Biophys Res Commun*. 2019 Aug 27;516(3):632-638.

[1087] Wu C, Guo Y, Su Y, et al. Cordycepin activates AMP-activated protein kinase (AMPK) via interaction with the γ1 subunit. *J Cell Mol Med*. 2014 Feb;18(2):293-304.

[1088] Lan T, Yu Y, Zhang J, et al. Cordycepin Ameliorates Nonalcoholic Steatohepatitis by Activation of the AMP-Activated Protein Kinase Signaling Pathway. *Hepatology*. 2021 Aug;74(2):686-703.

[1089] Gong X, Li T, Wan R, et al. Cordycepin attenuates high-fat diet-induced non-alcoholic fatty liver disease via down-regulation of lipid metabolism and inflammatory responses. *Int Immunopharmacol*. 2021 Feb;91:107173.

[1090] Chen Y, Wu Y, Li S, et al. Large-scale isolation and antitumor mechanism evaluation of compounds from the traditional Chinese medicine Cordyceps Militaris. *Eur J Med Chem*. 2021 Feb 15;212:113142.

[1091] Liu S, Tang J, Huang L, et al. Cordyceps Militaris Alleviates Severity of Murine Acute Lung Injury Through miRNAs-Mediated CXCR2 Inhibition. *Cell Physiol Biochem*. 2015;36(5):2003-11.

[1092] Lei J, Wei Y, Song P, et al. Cordycepin inhibits LPS-induced acute lung injury by inhibiting inflammation and oxidative stress. *Eur J Pharmacol*. 2018 Jan 5;818:110-114.

[1093] Yue GG, Lau CB, Fung KP, et al. Effects of Cordyceps sinensis, Cordyceps militaris and their isolated compounds on ion transport in Calu-3 human airway epithelial cells. *J Ethnopharmacol*. 2008 Apr 17;117(1):92-101.

[1094] Fung JC, Yue GG, Fung KP, et al. Cordyceps militaris extract stimulates Cl(-) secretion across human bronchial epithelia by both Ca(2+)(-) and cAMP-dependent pathways. *J Ethnopharmacol*. 2011 Oct 31;138(1):201-11.

[1095] Kim JH, Park DK, Lee CH, et al. A new isoflavone glycitein 7-O-beta-D-glucoside 4''-O-methylate, isolated from Cordyceps militaris grown on germinated soybeans extract, inhibits EGF-induced mucus hypersecretion in the human lung mucoepidermoid cells. *Phytother Res*. 2012 Dec;26(12):1807-12.

[1096] Song L, Yang J, Kong W, et al. Cordyceps militaris polysaccharide alleviates ovalbumin-induced allergic asthma through the Nrf2/HO-1 and NF-κB signaling pathways and regulates the gut microbiota. *Int J Biol Macromol*. 2023 May 31;238:124333.

[1097] Hsu CH, Sun HL, Sheu JN, et al. Effects of the immunomodulatory agent Cordyceps militaris on airway inflammation in a mouse asthma model. *Pediatr Neonatol*. 2008 Oct;49(5):171-8.

[1098] Han JY, Im J, Choi JN, et al. Induction of IL-8 expression by Cordyceps militaris grown on germinated soybeans through lipid rafts formation and signaling pathways via ERK and JNK in A549 cells. *J Ethnopharmacol*. 2010 Jan 8;127(1):55-61.

[1099] Fung JC, Yue GG, Fung KP, et al. Cordyceps militaris extract stimulates Cl(-) secretion across human bronchial epithelia by both Ca(2+)(-) and cAMP-dependent pathways. *J Ethnopharmacol*. 2011 Oct 31;138(1):201-11.

[1100] Yang X, Li Y, He Y, et al. Cordycepin alleviates airway hyperreactivity in a murine model of asthma by attenuating the inflammatory process. *Int Immunopharmacol*. 2015 Jun;26(2):401-8.

[1101] Fung JC, Yue GG, Fung KP, et al. Cordyceps militaris extract stimulates Cl(-) secretion across human bronchial epithelia by both Ca(2+)(-) and cAMP-dependent pathways. *J Ethnopharmacol*. 2011 Oct 31;138(1):201-11.

[1102] Phull AR, Dhong KR, Park HJ. Lactic Acid Bacteria Fermented Cordyceps militaris (GRC-SC11) Suppresses IgE Mediated Mast Cell Activation and Type I Hypersensitive Allergic Murine Model. *Nutrients*. 2021 Oct 28;13(11):3849.

[1103] Wu TF, Shi WY, Chiu YC, et al. Investigation of the molecular mechanism underlying the inhibitory activities of ethanol extract of Bombyx mori pupa-incubated Cordyceps militaris fruiting bodies toward allergic rhinitis. *Biomed Pharmacother*. 2021 Mar;135:111248.

[1104] Wu TF, Chan YY, Shi WY, et al. Uncovering the Molecular Mechanism of Anti-Allergic Activity of Silkworm Pupa-Grown Cordyceps militaris Fruit Body. *Am J Chin Med*. 2017;45(3):497-513.

[1105] Oh JY, Choi WS, Lee CH, et al. The ethyl acetate extract of Cordyceps militaris inhibits IgE-mediated allergic responses in mast cells and passive cutaneous anaphylaxis reaction in mice. *J Ethnopharmacol*. 2011 May 17;135(2):422-9.

[1106] Park DK, Choi WS, Park HJ. Antiallergic activity of novel isoflavone methyl-glycosides from Cordyceps militaris grown on germinated soybeans in antigen-stimulated mast cells. *J Agric Food Chem*. 2012 Mar 7;60(9):2309-15.

[1107] Oh JY, Choi WS, Lee CH, et al. The ethyl acetate extract of Cordyceps militaris inhibits IgE-mediated allergic responses in mast cells and passive cutaneous anaphylaxis reaction in mice. *J Ethnopharmacol*. 2011 May 17;135(2):422-9.

[1108] Kim HY, Jee H, Yeom JH, et al. The ameliorative effect of AST2017-01 in an ovalbumin-induced allergic rhinitis animal model. *Inflamm Res*. 2019 May;68(5):387-395.

[1109] Yoou MS, Jin MH, Lee SY, et al. Cordycepin Suppresses Thymic Stromal Lymphopoietin Expression via Blocking Caspase-1 and Receptor-Interacting Protein 2 Signaling Pathways in Mast Cells. *Biol Pharm Bull*. 2016;39(1):90-6.

[1110] Fan HB, Zou Y, Han Q, et al. Cordyceps militaris Immunomodulatory Protein Promotes the Phagocytic Ability of Macrophages through the TLR4-NF-κB Pathway. *Int J Mol Sci*. 2021 Nov 11;22(22):12188.

[1111] Kim CS, Lee SY, Cho SH, et al. Cordyceps militaris induces the IL-18 expression via its promoter activation for IFN-gamma production. *J Ethnopharmacol*. 2008 Dec 8;120(3):366-71.

[1112] Sun Y, Du X, Li S, et al. Dietary Cordyceps militaris protects against Vibrio splendidus infection in sea cucumber Apostichopus japonicus. *Fish Shellfish Immunol*. 2015 Aug;45(2):964-71.

[1113] Yu Y, Wen Q, Song A, et al. Isolation and immune activity of a new acidic Cordyceps militaris exopolysaccharide. *Int J Biol Macromol*. 2022 Jan 1;194:706-714.

[1114] Liu JY, Feng CP, Li X, et al. Immunomodulatory and antioxidative activity of Cordyceps militaris polysaccharides in mice. *Int J Biol Macromol*. 2016 May;86:594-8.

[1115] He BL, Zheng QW, Guo LQ, et al. Structural characterization and immune-enhancing activity of a novel high-molecular-weight polysaccharide from Cordyceps militaris. *Int J Biol Macromol*. 2020 Feb 15;145:11-20.

[1116] Bi S , Jing Y , Zhou Q , et al. Structural elucidation and immunostimulatory activity of a new polysaccharide from Cordyceps militaris. *Food Funct*. 2018 Jan 24;9(1):279-293.

[1117] Pei H, He Z, Chen W, et al. Network pharmacology and molecular docking analysis on the mechanism of Cordyceps militaris polysaccharide regulating immunity through TLR4/TNF-α pathways. *J Biochem Mol Toxicol*. 2023 Jun;37(6):e23345.

[1118] Zhu SJ, Pan J, Zhao B, et al. Comparisons on enhancing the immunity of fresh and dry Cordyceps militaris in vivo and in vitro. *J Ethnopharmacol*. 2013 Oct 7;149(3):713-9.

[1119] Shin JS, Chung SH, Lee WS, et al. Immunostimulatory effects of cordycepin-enriched WIB-801CE from Cordyceps militaris in splenocytes and cyclophosphamide-induced immunosuppressed mice. *Phytother Res*. 2018 Jan;32(1):132-139.

[1120] Lee JS, Hong EK. Immunostimulating activity of the polysaccharides isolated from Cordyceps militaris. *Int Immunopharmacol*. 2011 Sep;11(9):1226-33.

[1121] Zhang Y, Zeng Y, Cui Y, et al. Structural characterization, antioxidant and immunomodulatory activities of a neutral polysaccharide from Cordyceps militaris cultivated on hull-less barley. *Carbohydr Polym*. 2020 May 1;235:115969.

[1122] Jeong MH, Seo MJ, Park JU, et al. Effect of cordycepin purified from Cordyceps militaris on Th1 and Th2 cytokines in mouse splenocytes. *J Microbiol Biotechnol*. 2012 Aug;22(8):1161-4.

[1123] Luo X, Duan Y, Yang W, et al. Structural elucidation and immunostimulatory activity of polysaccharide isolated by subcritical water extraction from Cordyceps militaris. *Carbohydr Polym*. 2017 Feb 10;157:794-802.

[1124] Lee JS, Kwon DS, Lee KR, et al. Mechanism of macrophage activation induced by polysaccharide from Cordyceps militaris culture broth. *Carbohydr Polym*. 2015 Apr 20;120:29-37.

[1125] Kim HS, Kim JY, Kang JS, et al. Cordlan polysaccharide isolated from mushroom Cordyceps militaris induces dendritic cell maturation through toll-like receptor 4 signalings. *Food Chem Toxicol*. 2010 Jul;48(7):1926-33.

[1126] Zhang M, Shan Y, Gao H, et al. Expression of a recombinant hybrid antimicrobial peptide magainin II-cecropin B in the mycelium of the medicinal fungus Cordyceps militaris and its validation in mice. *Microb Cell Fact*. 2018 Feb 5;17(1):18.

[1127] Kim GY, Ko WS, Lee JY, et al. Water extract of Cordyceps militaris enhances maturation of murine bone marrow-derived dendritic cells in vitro. *Biol Pharm Bull*. 2006 Feb;29(2):354-60.

[1128] Zhu L, Tang Q, Zhou S, et al. Isolation and purification of a polysaccharide from the caterpillar medicinal mushroom Cordyceps militaris (Ascomycetes) fruit bodies and its immunomodulation of RAW 264.7 macrophages. *Int J Med Mushrooms*. 2014;16(3):247-57.

[1129] Yang Q, Jia B, Liu X, et al. Molecular Cloning, Expression and Macrophage Activation of an Immunoregulatory Protein from Cordyceps militaris. *Molecules*. 2021 Nov 24;26(23):7107.

[1130] Lee JS, Kwon JS, Won DP, et al. Study of macrophage activation and structural characteristics of purified polysaccharide from the fruiting body of Cordyceps militaris. *J Microbiol Biotechnol*. 2010 Jul;20(7):1053-60.

[1131] Kwon HK, Jo WR, Park HJ. Immune-enhancing activity of C. militaris fermented with Pediococcus pentosaceus (GRC-ON89A) in CY-induced immunosuppressed model. *BMC Complement Altern Med*. 2018 Feb 23;18(1):75.

[1132] Wang M, Meng XY, Yang RL, et al. Cordyceps militaris polysaccharides can enhance the immunity and antioxidation activity in immunosuppressed mice. *Carbohydr Polym*. 2012 Jun 20;89(2):461-6.

[1133] Xu G, Yuan G, Lu X, et al. Study on the effect of regulation of Cordyceps militaris polypeptide on the immune function of mice based on a transcription factor regulatory network. *Food Funct*. 2020 Jul 22;11(7):6066-6077.

[1134] Shin S, Kwon J, Lee S, et al. Immunostimulatory Effects of Cordyceps militaris on Macrophages through the Enhanced Production of Cytokines via the Activation of NF-kappaB. *Immune Netw*. 2010 Apr;10(2):55-63.

[1135] Shin S, Park Y, Kim S, et al. Cordyceps militaris Enhances MHC-restricted Antigen Presentation via the Induced Expression of MHC Molecules and Production of Cytokines. *Immune Netw*. 2010 Aug;10(4):135-43.

[1136] Jeong SC, Koyyalamudi SR, Hughes J, et al. Antioxidant and immunomodulating activities of exo-and endopolysaccharide fractions from submerged mycelia cultures of culinary-medicinal mushrooms. *Int J Med Mushrooms*. 2013;15(3):251-66.

[1137] Woolley VC, Teakle GR, Prince G, et al. Cordycepin, a metabolite of Cordyceps militaris, reduces immune-related gene expression in insects. *J Invertebr Pathol*. 2020 Nov;177:107480.

[1138] Xiong Y, Zhang S, Xu L, et al. Suppression of T-cell activation in vitro and in vivo by cordycepin from Cordyceps militaris. *J Surg Res*. 2013 Dec;185(2):912-22.

[1139] Sun Y, Shao Y, Zhang Z, et al. Regulation of human cytokines by Cordyceps militaris. *J Food Drug Anal*. 2014 Dec;22(4):463-467.

[1140] Yu R, Song L, Zhao Y, et al. Isolation and biological properties of polysaccharide CPS-1 from cultured Cordyceps militaris. *Fitoterapia*. 2004 Jul;75(5):465-72.

[1141] Shin S, Lee S, Kwon J, et al. Cordycepin Suppresses Expression of Diabetes Regulating Genes by Inhibition of Lipopolysaccharide-induced Inflammation in Macrophages. *Immune Netw*. 2009 Jun;9(3):98-105.

[1142] Li XT, Li HC, Li CB, et al. Protective effects on mitochondria and anti-aging activity of polysaccharides from cultivated fruiting bodies of Cordyceps militaris. *Am J Chin Med*. 2010;38(6):1093-106.

[1143] Liu Y, E Q, Zuo J, et al. Protective effect of Cordyceps polysaccharide on hydrogen peroxide-induced mitochondrial dysfunction in HL-7702 cells. *Mol Med Rep*. 2013 Mar;7(3):747-54.

[1144] Chueaphromsri P, Kunhorm P, Phonchai R, et al. Cordycepin Enhances SIRT1 Expression and Maintains Stemness of Human Mesenchymal Stem Cells. *In Vivo*. 2023 Mar-Apr;37(2):596-610.

[1145] Hawley SA, Ross FA, Russell FM, et al. Mechanism of Activation of AMPK by Cordycepin. *Cell Chem Biol*. 2020 Feb 20;27(2):214-222.e4.

[1146] Chen BY, Huang HS, Tsai KJ, et al. Protective Effect of a Water-Soluble Carotenoid-Rich Extract of Cordyceps militaris against Light-Evoked Functional Vision Deterioration in Mice. *Nutrients*. 2022 Apr 18;14(8):1675.

[1147] Lan L, Wang S, Duan S, et al. Cordyceps militaris Carotenoids Protect Human Retinal Endothelial Cells against the Oxidative Injury and Apoptosis Resulting from H2O2. *Evid Based Complement Alternat Med*. 2022 Sep 30;2022:1259093.

[1148] Cheng C, Zhang S, Gong Y, et al. Cordycepin inhibits myogenesis via activating the ERK1/2 MAPK signalling pathway in C2C12 cells. *Biomed Pharmacother*. 2023 Sep;165:115163.

[1149] Molecules. 2020 Dec 4;25(23):5733. Cordyceps militaris Fungus Extracts-Mediated Nanoemulsion for Improvement Antioxidant, Antimicrobial, and Anti-Inflammatory Activities. *Molecules.* 2020 Dec 4;25(23):5733.

[1150] Huang S, Zou Y, Tang H, et al. Cordyceps militaris polysaccharides modulate gut microbiota and improve metabolic disorders in mice with diet-induced obesity. *J Sci Food Agric.* 2023 Mar 15;103(4):1885-1894.

[1151] Chiu CP, Liu SC, Tang CH, et al. Anti-inflammatory Cerebrosides from Cultivated Cordyceps militaris. *J Agric Food Chem.* 2016 Feb 24;64(7):1540-8.

[1152] Zhang D, Tang Q, He X, et al. Antimicrobial, antioxidant, anti-inflammatory, and cytotoxic activities of Cordyceps militaris spent substrate. *PLoS One.* 2023 Sep 8;18(9):e0291363.

[1153] Rao YK, Fang SH, Wu WS, et al. Constituents isolated from Cordyceps militaris suppress enhanced inflammatory mediator's production and human cancer cell proliferation. *J Ethnopharmacol.* 2010 Sep 15;131(2):363-7.

[1154] Smiderle FR, Baggio CH, Borato DG, et al. Anti-inflammatory properties of the medicinal mushroom Cordyceps militaris might be related to its linear $(1{\rightarrow}3)$-β-D-glucan. *PLoS One.* 2014 Oct 17;9(10):e110266.

[1155] Won SY, Park EH. Anti-inflammatory and related pharmacological activities of cultured mycelia and fruiting bodies of Cordyceps militaris. *J Ethnopharmacol.* 2005 Jan 15;96(3):555-61.

[1156] Chien RC, Lin LM, Chang YH, et al. Anti-Inflammation Properties of Fruiting Bodies and Submerged Cultured Mycelia of Culinary-Medicinal Higher Basidiomycetes Mushrooms. *Int J Med Mushrooms.* 2016;18(11):999-1009.

[1157] Sun Y, Shao Y, Zhang Z, et al. Regulation of human cytokines by Cordyceps militaris. *J Food Drug Anal.* 2014 Dec;22(4):463-467.

[1158] Jo WS, Choi YJ, Kim HJ, et al. The Anti-inflammatory Effects of Water Extract from Cordyceps militaris in Murine Macrophage. *Mycobiology.* 2010 Mar;38(1):46-51.

[1159] Yu R, Song L, Zhao Y, et al. Isolation and biological properties of polysaccharide CPS-1 from cultured Cordyceps militaris. *Fitoterapia.* 2004 Jul;75(5):465-72.

[1160] Kwon HK, Song MJ, Lee HJ, et al. Pediococcus pentosaceus-Fermented Cordyceps militaris Inhibits Inflammatory Reactions and Alleviates Contact Dermatitis. *Int J Mol Sci.* 2018 Nov 7;19(11):3504.

[1161] Yoon JY, Kim JH, Baek KS, et al. A direct protein kinase B-targeted anti-inflammatory activity of cordycepin from artificially cultured fruit body of Cordyceps militaris. *Pharmacogn Mag.* 2015 Jul-Sep;11(43):477-85.

[1162] Huang YP, Chen DR, Lin WJ, et al. Ergosta-7,9(11),22-trien-3β-ol Attenuates Inflammatory Responses via Inhibiting MAPK/AP-1 Induced IL-6/JAK/STAT Pathways and Activating Nrf2/HO-1 Signaling in LPS-Stimulated Macrophage-like Cells. *Antioxidants (Basel).* 2021 Sep 8;10(9):1430.

[1163] Kim HG, Shrestha B, Lim SY, et al. Cordycepin inhibits lipopolysaccharide-induced inflammation by the suppression of NF-kappaB through Akt and p38 inhibition in RAW 264.7 macrophage cells. *Eur J Pharmacol.* 2006 Sep 18;545(2-3):192-9.

[1164] Tan L, Song X, Ren Y, et al. Anti-inflammatory effects of cordycepin: A review. *Phytother Res.* 2020 Oct 8.

[1165] Jeong JW, Jin CY, Kim GY, et al. Anti-inflammatory effects of cordycepin via suppression of inflammatory mediators in BV2 microglial cells. *Int Immunopharmacol.* 2010 Dec;10(12):1580-6.

[1166] Yu T, Shim J, Yang Y, et al. 3-(4-(tert-Octyl)phenoxy)propane-1,2-diol suppresses inflammatory responses via inhibition of multiple kinases. *Biochem Pharmacol.* 2012 Jun 1;83(11):1540-51.

[1167] Yong T, Zhang M, Chen D, et al. Actions of water extract from Cordyceps militaris in hyperuricemic mice induced by potassium oxonate combined with hypoxanthine. *J Ethnopharmacol.* 2016 Dec 24;194:403-411.

[1168] Ma L, Zhang S, Yuan Y, et al. Hypouricemic actions of exopolysaccharide produced by Cordyceps militaris in potassium oxonate-induced hyperuricemic mice. *Curr Microbiol.* 2014 Dec;69(6):852-7.

[1169] Quy TN, Xuan TD. Xanthine Oxidase Inhibitory Potential, Antioxidant and Antibacterial Activities of Cordyceps militaris (L.) Link Fruiting Body. *Medicines (Basel).* 2019 Jan 29;6(1):20.

[1170] Jiao C, Liang H, Liu L, et al. Transcriptomic analysis of the anti-inflammatory effect of Cordyceps militaris extract on acute gouty arthritis. *Front Pharmacol.* 2022 Oct 14;13:1035101.

[1171] Yong T, Chen S, Xie Y, et al. Cordycepin, a Characteristic Bioactive Constituent in Cordyceps militaris, Ameliorates Hyperuricemia through URAT1 in Hyperuricemic Mice. *Front Microbiol.* 2018 Jan 25;9:58.

[1172] Liu SC, Chiu CP, Tsai CH, et al. Soya-cerebroside, an extract of Cordyceps militaris, suppresses monocyte migration and prevents cartilage degradation in inflammatory animal models. *Sci Rep.* 2017 Feb 22;7:43205.

[1173] Li Y, Li K, Mao L, et al. Cordycepin inhibits LPS-induced inflammatory and matrix degradation in the intervertebral disc. *PeerJ.* 2016 May 10;4:e1992.

[1174] Lu HY, Tsai WC, Liu JS, et al. Preparation and evaluation of Cordyceps militaris polysaccharide- and sesame oil-loaded nanoemulsion for the treatment of candidal vaginitis in mice. *Biomed Pharmacother.* 2023 Sep 14;167:115506.

[1175] Lin S, Hsu WK, Tsai MS, et al. Effects of Cordyceps militaris fermentation products on reproductive development in juvenile male mice. *Sci Rep.* 2022 Aug 12;12(1):13720.

[1176] Chang Y, Jeng KC, Huang KF, et al. Effect of Cordyceps militaris supplementation on sperm production, sperm motility and hormones in Sprague-Dawley rats. *Am J Chin Med.* 2008;36(5):849-59.

[1177] Lin WH, Tsai MT, Chen YS, et al. Improvement of sperm production in subfertile boars by Cordyceps militaris supplement. *Am J Chin Med.* 2007;35(4):631-41.

[1178] Sohn SH, Lee SC, Hwang SY, et al. Effect of long-term administration of cordycepin from Cordyceps militaris on testicular function in middle-aged rats. *Planta Med.* 2012 Oct;78(15):1620-5.

[1179] Kopalli SR, Cha KM, Cho JY, et al. Cordycepin mitigates spermatogenic and redox related expression in H2O2-exposed Leydig cells and regulates testicular oxidative apoptotic signalling in aged rats. *Pharm Biol.* 2022 Dec;60(1):404-416.

[1180] Kopalli SR, Cha KM, Lee SH, et al. Cordycepin, an Active Constituent of Nutrient Powerhouse and Potential Medicinal Mushroom Cordyceps militaris Linn., Ameliorates Age-Related Testicular Dysfunction in Rats. *Nutrients.* 2019 Apr 23;11(4):906.

[1181] Pohsa S, Hanchang W, Singpoonga N, et al. Effects of Cultured Cordycep militaris on Sexual Performance and Erectile Function in Streptozotocin-Induced Diabetic Male Rats. *Biomed Res Int.* 2020 Nov 13;2020:4198397.

[1182] Nguyen TV, Chumnanpuen P, Parunyakul K, et al. A study of the aphrodisiac properties of Cordyceps militaris in streptozotocin-induced diabetic male rats. *Vet World*. 2021 Feb;14(2):537-544.

[1183] Kopalli SR, Cha KM, Cho JY, et al. Cordycepin from Medicinal Fungi Cordyceps militaris Mitigates Inflammaging-Associated Testicular Damage via Regulating NF-κB/MAPKs Signaling in Naturally Aged Rats. *Mycobiology*. 2022 Feb 17;50(1):89-98.

[1184] Kusama K, Miyagawa M, Ota K, et al. Cordyceps militaris Fruit Body Extract Decreases Testosterone Catabolism and Testosterone-Stimulated Prostate Hypertrophy. *Nutrients*. 2020 Dec 26;13(1):50.

[1185] Liu J, Yang S, Yang X, et al. [Anticarcinogenic effect and hormonal effect of Cordyceps militaris Link]. *Zhongguo Zhong Yao Za Zhi*. 1997 Feb;22(2):111-3, inside back cover.

[1186] Verma AK. Cordycepin: a bioactive metabolite of Cordyceps militaris and polyadenylation inhibitor with therapeutic potential against COVID-19. *J Biomol Struct Dyn*. 2022 May;40(8):3745-3752.

[1187] Singh M, Verma H, Gera N, et al. Evaluation of Cordyceps militaris steroids as anti-inflammatory agents to combat the Covid-19 cytokine storm: a bioinformatics and structure-based drug designing approach. *J Biomol Struct Dyn*. 2023 Aug 7:1-19.

[1188] Lee S, Lee HH, Kim J, et al. Anti-tumor effect of Cordyceps militaris in HCV-infected human hepatocarcinoma 7.5 cells. *J Microbiol*. 2015 Jul;53(7):468-74.

[1189] Ueda Y, Mori K, Satoh S, et al. Anti-HCV activity of the Chinese medicinal fungus Cordyceps militaris. *Biochem Biophys Res Commun*. 2014 May 2;447(2):341-5.

[1190] Lee HH, Park H, Sung GH, et al. Anti-influenza effect of Cordyceps militaris through immunomodulation in a DBA/2 mouse model. *J Microbiol*. 2014 Aug;52(8):696-701.

[1191] Ohta Y, Lee JB, Hayashi K, et al. In vivo anti-influenza virus activity of an immunomodulatory acidic polysaccharide isolated from Cordyceps militaris grown on germinated soybeans. *J Agric Food Chem*. 2007 Dec 12;55(25):10194-9.

[1192] Jiang Y, Wong JH, Fu M, et al. Isolation of adenosine, iso-sinensetin and dimethylguanosine with antioxidant and HIV-1 protease inhibiting activities from fruiting bodies of Cordyceps militaris. *Phytomedicine*. 2011 Jan 15;18(2-3):189-93.

[1193] Han NR, Moon PD, Yoo MS, et al. Regulatory effects of chrysophanol, a bioactive compound of AST2017-01 in a mouse model of 2,4-dinitrofluorobenzene-induced atopic dermatitis. *Int Immunopharmacol*. 2018 Sep;62:220-226.

[1194] Kwon HK, Song MJ, Lee HJ, et al. Pediococcus pentosaceus-Fermented Cordyceps militaris Inhibits Inflammatory Reactions and Alleviates Contact Dermatitis. *Int J Mol Sci*. 2018 Nov 7;19(11):3504.

[1195] Choi EJ, Park B, Lee J, et al. Anti-atopic dermatitis properties of Cordyceps militaris on TNFα/IFNγ-stimulated HaCaT cells and experimentally induced atopic dermatitis in mice. *Phys Act Nutr*. 2020 Dec;24(4):7-14.

[1196] Hwang SH, Yang Y, Jeong Y, et al. Ovalicin attenuates atopic dermatitis symptoms by inhibiting IL-31 signaling and intracellular calcium influx. *J Biomed Res*. 2021 Jun 16;35(6):448-458.

[1197] Upatcha N, Kaokaen P, Sorraksa N, et al. Nanoencapsulated cordyceps extract enhances collagen synthesis and skin cell regeneration through antioxidation and autophagy. *J Microencapsul*. 2023 Dec;40(5):303-317.

[1198] Cha JY, Yang HJ, Park MY, et al. Melanogenesis effect of Cordyceps militaris culture broth on the melanin formation of B16F0 melanoma cells. *Immunopharmacol Immunotoxicol*. 2011 Oct 13.

[1199] Molecules. 2020 Dec 4;25(23):5733. Cordyceps militaris Fungus Extracts-Mediated Nanoemulsion for Improvement Antioxidant, Antimicrobial, and Anti-Inflammatory Activities. *Molecules*. 2020 Dec 4;25(23):5733.

[1200] Reis FS, Barros L, Calhelha RC, et al. The methanolic extract of Cordyceps militaris (L.) Link fruiting body shows antioxidant, antibacterial, antifungal and antihuman tumor cell lines properties. *Food Chem Toxicol*. 2013 Dec;62:91-8.

[1201] Wong JH, Ng TB, Wang H, et al. Cordymin, an antifungal peptide from the medicinal fungus Cordyceps militaris. *Phytomedicine*. 2011 Mar 15;18(5):387-92.

[1202] Dong CH, Yang T, Lian T. A comparative study of the antimicrobial, antioxidant, and cytotoxic activities of methanol extracts from fruit bodies and fermented mycelia of caterpillar medicinal mushroom Cordyceps militaris (Ascomycetes). *Int J Med Mushrooms*. 2014;16(5):485-95.

[1203] Ding K, Wang Y, Han C. Polysaccharide Elicitors Affect the Yield, Polysaccharide Synthase and Antibacterial Activity of Intracellular Polysaccharides from Submerged Culture of Cordyceps milifaris (Ascomycetes). *Int J Med Mushrooms*. 2023;25(2):35-48.

[1204] Quy TN, Xuan TD. Xanthine Oxidase Inhibitory Potential, Antioxidant and Antibacterial Activities of Cordyceps militaris (L.) Link Fruiting Body. *Medicines (Basel)*. 2019 Jan 29;6(1):20.

[1205] Park BT, Na KH, Jung EC, et al. Antifungal and Anticancer Activities of a Protein from the Mushroom Cordyceps militaris. *Korean J Physiol Pharmacol*. 2009 Feb;13(1):49-54.

[1206] Eiamthaworn K, Kaewkod T, Bovonsombut S, et al. Efficacy of Cordyceps militaris Extracts against Some Skin Pathogenic Bacteria and Antioxidant Activity. *J Fungi (Basel)*. 2022 Mar 22;8(4):327.

[1207] Zhou X, Cai G, He Y, et al. Separation of cordycepin from Cordyceps militaris fermentation supernatant using preparative HPLC and evaluation of its antibacterial activity as an NAD+-dependent DNA ligase inhibitor. *Exp Ther Med*. 2016 Sep;12(3):1812-1816.

[1208] Molecules. 2020 Dec 4;25(23):5733. Cordyceps militaris Fungus Extracts-Mediated Nanoemulsion for Improvement Antioxidant, Antimicrobial, and Anti-Inflammatory Activities. *Molecules*. 2020 Dec 4;25(23):5733.

[1209] Zhang X, Zhang X, Gu S, et al. Structure analysis and antioxidant activity of polysaccharide-iron (III) from Cordyceps militaris mycelia. *Int J Biol Macromol*. 2021 May 1;178:170-179.

[1210] Zhang D, Tang Q, He X, et al. Antimicrobial, antioxidant, anti-inflammatory, and cytotoxic activities of Cordyceps militaris spent substrate. *PLoS One*. 2023 Sep 8;18(9):e0291363.

[1211] Wang L, Xu N, Zhang J, et al. Antihyperlipidemic and hepatoprotective activities of residue polysaccharide from Cordyceps militaris SU-12. *Carbohydr Polym*. 2015 Oct 20;131:355-62.

[1212] Zhang Y, Zeng Y, Cui Y, et al. Structural characterization, antioxidant and immunomodulatory activities of a neutral polysaccharide from Cordyceps militaris cultivated on hull-less barley. *Carbohydr Polym*. 2020 May 1;235:115969.

[1213] Reis FS, Barros L, Calhelha RC, et al. The methanolic extract of Cordyceps militaris (L.) Link fruiting body shows antioxidant, antibacterial, antifungal and antihuman tumor cell lines properties. *Food Chem Toxicol*. 2013 Dec;62:91-8.

[1214] Liu Y, Li Y, Zhang H, Li C, et al. Polysaccharides from Cordyceps miltaris cultured at different pH: Sugar composition and antioxidant activity. *Int J Biol Macromol*. 2020 Nov 1;162:349-358.

[1215] Chen X, Wu G, Huang Z. Structural analysis and antioxidant activities of polysaccharides from cultured Cordyceps militaris. *Int J Biol Macromol*. 2013 Jul;58:18-22.

[1216] Zhao H, Lai Q, Zhang J, et al. Antioxidant and Hypoglycemic Effects of Acidic-Extractable Polysaccharides from Cordyceps militaris on Type 2 Diabetes Mice. *Oxid Med Cell Longev*. 2018 Nov 25;2018:9150807.

[1217] Jing Y, Zhu J, Liu T, et al. Structural characterization and biological activities of a novel polysaccharide from cultured Cordyceps militaris and its sulfated derivative. *J Agric Food Chem*. 2015 Apr 8;63(13):3464-71.

[1218] Wu HC, Chen ST, Chang JC, et al. Radical Scavenging and Antiproliferative Effects of Cordycepin-Rich Ethanol Extract from Brown Rice-Cultivated Cordyceps militaris (Ascomycetes) Mycelium on Breast Cancer Cell Lines. *Int J Med Mushrooms*. 2019;21(7):657-669.

[1219] Jiang Y, Wong JH, Fu M, et al. Isolation of adenosine, iso-sinensetin and dimethylguanosine with antioxidant and HIV-1 protease inhibiting activities from fruiting bodies of Cordyceps militaris. *Phytomedicine*. 2011 Jan 15;18(2-3):189-93.

[1220] Lin R, Liu H, Wu S, et al. Production and in vitro antioxidant activity of exopolysaccharide by a mutant, Cordyceps militaris SU5-08. *Int J Biol Macromol*. 2012 Jul-Aug;51(1-2):153-7.

[1221] Huang SJ, Lin CP, Mau JL, et al. Effect of UV-B Irradiation on Physiologically Active Substance Content and Antioxidant Properties of the Medicinal Caterpillar Fungus Cordyceps militaris (Ascomycetes). *Int J Med Mushrooms*. 2015;17(3):241-53.

[1222] Dong CH, Yang T, Lian T. A comparative study of the antimicrobial, antioxidant, and cytotoxic activities of methanol extracts from fruit bodies and fermented mycelia of caterpillar medicinal mushroom Cordyceps militaris (Ascomycetes). *Int J Med Mushrooms*. 2014;16(5):485-95.

[1223] Gu YX, Song YW, Fan LQ, et al. [Antioxidant activity of natural and cultured Cordyceps sp]. *Zhongguo Zhong Yao Za Zhi*. 2007 Jun;32(11):1028-31.

[1224] Gao Q, Zhang D, Ding W, et al. Effects of Exogenous Lanthanum Nitrate on the Active Substance Content and Antioxidant Activity of Caterpillar Medicinal Mushroom Cordyceps militaris (Ascomycetes). *Int J Med Mushrooms*. 2023;25(6):41-54.

[1225] Quy TN, Xuan TD. Xanthine Oxidase Inhibitory Potential, Antioxidant and Antibacterial Activities of Cordyceps militaris (L.) Link Fruiting Body. *Medicines (Basel)*. 2019 Jan 29;6(1):20.

[1226] Shi K, Yang G, He L, et al. Purification, characterization, antioxidant, and antitumor activity of polysaccharides isolated from silkworm cordyceps. *J Food Biochem*. 2020 Nov;44(11):e13482.

[1227] Eiamthaworn K, Kaewkod T, Bovonsombut S, et al. Efficacy of Cordyceps militaris Extracts against Some Skin Pathogenic Bacteria and Antioxidant Activity. *J Fungi (Basel)*. 2022 Mar 22;8(4):327.

[1228] Xu L, Wang F, Zhang Z, et al. Optimization of Polysaccharide Production from Cordyceps militaris by Solid-State Fermentation on Rice and Its Antioxidant Activities. *Foods*. 2019 Nov 19;8(11):590.

[1229] Jeong SC, Koyyalamudi SR, Hughes J, et al. Antioxidant and immunomodulating activities of exo-and endopolysaccharide fractions from submerged mycelia cultures of culinary-medicinal mushrooms. *Int J Med Mushrooms*. 2013;15(3):251-66.

[1230] Liu YM, Lai YH, Hsieh FM, et al. Antioxidant Activities of Selected Medicinal Mushroom Submerged Cultivated Mycelia. *Int J Med Mushrooms*. 2020;22(4):367-377.

[1231] Park JM, Lee JS, Lee KR, et al. Cordyceps militaris extract protects human dermal fibroblasts against oxidative stress-induced apoptosis and premature senescence. *Nutrients*. 2014 Sep 16;6(9):3711-26.

[1232] Veena RK, Carmel EJ, Ramya H, et al. Caterpillar Medicinal Mushroom, Cordyceps militaris (Ascomycetes), Mycelia Attenuates Doxorubicin-Induced Oxidative Stress and Upregulates Krebs Cycle Dehydrogenases Activity and ATP Level in Rat Brain. *Int J Med Mushrooms*. 2020;22(6):593-604.

[1233] Yu HM, Wang BS, Huang SC, et al. Comparison of protective effects between cultured Cordyceps militaris and natural Cordyceps sinensis against oxidative damage. *J Agric Food Chem*. 2006 Apr 19;54(8):3132-8.

[1234] Shen Q, Chen S. [Effect of Cordyceps militaris on the damage of rats induced by n-hexane]. *Zhong Yao Cai*. 2001 Feb;24(2):112-6.

[1235] Lan YH, Lu YS, Wu JY, et al. Cordyceps militaris Reduces Oxidative Stress and Regulates Immune T Cells to Inhibit Metastatic Melanoma Invasion. *Antioxidants (Basel)*. 2022 Jul 30;11(8):1502.

[1236] He MT, Lee AY, Park CH, et al. Protective effect of Cordyceps militaris against hydrogen peroxide-induced oxidative stress in vitro. *Nutr Res Pract*. 2019 Aug;13(4):279-285.

[1237] Kim JR, Yeon SH, Kim HS, et al. Larvicidal activity against Plutella xylostella of cordycepin from the fruiting body of Cordyceps militaris. *Pest Manag Sci*. 2002 Jul;58(7):713-7.

[1238] Kriukov VIu, Iaroslavtseva ON, Dubovskiĭ IM, et al. [Insecticidal and immunosuppressive effect of ascomycete Cordyceps militaris on the larvae of the Colorado potato beetle Leptinotarsa decemlineata]. *Izv Akad Nauk Ser Biol*. 2014 May-Jun;(3):296-303.

[1239] Quy TN, Xuan TD, Andriana Y, et al. Cordycepin Isolated from Cordyceps militaris: Its Newly Discovered Herbicidal Property and Potential Plant-Based Novel Alternative to Glyphosate. *Molecules*. 2019 Aug 9;24(16):2901.

[1240] Hirsch KR, Smith-Ryan AE, Roelofs EJ, et al. Cordyceps militaris Improves Tolerance to High-Intensity Exercise After Acute and Chronic Supplementation. *J Diet Suppl*. 2017 Jan;14(1):42-53.

[1241] Dubhashi S, Sinha S, Dwivedi S, et al. Early Trends to Show the Efficacy of Cordyceps militaris in Mild to Moderate COVID Inflammation. *Cureus*. 2023 Aug 18;15(8):e43731.

[1242] Kang HJ, Baik HW, Kim SJ, et al. Cordyceps militaris Enhances Cell-Mediated Immunity in Healthy Korean Men. *J Med Food*. 2015 Oct;18(10):1164-72.

[1243] Ding M, Lv K, Zhang D, et al. Effect of Flammulina velutipes polysaccharides on endoplasmic reticulum stress-mediated apoptosis by activating PLC-IP3 pathway in HepG2 cells. *J Food Sci*. 2023 Jan;88(1):523-536.

[1244] Xu H, Hu Y, Hu Q, et al. Isolation, characterization and HepG-2 inhibition of a novel proteoglycan from Flammulina velutipes. *Int J Biol Macromol*. 2021 Oct 31;189:11-17.

[1245] Chen CC, Tang CT, Lai CY, et al. In Vitro Assessment of the Antioxidant and Anticancer Properties of Flammulina velutipes Stipe Extracts. *Anticancer Res*. 2023 Jul;43(7):3057-3067.

[1246] Yi C, Sun C, Tong S, et al. Cytotoxic effect of novel Flammulina velutipes sterols and its oral bioavailability via mixed micellar nanoformulation. *Int J Pharm*. 2013 May 1;448(1):44-50.

[1247] Yi C, Zhong H, Tong S, et al. Enhanced oral bioavailability of a sterol-loaded microemulsion formulation of Flammulina velutipes, a potential antitumor drug. *Int J Nanomedicine*. 2012;7:5067-78.

[1248] Chang YC, Hsiao YM, Wu MF, et al. Interruption of lung cancer cell migration and proliferation by fungal immunomodulatory protein FIP-fve from Flammulina velutipes. *J Agric Food Chem*. 2013 Dec 11;61(49):12044-52.

[1249] Gu YH, Leonard J. In vitro effects on proliferation, apoptosis and colony inhibition in ER-dependent and ER-independent human breast cancer cells by selected mushroom species. *Oncol Rep*. 2006 Feb;15(2):417-23.

[1250] Jia W, Feng J, Zhang JS, et al. Structural Characteristics of the Novel Polysaccharide FVPA1 from Winter Culinary-Medicinal Mushroom, Flammulina velutipes (Agaricomycetes), Capable of Enhancing Natural Killer Cell Activity against K562 Tumor Cells. *Int J Med Mushrooms*. 2017;19(6):535-546.

[1251] Chou YN, Lee MM, Deng JS, et al. Water Extract from Brown Strain of Flammulina velutipes Alleviates Cisplatin-Induced Acute Kidney Injury by Attenuating Oxidative Stress, Inflammation, and Autophagy via PI3K/AKT Pathway Regulation. *Int J Mol Sci*. 2023 May 29;24(11):9448.

[1252] Chen GT, Fu YX, Yang WJ, et al. Effects of polysaccharides from the base of Flammulina Velutipes stipe on growth of murine RAW264.7, B16F10 and L929 cells. *Int J Biol Macromol*. 2018 Feb;107(Pt B):2150-2156.

[1253] Ng TB, Ngai PH, Xia L. An agglutinin with mitogenic and antiproliferative activities from the mushroom Flammulina velutipes. *Mycologia*. 2006 Mar-Apr;98(2):167-71.

[1254] Krasnopolskaya LM, Shuktueva MI, Avtonomova AV, et al. Antitumor and Antioxidant Properties of Water-Soluble Polysaccharides from Submerged Mycelium of Flammulina velutipes. *Antibiot Khimioter*. 2016;61(11-12):16-20.

[1255] Otagiri K, Ohkuma T, Ikekawa T, et al. Intensification of antitumor-immunity by protein-bound polysaccharide, EA6, derived from Flammulina velutipes (Curt. ex Fr.) Sing. combined with murine leukemia L1210 vaccine in animal experiments. *J Pharmacobiodyn*. 1983 Feb;6(2):96-104.

[1256] Leung MY, Fung KP, Choy YM. The isolation and characterization of an immunomodulatory and anti-tumor polysaccharide preparation from Flammulina velutipes. *Immunopharmacology*. 1997 Jan;35(3):255-63.

[1257] Chang HH, Hsieh KY, Yeh CH, et al. Oral administration of an Enoki mushroom protein FVE activates innate and adaptive immunity and induces anti-tumor activity against murine hepatocellular carcinoma. *Int Immunopharmacol*. 2010 Feb;10(2):239-46.

[1258] Hu Q, Yu J, Yang W, et al. Identification of flavonoids from Flammulina velutipes and its neuroprotective effect on pheochromocytoma-12 cells. *Food Chem*. 2016 Aug 1;204:274-282.

[1259] Su A, Yang W, Zhao L, et al. Flammulina velutipes polysaccharides improve scopolamine-induced learning and memory impairment in mice by modulating gut microbiota composition. *Food Funct*. 2018 Mar 1;9(3):1424-1432.

[1260] Chen F, Wu M, Wu P, et al. Natural Flammulina velutipes-Based Nerve Guidance Conduit as a Potential Biomaterial for Peripheral Nerve Regeneration: In Vitro and In Vivo Studies. *ACS Biomater Sci Eng*. 2021 Aug 9;7(8):3821-3834.

[1261] Su A, Yang W, Zhao L, et al. Flammulina velutipes polysaccharides improve scopolamine-induced learning and memory impairment in mice by modulating gut microbiota composition. *Food Funct*. 2018 Mar 1;9(3):1424-1432.

[1262] Zhang Y, Li H, Yang X, et al. Cognitive-enhancing effect of polysaccharides from Flammulina velutipes on Alzheimer's disease by compatibilizing with ginsenosides. *Int J Biol Macromol*. 2018 Jun;112:788-795.

[1263] Yamashina K, Yamamoto S, Matsumoto M, et al. Suppressive Effect of Fruiting Bodies of Medicinal Mushrooms on Demyelination and Motor Dysfunction in a Cuprizone-Induced Multiple Sclerosis Mouse Model. *Int J Med Mushrooms*. 2022;24(9):15-24.

[1264] Liang Q, Zhao Q, Hao X, et al. The Effect of Flammulina velutipes Polysaccharide on Immunization Analyzed by Intestinal Flora and Proteomics. *Front Nutr*. 2022 Jan 28;9:841230.

[1265] Xu Y, Zhang Z, Wang B, He X, et al. Flammulina velutipes Polysaccharides Modulate Gut Microbiota and Alleviate Carbon Tetrachloride-Induced Hepatic Oxidative Injury in Mice. *Front Microbiol*. 2022 Mar 23;13:847653.

[1266] Hao Y, Wang X, Yuan S, et al. Flammulina velutipes polysaccharide improves C57BL/6 mice gut health through regulation of intestine microbial metabolic activity. *Int J Biol Macromol*. 2021 Jan 15;167:1308-1318.

[1267] Luo Z, Gao Q, Li Y, et al. Flammulina velutipes Mycorrhizae Attenuate High Fat Diet-Induced Lipid Disorder, Oxidative Stress and Inflammation in the Liver and Perirenal Adipose Tissue of Mice. *Nutrients*. 2022 Sep 16;14(18):3830.

[1268] Su A, Ma G, Ma N, et al. Effects of Flammulina velutipes polysaccharides on gut microbiota composition and metabolism in vitro fermentation. *Food Sci Biotechnol*. 2022 Nov 22;32(3):361-369.

[1269] Liu Y, Li H, Ren P, et al. Polysaccharide from Flammulina velutipes residues protects mice from Pb poisoning by activating Akt/GSK3β/Nrf-2/HO-1 signaling pathway and modulating gut microbiota. *Int J Biol Macromol*. 2023 Mar 1;230:123154.

[1270] Su A, Yang W, Zhao L, et al. Flammulina velutipes polysaccharides improve scopolamine-induced learning and memory impairment in mice by modulating gut microbiota composition. *Food Funct*. 2018 Mar 1;9(3):1424-1432.

[1271] Zhao R, Ji Y, Chen X, et al. Polysaccharide from Flammulina velutipes attenuates markers of metabolic syndrome by modulating the gut microbiota and lipid metabolism in high fat diet-fed mice. *Food Funct*. 2021 Aug 2;12(15):6964-6980.

[1272] Hao Y, Liao X, Wang X, et al. The biological regulatory activities of Flammulina velutipes polysaccharide in mice intestinal microbiota, immune repertoire and heart transcriptome. *Int J Biol Macromol*. 2021 Aug 31;185:582-591.

[1273] Liu X, Zhao J, Zhang G, et al. Dietary Supplementation with Flammulina velutipes Stem Waste on Growth Performance, Fecal Short Chain Fatty Acids and Serum Profile in Weaned Piglets. *Animals (Basel)*. 2020 Jan 3;10(1):82.

[1274] Wei J, Xiao H, Wei Y, et al. Longitudinal Study of the Effects of Flammulina velutipes Stipe Wastes on the Cecal Microbiota of Laying Hens. *mSystems*. 2023 Feb 23;8(1):e0083522.

[1275] Ye J, Wang X, Wang K, et al. A novel polysaccharide isolated from Flammulina velutipes, characterization, macrophage immunomodulatory activities and its impact on gut microbiota in rats. *J Anim Physiol Anim Nutr (Berl)*. 2020 Mar;104(2):735-748.

[1276] Zhao R, Ji Y, Chen X, et al. Effects of a β-type glycosidic polysaccharide from Flammulina velutipes on anti-inflammation and gut microbiota modulation in colitis mice. *Food Funct*. 2020 May 1;11(5):4259-4274.

[1277] Ma S, Xu J, Lai T, et al. Inhibitory Effect of Fermented Flammulina velutipes Polysaccharides on Mice Intestinal Inflammation. *Front Nutr*. 2022 Jun 21;9:934073.

[1278] Hao R, Zhou X, Zhao X, et al. Flammulina velutipes polysaccharide counteracts cadmium-induced gut injury in mice via modulating gut inflammation, gut microbiota and intestinal barrier. *Sci Total Environ*. 2023 Jun 15;877:162910.

[1279] Ye J, Wang X, Wang K, et al. A novel polysaccharide isolated from Flammulina velutipes, characterization, macrophage immunomodulatory activities and its impact on gut microbiota in rats. *J Anim Physiol Anim Nutr (Berl)*. 2020 Mar;104(2):735-748.

[1280] Watanabe H, Narai A, Shimizu M. Purification and cDNA cloning of a protein derived from Flammulina velutipes that increases the permeability of the intestinal Caco-2 cell monolayer. *Eur J Biochem*. 1999 Jun;262(3):850-7.

[1281] Zhao R, Ji Y, Chen X, et al. Effects of a β-type glycosidic polysaccharide from Flammulina velutipes on anti-inflammation and gut microbiota modulation in colitis mice. *Food Funct*. 2020 May 1;11(5):4259-4274.

[1282] Liang Q, Zhao Q, Hao X, et al. The Effect of Flammulina velutipes Polysaccharide on Immunization Analyzed by Intestinal Flora and Proteomics. *Front Nutr*. 2022 Jan 28;9:841230.

[1283] Zhang J, Ma N, Ma G, et al. Characterization of soy protein isolate/Flammulina velutipes polysaccharide hydrogel and its immunostimulatory effects on RAW264.7 cells. *Food Chem Toxicol*. 2021 May;151:112126.

[1284] Yan ZF, Liu NX, Mao XX, et al. Activation effects of polysaccharides of Flammulina velutipes mycorrhizae on the T lymphocyte immune function. *J Immunol Res*. 2014;2014:285421.

[1285] Ye J, Wang X, Wang K, et al. A novel polysaccharide isolated from Flammulina velutipes, characterization, macrophage immunomodulatory activities and its impact on gut microbiota in rats. *J Anim Physiol Anim Nutr (Berl)*. 2020 Mar;104(2):735-748.

[1286] Wu M, Luo X, Xu X, et al. Antioxidant and immunomodulatory activities of a polysaccharide from Flammulina velutipes. *J Tradit Chin Med*. 2014 Dec;34(6):733-40.

[1287] Wang WH, Zhang JS, Feng T, et al. Structural elucidation of a polysaccharide from Flammulina velutipes and its immunomodulation activities on mouse B lymphocytes. *Sci Rep*. 2018 Feb 15;8(1):3120.

[1288] Mahfuz S, Song H, Miao Y, et al. Dietary inclusion of mushroom (Flammulina velutipes) stem waste on growth performance and immune responses in growing layer hens. *J Sci Food Agric*. 2019 Jan 30;99(2):703-710.

[1289] Mahfuz S, He T, Liu S, et al. Dietary Inclusion of Mushroom (Flammulina velutipes) Stem Waste on Growth Performance, Antibody Response, Immune Status, and Serum Cholesterol in Broiler Chickens. *Animals (Basel)*. 2019 Sep 17;9(9):692.

[1290] Mahfuz S, Song H, Liu Z, et al. Effect of golden needle mushroom (Flammulina velutipes) stem waste on laying performance, calcium utilization, immune response and serum immunity at early phase of production. *Asian-Australas J Anim Sci*. 2018 May;31(5):705-711.

[1291] Yin H, Wang Y, Wang Y, et al. Purification, characterization and immuno-modulating properties of polysaccharides isolated from Flammulina velutipes mycelium. *Am J Chin Med*. 2010;38(1):191-204.

[1292] Kashina S, Villavicencio LL, Zaina S, et al. Activity of Extracts from Submerged Cultured Mycelium of Winter Mushroom, Flammulina velutipes (Agaricomycetes), on the Immune System In Vitro. *Int J Med Mushrooms*. 2016;18(1):49-57.

[1293] Leung MY, Fung KP, Choy YM. The isolation and characterization of an immunomodulatory and anti-tumor polysaccharide preparation from Flammulina velutipes. *Immunopharmacology*. 1997 Jan;35(3):255-63.

[1294] Feng T, Jia W, Wang WH, et al. Structural Characterization and Immunological Activities of a Novel Water-Soluble Polysaccharide from the Fruiting Bodies of Culinary-Medicinal Winter Mushroom, Flammulina velutipes (Agaricomycetes). *Int J Med Mushrooms*. 2016;18(9):807-819.

[1295] Wang PH, Hsu CI, Tang SC, et al. Fungal immunomodulatory protein from Flammulina velutipes induces interferon-gamma production through p38 mitogen-activated protein kinase signaling pathway. *J Agric Food Chem*. 2004 May 5;52(9):2721-5.

[1296] Xu J, Xu D, Hu Q, et al. Immune regulatory functions of biologically active proteins from edible fungi. *Front Immunol*. 2023 Jan 12;13:1034545.

[1297] Gu K, Wang T, Peng L, et al. FIP-fve Stimulates Cell Proliferation and Enhances IL-2 Release by Activating MAP2K3/p38α (MAPK14) Signaling Pathway in Jurkat E6-1 Cells. *Front Nutr*. 2022 May 9;9:881924.

[1298] Ou CC, Hsiao YM, Wu WJ, et al. FIP-fve stimulates interferon-gamma production via modulation of calcium release and PKC-alpha activation. *J Agric Food Chem*. 2009 Nov 25;57(22):11008-13.

[1299] Bastiaan-Net S, Chanput W, Hertz A, et al. Biochemical and functional characterization of recombinant fungal immunomodulatory proteins (rFIPs). *Int Immunopharmacol*. 2013 Jan;15(1):167-75.

[1300] Chang HL, Lei LS, Yu CL, et al. [Effect of Flammulina velutipes polysaccharides on production of cytokines by murine immunocytes and serum levels of cytokines in tumor-bearing mice]. *Zhong Yao Cai*. 2009 Apr;32(4):561-3.

[1301] Zhang J, Tyler HL, Haron MH, et al. Macrophage activation by edible mushrooms is due to the collaborative interaction of toll-like receptor agonists and dectin-1b activating beta glucans derived from colonizing microorganisms. *Food Funct*. 2019 Dec 11;10(12):8208-8217.

[1302] Jeurink PV, Noguera CL, Savelkoul HF, et al. Immunomodulatory capacity of fungal proteins on the cytokine production of human peripheral blood mononuclear cells. *Int Immunopharmacol*. 2008 Aug;8(8):1124-33.

[1303] Chen X, Fang D, Zhao R, et al. Effects of ultrasound-assisted extraction on antioxidant activity and bidirectional immunomodulatory activity of Flammulina velutipes polysaccharide. *Int J Biol Macromol*. 2019 Nov 1;140:505-514.

[1304] Ma S, Zhang H, Xu J. Characterization, Antioxidant and Anti-Inflammation Capacities of Fermented Flammulina velutipes Polyphenols. *Molecules*. 2021 Oct 14;26(20):6205.

[1305] Chen X, Fang D, Zhao R, et al. Effects of ultrasound-assisted extraction on antioxidant activity and bidirectional immunomodulatory activity of Flammulina velutipes polysaccharide. *Int J Biol Macromol*. 2019 Nov 1;140:505-514.

[1306] Zhao R, Ji Y, Chen X, et al. Effects of a β-type glycosidic polysaccharide from Flammulina velutipes on anti-inflammation and gut microbiota modulation in colitis mice. *Food Funct*. 2020 May 1;11(5):4259-4274.

[1307] Gunawardena D, Bennett L, Shanmugam K, et al. Anti-inflammatory effects of five commercially available mushroom species determined in lipopolysaccharide and interferon-γ activated murine macrophages. *Food Chem*. 2014 Apr 1;148:92-6.

[1308] Chu PY, Sun HL, Ko JL, et al. Oral fungal immunomodulatory protein-Flammulina velutipes has influence on pulmonary inflammatory process and potential treatment for allergic airway disease: A mouse model. *J Microbiol Immunol Infect*. 2017 Jun;50(3):297-306.

[1309] Chang YC, Hsiao YM, Hung SC, et al. Alleviation of Dermatophagoides microceras-induced allergy by an immunomodulatory protein, FIP-fve, from Flammulina velutipes in mice. *Biosci Biotechnol Biochem*. 2015;79(1):88-96.

[1310] Lee YT, Lee SS, Sun HL, et al. Effect of the fungal immunomodulatory protein FIP-fve on airway inflammation and cytokine production in mouse asthma model. *Cytokine*. 2013 Jan;61(1):237-44.

[1311] Pan HH, Ko JL, Wu CT, et al. Effect of the Fungal Immunomodulatory Protein FIP-fve in the Neutrophilic Asthma Animal Model. *Int Arch Allergy Immunol*. 2021;182(12):1143-1154.

[1312] Lee YT, Wu CT, Sun HL, et al. Fungal immunomodulatory protein-fve could modulate airway remodel through by affect IL17 cytokine. *J Microbiol Immunol Infect*. 2018 Oct;51(5):598-607.

[1313] Wu CT, Lee YT, Ku MS, et al. Role of biomarkers and effect of FIP-fve in acute and chronic animal asthma models. *J Microbiol Immunol Infect*. 2020 Dec;53(6):996-1007.

[1314] Hsieh KY, Hsu CI, Lin JY, et al. Oral administration of an edible-mushroom-derived protein inhibits the development of food-allergic reactions in mice. *Clin Exp Allergy*. 2003 Nov;33(11):1595-602.

[1315] Yuan F, Gao Z, Liu W, et al. Characterization, Antioxidant, Anti-Aging and Organ Protective Effects of Sulfated Polysaccharides from Flammulina velutipes. *Molecules*. 2019 Sep 28;24(19):3517.

[1316] Ma Z, Cui F, Gao X, et al. Purification, characterization, antioxidant activity and anti-aging of exopolysaccharides by Flammulina velutipes SF-06. *Antonie Van Leeuwenhoek*. 2015 Jan;107(1):73-82.

[1317] Iguchi K, Nagashima K, Mochizuki J, et al. Enokitake Mushroom and Its Active Component, Adenosine, Which Restores Testosterone Production in Impaired and Fatigued Mouse Models. *Nutrients*. 2023 Apr 29;15(9):2142.

[1318] Xu Y, Zhang Z, Wang B, He X, et al. Flammulina velutipes Polysaccharides Modulate Gut Microbiota and Alleviate Carbon Tetrachloride-Induced Hepatic Oxidative Injury in Mice. *Front Microbiol*. 2022 Mar 23;13:847653.

[1319] Luo Z, Gao Q, Li Y, et al. Flammulina velutipes Mycorrhizae Attenuate High Fat Diet-Induced Lipid Disorder, Oxidative Stress and Inflammation in the Liver and Perirenal Adipose Tissue of Mice. *Nutrients*. 2022 Sep 16;14(18):3830.

[1320] Nguepi Tsopmejio IS, Yuan J, Diao Z, et al. Auricularia polytricha and Flammulina velutipes reduce liver injury in DSS-induced Inflammatory Bowel Disease by improving inflammation, oxidative stress, and apoptosis through the regulation of TLR4/NF-κB signaling pathways. *J Nutr Biochem*. 2023 Jan;111:109190.

[1321] Kim JS, Chung HY, Na K. Cytoprotective effect of polysaccharide isolated from different mushrooms against 7-ketocholesterol induced damage in mouse liver cell line (BNL CL. 2). *Nutr Res Pract*. 2007 Fall;1(3):180-3.

[1322] Zhao R, Ji Y, Chen X, et al. Flammulina velutipes polysaccharides regulate lipid metabolism disorders in HFD-fed mice via bile acids metabolism. *Int J Biol Macromol*. 2023 Oct 11;253(Pt 6):127308.

[1323] Yeh MY, Ko WC, Lin LY. Hypolipidemic and antioxidant activity of enoki mushrooms (Flammulina velutipes). *Biomed Res Int*. 2014;2014:352385.

[1324] Mahfuz S, He T, Liu S, et al. Dietary Inclusion of Mushroom (Flammulina velutipes) Stem Waste on Growth Performance, Antibody Response, Immune Status, and Serum Cholesterol in Broiler Chickens. *Animals (Basel)*. 2019 Sep 17;9(9):692.

[1325] Rahman MA, Abdullah N, Aminudin N. Antioxidative Effects and Inhibition of Human Low Density Lipoprotein Oxidation In Vitro of Polyphenolic Compounds in Flammulina velutipes (Golden Needle Mushroom). *Oxid Med Cell Longev*. 2015;2015:403023.

[1326] Fukushima M, Ohashi T, Fujiwara Y, et al. Cholesterol-lowering effects of maitake (Grifola frondosa) fiber, shiitake (Lentinus edodes) fiber, and enokitake (Flammulina velutipes) fiber in rats. *Exp Biol Med (Maywood)*. 2001 Sep;226(8):758-65.

[1327] Zhao R, Ji Y, Chen X, et al. Polysaccharide from Flammulina velutipes attenuates markers of metabolic syndrome by modulating the gut microbiota and lipid metabolism in high fat diet-fed mice. *Food Funct*. 2021 Aug 2;12(15):6964-6980.

[1328] Hao Y, Liao X, Wang X, et al. The biological regulatory activities of Flammulina velutipes polysaccharide in mice intestinal microbiota, immune repertoire and heart transcriptome. *Int J Biol Macromol*. 2021 Aug 31;185:582-591.

[1329] Kim JM, Ra KS, Noh DO, et al. Optimization of submerged culture conditions for the production of angiotensin converting enzyme inhibitor from Flammulina velutipes. *J Ind Microbiol Biotechnol*. 2002 Nov;29(5):292-5.

[1330] Lin L, Cui F, Zhang J, et al. Antioxidative and renoprotective effects of residue polysaccharides from Flammulina velutipes. *Carbohydr Polym*. 2016 Aug 1;146:388-95.

[1331] Wu H, Yuan J, Yin H, et al. Flammulina velutipes stem regulates oxidative damage and synthesis of yolk precursors in aging laying hens by regulating the liver-blood-ovary axis. *Poult Sci*. 2023 Jan;102(1):102261.

[1332] Liu Y, Li H, Ren P, et al. Polysaccharide from Flammulina velutipes residues protects mice from Pb poisoning by activating Akt/GSK3β/Nrf-2/HO-1 signaling pathway and modulating gut microbiota. *Int J Biol Macromol*. 2023 Mar 1;230:123154.

[1333] Liang Q, Zhao Q, Hao X, et al. The Effect of Flammulina velutipes Polysaccharide on Immunization Analyzed by Intestinal Flora and Proteomics. *Front Nutr*. 2022 Jan 28;9:841230.

[1334] Lin L, Cui F, Zhang J, et al. Antioxidative and renoprotective effects of residue polysaccharides from Flammulina velutipes. *Carbohydr Polym*. 2016 Aug 1;146:388-95.

[1335] Ma Z, Cui F, Gao X, et al. Purification, characterization, antioxidant activity and anti-aging of exopolysaccharides by Flammulina velutipes SF-06. *Antonie Van Leeuwenhoek*. 2015 Jan;107(1):73-82.

[1336] Ma S, Zhang H, Xu J. Characterization, Antioxidant and Anti-Inflammation Capacities of Fermented Flammulina velutipes Polyphenols. *Molecules*. 2021 Oct 14;26(20):6205.

[1337] Xia Z. Preparation of the oligosaccharides derived from Flammulina velutipes and their antioxidant activities. *Carbohydr Polym*. 2015 Mar 15;118:41-3.

[1338] Dong YR, Cheng SJ, Qi GH, et al. Antimicrobial and antioxidant activities of Flammulina velutipes polysaccharides and polysaccharide-iron(III) complex [corrected]. *Carbohydr Polym*. 2017 Apr 1;161:26-32.

[1339] Chen CC, Tang CT, Lai CY, et al. In Vitro Assessment of the Antioxidant and Anticancer Properties of Flammulina velutipes Stipe Extracts. *Anticancer Res*. 2023 Jul;43(7):3057-3067.

[1340] Wu M, Luo X, Xu X, et al. Antioxidant and immunomodulatory activities of a polysaccharide from Flammulina velutipes. *J Tradit Chin Med*. 2014 Dec;34(6):733-40.

[1341] Liu Y, Zhang B, Ibrahim SA, et al. Purification, characterization and antioxidant activity of polysaccharides from Flammulina velutipes residue. *Carbohydr Polym*. 2016 Jul 10;145:71-7.

[1342] Hu YN, Sung TJ, Chou CH, et al. Characterization and Antioxidant Activities of Yellow Strain Flammulina velutipes (Jinhua Mushroom) Polysaccharides and Their Effects on ROS Content in L929 Cell. *Antioxidants (Basel)*. 2019 Aug 10;8(8):298.

[1343] Yuan F, Gao Z, Liu W, et al. Characterization, Antioxidant, Anti-Aging and Organ Protective Effects of Sulfated Polysaccharides from Flammulina velutipes. *Molecules*. 2019 Sep 28;24(19):3517.

[1344] Sun M, Ni L, Huang Y, et al. Effects of different drying treatments on the microstructure, free amino acids, volatile compounds and antioxidant activity of Flammulina velutipes root. *Food Chem X*. 2023 Mar 21;18:100656.

[1345] Krsmanović N, Rašeta M, Mišković J, et al. Effects of UV Stress in Promoting Antioxidant Activities in Fungal Species Trametes versicolor (L.) Lloyd and Flammulina velutipes (Curtis) Singer. *Antioxidants (Basel)*. 2023 Jan 28;12(2):302.

[1346] Chen X, Fang D, Zhao R, et al. Effects of ultrasound-assisted extraction on antioxidant activity and bidirectional immunomodulatory activity of Flammulina velutipes polysaccharide. *Int J Biol Macromol*. 2019 Nov 1;140:505-514.

[1347] Zhang Z, Lv G, He W, et al. Effects of extraction methods on the antioxidant activities of polysaccharides obtained from Flammulina velutipes. *Carbohydr Polym*. 2013 Nov 6;98(2):1524-31.

[1348] Guo Z, Zhao L, Zhen D, et al. The Effects of Ethanol Concentration during Isolation and Purity on the In Vitro Antioxidant Properties of Polysaccharides from the Winter Culinary-Medicinal Mushroom, Flammulina velutipes (Agaricomycetes) Stembase. *Int J Med Mushrooms*. 2019;21(9):895-908.

[1349] Bao HN, Ochiai Y, Ohshima T. Antioxidative activities of hydrophilic extracts prepared from the fruiting body and spent culture medium of Flammulina velutipes. *Bioresour Technol*. 2010 Aug;101(15):6248-55.

[1350] Zeng X, Suwandi J, Fuller J, et al. Antioxidant capacity and mineral contents of edible wild Australian mushrooms. *Food Sci Technol Int*. 2012 Aug;18(4):367-79.

[1351] He JZ, Ru QM, Dong DD, et al. Chemical characteristics and antioxidant properties of crude water soluble polysaccharides from four common edible mushrooms. *Molecules*. 2012 Apr 11;17(4):4373-87.

[1352] Miyazawa N, Yoshimoto H, Kurihara S, et al. Improvement of Diet-induced Obesity by Ingestion of Mushroom Chitosan Prepared from Flammulina velutipes. *J Oleo Sci*. 2018 Feb 1;67(2):245-254.

[1353] Park HJ, Lee S, Ye M, et al. Anti-Obesity Effect of Chitoglucan in High-Fat-Induced Obesity Mice. *Int J Environ Res Public Health*. 2022 Dec 24;20(1):281.

[1354] Zhu Y, Chen F, Wu M, et al. Biocompatible and antibacterial Flammulina velutipes-based natural hybrid cryogel to treat noncompressible hemorrhages and skin defects. *Front Bioeng Biotechnol*. 2022 Oct 11;10:960407.

[1355] Chen F, Zhang Q, Wu P, et al. Green fabrication of seedbed-like Flammulina velutipes polysaccharides-derived scaffolds accelerating full-thickness skin wound healing accompanied by hair follicle regeneration. *Int J Biol Macromol*. 2021 Jan 15;167:117-129.

[1356] Xu H, Zhang Y, Liu L, et al. Residues of Culinary-Medicinal Winter Mushroom, Flammulina velutipes (Agaricomycetes), Cultivation as a Potential Source of Functional Skin Substitute with Multiple Bioactivities. *Int J Med Mushrooms*. 2022;24(2):75-84.

[1357] Xu H, Liu L, Cao C, et al. Wound Healing Activity of a Skin Substitute from Residues of Culinary-Medicinal Winter Mushroom Flammulina velutipes (Agaricomycetes) Cultivation. *Int J Med Mushrooms*. 2019;21(7):683-691.

[1358] Jang SG, Jeon KS, Lee EH, et al. Isolation of 1',3'-dilinolenoyl'-2'-linoleoylglycerol with tyrosinase inhibitory activity from Flammulina velutipes. *J Microbiol Biotechnol*. 2009 Jul;19(7):681-4.

[1359] Huang LH, Lin HY, Lyu YT, et al. Development of a Transgenic Flammulina velutipes Oral Vaccine for Hepatitis B. *Food Technol Biotechnol*. 2019 Mar;57(1):105-112.

[1360] Chang YC, Chow YH, Sun HL, et al. Alleviation of respiratory syncytial virus replication and inflammation by fungal immunomodulatory protein FIP-fve from Flammulina velutipes. *Antiviral Res*. 2014 Oct;110:124-31.

[1361] Hou FH, Chia MY, Liao JW, et al. Efficacy of fungal immunomodulatory protein to promote swine immune responses against porcine reproductive and respiratory syndrome virus infection. *Vet Immunol Immunopathol*. 2020 Apr 27;224:110056.

[1362] Krupodorova T, Rybalko S, Barshteyn V. Antiviral activity of Basidiomycete mycelia against influenza type A (serotype H1N1) and herpes simplex virus type 2 in cell culture. *Virol Sin*. 2014 Oct;29(5):284-90.

[1363] Zhu Y, Chen F, Wu M, et al. Biocompatible and antibacterial Flammulina velutipes-based natural hybrid cryogel to treat noncompressible hemorrhages and skin defects. *Front Bioeng Biotechnol*. 2022 Oct 11;10:960407.

[1364] Kashina S, Flores Villavicencio LL, Balleza M, et al. Extracts from Flammulina velutipes Inhibit the Adhesion of Pathogenic Fungi to Epithelial Cells. *Pharmacognosy Res*. 2016 Mar;8(Suppl 1):S56-60.

[1365] Dong YR, Cheng SJ, Qi GH, et al. Antimicrobial and antioxidant activities of Flammulina velutipes polysaccharides and polysaccharide-iron(III) complex [corrected]. *Carbohydr Polym*. 2017 Apr 1;161:26-32.

[1366] Cui C, Xu H, Yang H, et al. Antibacterial Activity of Fruiting Body Extracts from Culinary-Medicinal Winter Mushroom, Flammulina velutipes (Agaricomycetes) against Oral Pathogen Streptococcus mutans. *Int J Med Mushrooms*. 2020;22(2):115-124.

[1367] Ishikawa NK, Fukushi Y, Yamaji K, et al. Antimicrobial cuparene-type sesquiterpenes, enokipodins C and D, from a mycelial culture of Flammulina velutipes. *J Nat Prod*. 2001 Jul;64(7):932-4.

[1368] Ferreira JM, Carreira DN, Braga FR, et al. First report of the nematicidal activity of Flammulina velutipes, its spent mushroom compost and metabolites. *3 Biotech*. 2019 Nov;9(11):410.

[1369] Tso KH, Lumsangkul C, Ju JC, et al. The Potential of Peroxidases Extracted from the Spent Mushroom (Flammulina velutipes) Substrate Significantly Degrade Mycotoxin Deoxynivalenol. *Toxins (Basel)*. 2021 Jan 19;13(1):72.

[1370] Tsujiyama S, Nitta T, Maoka T. Biodegradation of polyvinyl alcohol by Flammulina velutipes in an unsubmerged culture. *J Biosci Bioeng*. 2011 Jul;112(1):58-62.

[1371] Chen YJ, Chen CC, Huang HL. Induction of apoptosis by Armillaria mellea constituent armillarikin in human hepatocellular carcinoma. *Onco Targets Ther*. 2016 Aug 1;9:4773-83.

[1372] Leu YS, Chen YJ, Chen CC, et al. Induction of Autophagic Death of Human Hepatocellular Carcinoma Cells by Armillaridin from Armillaria mellea. *Am J Chin Med*. 2019;47(6):1365-1380.

[1373] Li Z, Wang Y, Jiang B, et al. Structure, cytotoxic activity and mechanism of protoilludane sesquiterpene aryl esters from the mycelium of Armillaria mellea. *J Ethnopharmacol*. 2016 May 26;184:119-27.

[1374] Wu J, Zhou J, Lang Y, et al. A polysaccharide from Armillaria mellea exhibits strong in vitro anticancer activity via apoptosis-involved mechanisms. *Int J Biol Macromol*. 2012 Nov;51(4):663-7.

[1375] Misiek M, Williams J, Schmich K, et al. Structure and cytotoxicity of arnamial and related fungal sesquiterpene aryl esters. *J Nat Prod*. 2009 Oct;72(10):1888-91.

[1376] Bohnert M, Scherer O, Wiechmann K, et al. Melleolides induce rapid cell death in human primary monocytes and cancer cells. *Bioorg Med Chem*. 2014 Aug 1;22(15):3856-61.

[1377] Misiek M, Williams J, Schmich K, et al. Structure and cytotoxicity of arnamial and related fungal sesquiterpene aryl esters. *J Nat Prod*. 2009 Oct;72(10):1888-91.

[1378] Chang WH, Huang HL, Huang WP, et al. Armillaridin induces autophagy-associated cell death in human chronic myelogenous leukemia K562 cells. *Tumour Biol*. 2016 Oct;37(10):14291-14300.

[1379] Bohnert M, Scherer O, Wiechmann K, et al. Melleolides induce rapid cell death in human primary monocytes and cancer cells. *Bioorg Med Chem*. 2014 Aug 1;22(15):3856-61.

[1380] Misiek M, Williams J, Schmich K, et al. Structure and cytotoxicity of arnamial and related fungal sesquiterpene aryl esters. *J Nat Prod*. 2009 Oct;72(10):1888-91.

[1381] Chi CW, Chen CC, Chen YJ. Therapeutic and radiosensitizing effects of armillaridin on human esophageal cancer cells. *Evid Based Complement Alternat Med*. 2013;2013:459271.

[1382] Li YP, Wu KF, Liu Y. [Protective effect of Armillaria mellea polysaccharide on mice bone marrow cell damage caused by cyclophosphamide]. *Zhongguo Zhong Yao Za Zhi*. 2005 Feb;30(4):283-6.

[1383] Yao L, Lv J, Duan C, et al. Armillaria mellea fermentation liquor ameliorates p-chlorophenylalanine-induced insomnia associated with the modulation of serotonergic system and gut microbiota in rats. *J Food Biochem*. 2022 Feb;46(2):e14075.

[1384] Gual-Grau A, Guirro M, Crescenti A, et al. In vitro fermentability of a broad range of natural ingredients by fecal microbiota from lean and obese individuals: potential health benefits. *Int J Food Sci Nutr*. 2022 Mar;73(2):195-209.

[1385] Li H, Xu G, Yuan G. Effects of an Armillaria mellea Polysaccharide on Learning and Memory of D-Galactose-Induced Aging Mice. *Front Pharmacol*. 2022 Jul 18;13:919920.

[1386] An S, Lu W, Zhang Y, et al. Pharmacological Basis for Use of Armillaria mellea Polysaccharides in Alzheimer's Disease: Antiapoptosis and Antioxidation. *Oxid Med Cell Longev*. 2017;2017:4184562.

[1387] Petrovic N, Kosanic M, Tosti T, et al. Chemical Characterization and Bioactive Properties of the Edible and Medicinal Honey Mushroom Armillaria mellea (Agaricomycetes) from Serbia. *Int J Med Mushrooms*. 2023;25(4):1-15.

[1388] Watanabe N, Obuchi T, Tamai M, et al. A novel N6-substituted adenosine isolated from mi huan jun (Armillaria mellea) as a cerebral-protecting compound. *Planta Med*. 1990 Feb;56(1):48-52.

[1389] Geng Y, Zhu S, Cheng P, et al. Bioassay-guided fractionation of ethyl acetate extract from Armillaria mellea attenuates inflammatory response in lipopolysaccharide (LPS) stimulated BV-2 microglia. *Phytomedicine*. 2017 Mar 15;26:55-61.

[1390] Lin YE, Wang HL, Lu KH, et al. Water extract of Armillaria mellea (Vahl) P. Kumm. Alleviates the depression-like behaviors in acute- and chronic mild stress-induced rodent models via anti-inflammatory action. *J Ethnopharmacol*. 2021 Jan 30;265:113395.

[1391] Zhang T, Du Y, Liu X, et al. Study on antidepressant-like effect of protoilludane sesquiterpenoid aromatic esters from Armillaria Mellea. *Nat Prod Res*. 2021 Mar;35(6):1042-1045.

[1392] Yao L, Lv J, Duan C, et al. Armillaria mellea fermentation liquor ameliorates p-chlorophenylalanine-induced insomnia associated with the modulation of serotonergic system and gut microbiota in rats. *J Food Biochem*. 2022 Feb;46(2):e14075.

[1393] Li IC, Lin TW, Lee TY, et al. Oral Administration of Armillaria mellea Mycelia Promotes Non-Rapid Eye Movement and Rapid Eye Movement Sleep in Rats. *J Fungi (Basel)*. 2021 May 10;7(5):371.

[1394] Chen R, Ren X, Yin W, et al. Ultrasonic disruption extraction, characterization and bioactivities of polysaccharides from wild Armillaria mellea. *Int J Biol Macromol*. 2020 Aug 1;156:1491-1502.

[1395] Sun Y, Liang H, Zhang X, et al. Structural elucidation and immunological activity of a polysaccharide from the fruiting body of Armillaria mellea. *Bioresour Technol*. 2009 Mar;100(5):1860-3.

[1396] Lee JS, Oka K, Watanabe O, et al. Immunomodulatory effect of mushrooms on cytotoxic activity and cytokine production of intestinal lamina propria leukocytes does not necessarily depend on β-glucan contents. *Food Chem*. 2011 Jun 15;126(4):1521-6.

[1397] Liu TP, Chen CC, Shiao PY, et al. Armillaridin, a Honey Medicinal Mushroom, Armillaria mellea (Higher Basidiomycetes) Component, Inhibits Differentiation and Activation of Human Macrophages. *Int J Med Mushrooms*. 2015;17(2):161-8.

[1398] Li X, Zhu J, Wang T, et al. Antidiabetic activity of Armillaria mellea polysaccharides: Joint ultrasonic and enzyme assisted extraction. *Ultrason Sonochem*. 2023 Mar 18;95:106370.

[1399] Zavastin DE, Mircea C, Aprotosoaie AC, et al. Armillaria mellea: phenolic content, in vitro antioxidant and antihyperglycemic effects. *Rev Med Chir Soc Med Nat Iasi*. 2015 Jan-Mar;119(1):273-80.

[1400] Petrovic N, Kosanic M, Tosti T, et al. Chemical Characterization and Bioactive Properties of the Edible and Medicinal Honey Mushroom Armillaria mellea (Agaricomycetes) from Serbia. *Int J Med Mushrooms*. 2023;25(4):1-15.

[1401] Geng Y, Wang J, Xie M, et al. Screening and isolation for anti-hepatofibrotic components from medicinal mushrooms using TGF-(β1-induced live fibrosis in hepatic stellate cells. *Int J Med Mushrooms*. 2014;16(6):529-39.

[1402] Chang CC, Cheng JJ, Lee IJ, et al. Purification, structural elucidation, and anti-inflammatory activity of xylosyl galactofucan from Armillaria mellea. *Int J Biol Macromol*. 2018 Jul 15;114:584-591.

[1403] Lai MN, Ng LT. Antioxidant and antiedema properties of solid-state cultured honey mushroom, Armillaria mellea (higher Basidiomycetes), extracts and their polysaccharide and polyphenol contents. *Int J Med Mushrooms*. 2013;15(1):1-8.

[1404] Li ZL, Wang SM, Wang H. Honey Mushroom, Armillaria mellea (Agaricomycetes) and Its Fermentation Products Target Regulation of OAT1/OAT3 Proteins to Reduce Hyperuricemia in Mice. *Front Biosci (Landmark Ed)*. 2023 Sep 27;28(9):228.

[1405] Yong T, Chen S, Xie Y, et al. Hypouricemic Effects of Armillaria mellea on Hyperuricemic Mice Regulated through OAT1 and CNT2. *Am J Chin Med*. 2018;46(3):585-599.

[1406] Yao L, Lv J, Duan C, et al. Armillaria mellea fermentation liquor ameliorates p-chlorophenylalanine-induced insomnia associated with the modulation of serotonergic system and gut microbiota in rats. *J Food Biochem*. 2022 Feb;46(2):e14075.

[1407] Zavastin DE, Mircea C, Aprotosoaie AC, et al. Armillaria mellea: phenolic content, in vitro antioxidant and antihyperglycemic effects. *Rev Med Chir Soc Med Nat Iasi*. 2015 Jan-Mar;119(1):273-80.

[1408] Lung MY, Chang YC. Antioxidant properties of the edible Basidiomycete Armillaria mellea in submerged cultures. *Int J Mol Sci*. 2011;12(10):6367-84.

[1409] Erbiai EH, da Silva LP, Saidi R, et al. Chemical Composition, Bioactive Compounds, and Antioxidant Activity of Two Wild Edible Mushrooms Armillaria mellea and Macrolepiota procera from Two Countries (Morocco and Portugal). *Biomolecules*. 2021 Apr 14;11(4):575.

[1410] Chen R, Ren X, Yin W, et al. Ultrasonic disruption extraction, characterization and bioactivities of polysaccharides from wild Armillaria mellea. *Int J Biol Macromol*. 2020 Aug 1;156:1491-1502.

[1411] Petrovic N, Kosanic M, Tosti T, et al. Chemical Characterization and Bioactive Properties of the Edible and Medicinal Honey Mushroom Armillaria mellea (Agaricomycetes) from Serbia. *Int J Med Mushrooms*. 2023;25(4):1-15.

[1412] Zhang S, Liu X, Yan L, et al. Chemical compositions and antioxidant activities of polysaccharides from the sporophores and cultured products of Armillaria mellea. *Molecules*. 2015 Mar 31;20(4):5680-97.

[1413] Lai MN, Ng LT. Antioxidant and antiedema properties of solid-state cultured honey mushroom, Armillaria mellea (higher Basidiomycetes), extracts and their polysaccharide and polyphenol contents. *Int J Med Mushrooms*. 2013;15(1):1-8.

[1414] Radzki W, Slawinska A, Skrzypczak K, et al. The Impact of Drying of Wild-Growing Mushrooms on the Content and Antioxidant Capacity of Water- Soluble Polysaccharides. *Int J Med Mushrooms*. 2019;21(4):393-400.

[1415] Prasad R, Varshney VK, Harsh NS, et al. Antioxidant Capacity and Total Phenolics Content of the Fruiting Bodies and Submerged Cultured Mycelia of Sixteen Higher Basidiomycetes Mushrooms from India. *Int J Med Mushrooms*. 2015;17(10):933-41.

[1416] Donnelly DM, Abe F, Coveney D, et al. Antibacterial sesquiterpene aryl esters from Armillaria mellea. *J Nat Prod*. 1985 Jan-Feb;48(1):10-6.

[1417] Petrovic N, Kosanic M, Tosti T, et al. Chemical Characterization and Bioactive Properties of the Edible and Medicinal Honey Mushroom Armillaria mellea (Agaricomycetes) from Serbia. *Int J Med Mushrooms*. 2023;25(4):1-15.

[1418] Obuchi T, Kondoh H, Watanabe N, et al. Armillaric acid, a new antibiotic produced by Armillaria mellea. *Planta Med*. 1990 Apr;56(2):198-201.

[1419] Kózka B, Sośnicka A, Nałęcz-Jawecki G, et al. Various species of Basidiomycota fungi reveal different abilities to degrade pharmaceuticals and also different pathways of degradation. *Chemosphere*. 2023 Oct;338:139481.

[1420] Ren D, Wang N, Guo J, et al. Chemical characterization of Pleurotus eryngii polysaccharide and its tumor-inhibitory effects against human hepatoblastoma HepG-2 cells. *Carbohydr Polym*. 2016 Mar 15;138:123-33.

[1421] Mariga AM, Yang WJ, Mugambi DK, et al. Antiproliferative and immunostimulatory activity of a protein from Pleurotus eryngii. *J Sci Food Agric*. 2014 Dec;94(15):3152-62.

[1422] Ma G, Yang W, Mariga AM, et al. Purification, characterization and antitumor activity of polysaccharides from Pleurotus eryngii residue. *Carbohydr Polym*. 2014 Dec 19;114:297-305.

[1423] Cui F, Li Y, Yang Y, et al. Changes in chemical components and cytotoxicity at different maturity stages of Pleurotus eryngii fruiting body. *J Agric Food Chem*. 2014 Dec 31;62(52):12631-40.

[1424] Mariga AM, Yang WJ, Mugambi DK, et al. Antiproliferative and immunostimulatory activity of a protein from Pleurotus eryngii. *J Sci Food Agric*. 2014 Dec;94(15):3152-62.

[1425] Sun Y, Hu X, Li W. Antioxidant, antitumor and immunostimulatory activities of the polypeptide from Pleurotus eryngii mycelium. *Int J Biol Macromol*. 2017 Apr;97:323-330.

[1426] Mariga AM, Yang WJ, Mugambi DK, et al. Antiproliferative and immunostimulatory activity of a protein from Pleurotus eryngii. *J Sci Food Agric*. 2014 Dec;94(15):3152-62.

[1427] Cui F, Li Y, Yang Y, et al. Changes in chemical components and cytotoxicity at different maturity stages of Pleurotus eryngii fruiting body. *J Agric Food Chem*. 2014 Dec 31;62(52):12631-40.

[1428] Hu Q, Yuan B, Xiao H, et al. Polyphenols-rich extract from Pleurotus eryngii with growth inhibitory of HCT116 colon cancer cells and anti-inflammatory function in RAW264.7 cells. *Food Funct*. 2018 Mar 1;9(3):1601-1611.

[1429] Yuan B, Ma N, Zhao L, et al. In vitro and in vivo inhibitory effects of a Pleurotus eryngii protein on colon cancer cells. *Food Funct*. 2017 Oct 18;8(10):3553-3562.

[1430] Fontana S, Flugy A, Schillaci O, et al. In vitro antitumor effects of the cold-water extracts of Mediterranean species of genus Pleurotus (higher Basidiomycetes) on human colon cancer cells. *Int J Med Mushrooms*. 2014;16(1):49-63.

[1431] Mariga AM, Yang WJ, Mugambi DK, et al. Antiproliferative and immunostimulatory activity of a protein from Pleurotus eryngii. *J Sci Food Agric*. 2014 Dec;94(15):3152-62.

[1432] Yang Z, Xu J, Fu Q, et al. Antitumor activity of a polysaccharide from Pleurotus eryngii on mice bearing renal cancer. *Carbohydr Polym*. 2013 Jun 20;95(2):615-20.

[1433] Sun Y, Hu X, Li W. Antioxidant, antitumor and immunostimulatory activities of the polypeptide from Pleurotus eryngii mycelium. *Int J Biol Macromol*. 2017 Apr;97:323-330.

[1434] Chen P, Yong Y, Gu Y, et al. Comparison of antioxidant and antiproliferation activities of polysaccharides from eight species of medicinal mushrooms. *Int J Med Mushrooms*. 2015;17(3):287-95.

[1435] Bae JS, Park JW, Park SH, et al. Apoptotic cell death of human leukaemia U937 cells by ubiquinone-9 purified from Pleurotus eryngii. *Nat Prod Res*. 2009;23(12):1112-9.

[1436] Sun Y, Hu X, Li W. Antioxidant, antitumor and immunostimulatory activities of the polypeptide from Pleurotus eryngii mycelium. *Int J Biol Macromol*. 2017 Apr;97:323-330.

[1437] Xue Z, Li J, Cheng A, Yu W, et al. Structure Identification of Triterpene from the Mushroom Pleurotus eryngii with Inhibitory Effects Against Breast Cancer. *Plant Foods Hum Nutr*. 2015 Sep;70(3):291-6.

[1438] Chen P, Yong Y, Gu Y, et al. Comparison of antioxidant and antiproliferation activities of polysaccharides from eight species of medicinal mushrooms. *Int J Med Mushrooms*. 2015;17(3):287-95.

[1439] Kikuchi T, Motoyashiki N, Yamada T, et al. Ergostane-Type Sterols from King Trumpet Mushroom (Pleurotus eryngii) and Their Inhibitory Effects on Aromatase. *Int J Mol Sci*. 2017 Nov 21;18(11):2479.

[1440] Shenbhagaraman R, Jagadish LK, Premalatha K, et al. Optimization of extracellular glucan production from Pleurotus eryngii and its impact on angiogenesis. *Int J Biol Macromol*. 2012 May 1;50(4):957-64.

[1441] Boulaka A, Mantellou P, Stanc GM, et al. Genoprotective activity of the Pleurotus eryngii mushrooms following their in vitro and in vivo fermentation by fecal microbiota. *Front Nutr*. 2022 Aug 23;9:988517.

[1442] Tektemur NK, Tektemur A, Güzel EE. King Oyster Mushroom, Pleurotus eryngii (Agaricomycetes), Extract Can Attenuate Doxorubicin-Induced Lung Damage by Inhibiting Oxidative Stress in Rats. *Int J Med Mushrooms*. 2023;25(1):1-12.

[1443] Erdem Guzel E, Kaya Tektemur N, Tektemur A, et al. The antioxidant and anti-apoptotic potential of Pleurotus eryngii extract and its chitosan-loaded nanoparticles against doxorubicin-induced testicular toxicity in male rats. *Andrologia*. 2021 Dec;53(11):e14225.

[1444] Barone R, Caruso Bavisotto C, Rappa F, et al. JNK pathway and heat shock response mediate the survival of C26 colon carcinoma bearing mice fed with the mushroom Pleurotus eryngii var. eryngii without affecting tumor growth or cachexia. *Food Funct*. 2021 Apr 7;12(7):3083-3095.

[1445] Biscaia SMP, Carbonero ER, Bellan DL, et al. Safe therapeutics of murine melanoma model using a novel antineoplasic, the partially methylated mannogalactan from Pleurotus eryngii. *Carbohydr Polym*. 2017 Dec 15;178:95-104.

[1446] Jeong YT, Yang BK, Li CR, et al. Anti-tumor Effects of Exo- and Endo-biopolymers Produced from Submerged Cultures of Three Different Mushrooms. *Mycobiology*. 2008 Jun;36(2):106-9.

[1447] Wang X, Qu Y, Wang Y, et al. β-1,6-Glucan From Pleurotus eryngii Modulates the Immunity and Gut Microbiota. *Front Immunol*. 2022 May 2;13:859923.

[1448] Nakahara D, Nan C, Mori K, et al. Effect of mushroom polysaccharides from Pleurotus eryngii on obesity and gut microbiota in mice fed a high-fat diet. *Eur J Nutr*. 2020 Oct;59(7):3231-3244.

[1449] Mitsou EK, Saxami G, Stamoulou E, et al. Effects of Rich in B-Glucans Edible Mushrooms on Aging Gut Microbiota Characteristics: An In Vitro Study. *Molecules*. 2020 Jun 18;25(12):2806.

[1450] Li S, Shah NP. Characterization, antioxidative and bifidogenic effects of polysaccharides from Pleurotus eryngii after heat treatments. *Food Chem*. 2016 Apr 15;197(Pt A):240-9.

[1451] Ma G, Kimatu BM, Zhao L, et al. In vivo fermentation of a Pleurotus eryngii polysaccharide and its effects on fecal microbiota composition and immune response. *Food Funct*. 2017 May 24;8(5):1810-1821.

[1452] Chou WT, Sheih IC, Fang TJ. The applications of polysaccharides from various mushroom wastes as prebiotics in different systems. *J Food Sci*. 2013 Jul;78(7):M1041-8.

[1453] Saxami G, Mitsou EK, Kerezoudi EN, et al. In Vitro Fermentation of Edible Mushrooms: Effects on Faecal Microbiota Characteristics of Autistic and Neurotypical Children. *Microorganisms*. 2023 Feb 6;11(2):414.

[1454] Nakahara D, Nan C, Mori K, et al. Effect of mushroom polysaccharides from Pleurotus eryngii on obesity and gut microbiota in mice fed a high-fat diet. *Eur J Nutr*. 2020 Oct;59(7):3231-3244.

[1455] Saxami G, Kerezoudi EN, Mitsou EK, et al. Fermentation Supernatants of Pleurotus eryngii Mushroom Ameliorate Intestinal Epithelial Barrier Dysfunction in Lipopolysaccharide-Induced Caco-2 Cells via Upregulation of Tight Junctions. *Microorganisms*. 2021 Oct 1;9(10):2071.

[1456] Ma G, Kimatu BM, Zhao L, et al. Impacts of Dietary Pleurotus eryngii Polysaccharide on Nutrient Digestion, Metabolism, and Immune Response of the Small Intestine and Colon-An iTRAQ-Based Proteomic Analysis. *Proteomics*. 2018 Apr;18(7):e1700443.

[1457] Hu Q, Yuan B, Wu X, et al. Dietary Intake of Pleurotus eryngii Ameliorated Dextran-Sodium-Sulfate-Induced Colitis in Mice. *Mol Nutr Food Res*. 2019 Sep;63(17):e1801265.

[1458] Ma G, Hu Q, Han Y, et al. Inhibitory effects of β-type glycosidic polysaccharide from Pleurotus eryngii on dextran sodium sulfate-induced colitis in mice. *Food Funct*. 2021 May 11;12(9):3831-3841.

[1459] Vetvicka V, Gover O, Hayby H, et al. Immunomodulating Effects Exerted by Glucans Extracted from the King Oyster Culinary-Medicinal Mushroom Pleurotus eryngii (Agaricomycetes) Grown in Substrates Containing Various Concentrations of Olive Mill Waste. *Int J Med Mushrooms*. 2019;21(8):765-781.

[1460] Park YS, Jang S, Lee H, et al. Identification of the Antidepressant Function of the Edible Mushroom Pleurotus eryngii. *J Fungi (Basel)*. 2021 Mar 8;7(3):190.

[1461] Minami A, Matsushita H, Horii Y, et al. Improvement of depression-like behavior and memory impairment with the ethanol extract of Pleurotus eryngii in ovariectomized rats. *Biol Pharm Bull*. 2013;36(12):1990-5.

[1462] Kushairi N, Phan CW, Sabaratnam V et al. Comparative Neuroprotective, Anti-Inflammatory and Neurite Outgrowth Activities of Extracts of King Oyster Mushroom, Pleurotus eryngii (Agaricomycetes). *Int J Med Mushrooms*. 2020;22(12):1171-1181.

[1463] Minami A, Matsushita H, Horii Y, et al. Improvement of depression-like behavior and memory impairment with the ethanol extract of Pleurotus eryngii in ovariectomized rats. *Biol Pharm Bull*. 2013;36(12):1990-5.

[1464] Liang CH, Huang PC, Mau JL, et al. Effect of the King Oyster Culinary-Medicinal Mushroom Pleurotus eryngii (Agaricomycetes) Basidiocarps Powder to Ameliorate Memory and Learning Deficit in Ability in Aβ-Induced Alzheimer's Disease C57BL/6J Mice Model. *Int J Med Mushrooms*. 2020;22(2):145-159.

[1465] Zhang CJ, Guo JY, Cheng H, et al. Protective Effects of the King Oyster Culinary-Medicinal Mushroom, Pleurotus eryngii (Agaricomycetes), Polysaccharides on β-Amyloid-Induced Neurotoxicity in PC12 Cells and Aging Rats, In Vitro and In Vivo Studies. *Int J Med Mushrooms*. 2020;22(4):325-333.

[1466] Poniedziałek B, Siwulski M, Wiater A, et al. The Effect of Mushroom Extracts on Human Platelet and Blood Coagulation: In vitro Screening of Eight Edible Species. *Nutrients*. 2019 Dec 12;11(12):3040.

[1467] Mori K, Kobayashi C, Tomita T, et al. Antiatherosclerotic effect of the edible mushrooms Pleurotus eryngii (Eringi), Grifola frondosa (Maitake), and Hypsizygus marmoreus (Bunashimeji) in apolipoprotein E-deficient mice. *Nutr Res*. 2008 May;28(5):335-42.

[1468] Zhao Y, Zhang Z, Wang L, et al. Hypolipidemic mechanism of Pleurotus eryngii polysaccharides in high-fat diet-induced obese mice based on metabolomics. *Front Nutr*. 2023 Jan 25;10:1118923.

[1469] Nakahara D, Nan C, Mori K, et al. Effect of mushroom polysaccharides from Pleurotus eryngii on obesity and gut microbiota in mice fed a high-fat diet. *Eur J Nutr*. 2020 Oct;59(7):3231-3244.

[1470] Zhao Y, Chen X, Zhao Y, et al. Optimization of extraction parameters of Pleurotus eryngii polysaccharides and evaluation of the hypolipidemic effect. *RSC Adv*. 2020 Mar 24;10(20):11918-11928.

[1471] Chen L, Zhang Y, Sha O, et al. Hypolipidaemic and hypoglycaemic activities of polysaccharide from Pleurotus eryngii in Kunming mice. *Int J Biol Macromol*. 2016 Dec;93(Pt A):1206-1209.

[1472] Alam N, Yoon KN, Lee JS, et al. Dietary effect of Pleurotus eryngii on biochemical function and histology in hypercholesterolemic rats. *Saudi J Biol Sci*. 2011 Oct;18(4):403-9.

[1473] Wei H, Yue S, Zhang S, et al. Lipid-Lowering Effect of the Pleurotus eryngii (King Oyster Mushroom) Polysaccharide from Solid-State Fermentation on Both Macrophage-Derived Foam Cells and Zebrafish Models. *Polymers (Basel)*. 2018 May 3;10(5):492.

[1474] Mizutani T, Inatomi S, Inazu A, et al. Hypolipidemic effect of Pleurotus eryngii extract in fat-loaded mice. *J Nutr Sci Vitaminol (Tokyo)*. 2010;56(1):48-53.

[1475] Ren Z, Li J, Xu N, et al. Anti-hyperlipidemic and antioxidant effects of alkali-extractable mycelia polysaccharides by Pleurotus eryngii var. tuolensis. *Carbohydr Polym*. 2017 Nov 1;175:282-292.

[1476] Xu N, Ren Z, Zhang J, et al. Antioxidant and anti-hyperlipidemic effects of mycelia zinc polysaccharides by Pleurotus eryngii var. tuoliensis. *Int J Biol Macromol*. 2017 Feb;95:204-214.

[1477] Zhang C, Li J, Wang J, et al. Antihyperlipidaemic and hepatoprotective activities of acidic and enzymatic hydrolysis exopolysaccharides from Pleurotus eryngii SI-04. *BMC Complement Altern Med*. 2017 Aug 14;17(1):403.

[1478] Chen J, Yong Y, Xing M, et al. Characterization of polysaccharides with marked inhibitory effect on lipid accumulation in Pleurotus eryngii. *Carbohydr Polym*. 2013 Sep 12;97(2):604-13.

[1479] Choi JH, Kim DW, Kim S, et al. In Vitro Antioxidant and In Vivo Hypolipidemic Effects of the King Oyster Culinary-Medicinal Mushroom, Pleurotus eryngii var. ferulae DDL01 (Agaricomycetes), in Rats with High-Fat Diet-Induced Fatty Liver and Hyperlipidemia. *Int J Med Mushrooms*. 2017;19(2):107-119.

[1480] Huang JF, Zhan T, Yu XL, et al. Therapeutic effect of Pleurotus eryngii cellulose on experimental fatty liver in rats. *Genet Mol Res*. 2016 Feb 26;15(1):15017805.

[1481] Huang J, Wu Q, Lin Z, et al. Therapeutic effects of chitin from Pleurotus eryngii on high-fat diet induced obesity in rats. *Acta Sci Pol Technol Aliment*. 2020 Jul-Sep;19(3):279-289.

[1482] Nakahara D, Nan C, Mori K, et al. Effect of mushroom polysaccharides from Pleurotus eryngii on obesity and gut microbiota in mice fed a high-fat diet. *Eur J Nutr*. 2020 Oct;59(7):3231-3244.

[1483] Jo KJ, Ghim J, Kim J, et al. Water Extract of Pleurotus eryngii var. ferulae Prevents High-Fat Diet-Induced Obesity by Inhibiting Pancreatic Lipase. *J Med Food*. 2019 Feb;22(2):178-185.

[1484] Kang MJ, Kim KK, Son BY, et al. The Anti-Adipogenic Activity of a New Cultivar, Pleurotus eryngii var. ferulae 'Beesan No. 2', through Down-Regulation of PPAR γ and C/EBP α in 3T3-L1 Cells. *J Microbiol Biotechnol*. 2016 Nov 28;26(11):1836-1844.

[1485] Kim DH, Park YH, Lee JS, et al. Anti-Obesity Effect of DKB-117 through the Inhibition of Pancreatic Lipase and α-Amylase Activity. *Nutrients*. 2020 Oct 6;12(10):3053.

[1486] Ren D, Zhao Y, Nie Y, et al. Chemical composition of Pleurotus eryngii polysaccharides and their inhibitory effects on high-fructose diet-induced insulin resistance and oxidative stress in mice. *Food Funct*. 2014 Oct;5(10):2609-20.

[1487] Gong P, Long H, Guo Y, et al. Isolation, Structural Characterization, and Hypoglycemic Activities In Vitro of Polysaccharides from Pleurotus eryngii. *Molecules*. 2022 Oct 21;27(20):7140.

[1488] Chen L, Zhang Y, Sha O, et al. Hypolipidaemic and hypoglycaemic activities of polysaccharide from Pleurotus eryngii in Kunming mice. *Int J Biol Macromol*. 2016 Dec;93(Pt A):1206-1209.

[1489] Zhang C, Zhang L, Liu H, et al. Antioxidation, anti-hyperglycaemia and renoprotective effects of extracellular polysaccharides from Pleurotus eryngii SI-04. *Int J Biol Macromol*. 2018 May;111:219-228.

[1490] Li JP, Lei YL, Zhan H. The effects of the king oyster mushroom Pleurotus eryngii (higher Basidiomycetes) on glycemic control in alloxan-induced diabetic mice. *Int J Med Mushrooms*. 2014;16(3):219-25.

[1491] Zhang C, Zhang L, Liu H, et al. Antioxidation, anti-hyperglycaemia and renoprotective effects of extracellular polysaccharides from Pleurotus eryngii SI-04. *Int J Biol Macromol*. 2018 May;111:219-228.

[1492] Liu M, Yao W, Zhao F, et al. Characterization and Attenuation of Streptozotocin-Induced Diabetic Organ Damage by Polysaccharides from Spent Mushroom Substrate (Pleurotus eryngii). *Oxid Med Cell Longev*. 2018 Sep 30;2018:4285161.

[1493] Wang X, Qu Y, Wang Y, et al. β-1,6-Glucan From Pleurotus eryngii Modulates the Immunity and Gut Microbiota. *Front Immunol*. 2022 May 2;13:859923.

[1494] Chen L, Ren A, Wang Y, et al. Heterogalactan WPEP-N-b from Pleurotus eryngii enhances immunity in immunocompromised mice. *Int J Biol Macromol*. 2023 Jan 15;225:1010-1020.

[1495] Abreu H, Zavadinack M, Smiderle FR, et al. Polysaccharides from Pleurotus eryngii: Selective extraction methodologies and their modulatory effects on THP-1 macrophages. *Carbohydr Polym*. 2021 Jan 15;252:117177.

[1496] Vlassopoulou M, Paschalidis N, Savvides AL, et al. Immunomodulating Activity of Pleurotus eryngii Mushrooms Following Their In Vitro Fermentation by Human Fecal Microbiota. *J Fungi (Basel)*. 2022 Mar 22;8(4):329.

[1497] Mariga AM, Pei F, Yang WJ, et al. Immunopotentiation of Pleurotus eryngii (DC. ex Fr.) Quel. *J Ethnopharmacol*. 2014 May 14;153(3):604-14.

[1498] Yan J, Meng Y, Zhang M, et al. A 3-O-methylated heterogalactan from Pleurotus eryngii activates macrophages. *Carbohydr Polym*. 2019 Feb 15;206:706-715.

[1499] Ellefsen CF, Wold CW, Wilkins AL, et al. Water-soluble polysaccharides from Pleurotus eryngii fruiting bodies, their activity and affinity for Toll-like receptor 2 and dectin-1. *Carbohydr Polym*. 2021 Jul 15;264:117991.

[1500] Xu D, Wang H, Zheng W, et al. Charaterization and immunomodulatory activities of polysaccharide isolated from Pleurotus eryngii. *Int J Biol Macromol*. 2016 Nov;92:30-36.

[1501] Ma N, Du H, Ma G, et al. Characterization of the Immunomodulatory Mechanism of a Pleurotus eryngii Protein by Isobaric Tags for Relative and Absolute Quantitation Proteomics. *J Agric Food Chem*. 2020 Nov 18;68(46):13189-13199.

[1502] Sun Y, Hu X, Li W. Antioxidant, antitumor and immunostimulatory activities of the polypeptide from Pleurotus eryngii mycelium. *Int J Biol Macromol*. 2017 Apr;97:323-330.

[1503] Hu Q, Du H, Ma G, et al. Purification, identification and functional characterization of an immunomodulatory protein from Pleurotus eryngii. *Food Funct*. 2018 Jul 17;9(7):3764-3775.

[1504] Xu J, Xu D, Hu Q, et al. Immune regulatory functions of biologically active proteins from edible fungi. *Front Immunol*. 2023 Jan 12;13:1034545.

[1505] Ike K, Kameyama N, Ito A, et al. Induction of a T-Helper 1 (Th1) immune response in mice by an extract from the Pleurotus eryngii (Eringi) mushroom. *J Med Food*. 2012 Dec;15(12):1124-8.

[1506] Kim YH, Jung EG, Han KI, et al. Immunomodulatory Effects of Extracellular β-Glucan Isolated from the King Oyster Mushroom Pleurotus eryngii (Agaricomycetes) and Its Sulfated Form on Signaling Molecules Involved in Innate Immunity. *Int J Med Mushrooms*. 2017;19(6):521-533.

[1507] Li S, Shah NP. Effects of Pleurotus eryngii polysaccharides on bacterial growth, texture properties, proteolytic capacity, and angiotensin-I-converting enzyme-inhibitory activities of fermented milk. *J Dairy Sci*. 2015 May;98(5):2949-61.

[1508] Sides R, Griess-Fishheimer S, Zaretsky J, et al. The Use of Mushrooms and Spirulina Algae as Supplements to Prevent Growth Inhibition in a Pre-Clinical Model for an Unbalanced Diet. *Nutrients*. 2021 Nov 29;13(12):4316.

[1509] Yokoyama S, Bang TH, Shimizu K, et al. Osteoclastogenesis inhibitory effect of ergosterol peroxide isolated from Pleurotus eryngii. *Nat Prod Commun*. 2012 Sep;7(9):1163-4.

[1510] Kim SW, Kim HG, Lee BE, et al. Effects of mushroom, Pleurotus eryngii, extracts on bone metabolism. *Clin Nutr*. 2006 Feb;25(1):166-70.

[1511] Ohyama Y, Matsushita H, Minami A, et al. Effect of the ethanol extract of Pleurotus eryngii on bone metabolism in ovariectomized rats. *Climacteric*. 2014 Aug;17(4):492-9.

[1512] Shimizu K, Yamanaka M, Gyokusen M, et al. Estrogen-like activity and prevention effect of bone loss in calcium deficient ovariectomized rats by the extract of Pleurotus eryngii. *Phytother Res*. 2006 Aug;20(8):659-64.

[1513] Han EH, Hwang YP, Kim HG, et al. Inhibitory effect of Pleurotus eryngii extracts on the activities of allergic mediators in antigen-stimulated mast cells. *Food Chem Toxicol*. 2011 Jun;49(6):1416-25.

[1514] Yamashina K, Yamamoto S, Matsumoto M, et al. Suppressive Effect of Fruiting Bodies of Medicinal Mushrooms on Demyelination and Motor Dysfunction in a Cuprizone-Induced Multiple Sclerosis Mouse Model. *Int J Med Mushrooms*. 2022;24(9):15-24.

[1515] Ma G, Kimatu BM, Yang W, et al. Preparation of newly identified polysaccharide from Pleurotus eryngii and its anti-inflammation activities potential. *J Food Sci*. 2020 Sep;85(9):2822-2831.

[1516] Yuan B, Zhao L, Rakariyatham K, et al. Isolation of a novel bioactive protein from an edible mushroom Pleurotus eryngii and its anti-inflammatory potential. *Food Funct*. 2017 Jun 21;8(6):2175-2183.

[1517] Hu Q, Yuan B, Xiao H, et al. Polyphenols-rich extract from Pleurotus eryngii with growth inhibitory of HCT116 colon cancer cells and anti-inflammatory function in RAW264.7 cells. *Food Funct*. 2018 Mar 1;9(3):1601-1611.

[1518] Kikuchi T, Maekawa Y, Tomio A, et al. Six new ergostane-type steroids from king trumpet mushroom (Pleurotus eryngii) and their inhibitory effects on nitric oxide production. *Steroids*. 2016 Nov;115:9-17.

[1519] Kikuchi T, Horii Y, Maekawa Y, et al. Pleurocins A and B: Unusual 11(9 → 7)-abeo-Ergostanes and Eringiacetal B: A 13,14-seco-13,14-Epoxyergostane from Fruiting Bodies of Pleurotus eryngii and Their Inhibitory Effects on Nitric Oxide Production. *J Org Chem*. 2017 Oct 6;82(19):10611-10616.

[1520] Souilem F, Fernandes Â, Calhelha RC, et al. Wild mushrooms and their mycelia as sources of bioactive compounds: Antioxidant, anti-inflammatory and cytotoxic properties. *Food Chem*. 2017 Sep 1;230:40-48.

[1521] Kawai J, Andoh T, Ouchi K, et al. Pleurotus eryngii Ameliorates Lipopolysaccharide-Induced Lung Inflammation in Mice. *Evid Based Complement Alternat Med*. 2014;2014:532389.

[1522] Zhang C, Li S, Zhang J, et al. Antioxidant and hepatoprotective activities of intracellular polysaccharide from Pleurotus eryngii SI-04. *Int J Biol Macromol*. 2016 Oct;91:568-77.

[1523] Zhang C, Li J, Wang J, et al. Antihyperlipidaemic and hepatoprotective activities of acidic and enzymatic hydrolysis exopolysaccharides from Pleurotus eryngii SI-04. *BMC Complement Altern Med*. 2017 Aug 14;17(1):403.

[1524] Zhang C, Song X, Cui W, et al. Antioxidant and anti-ageing effects of enzymatic polysaccharide from Pleurotus eryngii residue. *Int J Biol Macromol*. 2021 Mar 15;173:341-350.

[1525] Lee TT, Ciou JY, Chiang CJ, et al. Effect of Pleurotus eryngii stalk residue on the oxidative status and meat quality of broiler chickens. *J Agric Food Chem*. 2012 Nov 7;60(44):11157-63.

[1526] Ren D, Zhao Y, Nie Y, et al. Chemical composition of Pleurotus eryngii polysaccharides and their inhibitory effects on high-fructose diet-induced insulin resistance and oxidative stress in mice. *Food Funct*. 2014 Oct;5(10):2609-20.

[1527] Gao Z, Lai Q, Yang Q, et al. The characteristic, antioxidative and multiple organ protective of acidic-extractable mycelium polysaccharides by Pleurotus eryngii var. tuoliensis on high-fat emulsion induced-hypertriglyceridemic mice. *Sci Rep*. 2018 Nov 30;8(1):17500.

[1528] Petraglia T, Latronico T, Fanigliulo A, et al. Antioxidant Activity of Polysaccharides from the Edible Mushroom Pleurotus eryngii. *Molecules*. 2023 Feb 26;28(5):2176.

[1529] Liu L, Wang L, Li X, et al. Effects of Different Bud Thinning Methods on Nutritional Quality and Antioxidant Activities of Fruiting Bodies of Pleurotus eryngii. *Front Plant Sci*. 2022 Jun 16;13:917010.

[1530] Santana RDS, Mendes FS, Paula da Silva BJ, et al. Recovery and partial purification of fibrinolytic protease from Pleurotus ostreatus and P. eryngii and cytotoxic and antioxidant activity of their extracts. *Prep Biochem Biotechnol*. 2023 Sep 5:1-8.

[1531] Sun Y, Hu X, Li W. Antioxidant, antitumor and immunostimulatory activities of the polypeptide from Pleurotus eryngii mycelium. *Int J Biol Macromol*. 2017 Apr;97:323-330.

[1532] Zhang A, Li X, Xing C, et al. Antioxidant activity of polysaccharide extracted from Pleurotus eryngii using response surface methodology. *Int J Biol Macromol*. 2014 Apr;65:28-32.

[1533] Li S, Shah NP. Characterization, antioxidative and bifidogenic effects of polysaccharides from Pleurotus eryngii after heat treatments. *Food Chem*. 2016 Apr 15;197(Pt A):240-9.

[1534] Sun X, Hao L, Ma H, et al. Extraction and in vitro antioxidant activity of exopolysaccharide by Pleurotus eryngii SI-02. *Braz J Microbiol*. 2014 Mar 10;44(4):1081-8.

[1535] Li S, Shah NP. Sulphonated modification of polysaccharides from Pleurotus eryngii and Streptococcus thermophilus ASCC 1275 and antioxidant activities investigation using CCD and Caco-2 cell line models. *Food Chem*. 2017 Jun 15;225:246-257.

[1536] Mishra KK, Pal RS, Arunkumar R, et al. Antioxidant properties of different edible mushroom species and increased bioconversion efficiency of Pleurotus eryngii using locally available casing materials. *Food Chem*. 2013 Jun 1;138(2-3):1557-63.

[1537] Li S, Shah NP. Antioxidant and antibacterial activities of sulphated polysaccharides from Pleurotus eryngii and Streptococcus thermophilus ASCC 1275. *Food Chem*. 2014 Dec 15;165:262-70.

[1538] Li S, Shah NP. Effects of various heat treatments on phenolic profiles and antioxidant activities of Pleurotus eryngii extracts. *J Food Sci*. 2013 Aug;78(8):C1122-9.

[1539] Jia X, Wang C, Bai Y, et al. Sulfation of the Extracellular Polysaccharide Produced by the King Oyster Culinary-Medicinal Mushroom, Pleurotus eryngii (Agaricomycetes), and Its Antioxidant Properties In Vitro. *Int J Med Mushrooms*. 2017;19(4):355-362.

[1540] Choi JH, Kim DW, Kim S, et al. In Vitro Antioxidant and In Vivo Hypolipidemic Effects of the King Oyster Culinary-Medicinal Mushroom, Pleurotus eryngii var. ferulae DDL01 (Agaricomycetes), in Rats with High-Fat Diet-Induced Fatty Liver and Hyperlipidemia. *Int J Med Mushrooms*. 2017;19(2):107-119.

[1541] Liang CH, Ho KJ, Huang LY, et al. Antioxidant properties of fruiting bodies, mycelia, and fermented products of the culinary-medicinal king oyster mushroom, Pleurotus eryngii (higher Basidiomycetes), with high ergothioneine content. *Int J Med Mushrooms*. 2013;15(3):267-75.

[1542] Liu X, Zhou B, Lin R, et al. Extraction and antioxidant activities of intracellular polysaccharide from Pleurotus sp. mycelium. *Int J Biol Macromol*. 2010 Aug 1;47(2):116-9.

[1543] Zeng X, Suwandi J, Fuller J, et al. Antioxidant capacity and mineral contents of edible wild Australian mushrooms. *Food Sci Technol Int*. 2012 Aug;18(4):367-79.

[1544] Roncero-Ramos I, Mendiola-Lanao M, Pérez-Clavijo M, et al. Effect of different cooking methods on nutritional value and antioxidant activity of cultivated mushrooms. *Int J Food Sci Nutr*. 2017 May;68(3):287-297.

[1545] Chen P, Yong Y, Gu Y, et al. Comparison of antioxidant and antiproliferation activities of polysaccharides from eight species of medicinal mushrooms. *Int J Med Mushrooms*. 2015;17(3):287-95.

[1546] Reis FS, Martins A, Barros L, et al. Antioxidant properties and phenolic profile of the most widely appreciated cultivated mushrooms: a comparative study between in vivo and in vitro samples. *Food Chem Toxicol*. 2012 May;50(5):1201-7.

[1547] Kim MY, Seguin P, Ahn JK, et al. Phenolic compound concentration and antioxidant activities of edible and medicinal mushrooms from Korea. *J Agric Food Chem*. 2008 Aug 27;56(16):7265-70.

[1548] Choi JH, Kim HG, Jin SW, et al. Topical application of Pleurotus eryngii extracts inhibits 2,4-dinitrochlorobenzene-induced atopic dermatitis in NC/Nga mice by the regulation of Th1/Th2 balance. *Food Chem Toxicol*. 2013 Mar;53:38-45.

[1549] Lee IS, Ryoo IJ, Kwon KY, et al. Pleurone, a novel human neutrophil elastase inhibitor from the fruiting bodies of the mushroom Pleurotus eryngii var. ferulae. *J Antibiot (Tokyo)*. 2011 Aug;64(8):587-9.

[1550] Krupodorova T, Rybalko S, Barshteyn V. Antiviral activity of Basidiomycete mycelia against influenza type A (serotype H1N1) and herpes simplex virus type 2 in cell culture. *Virol Sin*. 2014 Oct;29(5):284-90.

[1551] Acay H, Yildirim A, Erdem Güzel E, et al. Evaluation and characterization of Pleurotus eryngii extract-loaded chitosan nanoparticles as antimicrobial agents against some human pathogens. *Prep Biochem Biotechnol*. 2020;50(9):897-906.

[1552] Li S, Shah NP. Antioxidant and antibacterial activities of sulphated polysaccharides from Pleurotus eryngii and Streptococcus thermophilus ASCC 1275. *Food Chem*. 2014 Dec 15;165:262-70.

[1553] Wang H, Ng TB. Eryngin, a novel antifungal peptide from fruiting bodies of the edible mushroom Pleurotus eryngii. *Peptides*. 2004 Jan;25(1):1-5.

[1554] Schillaci D, Arizza V, Gargano ML, et al. Antibacterial activity of Mediterranean Oyster mushrooms, species of genus Pleurotus (higher Basidiomycetes). *Int J Med Mushrooms*. 2013;15(6):591-4

[1555] Kalyoncu F, Oskay M, Sağlam H, et al. Antimicrobial and antioxidant activities of mycelia of 10 wild mushroom species. *J Med Food*. 2010 Apr;13(2):415-9.

[1556] Shang X, Tan Q, Liu R, et al. In vitro anti-Helicobacter pylori effects of medicinal mushroom extracts, with special emphasis on the Lion's Mane mushroom, Hericium erinaceus (higher Basidiomycetes). *Int J Med Mushrooms*. 2013;15(2):165-74.

[1557] Cruz-Arévalo J, Sánchez JE, González-Cortázar M, et al. Chemical Composition of an Anthelmintic Fraction of Pleurotus eryngii against Eggs and Infective Larvae (L3) of Haemonchus contortus. *Biomed Res Int*. 2020 Aug 6;2020:4138950.

[1558] Haidukowski M, Casamassima E, Cimmarusti MT, et al. Aflatoxin B1-Adsorbing Capability of Pleurotus eryngii Mycelium: Efficiency and Modeling of the Process. *Front Microbiol*. 2019 Jun 25;10:1386.

[1559] Branà MT, Cimmarusti MT, Haidukowski M, et al. Bioremediation of aflatoxin B1-contaminated maize by king oyster mushroom (Pleurotus eryngii). *PLoS One*. 2017 Aug 3;12(8):e0182574.

[1560] Branà MT, Sergio L, Haidukowski M, et al. Degradation of Aflatoxin B1 by a Sustainable Enzymatic Extract from Spent Mushroom Substrate of Pleurotus eryngii. *Toxins (Basel)*. 2020 Jan 14;12(1):49.

[1561] Baran W, Adamek E, Włodarczyk A, et al. The remediation of sulfonamides from the environment by Pleurotus eryngii mycelium. Efficiency, products and mechanisms of mycodegradation. *Chemosphere*. 2021 Jan;262:128026.

[1562] Tang X, Dong S, Shi W, et al. Fates of nickel and fluoranthene during the bioremediation by Pleurotus eryngii in three different soils. *J Basic Microbiol*. 2016 Nov;56(11):1194-1202.

241

1563 Amin F, Talpur FN, Balouch A, et al. Utilization of Pleurotus eryngii biosorbent as an environmental bioremedy for the decontamination of trace cadmium(II) ions from water system. *Water Sci Technol*. 2018 Oct;78(5-6):1148-1158.

1564 Hadibarata T, Kristanti RA, Hamdzah M. Biosorption and biotransformation of fluoranthene by the white-rot fungus Pleurotus eryngii F032. *Biotechnol Appl Biochem*. 2014 Mar-Apr;61(2):126-33.

1565 Wu J, Xia A, Chen C, et al. Adsorption Thermodynamics and Dynamics of Three Typical Dyes onto Bio-adsorbent Spent Substrate of Pleurotus eryngii. *Int J Environ Res Public Health*. 2019 Feb 26;16(5):679.

1566 Gómez-Toribio V, García-Martín AB, Martínez MJ, et al. Enhancing the production of hydroxyl radicals by Pleurotus eryngii via quinone redox cycling for pollutant removal. *Appl Environ Microbiol*. 2009 Jun;75(12):3954-62.

1567 Hadibarata T, Kristanti RA. Potential of a white-rot fungus Pleurotus eryngii F032 for degradation and transformation of fluorene. *Fungal Biol*. 2014 Feb;118(2):222-7.

1568 Chang BV, Fan SN, Tsai YC, et al. Removal of emerging contaminants using spent mushroom compost. *Sci Total Environ*. 2018 Sep 1;634:922-933.

1569 Zhou J, Ge W, Zhang X, et al. Effects of spent mushroom substrate on the dissipation of polycyclic aromatic hydrocarbons in agricultural soil. *Chemosphere*. 2020 Nov;259:127462.

1570 Kleftaki SA, Amerikanou C, Gioxari A, et al. A Randomized Controlled Trial on Pleurotus eryngii Mushrooms with Antioxidant Compounds and Vitamin D2 in Managing Metabolic Disorders. *Antioxidants (Basel)*. 2022 Oct 26;11(11):2113.

1571 Kleftaki SA, Simati S, Amerikanou C, et al. Pleurotus eryngii improves postprandial glycaemia, hunger and fullness perception, and enhances ghrelin suppression in people with metabolically unhealthy obesity. *Pharmacol Res*. 2022 Jan;175:105979.

1572 Ghosh S, Nandi S, Banerjee A, et al. Prospecting medicinal properties of Lion's mane mushroom. *J Food Biochem*. 2021 Jun 24:e13833.

1573 Sangtitanu T, Sangtanoo P, Srimongkol P, et al. Peptides obtained from edible mushrooms: Hericium erinaceus offers the ability to scavenge free radicals and induce apoptosis in lung cancer cells in humans. *Food Funct*. 2020 Jun 24;11(6):4927-4939.

1574 Zan X, Cui F, Li Y, et al. Hericium erinaceus polysaccharide-protein HEG-5 inhibits SGC-7901 cell growth via cell cycle arrest and apoptosis. *Int J Biol Macromol*. 2015 May;76:242-53.

1575 Li G, Yu K, Li F, et al. Anticancer potential of Hericium erinaceus extracts against human gastrointestinal cancers. *J Ethnopharmacol*. 2014 Apr 28;153(2):521-30.

1576 Tung SY, Lee KC, Lee KF, et al. Apoptotic mechanisms of gastric cancer cells induced by isolated erinacine S through epigenetic histone H3 methylation of FasL and TRAIL. *Food Funct*. 2021 Apr 21;12(8):3455-3468.

1577 Kuo HC, Kuo YR, Lee KF, et al. A Comparative Proteomic Analysis of Erinacine A's Inhibition of Gastric Cancer Cell Viability and Invasiveness. *Cell Physiol Biochem*. 2017;43(1):195-208.

1578 Wang M, Zhang Y, Xiao X, et al. A Polysaccharide Isolated from Mycelia of the Lion's Mane Medicinal Mushroom Hericium erinaceus (Agaricomycetes) Induced Apoptosis in Precancerous Human Gastric Cells. *Int J Med Mushrooms*. 2017;19(12):1053-1060.

1579 Zhang F, Lv H, Zhang X. Erinacerins, Novel Glioma Inhibitors from Hericium erinaceus, Induce Apoptosis of U87 Cells through Bax/Capase-2 Pathway. *Anticancer Agents Med Chem*. 2020;20(17):2082-2088.

1580 Chang HC, Yang HL, Pan JH, et al. Hericium erinaceus Inhibits TNF-α-Induced Angiogenesis and ROS Generation through Suppression of MMP-9/NF-κB Signaling and Activation of Nrf2-Mediated Antioxidant Genes in Human EA.hy926 Endothelial Cells. *Oxid Med Cell Longev*. 2016;2016:8257238.

1581 Hou XX, Liu JY, Li ZY, et al. Fruiting body polysaccharides of Hericium erinaceus induce apoptosis in human colorectal cancer cells via ROS generation mediating caspase-9-dependent signaling pathways. *Food Funct*. 2020 Jul 22;11(7):6128-6138.

1582 Ruan Y, Han C, Wang D, et al. New benzaldehyde derivatives from the fruiting bodies of Hericium erinaceus with cytotoxic activity. *Nat Prod Res*. 2023 Jan 20:1-10.

1583 Cao Z, Zhang Z, Wei D, et al. Enrichment Extraction and Activity Study of the Different Varieties of Hericium erinaceus against HCT-8 Colon Cancer Cells. *Molecules*. 2023 Aug 28;28(17):6288.

1584 Liu JY, Hou XX, Li ZY, et al. Isolation and structural characterization of a novel polysaccharide from Hericium erinaceus fruiting bodies and its arrest of cell cycle at S-sphage in colon cancer cells. *Int J Biol Macromol*. 2020 Aug 15;157:288-295.

1585 Kim SP, Kang MY, Kim JH, et al. Composition and mechanism of antitumor effects of Hericium erinaceus mushroom extracts in tumor-bearing mice. *J Agric Food Chem*. 2011 Sep 28;59(18):9861-9.

1586 Lee KC, Kuo HC, Shen CH, et al. A proteomics approach to identifying novel protein targets involved in erinacine A-mediated inhibition of colorectal cancer cells' aggressiveness.

1587 Ruan Y, Han C, Wang D, et al. New benzaldehyde derivatives from the fruiting bodies of Hericium erinaceus with cytotoxic activity. *Nat Prod Res*. 2023 Jan 20:1-10.

1588 Zhou LJ, Mo YB, Bu X, et al. Erinacine Facilitates the Opening of the Mitochondrial Permeability Transition Pore Through the Inhibition of the PI3K/ Akt/GSK-3β Signaling Pathway in Human Hepatocellular Carcinoma. *Cell Physiol Biochem*. 2018;50(3):851-867.

1589 Chen ZY, Yan RQ, Qin GZ, et al. [Effect of six edible plants on the development of AFB1-induced gamma-glutamyltranspeptidase-positive hepatocyte foci in rats]. *Zhonghua Zhong Liu Za Zhi*. 1987 Mar;9(2):109-11.

1590 Kim SP, Kang MY, Choi YH, et al. Mechanism of Hericium erinaceus (Yamabushitake) mushroom-induced apoptosis of U937 human monocytic leukemia cells. *Food Funct*. 2011 Jun;2(6):348-56.

1591 Kim SP, Nam SH, Friedman M. Hericium erinaceus (Lion's Mane) mushroom extracts inhibit metastasis of cancer cells to the lung in CT-26 colon cancer-tansplanted mice. *J Agric Food Chem*. 2013 May 22;61(20):4898-904.

1592 Wang JC, Hǔ SH, Su CH, et al. Antitumor and immunoenhancing activities of polysaccharide from culture broth of Hericium spp. *Kaohsiung J Med Sci*. 2001 Sep;17(9):461-7.

1593 Lee JS, Hong EK. Hericium erinaceus enhances doxorubicin-induced apoptosis in human hepatocellular carcinoma cells. *Cancer Lett*. 2010 Nov 28;297(2):144-54.

1594 Wang D, Zhu X, Tang X, et al. Auxiliary antitumor effects of fungal proteins from Hericium erinaceus by target on the gut microbiota. *J Food Sci*. 2020 Jun;85(6):1872-1890.

[1595] Lee SR, Jung K, Noh HJ, et al. A new cerebroside from the fruiting bodies of Hericium erinaceus and its applicability to cancer treatment. *Bioorg Med Chem Lett.* 2015 Dec 15;25(24):5712-5.

[1596] Yang PP, Chueh SH, Shie HL, et al. Effects of Hericium erinaceus Mycelium Extracts on the Functional Activity of Purinoceptors and Neuropathic Pain in Mice with L5 Spinal Nerve Ligation. *Evid Based Complement Alternat Med.* 2020 May 13;2020:2890194.

[1597] Yeh CH, Sun LW, Lai CM, et al. Effect of ethanol extracts of Hericium erinaceus mycelium on morphine-induced microglial migration. *Mol Med Rep.* 2019 Dec;20(6):5279-5285.

[1598] Liu PS, Chueh SH, Chen CC, et al. Lion's Mane Medicinal Mushroom, Hericium erinaceus (Agaricomycetes), Modulates Purinoceptor-Coupled Calcium Signaling and Murine Nociceptive Behavior. *Int J Med Mushrooms.* 2017;19(6):499-507.

[1599] Lai PL, Naidu M, Sabaratnam V, et al. Neurotrophic properties of the Lion's mane medicinal mushroom, Hericium erinaceus (Higher Basidiomycetes) from Malaysia. *Int J Med Mushrooms.* 2013;15(6):539-54.

[1600] Jung JK, Kim SY, Lee MK. Neurotrophic isoindolinones from the fruiting bodies of Hericium erinaceus. *Bioorg Med Chem Lett.* 2021 Jan 1;31:127714.

[1601] Ratto D, Corana F, Mannucci B, et al. Hericium erinaceus Improves Recognition Memory and Induces Hippocampal and Cerebellar Neurogenesis in Frail Mice during Aging. *Nutrients.* 2019 Mar 27;11(4):715.

[1602] Ryu S, Kim HG, Kim JY, et al. Hericium erinaceus Extract Reduces Anxiety and Depressive Behaviors by Promoting Hippocampal Neurogenesis in the Adult Mouse Brain. *J Med Food.* 2018 Feb;21(2):174-180.

[1603] Phan CW, Lee GS, Hong SL, et al. Hericium erinaceus (Bull.: Fr) Pers. cultivated under tropical conditions: isolation of hericenones and demonstration of NGF-mediated neurite outgrowth in PC12 cells via MEK/ERK and PI3K-Akt signaling pathways. *Food Funct.* 2014 Dec;5(12):3160-9.

[1604] Zhang CC, Cao CY, Kubo M, et al. Chemical Constituents from Hericium erinaceus Promote Neuronal Survival and Potentiate Neurite Outgrowth via the TrkA/Erk1/2 Pathway. *Int J Mol Sci.* 2017 Jul 30;18(8):1659.

[1605] Zhang CC, Yin X, Cao CY, et al. Chemical constituents from Hericium erinaceus and their ability to stimulate NGF-mediated neurite outgrowth on PC12 cells. *Bioorg Med Chem Lett.* 2015 Nov 15;25(22):5078-82.

[1606] Mori K, Obara Y, Hirota M, et al. Nerve growth factor-inducing activity of Hericium erinaceus in 1321N1 human astrocytoma cells. *Biol Pharm Bull.* 2008 Sep;31(9):1727-32.

[1607] Zhang Y, Liu L, Bao L, et al. Three new cyathane diterpenes with neurotrophic activity from the liquid cultures of Hericium erinaceus. *J Antibiot (Tokyo).* 2018 Sep;71(9):818-821.

[1608] Samberkar S, Gandhi S, Naidu M, et al. Lion's Mane, Hericium erinaceus and Tiger Milk, Lignosus rhinocerotis (Higher Basidiomycetes) Medicinal Mushrooms Stimulate Neurite Outgrowth in Dissociated Cells of Brain, Spinal Cord, and Retina: An In Vitro Study. *Int J Med Mushrooms.* 2015;17(11):1047-54.

[1609] Raman J, Lakshmanan H, John PA, et al. Neurite outgrowth stimulatory effects of myco synthesized AuNPs from Hericium erinaceus (Bull.: Fr.) Pers. on pheochromocytoma (PC-12) cells. *Int J Nanomedicine.* 2015 Sep 18;10:5853-63.

[1610] Park YS, Lee HS, Won MH, et al. Effect of an exo-polysaccharide from the culture broth of Hericium erinaceus on enhancement of growth and differentiation of rat adrenal nerve cells. *Cytotechnology.* 2002 Sep;39(3):155-62.

[1611] Huang HT, Ho CH, Sung HY, et al. Hericium erinaceus mycelium and its small bioactive compounds promote oligodendrocyte maturation with an increase in myelin basic protein. *Sci Rep.* 2021 Mar 22;11(1):6551.

[1612] Kolotushkina EV, Moldavan MG, Voronin KY, et al. The influence of Hericium erinaceus extract on myelination process in vitro. *Fiziol Zh (1994).* 2003;49(1):38-45.

[1613] Wong KH, Naidu M, David RP, et al. Neuroregenerative potential of lion's mane mushroom, Hericium erinaceus (Bull.: Fr.) Pers. (higher Basidiomycetes), in the treatment of peripheral nerve injury (review). *Int J Med Mushrooms.* 2012;14(5):427-46.

[1614] Wong KH, Kanagasabapathy G, Naidu M, et al. Hericium erinaceus (Bull.: Fr.) Pers., a medicinal mushroom, activates peripheral nerve regeneration. *Chin J Integr Med.* 2016 Oct;22(10):759-67.

[1615] Üstün R, Ayhan P. Regenerative activity of Hericium erinaceus on axonal injury model using in vitro laser microdissection technique. *Neurol Res.* 2019 Mar;41(3):265-274.

[1616] Wong KH, Naidu M, David P, et al. Peripheral Nerve Regeneration Following Crush Injury to Rat Peroneal Nerve by Aqueous Extract of Medicinal Mushroom Hericium erinaceus (Bull.: Fr) Pers. (Aphyllophoromycetideae). *Evid Based Complement Alternat Med.* 2011;2011:580752.

[1617] Lin CY, Chen YJ, Hsu CH, et al. Erinacine S from Hericium erinaceus mycelium promotes neuronal regeneration by inducing neurosteroids accumulation. *J Food Drug Anal.* 2023 Mar 15;31(1):32-54.

[1618] Kushairi N, Phan CW, Sabaratnam V, et al. Lion's Mane Mushroom, Hericium erinaceus (Bull.: Fr.) Pers. Suppresses H2O2-Induced Oxidative Damage and LPS-Induced Inflammation in HT22 Hippocampal Neurons and BV2 Microglia. *Antioxidants (Basel).* 2019 Aug 1;8(8):261.

[1619] Roda E, Priori EC, Ratto D, et al. Neuroprotective Metabolites of Hericium erinaceus Promote Neuro-Healthy Aging. *Int J Mol Sci.* 2021 Jun 15;22(12):6379.

[1620] Amara I, Scuto M, Zappalà A, et al. Hericium Erinaceus Prevents DEHP-Induced Mitochondrial Dysfunction and Apoptosis in PC12 Cells. *Int J Mol Sci.* 2020 Mar 20;21(6):2138.

[1621] Chong PS, Khairuddin S, Tse ACK, et al. Hericium erinaceus potentially rescues behavioural motor deficits through ERK-CREB-PSD95 neuroprotective mechanisms in rat model of 3-acetylpyridine-induced cerebellar ataxia. *Sci Rep.* 2020 Sep 10;10(1):14945.

[1622] Lew SY, Lim SH, Lim LW, et al. Neuroprotective effects of Hericium erinaceus (Bull.: Fr.) Pers. against high-dose corticosterone-induced oxidative stress in PC-12 cells. *BMC Complement Med Ther.* 2020 Nov 11;20(1):340.

[1623] Kuo HC, Lu CC, Shen CH, et al. Hericium erinaceus mycelium and its isolated erinacine A protection from MPTP-induced neurotoxicity through the ER stress, triggering an apoptosis cascade. *J Transl Med.* 2016 Mar 18;14:78.

[1624] Sun SK, Ho CY, Yen WY, et al. Effect of Water and Ethanol Extracts from Hericium erinaceus Solid-State Fermented Wheat Product on the Protection and Repair of Brain Cells in Zebrafish Embryos. *Molecules.* 2021 May 30;26(11):3297.

[1625] Cheng JH, Tsai CL, Lien YY, et al. High molecular weight of polysaccharides from Hericium erinaceus against amyloid beta-induced neurotoxicity. *BMC Complement Altern Med.* 2016 Jun 7;16:170.

[1626] Wu YL, Chen SC, Chang JC, et al. The protective effect of erinacine A-enriched Hericium erinaceus mycelium ethanol extract on oxidative Stress-Induced neurotoxicity in cell and Drosophila models of spinocerebellar ataxia type 3. *Free Radic Biol Med*. 2023 Feb 1;195:1-12.

[1627] Lee KF, Chen JH, Teng CC, et al. Protective effects of Hericium erinaceus mycelium and its isolated erinacine A against ischemia-injury-induced neuronal cell death via the inhibition of iNOS/p38 MAPK and nitrotyrosine. *Int J Mol Sci*. 2014 Aug 27;15(9):15073-89.

[1628] Zhang J, An S, Hu W, et al. The Neuroprotective Properties of Hericium erinaceus in Glutamate-Damaged Differentiated PC12 Cells and an Alzheimer's Disease Mouse Model. *Int J Mol Sci*. 2016 Nov 1;17(11):1810.

[1629] Liu Z, Wang Q, Cui J, et al. Systemic Screening of Strains of the Lion's Mane Medicinal Mushroom Hericium erinaceus (Higher Basidiomycetes) and Its Protective Effects on Aβ-Triggered Neurotoxicity in PC12 Cells. *Int J Med Mushrooms*. 2015;17(3):219-29.

[1630] Bailly C, Gao JM. Erinacine A and related cyathane diterpenoids: Molecular diversity and mechanisms underlying their neuroprotection and anticancer activities. *Pharmacol Res*. 2020 Sep;159:104953.

[1631] Vishwanath M, Chaudhary CL, Park Y, et al. Total Synthesis of Isohericerinol A and Its Analogues to Access Their Potential Neurotrophic Effects. *J Org Chem*. 2022 Aug 19;87(16):10836-10847.

[1632] Hsu PC, Lan YJ, Chen CC, et al. Erinacine A attenuates glutamate transporter 1 downregulation and protects against ischemic brain injury. *Life Sci*. 2022 Oct 1;306:120833.

[1633] Hsu CL, Wen YT, Hsu TC, et al. Neuroprotective Effects of Erinacine A on an Experimental Model of Traumatic Optic Neuropathy. *Int J Mol Sci*. 2023 Jan 12;24(2):1504.

[1634] Kobayashi S, Tamura T, Koshishiba M, et al. Total Synthesis, Structure Revision, and Neuroprotective Effect of Hericenones C-H and Their Derivatives. *J Org Chem*. 2021 Feb 5;86(3):2602-2620.

[1635] Tamrakar S, Wang D, Hiraki E, et al. Deacylated Derivative of Hericenone C Treated by Lipase Shows Enhanced Neuroprotective Properties Compared to Its Parent Compound. *Molecules*. 2023 Jun 5;28(11):4549.

[1636] Jang HJ, Kim JE, Jeong KH, et al. The Neuroprotective Effect of Hericium erinaceus Extracts in Mouse Hippocampus after Pilocarpine-Induced Status Epilepticus. *Int J Mol Sci*. 2019 Feb 16;20(4):859.

[1637] Sun SK, Ho CY, Yen WY, et al. Effect of Water and Ethanol Extracts from Hericium erinaceus Solid-State Fermented Wheat Product on the Protection and Repair of Brain Cells in Zebrafish Embryos. *Molecules*. 2021 May 30;26(11):3297.

[1638] Mori K, Obara Y, Moriya T, et al. Effects of Hericium erinaceus on amyloid β(25-35) peptide-induced learning and memory deficits in mice. *Biomed Res*. 2011 Feb;32(1):67-72.

[1639] Brandalise F, Cesaroni V, Gregori A, et al. Dietary Supplementation of Hericium erinaceus Increases Mossy Fiber-CA3 Hippocampal Neurotransmission and Recognition Memory in Wild-Type Mice. *Evid Based Complement Alternat Med*. 2017;2017:3864340.

[1640] Roda E, De Luca F, Ratto D, et al. Cognitive Healthy Aging in Mice: Boosting Memory by an Ergothioneine-Rich Hericium erinaceus Primordium Extract. *Biology (Basel)*. 2023 Jan 28;12(2):196.

[1641] Rossi P, Cesaroni V, Brandalise F, et al. Dietary Supplementation of Lion's Mane Medicinal Mushroom, Hericium erinaceus (Agaricomycetes), and Spatial Memory in Wild-Type Mice. *Int J Med Mushrooms*. 2018;20(5):485-494.

[1642] Martínez-Mármol R, Chai Y, Conroy JN, et al. Hericerin derivatives activates a pan-neurotrophic pathway in central hippocampal neurons converging to ERK1/2 signaling enhancing spatial memory. *J Neurochem*. 2023 Jun;165(6):791-808.

[1643] Li H, Zhao H, Liu W, et al. Liver and Brain Protective Effect of Sulfated Polysaccharides from Residue of Lion's Mane Medicinal Mushroom, Hericium erinaceus (Agaricomycetes), on D-Galactose-Induced Aging Mice. *Int J Med Mushrooms*. 2021;23(5):55-65.

[1644] Fijałkowska A, Rychlik M, Krakowska A, et al. Effects of Dietary Supplementation with In Vitro-Cultivated Arboreal Medicinal Mushrooms on Long-Term Memory and Anxiety-Like Behavior of Male Mice. *Int J Med Mushrooms*. 2023;25(5):49-60.

[1645] Kushairi N, Phan CW, Sabaratnam V, et al. Lion's Mane Mushroom, Hericium erinaceus (Bull.: Fr.) Pers. Suppresses H2O2-Induced Oxidative Damage and LPS-Induced Inflammation in HT22 Hippocampal Neurons and BV2 Microglia. *Antioxidants (Basel)*. 2019 Aug 1;8(8):261.

[1646] Chau SC, Chong PS, Jin H, et al. Hericium erinaceus Promotes Anti-Inflammatory Effects and Regulation of Metabolites in an Animal Model of Cerebellar Ataxia. *Int J Mol Sci*. 2023 Mar 23;24(7):6089.

[1647] Wei J, Li JY, Feng XL, et al. Unprecedented Neoverrucosane and Cyathane Diterpenoids with Anti-Neuroinflammatory Activity from Cultures of the Culinary-Medicinal Mushroom Hericium erinaceus. *Molecules*. 2023 Aug 31;28(17):6380.

[1648] Zhang J, An S, Hu W, et al. The Neuroprotective Properties of Hericium erinaceus in Glutamate-Damaged Differentiated PC12 Cells and an Alzheimer's Disease Mouse Model. *Int J Mol Sci*. 2016 Nov 1;17(11):1810.

[1649] Lee SL, Hsu JY, Chen TC, et al. Erinacine A Prevents Lipopolysaccharide-Mediated Glial Cell Activation to Protect Dopaminergic Neurons against Inflammatory Factor-Induced Cell Death In Vitro and In Vivo. *Int J Mol Sci*. 2022 Jan 12;23(2):810.

[1650] Wang LY, Huang CS, Chen YH, et al. Anti-Inflammatory Effect of Erinacine C on NO Production Through Down-Regulation of NF-κB and Activation of Nrf2-Mediated HO-1 in BV2 Microglial Cells Treated with LPS. *Molecules*. 2019 Sep 12;24(18):3317.

[1651] Valu MV, Soare LC, Ducu C, et al. Hericium erinaceus (Bull.) Pers. Ethanolic Extract with Antioxidant Properties on Scopolamine-Induced Memory Deficits in a Zebrafish Model of Cognitive Impairment. *J Fungi (Basel)*. 2021 Jun 12;7(6):477.

[1652] Furuta S, Kuwahara R, Hiraki E, et al. Hericium erinaceus extracts alter behavioral rhythm in mice. *Biomed Res*. 2016;37(4):227-32.

[1653] Cordaro M, Salinaro AT, Siracusa R, et al. Key Mechanisms and Potential Implications of Hericium erinaceus in NLRP3 Inflammasome Activation by Reactive Oxygen Species during Alzheimer's Disease. *Antioxidants (Basel)*. 2021 Oct 22;10(11):1664.

[1654] Tsai-Teng T, Chin-Chu C, Li-Ya L, et al. Erinacine A-enriched Hericium erinaceus mycelium ameliorates Alzheimer's disease-related pathologies in APPswe/PS1dE9 transgenic mice. *J Biomed Sci*. 2016 Jun 27;23(1):49.

[1655] Hu W, Song M, Wang C, et al. Structural characterization of polysaccharide purified from Hericium erinaceus fermented mycelium and its pharmacological basis for application in Alzheimer's disease: Oxidative stress related calcium homeostasis. *Int J Biol Macromol*. 2021 Dec 15;193(Pt A):358-369.

[1656] Tzeng TT, Chen CC, Chen CC, et al. The Cyanthin Diterpenoid and Sesterterpene Constituents of Hericium erinaceus Mycelium Ameliorate Alzheimer's Disease-Related Pathologies in APP/PS1 Transgenic Mice. *Int J Mol Sci*. 2018 Feb 17;19(2):598.

[1657] Diling C, Tianqiao Y, Jian Y, et al. Docking Studies and Biological Evaluation of a Potential β-Secretase Inhibitor of 3-Hydroxyhericenone F from Hericium erinaceus. *Front Pharmacol*. 2017 May 12;8:219.

[1658] Trovato A, Siracusa R, Di Paola R, et al. Redox modulation of cellular stress response and lipoxin A4 expression by Hericium Erinaceus in rat brain: relevance to Alzheimer's disease pathogenesis. *Immun Ageing*. 2016 Jul 9;13:23.

[1659] Furuta S, Kuwahara R, Hiraki E, et al. Hericium erinaceus extracts alter behavioral rhythm in mice. *Biomed Res*. 2016;37(4):227-32.

[1660] Lee LY, Chou W, Chen WP, et al. Erinacine A-Enriched Hericium erinaceus Mycelium Delays Progression of Age-Related Cognitive Decline in Senescence Accelerated Mouse Prone 8 (SAMP8) Mice. *Nutrients*. 2021 Oct 19;13(10):3659.

[1661] Cuzzocrea S, Di Paola R, Siracusa R, et al. Hericium erinaceus and Coriolus versicolor Modulate Molecular and Biochemical Changes after Traumatic Brain Injury. *Antioxidants (Basel)*. 2021 Jun 2;10(6):898.

[1662] Cordaro M, Modafferi S, D'Amico R, et al. Natural Compounds Such as Hericium erinaceus and Coriolus versicolor Modulate Neuroinflammation, Oxidative Stress and Lipoxin A4 Expression in Rotenone-Induced Parkinson's Disease in Mice. *Biomedicines*. 2022 Oct 7;10(10):2505.

[1663] Lee KF, Tung SY, Teng CC, et al. Post-Treatment with Erinacine A, a Derived Diterpenoid of H. erinaceus, Attenuates Neurotoxicity in MPTP Model of Parkinson's Disease. *Antioxidants (Basel)*. 2020 Feb 4;9(2):137.

[1664] Chong PS, Poon CH, Roy J, et al. Neurogenesis-dependent antidepressant-like activity of Hericium erinaceus in an animal model of depression. *Chin Med*. 2021 Dec 7;16(1):132.

[1665] Anuar AM, Minami A, Matsushita H, et al. Ameliorating Effect of the Edible Mushroom Hericium erinaceus on Depressive-Like Behavior in Ovariectomized Rats. *Biol Pharm Bull*. 2022;45(10):1438-1443.

[1666] Ryu S, Kim HG, Kim JY, et al. Hericium erinaceus Extract Reduces Anxiety and Depressive Behaviors by Promoting Hippocampal Neurogenesis in the Adult Mouse Brain. *J Med Food*. 2018 Feb;21(2):174-180.

[1667] Chiu CH, Chyau CC, Chen CC, et al. Erinacine A-Enriched Hericium erinaceus Mycelium Produces Antidepressant-Like Effects through Modulating BDNF/PI3K/Akt/GSK-3β Signaling in Mice. *Int J Mol Sci*. 2018 Jan 24;19(2):341.

[1668] Rodriguez MN, Lippi SLP. Lion's Mane (Hericium erinaceus) Exerts Anxiolytic Effects in the rTg4510 Tau Mouse Model. *Behav Sci (Basel)*. 2022 Jul 15;12(7):235.

[1669] Ryu S, Kim HG, Kim JY, et al. Hericium erinaceus Extract Reduces Anxiety and Depressive Behaviors by Promoting Hippocampal Neurogenesis in the Adult Mouse Brain. *J Med Food*. 2018 Feb;21(2):174-180.

[1670] Li TJ, Lee TY, Lo Y, et al. Hericium erinaceus mycelium ameliorate anxiety induced by continuous sleep disturbance in vivo. *BMC Complement Med Ther*. 2021 Dec 5;21(1):295.

[1671] Ren Z, Xu Z, Amakye WK, et al. Hericium erinaceus mycelium-Derived Polysaccharide Alleviates Ulcerative Colitis and Modulates Gut Microbiota in Cynomolgus Monkeys. *Mol Nutr Food Res*. 2023 Feb;67(3):e2200450.

[1672] Tian B, Geng Y, Xu T, et al. Digestive Characteristics of Hericium erinaceus Polysaccharides and Their Positive Effects on Fecal Microbiota of Male and Female Volunteers During in vitro Fermentation. *Front Nutr*. 2022 Mar 31;9:858585.

[1673] Cho HW, Choi S, Seo K, et al. Gut microbiota profiling in aged dogs after feeding pet food contained Hericium erinaceus. *J Anim Sci Technol*. 2022 Sep;64(5):937-949.

[1674] Tian B, Liu R, Xu T, et al. Modulating effects of Hericium erinaceus polysaccharides on the immune response by regulating gut microbiota in cyclophosphamide-treated mice. *J Sci Food Agric*. 2023 Apr;103(6):3050-3064.

[1675] Yang Y, Ye H, Zhao C, et al. Value added immunoregulatory polysaccharides of Hericium erinaceus and their effect on the gut microbiota. *Carbohydr Polym*. 2021 Jun 15;262:117668.

[1676] Yang Y, Zhao C, Diao M, et al. The Prebiotic Activity of Simulated Gastric and Intestinal Digesta of Polysaccharides from the Hericium erinaceus. *Molecules*. 2018 Nov 30;23(12):3158.

[1677] Wang XY, Yin JY, Nie SP, et al. Isolation, purification and physicochemical properties of polysaccharide from fruiting body of Hericium erinaceus and its effect on colonic health of mice. *Int J Biol Macromol*. 2018 Feb;107(Pt A):1310-1319.

[1678] Mitsou EK, Saxami G, Stamoulou E, et al. Effects of Rich in B-Glucans Edible Mushrooms on Aging Gut Microbiota Characteristics: An In Vitro Study. *Molecules*. 2020 Jun 18;25(12):2806.

[1679] Tian B, Wang P, Xu T, et al. Ameliorating effects of Hericium erinaceus polysaccharides on intestinal barrier injury in immunocompromised mice induced by cyclophosphamide. *Food Funct*. 2023 Mar 20;14(6):2921-2932.

[1680] Su Y, Cheng S, Ding Y, et al. A comparison of study on intestinal barrier protection of polysaccharides from Hericium erinaceus before and after fermentation. *Int J Biol Macromol*. 2023 Apr 1;233:123558.

[1681] Wu Y, Jiang H, Zhu E, et al. Hericium erinaceus polysaccharide facilitates restoration of injured intestinal mucosal immunity in Muscovy duck reovirus-infected Muscovy ducklings. *Int J Biol Macromol*. 2018 Feb;107(Pt A):1151-1161.

[1682] Liu Z, Li M, Yan P, et al. Transcriptome analysis of the effects of Hericium erinaceus polysaccharide on the lymphocyte homing in Muscovy duck reovirus-infected ducklings. *Int J Biol Macromol*. 2019 Nov 1;140:697-708.

[1683] Wang XY, Wang M, Yin JY, et al. Gastroprotective activity of polysaccharide from the fruiting body of Hericium erinaceus against acetic acid-induced gastric ulcer in rats and structure of one bioactive fraction. *Int J Biol Macromol*. 2022 Jun 15;210:455-464.

[1684] Zhu Y, Chen Y, Li Q, et al. Preparation, characterization, and anti-Helicobacter pylori activity of Bi3+-Hericium erinaceus polysaccharide complex. *Carbohydr Polym*. 2014 Sep 22;110:231-7.

[1685] Liu JH, Li L, Shang XD, et al. Anti-Helicobacter pylori activity of bioactive components isolated from Hericium erinaceus. *J Ethnopharmacol*. 2016 May 13;183:54-58.

[1686] Wang G, Zhang X, Maier SE, et al. In Vitro and In Vivo Inhibition of Helicobacter pylori by Ethanolic Extracts of Lion's Mane Medicinal Mushroom, Hericium erinaceus (Agaricomycetes). *Int J Med Mushrooms*. 2019;21(1):1-11.

[1687] Wang M, Kanako N, Zhang Y, et al. A unique polysaccharide purified from Hericium erinaceus mycelium prevents oxidative stress induced by H2O2 in human gastric mucosa epithelium cell. *PLoS One*. 2017 Jul 24;12(7):e0181546.

[1688] Liao B, Zhou C, Liu T, et al. A novel Hericium erinaceus polysaccharide: Structural characterization and prevention of H2O2-induced oxidative damage in GES-1 cells. *Int J Biol Macromol*. 2020 Jul 1;154:1460-1470.

[1689] Wang M, Konishi T, Gao Y, et al. Anti-Gastric Ulcer Activity of Polysaccharide Fraction Isolated from Mycelium Culture of Lion's Mane Medicinal Mushroom, Hericium erinaceus (Higher Basidiomycetes). *Int J Med Mushrooms*. 2015;17(11):1055-60.

[1690] Mao X, Lu ZM, Gong TT, et al. Therapeutic Effect and Potential Mechanisms of Lion's Mane Medicinal Mushroom, Hericium erinaceus (Agaricomycetes), Mycelia in Submerged Culture on Ethanol-Induced Chronic Gastric Injury. *Int J Med Mushrooms*. 2019;21(11):1137-1150.

[1691] Shang X, Tan Q, Liu R, et al. In vitro anti-Helicobacter pylori effects of medicinal mushroom extracts, with special emphasis on the Lion's Mane mushroom, Hericium erinaceus (higher Basidiomycetes). *Int J Med Mushrooms*. 2013;15(2):165-74.

[1692] Cui M, Ma Q, Zhang Z, et al. Semi-solid enzymolysis enhanced the protective effects of fruiting body powders and polysaccharides of Herinaceus erinaceus on gastric mucosal injury. *Int J Biol Macromol*. 2023 Aug 16;251:126388.

[1693] Hou C, Liu L, Ren J, et al. Structural characterization of two Hericium erinaceus polysaccharides and their protective effects on the alcohol-induced gastric mucosal injury. *Food Chem*. 2022 May 1;375:131896.

[1694] Chen W, Wu D, Jin Y, et al. Pre-protective effect of polysaccharides purified from Hericium erinaceus against ethanol-induced gastric mucosal injury in rats. *Int J Biol Macromol*. 2020 Sep 15;159:948-956.

[1695] Wang XY, Yin JY, Zhao MM, et al. Gastroprotective activity of polysaccharide from Hericium erinaceus against ethanol-induced gastric mucosal lesion and pylorus ligation-induced gastric ulcer, and its antioxidant activities. *Carbohydr Polym*. 2018 Apr 15;186:100-109.

[1696] Wong JY, Abdulla MA, Raman J, et al. Gastroprotective Effects of Lion's Mane Mushroom Hericium erinaceus (Bull.:Fr.) Pers. (Aphyllophoromycetideae) Extract against Ethanol-Induced Ulcer in Rats. *Evid Based Complement Alternat Med*. 2013;2013:492976.

[1697] Wang D, Xu D, Zhang Y, et al. A novel oligosaccharide isolated from Hericium erinaceus and its protection against LPS-induced Caco-2 cells via the TLR4/NF-κB pathway. *J Food Biochem*. 2020 Mar;44(3):e13135.

[1698] Qin T, Liu X, Luo Y, et al. Characterization of polysaccharides isolated from Hericium erinaceus and their protective effects on the DON-induced oxidative stress. *Int J Biol Macromol*. 2020 Jun 1;152:1265-1273.

[1699] Wang M, Gao Y, Xu D, et al. A polysaccharide from cultured mycelium of Hericium erinaceus and its anti-chronic atrophic gastritis activity. *Int J Biol Macromol*. 2015 Nov;81:656-61.

[1700] Ren Z, Xu Z, Amakye WK, et al. Hericium erinaceus mycelium-Derived Polysaccharide Alleviates Ulcerative Colitis and Modulates Gut Microbiota in Cynomolgus Monkeys. *Mol Nutr Food Res*. 2023 Feb;67(3):e2200450.

[1701] Ren Y, Sun Q, Gao R, et al. Low Weight Polysaccharide of Hericium erinaceus Ameliorates Colitis via Inhibiting the NLRP3 Inflammasome Activation in Association with Gut Microbiota Modulation. *Nutrients*. 2023 Feb 1;15(3):739.

[1702] Ren Y, Geng Y, Du Y, et al. Polysaccharide of Hericium erinaceus attenuates colitis in C57BL/6 mice via regulation of oxidative stress, inflammation-related signaling pathways and modulating the composition of the gut microbiota. *J Nutr Biochem*. 2018 Jul;57:67-76.

[1703] Shao S, Wang D, Zheng W, et al. A unique polysaccharide from Hericium erinaceus mycelium ameliorates acetic acid-induced ulcerative colitis rats by modulating the composition of the gut microbiota, short chain fatty acids levels and GPR41/43 receptors. *Int Immunopharmacol*. 2019 Jun;71:411-422.

[1704] Wang D, Zhang Y, Yang S, et al. A polysaccharide from cultured mycelium of Hericium erinaceus relieves ulcerative colitis by counteracting oxidative stress and improving mitochondrial function. *Int J Biol Macromol*. 2019 Mar 15;125:572-579.

[1705] Qin M, Geng Y, Lu Z, et al. Anti-Inflammatory Effects of Ethanol Extract of Lion's Mane Medicinal Mushroom, Hericium erinaceus (Agaricomycetes), in Mice with Ulcerative Colitis. *Int J Med Mushrooms*. 2016;18(3):227-34.

[1706] Diling C, Xin Y, Chaoqun Z, et al. Extracts from Hericium erinaceus relieve inflammatory bowel disease by regulating immunity and gut microbiota. *Oncotarget*. 2017 Sep 6;8(49):85838-85857.

[1707] Wang D, Xu D, Zhao D, et al. Screening and Comparison of Anti-Intestinal Inflammatory Activities of Three Polysaccharides from the Mycelium of Lion's Mane Culinary-Medicinal Mushroom, Hericium erinaceus (Agaricomycetes). *Int J Med Mushrooms*. 2021;23(9):63-71.

[1708] Tripodi F, Falletta E, Leri M, et al. Anti-Aging and Neuroprotective Properties of Grifola frondosa and Hericium erinaceus Extracts. *Nutrients*. 2022 Oct 18;14(20):4368.

[1709] Li IC, Lee LY, Chen YJ, et al. Erinacine A-enriched Hericium erinaceus mycelia promotes longevity in Drosophila melanogaster and aged mice. *PLoS One*. 2019 May 17;14(5):e0217226.

[1710] Roda E, Ratto D, De Luca F, et al. Searching for a Longevity Food, We Bump into Hericium erinaceus Primordium Rich in Ergothioneine: The "Longevity Vitamin" Improves Locomotor Performances during Aging. *Nutrients*. 2022 Mar 11;14(6):1177.

[1711] Kim SP, Moon E, Nam SH, et al. Hericium erinaceus mushroom extracts protect infected mice against Salmonella Typhimurium-Induced liver damage and mortality by stimulation of innate immune cells. *J Agric Food Chem*. 2012 Jun 6;60(22):5590-6.

[1712] Li H, Zhao H, Liu W, et al. Liver and Brain Protective Effect of Sulfated Polysaccharides from Residue of Lion's Mane Medicinal Mushroom, Hericium erinaceus (Agaricomycetes), on D-Galactose-Induced Aging Mice. *Int J Med Mushrooms*. 2021;23(5):55-65.

[1713] Cui F, Gao X, Zhang J, et al. Protective Effects of Extracellular and Intracellular Polysaccharides on Hepatotoxicity by Hericium erinaceus SG-02. *Curr Microbiol*. 2016 Sep;73(3):379-385.

[1714] Zhang Z, Lv G, Pan H, et al. Antioxidant and hepatoprotective potential of endo-polysaccharides from Hericium erinaceus grown on tofu whey. *Int J Biol Macromol*. 2012 Dec;51(5):1140-6.

[1715] Hao L, Xie Y, Wu G, et al. Protective Effect of Hericium erinaceus on Alcohol Induced Hepatotoxicity in Mice. *Evid Based Complement Alternat Med*. 2015;2015:418023.

[1716] Yang SY, Fang CJ, Chen YW, et al. Hericium erinaceus Mycelium Ameliorates In Vivo Progression of Osteoarthritis. *Nutrients*. 2022 Jun 23;14(13):2605.

[1717] Xie G, Tang L, Xie Y, et al. Secondary Metabolites from Hericium erinaceus and Their Anti-Inflammatory Activities. *Molecules*. 2022 Mar 27;27(7):2157.

[1718] Tada H, Kawahara K, Osawa H, et al. Hericium erinaceus ethanol extract and ergosterol exert anti-inflammatory activities by neutralizing lipopolysaccharide-induced pro-inflammatory cytokine production in human monocytes. *Biochem Biophys Res Commun*. 2022 Dec 25;636(Pt 2):1-9.

[1719] Kim YO, Lee SW, Oh CH, et al. Hericium erinaceus suppresses LPS-induced pro-inflammation gene activation in RAW264.7 macrophages. *Immunopharmacol Immunotoxicol*. 2012 Jun;34(3):504-12.

[1720] Geng Y, Zhu S, Lu Z, et al. Anti-inflammatory activity of mycelial extracts from medicinal mushrooms. *Int J Med Mushrooms*. 2014;16(4):319-25.

[1721] Yang Y, Li J, Hong Q, et al. Polysaccharides from Hericium erinaceus Fruiting Bodies: Structural Characterization, Immunomodulatory Activity and Mechanism. *Nutrients*. 2022 Sep 9;14(18):3721.

[1722] Han Y, Huang J, Zhao C, et al. Hericium erinaceus polysaccharide improves the microstructure, immune function, proliferation and reduces apoptosis of thymus and spleen tissue cells of immunosuppressed mice. *Biosci Biotechnol Biochem*. 2023 Feb 24;87(3):279-289.

[1723] Liu Z, Liao L, Chen Q, et al. Effects of Hericium erinaceus polysaccharide on immunity and apoptosis of the main immune organs in Muscovy duck reovirus-infected ducklings. *Int J Biol Macromol*. 2021 Feb 28;171:448-456.

[1724] Yang Y, Ye H, Zhao C, et al. Value added immunoregulatory polysaccharides of Hericium erinaceus and their effect on the gut microbiota. *Carbohydr Polym*. 2021 Jun 15;262:117668.

[1725] Liu X, Ren Z, Yu R, et al. Structural characterization of enzymatic modification of Hericium erinaceus polysaccharide and its immune-enhancement activity. *Int J Biol Macromol*. 2021 Jan 1;166:1396-1408.

[1726] Yu Y, Hu Q, Liu J, et al. Isolation, purification and identification of immunologically active peptides from Hericium erinaceus. *Food Chem Toxicol*. 2021 May;151:112111.

[1727] Ren Z, Qin T, Qiu F, et al. Immunomodulatory effects of hydroxyethylated Hericium erinaceus polysaccharide on macrophages RAW264.7. *Int J Biol Macromol*. 2017 Dec;105(Pt 1):879-885.

[1728] Wu F, Huang H. Surface morphology and protective effect of Hericium erinaceus polysaccharide on cyclophosphamide-induced immunosuppression in mice. *Carbohydr Polym*. 2021 Jan 1;251:116930.

[1729] Ren Z, Luo Y, Meng Z, et al. Multi-walled carbon nanotube polysaccharide modified Hericium erinaceus polysaccharide as an adjuvant to extend immune responses. *Int J Biol Macromol*. 2021 Jul 1;182:574-582.

[1730] Sheng X, Yan J, Meng Y, et al. Immunomodulatory effects of Hericium erinaceus derived polysaccharides are mediated by intestinal immunology. *Food Funct*. 2017 Mar 22;8(3):1020-1027.

[1731] Yu R, Sun M, Meng Z, et al. Immunomodulatory effects of polysaccharides enzymatic hydrolysis from Hericium erinaceus on the MODE-K/DCs co-culture model. *Int J Biol Macromol*. 2021 Sep 30;187:272-280.

[1732] Zhu L, Wu D, Zhang H, et al. Effects of Atmospheric and Room Temperature Plasma (ARTP) Mutagenesis on Physicochemical Characteristics and Immune Activity In Vitro of Hericium erinaceus Polysaccharides. *Molecules*. 2019 Jan 11;24(2):262.

[1733] Wu D, Tang C, Liu Y, et al. Structural elucidation and immunomodulatory activity of a β-D-glucan prepared by freeze-thawing from Hericium erinaceus. *Carbohydr Polym*. 2019 Oct 15;222:114996.

[1734] Wu D, Yang S, Tang C, et al. Structural Properties and Macrophage Activation of Cell Wall Polysaccharides from the Fruiting Bodies of Hericium erinaceus. *Polymers (Basel)*. 2018 Aug 1;10(8):850.

[1735] Diling C, Chaoqun Z, Jian Y, et al. Immunomodulatory Activities of a Fungal Protein Extracted from Hericium erinaceus through Regulating the Gut Microbiota. *Front Immunol*. 2017 Jun 12;8:666.

[1736] Wu F, Zhou C, Zhou D, et al. Structure characterization of a novel polysaccharide from Hericium erinaceus fruiting bodies and its immunomodulatory activities. *Food Funct*. 2018 Jan 24;9(1):294-306.

[1737] Li QZ, Wu D, Chen X, et al. Chemical Compositions and Macrophage Activation of Polysaccharides from Leon's Mane Culinary-Medicinal Mushroom Hericium erinaceus (Higher Basidiomycetes) in Different Maturation Stages. *Int J Med Mushrooms*. 2015;17(5):443-52.

[1738] Lee JS, Min KM, Cho JY, et al. Study of macrophage activation and structural characteristics of purified polysaccharides from the fruiting body of Hericium erinaceus. *J Microbiol Biotechnol*. 2009 Sep;19(9):951-9.

[1739] Xu HM, Xie ZH, Zhang WY. [Immunomodulatory function of polysaccharide of Hericium erinaceus]. *Zhongguo Zhong Xi Yi Jie He Za Zhi*. 1994 Jul;14(7):427-8.

[1740] Wang JC, Hu SH, Su CH, et al. Antitumor and immunoenhancing activities of polysaccharide from culture broth of Hericium spp. *Kaohsiung J Med Sci*. 2001 Sep;17(9):461-7.

[1741] Tian B, Wang P, Xu T, et al. Ameliorating effects of Hericium erinaceus polysaccharides on intestinal barrier injury in immunocompromised mice induced by cyclophosphamide. *Food Funct*. 2023 Mar 20;14(6):2921-2932.

[1742] Ma B, Feng T, Zhang S, et al. The Inhibitory Effects of Hericium erinaceus β-glucan on in vitro Starch Digestion. Front Nutr. 2021 Jan 21;7:621131.

[1743] Cui W, Song X, Li X, et al. Structural characterization of Hericium erinaceus polysaccharides and the mechanism of anti-T2DM by modulating the gut microbiota and metabolites. *Int J Biol Macromol*. 2023 Jul 1;242(Pt 4):125165.

[1744] Chen B, Han J, Bao L, et al. Identification and α-Glucosidase Inhibitory Activity of Meroterpenoids from Hericium erinaceus. *Planta Med*. 2020 May;86(8):571-578.

[1745] Lee SK, Ryu SH, Turk A, et al. Characterization of α-glucosidase inhibitory constituents of the fruiting body of lion's mane mushroom (Hericium erinaceus). *J Ethnopharmacol*. 2020 Nov 15;262:113197.

[1746] Yan JK, Ding ZC, Gao X, et al. Comparative study of physicochemical properties and bioactivity of Hericium erinaceus polysaccharides at different solvent extractions. *Carbohydr Polym*. 2018 Aug 1;193:373-382.

[1747] Yao F, Gao H, Yin CM, et al. Evaluation of In Vitro Antioxidant and Antihyperglycemic Activities of Extracts from the Lion's Mane Medicinal Mushroom, Hericium erinaceus (Agaricomycetes). *Int J Med Mushrooms*. 2021;23(3):55-66.

[1748] Liang B, Guo Z, Xie F, et al. Antihyperglycemic and antihyperlipidemic activities of aqueous extract of Hericium erinaceus in experimental diabetic rats. *BMC Complement Altern Med*. 2013 Oct 3;13:253.

[1749] Wang K, Bao L, Qi Q, et al. Erinacerins C-L, isoindolin-1-ones with α-glucosidase inhibitory activity from cultures of the medicinal mushroom Hericium erinaceus. *J Nat Prod.* 2015 Jan 23;78(1):146-54.

[1750] Zhang C, Li J, Hu C, et al. Antihyperglycaemic and organic protective effects on pancreas, liver and kidney by polysaccharides from Hericium erinaceus SG-02 in streptozotocin-induced diabetic mice. *Sci Rep.* 2017 Sep 7;7(1):10847.

[1751] Tsai YC, Lin YC, Huang CC, et al. Hericium erinaceus Mycelium and Its Isolated Compound, Erinacine A, Ameliorate High-Fat High-Sucrose Diet-Induced Metabolic Dysfunction and Spatial Learning Deficits in Aging Mice. *J Med Food.* 2019 May;22(5):469-478.

[1752] Yi Z, Shao-Long Y, Ai-Hong W, et al. Protective Effect of Ethanol Extracts of Hericium erinaceus on Alloxan-Induced Diabetic Neuropathic Pain in Rats. *Evid Based Complement Alternat Med.* 2015;2015:595480.

[1753] Zhang C, Li J, Hu C, et al. Antihyperglycaemic and organic protective effects on pancreas, liver and kidney by polysaccharides from Hericium erinaceus SG-02 in streptozotocin-induced diabetic mice. *Sci Rep.* 2017 Sep 7;7(1):10847.

[1754] Hiwatashi K, Kosaka Y, Suzuki N, et al. Yamabushitake mushroom (Hericium erinaceus) improved lipid metabolism in mice fed a high-fat diet. *Biosci Biotechnol Biochem.* 2010;74(7):1447-51.

[1755] Liang B, Guo Z, Xie F, et al. Antihyperglycemic and antihyperlipidemic activities of aqueous extract of Hericium erinaceus in experimental diabetic rats. *BMC Complement Altern Med.* 2013 Oct 3;13:253.

[1756] Yang BK, Park JB, Song CH. Hypolipidemic effect of an Exo-biopolymer produced from a submerged mycelial culture of Hericium erinaceus. *Biosci Biotechnol Biochem.* 2003 Jun;67(6):1292-8.

[1757] Rahman MA, Abdullah N, Aminudin N. Inhibitory effect on in vitro LDL oxidation and HMG Co-A reductase activity of the liquid-liquid partitioned fractions of Hericium erinaceus (Bull.) Persoon (lion's mane mushroom). *Biomed Res Int.* 2014;2014:828149.

[1758] Hiraki E, Furuta S, Kuwahara R, et al. Anti-obesity activity of Yamabushitake (Hericium erinaceus) powder in ovariectomized mice, and its potentially active compounds. *J Nat Med.* 2017 Jul;71(3):482-491.

[1759] Mori K, Ouchi K, Hirasawa N. et al. The Anti-Inflammatory Effects of Lion's Mane Culinary-Medicinal Mushroom, Hericium erinaceus (Higher Basidiomycetes) in a Coculture System of 3T3-L1 Adipocytes and RAW264 Macrophages. *Int J Med Mushrooms.* 2015;17(7):609-18.

[1760] Mori K, Kikuchi H, Obara Y, et al. Inhibitory effect of hericenone B from Hericium erinaceus on collagen-induced platelet aggregation. *Phytomedicine.* 2010 Dec 1;17(14):1082-5.

[1761] Liu J, DU C, Wang Y, et al. Anti-fatigue activities of polysaccharides extracted from Hericium erinaceus. *Exp Ther Med.* 2015 Feb;9(2):483-487.

[1762] Komiya Y, Nakamura T, Ishii M, et al. Increase in muscle endurance in mice by dietary Yamabushitake mushroom (Hericium erinaceus) possibly via activation of PPARδ. *Anim Sci J.* 2019 Jun;90(6):781-789.

[1763] Choi J, Song E, Gwon H, et al. Aqueous Extracts of Pleurotus ostreatus and Hericium erinaceus Protect against Ultraviolet A-Induced Damage in Human Dermal Fibroblasts. *Int J Med Mushrooms.* 2022;24(2):63-74.

[1764] Abdulla MA, Fard AA, Sabaratnam V, et al. Potential activity of aqueous extract of culinary-medicinal Lion's Mane mushroom, Hericium erinaceus (Bull.: Fr.) Pers. (Aphyllophoromycetideae) in accelerating wound healing in rats. *Int J Med Mushrooms.* 2011;13(1):33-9.

[1765] Ellan K, Thayan R, Phan CW, et al. Anti-inflammatory effect of mushrooms in dengue-infected human monocytes. *Trop Biomed.* 2019 Dec 1;36(4):1087-1098.

[1766] Ellan K, Thayan R, Raman J, et al. Anti-viral activity of culinary and medicinal mushroom extracts against dengue virus serotype 2: an in-vitro study. *BMC Complement Altern Med.* 2019 Sep 18;19(1):260.

[1767] Ghosh S, Nandi S, Banerjee A, et al. Prospecting medicinal properties of Lion's mane mushroom. *J Food Biochem.* 2021 Jun 24:e13833.

[1768] Darmasiwi S, Aramsirirujiwet Y, Kimkong I. Antibiofilm activity and bioactive phenolic compounds of ethanol extract from the Hericium erinaceus basidiome. *J Adv Pharm Technol Res.* 2022 Apr-Jun;13(2):111-116.

[1769] Qian Z, Mengxun Z, Yingchao W, et al. Natural Compound 2-Chloro-1,3-dimethoxy-5-methylbenzene, Isolated from Hericium Erinaceus, Inhibits Fungal Growth by Disrupting Membranes and Triggering Apoptosis. *J Agric Food Chem.* 2022 Jun 1;70(21):6444-6454.

[1770] Shen T, Morlock G, Zorn H. Production of cyathane type secondary metabolites by submerged cultures of Hericium erinaceus and evaluation of their antibacterial activity by direct bioautography. *Fungal Biol Biotechnol.* 2015 Dec 22;2:8.

[1771] Ghosh S, Nandi S, Banerjee A, et al. Prospecting medicinal properties of Lion's mane mushroom. *J Food Biochem.* 2021 Jun 24:e13833.

[1772] Tu JQ, Liu HP, Wen YH, et al. A novel polysaccharide from Hericium erinaceus: Preparation, structural characteristics, thermal stabilities, and antioxidant activities in vitro. *J Food Biochem.* 2021 Sep;45(9):e13871.

[1773] Hsu CH, Liao EC, Chiang WC, et al. Antioxidative Activities of Micronized Solid-State Cultivated Hericium erinaceus Rich in Erinacine A against MPTP-Induced Damages. *Molecules.* 2023 Apr 12;28(8):3386.

[1774] Jiang S, Wang Y, Zhang X. Comparative studies on extracts from Hericium erinaceus by different polarity reagents to gain higher antioxidant activities. *Exp Ther Med.* 2016 Jul;12(1):513-517.

[1775] Valu MV, Soare LC, Sutan NA, et al. Optimization of Ultrasonic Extraction to Obtain Erinacine A and Polyphenols with Antioxidant Activity from the Fungal Biomass of Hericium erinaceus. *Foods.* 2020 Dec 18;9(12):1889.

[1776] Yan JK, Ding ZC, Gao X, et al. Comparative study of physicochemical properties and bioactivity of Hericium erinaceus polysaccharides at different solvent extractions. *Carbohydr Polym.* 2018 Aug 1;193:373-382.

[1777] Gao Y, Zheng W, Wang M, et al. Molecular properties, structure, and antioxidant activities of the oligosaccharide Hep-2 isolated from cultured mycelium of Hericium erinaceus. *J Food Biochem.* 2019 Sep;43(9):e12985.

[1778] Hou Y, Ding X, Hou W. Composition and antioxidant activity of water-soluble oligosaccharides from Hericium erinaceus. *Mol Med Rep.* 2015 May;11(5):3794-9.

[1779] Ghosh S, Chakraborty N, Banerjee A, et al. Mycochemical Profiling and Antioxidant Activity of Two Different Tea Preparations from Lion's Mane Medicinal Mushroom, Hericium erinaceus (Agaricomycetes). *Int J Med Mushrooms.* 2021;23(11):59-70.

[1780] Kim S. Antioxidant Compounds for the Inhibition of Enzymatic Browning by Polyphenol Oxidases in the Fruiting Body Extract of the Edible Mushroom Hericium erinaceus. *Foods*. 2020 Jul 17;9(7):951.

[1781] Han ZH, Ye JM, Wang GF. Evaluation of in vivo antioxidant activity of Hericium erinaceus polysaccharides. *Int J Biol Macromol*. 2013 Jan;52:66-71.

[1782] Yao F, Gao H, Yin CM, et al. Evaluation of In Vitro Antioxidant and Antihyperglycemic Activities of Extracts from the Lion's Mane Medicinal Mushroom, Hericium erinaceus (Agaricomycetes). *Int J Med Mushrooms*. 2021;23(3):55-66.

[1783] Zhang Z, Lv G, Pan H, et al. Antioxidant and hepatoprotective potential of endo-polysaccharides from Hericium erinaceus grown on tofu whey. *Int J Biol Macromol*. 2012 Dec;51(5):1140-6.

[1784] Jiang S, Liu S, Qin M. Effects of Extraction Conditions on Crude Polysaccharides and Antioxidant Activities of the Lion's Mane Medicinal Mushroom, Hericium erinaceus (Agaricomycetes). *Int J Med Mushrooms*. 2019;21(10):1007-1018.

[1785] Abdullah N, Ismail SM, Aminudin N, et al. Evaluation of Selected Culinary-Medicinal Mushrooms for Antioxidant and ACE Inhibitory Activities. *Evid Based Complement Alternat Med*. 2012;2012:464238.

[1786] Di Paola D, Iaria C, Capparucci F, et al. Aflatoxin B1 Toxicity in Zebrafish Larva (Danio rerio): Protective Role of Hericium erinaceus. *Toxins (Basel)*. 2021 Oct 8;13(10):710.

[1787] Wang JC, Hu SH, Lee WL, et al. Antimutagenicity of extracts of Hericium erinaceus. *Kaohsiung J Med Sci*. 2001 May;17(5):230-8.

[1788] Saitsu Y, Nishide A, Kikushima K, et al. Improvement of cognitive functions by oral intake of Hericium erinaceus. *Biomed Res*. 2019;40(4):125-131.

[1789] Mori K, Inatomi S, Ouchi K, et al. Improving effects of the mushroom Yamabushitake (Hericium erinaceus) on mild cognitive impairment: a double-blind placebo-controlled clinical trial. *Phytother Res*. 2009 Mar;23(3):367-72.

[1790] Li IC, Chang HH, Lin CH, et al. Prevention of Early Alzheimer's Disease by Erinacine A-Enriched Hericium erinaceus Mycelia Pilot Double-Blind Placebo-Controlled Study. *Front Aging Neurosci*. 2020 Jun 3;12:155.

[1791] Nagano M, Shimizu K, Kondo R, et al. Reduction of depression and anxiety by 4 weeks Hericium erinaceus intake. *Biomed Res*. 2010 Aug;31(4):231-7.

[1792] Vigna L, Morelli F, Agnelli GM, et al. Hericium erinaceus Improves Mood and Sleep Disorders in Patients Affected by Overweight or Obesity: Could Circulating Pro-BDNF and BDNF Be Potential Biomarkers? *Evid Based Complement Alternat Med*. 2019 Apr 18;2019:7861297.

[1793] Okamura H, Anno N, Tsuda A, et al. The effects of Hericium erinaceus (Amyloban® 3399) on sleep quality and subjective well-being among female undergraduate students: A pilot study. *Pers Med Universe*. 2015;4:76–78.

[1794] Xie XQ, Geng Y, Guan Q, et al. Influence of Short-Term Consumption of Hericium erinaceus on Serum Biochemical Markers and the Changes of the Gut Microbiota: A Pilot Study. *Nutrients*. 2021 Mar 21;13(3):1008.

[1795] Xu CP, Liu WW, Liu FX, et al. A double-blind study of effectiveness of hericium erinaceus pers therapy on chronic atrophic gastritis. A preliminary report. *Chin Med J (Engl)*. 1985;98(6):455-6.

[1796] Zhang Y, Sun D, Meng Q, et al. [Corrigendum] Grifola frondosa polysaccharides induce breast cancer cell apoptosis via the mitochondrial-dependent apoptotic pathway. *Int J Mol Med*. 2022 Nov;50(5):136.

[1797] Zhang Y, Sun D, Meng Q, et al. Grifola frondosa polysaccharides induce breast cancer cell apoptosis via the mitochondrial-dependent apoptotic pathway. *Int J Mol Med*. 2017 Oct;40(4):1089-1095.

[1798] Alonso EN, Ferronato MJ, Gandini NA, et al. Antitumoral Effects of D-Fraction from Grifola Frondosa (Maitake) Mushroom in Breast Cancer. *Nutr Cancer*. 2017 Jan;69(1):29-43.

[1799] Cui FJ, Tao WY, Xu ZH, et al. Structural analysis of anti-tumor heteropolysaccharide GFPS1b from the cultured mycelia of Grifola frondosa GF9801. *Bioresour Technol*. 2007 Jan;98(2):395-401.

[1800] Alonso EN, Ferronato MJ, Fermento ME, et al. Antitumoral and antimetastatic activity of Maitake D-Fraction in triple-negative breast cancer cells. *Oncotarget*. 2018 May 4;9(34):23396-23412.

[1801] Roldan-Deamicis A, Alonso E, Brie B, et al. Maitake Pro4X has anti-cancer activity and prevents oncogenesis in BALBc mice. *Cancer Med*. 2016 Sep;5(9):2427-41.

[1802] Roda E, Luca F, Iorio CD, et al. Novel Medicinal Mushroom Blend as a Promising Supplement in Integrative Oncology: A Multi-Tiered Study using 4T1 Triple-Negative Mouse Breast Cancer Model. *Int J Mol Sci*. 2020 May 14;21(10):3479.

[1803] Bie N, Han L, Wang Y, et al. A polysaccharide from Grifola frondosa fruit body induces HT-29 cells apoptosis by PI3K/AKT-MAPKs and NF-κB-pathway. *Int J Biol Macromol*. 2020 Mar 15;147:79-88.

[1804] Zhao J, He R, Zhong H, et al. A cold-water extracted polysaccharide-protein complex from Grifola frondosa exhibited anti-tumor activity via TLR4-NF-κB signaling activation and gut microbiota modification in H22 tumor-bearing mice. *Int J Biol Macromol*. 2023 Jun 1;239:124291.

[1805] Zhao J, Liang K, Zhong H, et al. A cold-water polysaccharide-protein complex from Grifola frondosa exhibited antiproliferative activity via mitochondrial apoptotic and Fas/FasL pathways in HepG2 cells. *Int J Biol Macromol*. 2022 Oct 1;218:1021-1032.

[1806] Yu J, Liu C, Ji HY, et al. The caspases-dependent apoptosis of hepatoma cells induced by an acid-soluble polysaccharide from Grifola frondosa. *Int J Biol Macromol*. 2020 Sep 15;159:364-372.

[1807] Ji HY, Chen P, Yu J, et al. Effects of Heat Treatment on the Structural Characteristics and Antitumor Activity of Polysaccharides from Grifola frondosa. *Appl Biochem Biotechnol*. 2019 Jun;188(2):481-490.

[1808] Chen P, Liu HP, Ji HH, et al. A cold-water soluble polysaccharide isolated from Grifola frondosa induces the apoptosis of HepG2 cells through mitochondrial passway. *Int J Biol Macromol*. 2019 Mar 15;125:1232-1241.

[1809] Mao GH, Ren Y, Feng WW, et al. Antitumor and immunomodulatory activity of a water-soluble polysaccharide from Grifola frondosa. *Carbohydr Polym*. 2015 Dec 10;134:406-12.

[1810] Lin CH, Chang CY, Lee KR, et al. Cold-water extracts of Grifola frondosa and its purified active fraction inhibit hepatocellular carcinoma in vitro and in vivo. *Exp Biol Med (Maywood)*. 2016 Jul;241(13):1374-85.

[1811] Zhao F, Zhao J, Song L, et al. The induction of apoptosis and autophagy in human hepatoma SMMC-7721 cells by combined treatment with vitamin C and polysaccharides extracted from Grifola frondosa. *Apoptosis*. 2017 Nov;22(11):1461-1472.

[1812] Wang CL, Meng M, Liu SB, et al. A chemically sulfated polysaccharide from Grifola frondos induces HepG2 cell apoptosis by notch1-NF-κB pathway. *Carbohydr Polym*. 2013 Jun 5;95(1):282-7.

[1813] Lin JT, Liu WH. o-Orsellinaldehyde from the submerged culture of the edible mushroom Grifola frondosa exhibits selective cytotoxic effect against Hep 3B cells through apoptosis. *J Agric Food Chem*. 2006 Oct 4;54(20):7564-9.

[1814] Cui F, Zan X, Li Y, et al. Grifola frondosa Glycoprotein GFG-3a Arrests S phase, Alters Proteome, and Induces Apoptosis in Human Gastric Cancer Cells. *Nutr Cancer*. 2016;68(2):267-79.

[1815] Liu C, Ji HY, Wu P, et al. The preparation of a cold-water soluble polysaccharide from Grifola frondosa and its inhibitory effects on MKN-45 cells. *Glycoconj J*. 2020 Aug;37(4):413-422.

[1816] Shomori K, Yamamoto M, Arifuku I, et al. Antitumor effects of a water-soluble extract from Maitake (Grifola frondosa) on human gastric cancer cell lines. *Oncol Rep*. 2009 Sep;22(3):615-20.

[1817] Cui FJ, Li Y, Xu YY, et al. Induction of apoptosis in SGC-7901 cells by polysaccharide-peptide GFPS1b from the cultured mycelia of Grifola frondosa GF9801. *Toxicol In Vitro*. 2007 Apr;21(3):417-27.

[1818] Kodama N, Komuta K, Sakai N, et al. Effects of D-Fraction, a polysaccharide from Grifola frondosa on tumor growth involve activation of NK cells. *Biol Pharm Bull*. 2002 Dec;25(12):1647-50.

[1819] Vetchinkina E, Shirokov A, Bucharskaya A, et al. Antitumor Activity of Extracts from Medicinal Basidiomycetes Mushrooms. *Int J Med Mushrooms*. 2016;18(11):955-964.

[1820] Vetchinkina E, Shirokov A, Bucharskaya A, et al. Antitumor Activity of Extracts from Medicinal Basidiomycetes Mushrooms. *Int J Med Mushrooms*. 2016;18(11):955-964.

[1821] Zhao F, Wang YF, Song L, et al. Synergistic Apoptotic Effect of D-Fraction From Grifola frondosa and Vitamin C on Hepatocellular Carcinoma SMMC-7721 Cells. *Integr Cancer Ther*. 2017 Jun;16(2):205-214.

[1822] Mao GH, Zhang ZH, Fei F, et al. Effect of Grifola frondosa polysaccharide on anti-tumor activity in combination with 5-Fu in Heps-bearing mice. *Int J Biol Macromol*. 2019 Jan;121:930-935.

[1823] Masuda Y, Inoue M, Miyata A, et al. Maitake beta-glucan enhances therapeutic effect and reduces myelosupression and nephrotoxicity of cisplatin in mice. *Int Immunopharmacol*. 2009 May;9(5):620-6.

[1824] Lin H, de Stanchina E, Zhou XK, Hong F. Maitake beta-glucan promotes recovery of leukocytes and myeloid cell function in peripheral blood from paclitaxel hematotoxicity. *Cancer Immunol Immunother*. 2010 Jun;59(6):885-97.

[1825] Yu J, Ji HY, Liu C, et al. The structural characteristics of an acid-soluble polysaccharide from Grifola frondosa and its antitumor effects on H22-bearing mice. *Int J Biol Macromol*. 2020 May 10:S0141-8130(20)33200-1.

[1826] Masuda Y, Nakayama Y, Tanaka A, et al. Antitumor activity of orally administered maitake α-glucan by stimulating antitumor immune response in murine tumor. *PLoS One*. 2017 Mar 9;12(3):e0173621.

[1827] Harada N, Kodama N, Nanba H. Relationship between dendritic cells and the D-fraction-induced Th-1 dominant response in BALB/c tumor-bearing mice. *Cancer Lett*. 2003 Mar 31;192(2):181-7.

[1828] Masuda Y, Murata Y, Hayashi M, et al. Inhibitory effect of MD-Fraction on tumor metastasis: involvement of NK cell activation and suppression of intercellular adhesion molecule (ICAM)-1 expression in lung vascular endothelial cells. *Biol Pharm Bull*. 2008 Jun;31(6):1104-8.

[1829] Masuda Y, Nakayama Y, Tanaka A, et al. Antitumor activity of orally administered maitake α-glucan by stimulating antitumor immune response in murine tumor. *PLoS One*. 2017 Mar 9;12(3):e0173621.

[1830] Masuda Y, Murata Y, Hayashi M, et al. Inhibitory effect of MD-Fraction on tumor metastasis: involvement of NK cell activation and suppression of intercellular adhesion molecule (ICAM)-1 expression in lung vascular endothelial cells. *Biol Pharm Bull*. 2008 Jun;31(6):1104-8.

[1831] Zhao J, He R, Zhong H, et al. Synergistic Antitumor Effect of Grifola frondose Polysaccharide-Protein Complex in Combination with Cyclophosphamide in H22 Tumor-Bearing Mice. *Molecules*. 2023 Mar 26;28(7):2954.

[1832] Zhang H, Dong X, Ji H, et al. Preparation and structural characterization of acid-extracted polysaccharide from Grifola frondosa and antitumor activity on S180 tumor-bearing mice. *Int J Biol Macromol*. 2023 Apr 15;234:123302.

[1833] Nie X, Shi B, Ding Y, et al. Preparation of a chemically sulfated polysaccharide derived from Grifola frondosa and its potential biological activities. Preparation of a chemically sulfated polysaccharide derived from Grifola frondosa and its potential biological activities. *Int J Biol Macromol*. 2006 Nov 15;39(4-5):228-33.

[1834] Ohno N, Suzuki I, Oikawa S, et al. Antitumor activity and structural characterization of glucans extracted from cultured fruit bodies of Grifola frondose. *Chem Pharm Bull (Tokyo)*. 1984 Mar;32(3):1142-51.

[1835] Ohno N, Adachi Y, Suzuki I, et al. Antitumor activity of a beta-1,3-glucan obtained from liquid cultured mycelium of Grifola frondosa. *J Pharmacobiodyn*. 1986 Oct;9(10):861-4.

[1836] Suzuki I, Itani T, Ohno N, et al. Antitumor activity of a polysaccharide fraction extracted from cultured fruiting bodies of Grifola frondose. *J Pharmacobiodyn*. 1984 Jul;7(7):492-500.

[1837] Ohno N, Iino K, Takeyama T, et al. Structural characterization and antitumor activity of the extracts from matted mycelium of cultured Grifola frondose. *Chem Pharm Bull (Tokyo)*. 1985 Aug;33(8):3395-401.

[1838] Ohno N, Iino K, Suzuki I, et al. Neutral and acidic antitumor polysaccharides extracted from cultured fruit bodies of Grifola frondosa. *Chem Pharm Bull (Tokyo)*. 1985 Mar;33(3):1181-6.

[1839] Konno S. Synergistic potentiation of D-fraction with vitamin C as possible alternative approach for cancer therapy. *Int J Gen Med*. 2009 Jul 30;2:91-108.

[1840] Li X, Rong J, Wu M, et al. [Anti-tumor effect of polysaccharide from Grifola frondosa and its influence on immunological function]. *Zhong Yao Cai*. 2003 Jan;26(1):31-2.

[1841] Suzuki I, Takeyama T, Ohno N, et al. Antitumor effect of polysaccharide grifolan NMF-5N on syngeneic tumor in mice. *J Pharmacobiodyn*. 1987 Feb;10(2):72-7.

[1842] Lee JS, Park BC, Ko YJ, et al. Grifola frondosa (maitake mushroom) water extract inhibits vascular endothelial growth factor-induced angiogenesis through inhibition of reactive oxygen species and extracellular signal-regulated kinase phosphorylation. *J Med Food*. 2008 Dec;11(4):643-51.

[1843] Matsui K, Kodama N, Nanba H. Effects of maitake (Grifola frondosa) D-Fraction on the carcinoma angiogenesis. *Cancer Lett.* 2001 Oct 30;172(2):193-8.

[1844] Wang Y, Shen X, Liao W, et al. A heteropolysaccharide, L-fuco-D-manno-1,6-α-D-galactan extracted from Grifola frondosa and antiangiogenic activity of its sulfated derivative. *Carbohydr Polym.* 2014 Jan 30;101:631-41.

[1845] Lin H, Cheung SW, Nesin M, et al. Enhancement of umbilical cord blood cell hematopoiesis by maitake beta-glucan is mediated by granulocyte colony-stimulating factor production. *Clin Vaccine Immunol.* 2007 Jan;14(1):21-7.

[1846] Inoue A, Kodama N, Nanba H. Effect of maitake (Grifola frondosa) D-fraction on the control of the T lymph node Th-1/Th-2 proportion. *Biol Pharm Bull.* 2002 Apr;25(4):536-40.

[1847] Kodama N, Harada N, Nanba H. A polysaccharide, extract from Grifola frondosa, induces Th-1 dominant responses in carcinoma-bearing BALB/c mice. *Jpn J Pharmacol.* 2002 Dec;90(4):357-60.

[1848] Masuda Y, Ito K, Konishi M, et al. A polysaccharide extracted from Grifola frondosa enhances the anti-tumor activity of bone marrow-derived dendritic cell-based immunotherapy against murine colon cancer. *Cancer Immunol Immunother.* 2010 Oct;59(10):1531-41.

[1849] Masuda Y, Matsumoto A, Toida T, et al. Characterization and antitumor effect of a novel polysaccharide from Grifola frondosa. *J Agric Food Chem.* 2009 Nov 11;57(21):10143-9.

[1850] Suzuki I, Itani T, Ohno N, et al. Effect of a polysaccharide fraction from Grifola frondosa on immune response in mice. *J Pharmacobiodyn.* 1985 Mar;8(3):217-26.

[1851] Suzuki I, Hashimoto K, Oikawa S, et al. Antitumor and immunomodulating activities of a beta-glucan obtained from liquid-cultured Grifola frondosa. *Chem Pharm Bull (Tokyo).* 1989 Feb;37(2):410-3.

[1852] Kodama N, Mizuno S, Nanba H, et al. Potential antitumor activity of a low-molecular-weight protein fraction from Grifola frondosa through enhancement of cytokine production. *J Med Food.* 2010 Feb;13(1):20-30.

[1853] Masuda Y, Inoue H, Ohta H, et al. Oral administration of soluble β-glucans extracted from Grifola frondosa induces systemic antitumor immune response and decreases immunosuppression in tumor-bearing mice. *Int J Cancer.* 2013 Jul;133(1):108-19.

[1854] Takeyama T, Suzuki I, Ohno N, et al. Host-mediated antitumor effect of grifolan NMF-5N, a polysaccharide obtained from Grifola frondosa. *J Pharmacobiodyn.* 1987 Nov;10(11):644-51.

[1855] Adachi K, Nanba H, Kuroda H. Potentiation of host-mediated antitumor activity in mice by beta-glucan obtained from Grifola frondosa (maitake). *Chem Pharm Bull (Tokyo).* 1987 Jan;35(1):262-70.

[1856] Hishida I, Nanba H, Kuroda H. Antitumor activity exhibited by orally administered extract from fruit body of Grifola frondosa (maitake). *Chem Pharm Bull (Tokyo).* 1988 May;36(5):1819-27.

[1857] Sanzen I, Imanishi N, Takamatsu N, et al. Nitric oxide-mediated antitumor activity induced by the extract from Grifola frondosa (Maitake mushroom) in a macrophage cell line, RAW264.7. *J Exp Clin Cancer Res.* 2001 Dec;20(4):591-7.

[1858] Chen Z, Tang Y, Liu A, et al. Oral administration of Grifola frondosa polysaccharides improves memory impairment in aged rats via antioxidant action. *Mol Nutr Food Res.* 2017 Nov;61(11).

[1859] Fan L, Chen L, Liang Z, et al. A Polysaccharide Extract from Maitake Culinary-Medicinal Mushroom, Grifola frondosa (Agaricomycetes) Ameliorates Learning and Memory Function in Aluminum Chloride-Induced Amnesia in Mice. *Int J Med Mushrooms.* 2019;21(11):1065-1074.

[1860] Nishina A, Kimura H, Sekiguchi A, et al. Lysophosphatidylethanolamine in Grifola frondosa as a neurotrophic activator via activation of MAPK. *J Lipid Res.* 2006 Jul;47(7):1434-43.

[1861] Ling-Sing Seow S, Naidu M, David P, et al. Potentiation of neuritogenic activity of medicinal mushrooms in rat pheochromocytoma cells. *BMC Complement Altern Med.* 2013 Jul 4;13:157.

[1862] Phan CW, David P, Naidu M, et al. Neurite outgrowth stimulatory effects of culinary-medicinal mushrooms and their toxicity assessment using differentiating Neuro-2a and embryonic fibroblast BALB/3T3. *BMC Complement Altern Med.* 2013 Oct 11;13:261.

[1863] Patel DK, Seo YR, Dutta SD, et al. Influence of Maitake (Grifola frondosa) Particle Sizes on Human Mesenchymal Stem Cells and In Vivo Evaluation of Their Therapeutic Potential. *Biomed Res Int.* 2020 Mar 6;2020:8193971.

[1864] Erjavec I, Brkljacic J, Vukicevic S, et al. Mushroom Extracts Decrease Bone Resorption and Improve Bone Formation. *Int J Med Mushrooms.* 2016;18(7):559-69.

[1865] Sun R, Jin D, Fei F, et al. Mushroom polysaccharides from Grifola frondosa (Dicks.) Gray and Inonotus obliquus (Fr.) Pilat ameliorated dextran sulfate sodium-induced colitis in mice by global modulation of systemic metabolism and the gut microbiota. *Front Pharmacol.* 2023 Jun 7;14:1172963.

[1866] Lee JS, Park SY, Thapa D, et al. Grifola frondosa water extract alleviates intestinal inflammation by suppressing TNF-alpha production and its signaling. *Exp Mol Med.* 2010 Feb 28;42(2):143-54.

[1867] Liu X, Chen S, Liu H, et al. Structural properties and anti-inflammatory activity of purified polysaccharides from Hen-of-the-woods mushrooms (Grifola frondosa). *Front Nutr.* 2023 Feb 7;10:1078868.

[1868] Hou L, Meng M, Chen Y, et al. A water-soluble polysaccharide from Grifola frondosa induced macrophages activation via TLR4-MyD88-IKKβ-NF-κB p65 pathways. *Oncotarget.* 2017 Sep 23;8(49):86604-86614.

[1869] Ma XL, Meng M, Han LR, et al. Immunomodulatory activity of macromolecular polysaccharide isolated from Grifola frondosa. *Chin J Nat Med.* 2015 Dec;13(12):906-14.

[1870] Li Q, Zhang F, Chen G, et al. Purification, characterization and immunomodulatory activity of a novel polysaccharide from Grifola frondosa. *Int J Biol Macromol.* 2018 May;111:1293-1303.

[1871] Xu X, Liu Y, Pan C, et al. Antioxidant and Immunomodulatory Activities of Polysaccharides from Fermented Wheat Products of Grifola frondosa: In Vitro Methods. *Int J Food Sci.* 2023 Aug 9;2023:3820276.

[1872] Seo YR, Patel DK, Shin WC, et al. Structural Elucidation and Immune-Enhancing Effects of Novel Polysaccharide from Grifola frondosa. *Biomed Res Int.* 2019 Apr 16;2019:7528609.

[1873] Wang L, Ha CL, Cheng TL, et al. Oral administration of submerged cultivated Grifola frondosa enhances phagocytic activity in normal mice. *J Pharm Pharmacol.* 2008 Feb;60(2):237-43.

[1874] Vetvicka V, Vetvickova J. Immune-enhancing effects of Maitake (Grifola frondosa) and Shiitake (Lentinula edodes) extracts. *Ann Transl Med.* 2014 Feb;2(2):14.

[1875] Meng M, Guo M, Feng C et al. Water-soluble polysaccharides from Grifola Frondosa fruiting bodies protect against immunosuppression in cyclophosphamide-induced mice via JAK2/STAT3/SOCS signal transduction pathways. *Food Funct.* 2019 Aug 1;10(8):4998-5007.

[1876] Wu MJ, Cheng TL, Cheng SY, et al. Immunomodulatory properties of Grifola frondosa in submerged culture. *J Agric Food Chem.* 2006 Apr 19;54(8):2906-14.

[1877] Han L, Cheng D, Wang L, et al. [Structure and immunomodulatory activity of extracellular polysaccharide from Grifola frondosa]. *Sheng Wu Gong Cheng Xue Bao.* 2016 May 25;32(5):648-656.

[1878] Ma X, Meng M, Han L, et al. Structural characterization and immunomodulatory activity of Grifola frondosa polysaccharide via toll-like receptor 4-mitogen-activated protein kinases-nuclear factor κB pathways. *Food Funct.* 2016 Jun 15;7(6):2763-72.

[1879] Meng M, Cheng D, Han L, et al. Isolation, purification, structural analysis and immunostimulatory activity of water-soluble polysaccharides from Grifola Frondosa fruiting body. *Carbohydr Polym.* 2017 Feb 10;157:1134-1143.

[1880] Tsao YW, Kuan YC, Wang JL, et al. Characterization of a novel maitake (Grifola frondosa) protein that activates natural killer and dendritic cells and enhances antitumor immunity in mice. *J Agric Food Chem.* 2013 Oct 16;61(41):9828-38.

[1881] Masuda Y, Togo T, Mizuno S, et al. Soluble β-glucan from Grifola frondosa induces proliferation and Dectin-1/Syk signaling in resident macrophages via the GM-CSF autocrine pathway. *J Leukoc Biol.* 2012 Apr;91(4):547-56.

[1882] Svagelj M, Berovic M, Gregori A, et al. Immunomodulating activities of cultivated maitake medicinal mushroom Grifola frondosa (Dicks.: Fr.) S.F. Gray (higher Basidiomycetes) on peripheral blood mononuclear cells. *Int J Med Mushrooms.* 2012;14(4):377-83.

[1883] Vetvicka V, Vetvickova J. Immune enhancing effects of WB365, a novel combination of Ashwagandha (Withania somnifera) and Maitake (Grifola frondosa) extracts. *N Am J Med Sci.* 2011 Jul;3(7):320-4.

[1884] Kodama N, Murata Y, Nanba H. Administration of a polysaccharide from Grifola frondosa stimulates immune function of normal mice. *J Med Food.* 2004 Summer;7(2):141-5.

[1885] Yang BK, Gu YA, Jeong YT, et al. Chemical characteristics and immuno-modulating activities of exo-biopolymers produced by Grifola frondosa during submerged fermentation process. *Int J Biol Macromol.* 2007 Aug 1;41(3):227-33.

[1886] Kodama N, Asakawa A, Inui A, et al. Enhancement of cytotoxicity of NK cells by D-Fraction, a polysaccharide from Grifola frondosa. *Oncol Rep.* 2005 Mar;13(3):497-502.

[1887] Wang Y, Fang J, Ni X, et al. Inducement of cytokine release by GFPBW2, a novel polysaccharide from fruit bodies of Grifola frondosa, through dectin-1 in macrophages. *J Agric Food Chem.* 2013 Nov 27;61(47):11400-9.

[1888] Adachi Y, Okazaki M, Ohno N, et al. Enhancement of cytokine production by macrophages stimulated with (1-->3)-beta-D-glucan, grifolan (GRN), isolated from Grifola frondosa. *Biol Pharm Bull.* 1994 Dec;17(12):1554-60.

[1889] Li Q, Chen G, Wang W, et al. A novel Se-polysaccharide from Se-enriched G. frondosa protects against immunosuppression and low Se status in Se-deficient mice. *Int J Biol Macromol.* 2018 Oct 1;117:878-889.

[1890] Masuda Y, Nakayama Y, Shimizu R, et al. Maitake α-glucan promotes differentiation of monocytic myeloid-derived suppressor cells into M1 macrophages. *Life Sci.* 2023 Mar 15;317:121453.

[1891] Huyan T, Li Q, Yang H, et al. Protective effect of polysaccharides on simulated microgravity-induced functional inhibition of human NK cells. *Carbohydr Polym.* 2014 Jan 30;101:819-27.

[1892] Tada R, Tanioka A, Ishibashi K, et al. Involvement of branched units at position 6 in the reactivity of a unique variety of beta-D-glucan from Aureobasidium pullulans to antibodies in human sera. *Biosci Biotechnol Biochem.* 2009 Apr 23;73(4):908-11.

[1893] Yin Y, Fu W, Fu M, et al. The immune effects of edible fungus polysaccharides compounds in mice. *Asia Pac J Clin Nutr.* 2007;16 Suppl 1:258-60.

[1894] Ito K, Masuda Y, Yamasaki Y, et al. Maitake beta-glucan enhances granulopoiesis and mobilization of granulocytes by increasing G-CSF production and modulating CXCR4/SDF-1 expression. *Int Immunopharmacol.* 2009 Sep;9(10):1189-96.

[1895] Zhang J, Tyler HL, Haron MH, et al. Macrophage activation by edible mushrooms is due to the collaborative interaction of toll-like receptor agonists and dectin-1b activating beta glucans derived from colonizing microorganisms. *Food Funct.* 2019 Dec 11;10(12):8208-8217.

[1896] Ohno N, Asada N, Adachi Y, et al. Enhancement of LPS triggered TNF-alpha (tumor necrosis factor-alpha) production by (1-->3)-beta-D-glucans in mice. *Biol Pharm Bull.* 1995 Jan;18(1):126-33.

[1897] Adachi Y, Ohno N, Yadomae T. Activation of murine kupffer cells by administration with gel-forming (1-->3)-beta-D-glucan from Grifola frondosa. *Biol Pharm Bull.* 1998 Mar;21(3):278-83.

[1898] Ohno N, Egawa Y, Hashimoto T, et al. Effect of beta-glucans on the nitric oxide synthesis by peritoneal macrophage in mice. *Biol Pharm Bull.* 1996 Apr;19(4):608-12.

[1899] Kodama N, Murata Y, Asakawa A, et al. Maitake D-Fraction enhances antitumor effects and reduces immunosuppression by mitomycin-C in tumor-bearing mice. *Nutrition.* 2005 May;21(5):624-9.

[1900] Ishibashi K, Miura NN, Adachi Y, et al. Relationship between solubility of grifolan, a fungal 1,3-beta-D-glucan, and production of tumor necrosis factor by macrophages in vitro. *Biosci Biotechnol Biochem.* 2001 Sep;65(9):1993-2000.

[1901] Okazaki M, Adachi Y, Ohno N, et al. Structure-activity relationship of (1-->3)-beta-D-glucans in the induction of cytokine production from macrophages, in vitro. *Biol Pharm Bull.* 1995 Oct;18(10):1320-7.

[1902] Wu SJ, Lu TM, Lai MN, et al. Immunomodulatory activities of medicinal mushroom Grifola frondosa extract and its bioactive constituent. *Am J Chin Med.* 2013;41(1):131-44.

[1903] Zhang ZH, Liao TT, Deng CM, et al. Purification and characterization of Se-enriched Grifola frondosa glycoprotein, and evaluating its amelioration effect on As3+ -induced immune toxicity. *J Sci Food Agric.* 2022 Apr;102(6):2526-2537.

[1904] Hu R. Grifola frondosa may play an anti-obesity role by affecting intestinal microbiota to increase the production of short-chain fatty acids. *Front Endocrinol (Lausanne).* 2023 Jan 17;13:1105073.

[1905] Aranaz P, Peña A, Vettorazzi A, et al. Grifola frondosa (Maitake) Extract Reduces Fat Accumulation and Improves Health Span in C. elegans through the DAF-16/FOXO and SKN-1/NRF2 Signalling Pathways. *Nutrients.* 2021 Nov 7;13(11):3968.

[1906] Jiang X, Hao J, Zhu Y, et al. The anti-obesity effects of a water-soluble glucan from Grifola frondosa via the modulation of chronic inflammation. *Front Immunol.* 2022 Jul 28;13:962341.

[1907] Jiang X, Hao J, Liu Z, et al. Anti-obesity effects of Grifola frondosa through the modulation of lipid metabolism via ceramide in mice fed a high-fat diet. *Food Funct*. 2021 Aug 2;12(15):6725-6739.

[1908] Nakai R, Masui H, Horio H, et al. Effect of maitake (Grifola frondosa) water extract on inhibition of adipocyte conversion of C3H10T1/2B2C1 cells. *J Nutr Sci Vitaminol (Tokyo)*. 1999 Jun;45(3):385-9.

[1909] Minamino K, Yanaga Y, Ohtsuru M. Bioactive substance from Grifola frondosa (maitake) mushroom inhibits CCAAT enhancer binding protein beta and delta expression on C3H10T1/2 B2C1 adipocyte cells. *J Nutr Sci Vitaminol (Tokyo)*. 2008 Jun;54(3):250-4.

[1910] Minamino K, Nagasawa Y, Ohtsuru M. A water-soluble extract from Grifola frondosa, maitake mushroom, decreases lipid droplets in brown adipocyte tissue cells. *J Nutr Sci Vitaminol (Tokyo)*. 2008 Dec;54(6):497-500.

[1911] Ma X, Zhou F, Chen Y, et al. A polysaccharide from Grifola frondosa relieves insulin resistance of HepG2 cell by Akt-GSK-3 pathway. *Glycoconj J*. 2014 Jul;31(5):355-63.

[1912] Xu Q, Guo J. Activity and toxicity of Cr(III)-enriched Grifola frondosa in insulin-resistant mice. *Biol Trace Elem Res*. 2009 Dec;131(3):271-7.

[1913] Preuss HG, Echard B, Bagchi D, et al. Enhanced insulin-hypoglycemic activity in rats consuming a specific glycoprotein extracted from maitake mushroom. *Mol Cell Biochem*. 2007 Dec;306(1-2):105-13.

[1914] Aoki H, Hanayama M, Mori K, et al. Grifola frondosa (Maitake) extract activates PPARδ and improves glucose intolerance in high-fat diet-induced obese mice. *Biosci Biotechnol Biochem*. 2018 Sep;82(9):1550-1559.

[1915] Kou L, Du M, Liu P, et al. Anti-Diabetic and Anti-Nephritic Activities of Grifola frondosa Mycelium Polysaccharides in Diet-Streptozotocin-Induced Diabetic Rats Via Modulation on Oxidative Stress. *Appl Biochem Biotechnol*. 2019 Jan;187(1):310-322.

[1916] Jiang T, Wang L, Ma A, et al. The hypoglycemic and renal protective effects of Grifola frondosa polysaccharides in early diabetic nephropathy. *J Food Biochem*. 2020 Dec;44(12):e13515.

[1917] Li N, Gao X, Pan Y, et al. Effects of alkaloid-rich extracts obtained from Grifola frondosa on gut microbiota and glucose homeostasis in rats. *Food Funct*. 2022 Mar 7;13(5):2729-2742.

[1918] Wu SJ, Tung YJ, Ng LT. Anti-diabetic effects of Grifola frondosa bioactive compound and its related molecular signaling pathways in palmitate-induced C2C12 cells. *J Ethnopharmacol*. 2020 Oct 5;260:112962.

[1919] Guo WL, Deng JC, Pan YY, et al. Hypoglycemic and hypolipidemic activities of Grifola frondosa polysaccharides and their relationships with the modulation of intestinal microflora in diabetic mice induced by high-fat diet and streptozotocin. *Int J Biol Macromol*. 2020 Jun 15;153:1231-1240.

[1920] Chen S, Mu Z, Yong T, et al. Grifolamine A, a novel bis-γ-butyrolactone from Grifola frondosa exerted inhibitory effect on α-glucosidase and their binding interaction: Affinity and molecular dynamics simulation. *Curr Res Food Sci*. 2022 Oct 27;5:2045-2052.

[1921] Cui B, Han L, Qu J, et al. Hypoglycemic activity of Grifola frondosa rich in vanadium. *Biol Trace Elem Res*. 2009 Nov;131(2):186-91.

[1922] Guo WL, Shi FF, Li L, et al. Preparation of a novel Grifola frondosa polysaccharide-chromium (III) complex and its hypoglycemic and hypolipidemic activities in high fat diet and streptozotocin-induced diabetic mice. *Int J Biol Macromol*. 2019 Jun 15;131:81-88.

[1923] Su CH, Lu TM, Lai MN, et al. Inhibitory potential of Grifola frondosa bioactive fractions on α-amylase and α-glucosidase for management of hyperglycemia. *Biotechnol Appl Biochem*. 2013 Jul-Aug;60(4):446-52.

[1924] Shen KP, Su CH, Lu TM, et al. Effects of Grifola frondosa non-polar bioactive components on high-fat diet fed and streptozotocin-induced hyperglycemic mice. *Pharm Biol*. 2015 May;53(5):705-9.

[1925] Horio H, Ohtsuru M. Maitake (Grifola frondosa) improve glucose tolerance of experimental diabetic rats. *J Nutr Sci Vitaminol (Tokyo)*. 2001 Feb;47(1):57-63.

[1926] Chen Y, Liu Y, Sarker MMR, et al. Structural characterization and antidiabetic potential of a novel heteropolysaccharide from Grifola frondosa via IRS1/PI3K-JNK signaling pathways. *Carbohydr Polym*. 2018 Oct 15;198:452-461.

[1927] Xiao C, Wu Q, Xie Y, et al. Hypoglycemic effects of Grifola frondosa (Maitake) polysaccharides F2 and F3 through improvement of insulin resistance in diabetic rats. *Food Funct*. 2015 Nov;6(11):3567-75.

[1928] Lo HC, Hsu TH, Chen CY. Submerged culture mycelium and broth of Grifola frondosa improve glycemic responses in diabetic rats. *Am J Chin Med*. 2008;36(2):265-85.

[1929] Chen Y, Liu D, Wang D, Lai S, et al. Hypoglycemic activity and gut microbiota regulation of a novel polysaccharide from Grifola frondosa in type 2 diabetic mice. *Food Chem Toxicol*. 2019 Apr;126:295-302.

[1930] Kubo K, Aoki H, Nanba H. Anti-diabetic activity present in the fruit body of Grifola frondosa (Maitake). I. *Biol Pharm Bull*. 1994 Aug;17(8):1106-10.

[1931] Lei H, Zhang M, Wang Q, et al. MT-α-glucan from the fruit body of the maitake medicinal mushroom Grifola frondosa (higher Basidiomyetes) shows protective effects for hypoglycemic pancreatic β-cells. *Int J Med Mushrooms*. 2013;15(4):373-81.

[1932] Hong L, Xun M, Wutong W. Anti-diabetic effect of an alpha-glucan from fruit body of maitake (Grifola frondosa) on KK-Ay mice. *J Pharm Pharmacol*. 2007 Apr;59(4):575-82.

[1933] Matsuur H, Asakawa C, Kurimoto M, et al. Alpha-glucosidase inhibitor from the seeds of balsam pear (Momordica charantia) and the fruit bodies of Grifola frondosa. *Biosci Biotechnol Biochem*. 2002 Jul;66(7):1576-8.

[1934] Lei H, Guo S, Han J, et al. Hypoglycemic and hypolipidemic activities of MT-α-glucan and its effect on immune function of diabetic mice. *Carbohydr Polym*. 2012 Jun 5;89(1):245-50.

[1935] Hong L, Qin W, Shuzhen G, et al. The protective effect of MT-α-glucan against streptozotocin (STZ)-induced NIT-1 pancreatic β-cell damage. *Carbohydr Polym*. 2013 Feb 15;92(2):1211-7.

[1936] Han C, Liu T. A comparison of hypoglycemic activity of three species of basidiomycetes rich in vanadium. *Biol Trace Elem Res*. 2009 Feb;127(2):177-82.

[1937] Su CH, Lai MN, Ng LT. Inhibitory effects of medicinal mushrooms on α-amylase and α-glucosidase - enzymes related to hyperglycemia. *Food Funct*. 2013 Apr 25;4(4):644-9.

[1938] Jiang T, Shen S, Wang L, et al. Grifola frondosa Polysaccharide Ameliorates Early Diabetic Nephropathy by Suppressing the TLR4/NF-κB Pathway. *Appl Biochem Biotechnol*. 2022 Sep;194(9):4093-4104.

[1939] Kou L, Du M, Liu P, et al. Anti-Diabetic and Anti-Nephritic Activities of Grifola frondosa Mycelium Polysaccharides in Diet-Streptozotocin-Induced Diabetic Rats Via Modulation on Oxidative Stress. *Appl Biochem Biotechnol*. 2019 Jan;187(1):310-322.

[1940] Jiang T, Wang L, Ma A, et al. The hypoglycemic and renal protective effects of Grifola frondosa polysaccharides in early diabetic nephropathy. *J Food Biochem*. 2020 Dec;44(12):e13515.

[1941] Chen YH, Lee CH, Hsu TH, et al. Submerged-Culture Mycelia and Broth of the Maitake Medicinal Mushroom Grifola frondosa (Higher Basidiomycetes) Alleviate Type 2 Diabetes-Induced Alterations in Immunocytic Function. *Int J Med Mushrooms*. 2015;17(6):541-56.

[1942] Wu WT, Hsu TH, Chen WL, et al. Polysaccharides of Grifola frondosa ameliorate oxidative stress and hypercholesterolaemia in hamsters fed a high-fat, high-cholesterol diet. *J Pharm Pharmacol*. 2022 Sep 1;74(9):1296-1306.

[1943] Li L, Guo WL, Zhang W et al. Grifola frondosa polysaccharides ameliorate lipid metabolic disorders and gut microbiota dysbiosis in high-fat diet fed rats. *Food Funct*. 2019 May 22;10(5):2560-2572.

[1944] Ding Y, Xiao C, Wu Q, et al. The Mechanisms Underlying the Hypolipidaemic Effects of Grifola frondosa in the Liver of Rats. *Front Microbiol*. 2016 Aug 3;7:1186.

[1945] Pan Y, Wan X, Zeng F, et al. Regulatory effect of Grifola frondosa extract rich in polysaccharides and organic acids on glycolipid metabolism and gut microbiota in rats. *Int J Biol Macromol*. 2020 Jul 15;155:1030-1039.

[1946] Jiang X, Hao J, Liu Z, et al. Anti-obesity effects of Grifola frondosa through the modulation of lipid metabolism via ceramide in mice fed a high-fat diet. *Food Funct*. 2021 Aug 2;12(15):6725-6739.

[1947] Guo WL, Deng JC, Pan YY, et al. Hypoglycemic and hypolipidemic activities of Grifola frondosa polysaccharides and their relationships with the modulation of intestinal microflora in diabetic mice induced by high-fat diet and streptozotocin. *Int J Biol Macromol*. 2020 Jun 15;153:1231-1240.

[1948] Liu J, Wu Y, Cai Y, et al. Long-term consumption of different doses of Grifola frondosa affects immunity and metabolism: correlation with intestinal mucosal microbiota and blood lipids. *3 Biotech*. 2023 Jun;13(6):189.

[1949] Pan YY, Zeng F, Guo WL, et al. Effect of Grifola frondosa 95% ethanol extract on lipid metabolism and gut microbiota composition in high-fat diet-fed rats. *Food Funct*. 2018 Dec 13;9(12):6268-6278.

[1950] Guo WL, Shi FF, Li L, et al. Preparation of a novel Grifola frondosa polysaccharide-chromium (III) complex and its hypoglycemic and hypolipidemic activities in high fat diet and streptozotocin-induced diabetic mice. *Int J Biol Macromol*. 2019 Jun 15;131:81-88.

[1951] Sato M, Tokuji Y, Yoneyama S, et al. Effect of dietary Maitake (Grifola frondosa) mushrooms on plasma cholesterol and hepatic gene expression in cholesterol-fed mice. *J Oleo Sci*. 2013;62(12):1049-58.

[1952] Kubo K, Nanba H. Anti-hyperliposis effect of maitake fruit body (Grifola frondosa). I. *Biol Pharm Bull*. 1997 Jul;20(7):781-5.

[1953] Kabir Y, Yamaguchi M, Kimura S. Effect of shiitake (Lentinus edodes) and maitake (Grifola frondosa) mushrooms on blood pressure and plasma lipids of spontaneously hypertensive rats. *J Nutr Sci Vitaminol (Tokyo)*. 1987 Oct;33(5):341-6.

[1954] Fukushima M, Ohashi T, Fujiwara Y, et al. Cholesterol-lowering effects of maitake (Grifola frondosa) fiber, shiitake (Lentinus edodes) fiber, and enokitake (Flammulina velutipes) fiber in rats. *Exp Biol Med (Maywood)*. 2001 Sep;226(8):758-65.

[1955] Ding Y, Xiao C, Wu Q, et al. The Mechanisms Underlying the Hypolipidaemic Effects of Grifola frondosa in the Liver of Rats. *Front Microbiol*. 2016 Aug 3;7:1186.

[1956] Adachi K, Nanba H, Otsuka M, et al. Blood pressure-lowering activity present in the fruit body of Grifola frondosa (maitake). I. *Chem Pharm Bull (Tokyo)*. 1988 Mar;36(3):1000-6.

[1957] Martin KR. Both common and specialty mushrooms inhibit adhesion molecule expression and in vitro binding of monocytes to human aortic endothelial cells in a pro-inflammatory environment. *Nutr J*. 2010 Jul 16;9:29.

[1958] Hu R. Grifola frondosa may play an anti-obesity role by affecting intestinal microbiota to increase the production of short-chain fatty acids. *Front Endocrinol (Lausanne)*. 2023 Jan 17;13:1105073.

[1959] Zhao J, He R, Zhong H, et al. A cold-water extracted polysaccharide-protein complex from Grifola frondosa exhibited anti-tumor activity via TLR4-NF-κB signaling activation and gut microbiota modification in H22 tumor-bearing mice. *Int J Biol Macromol*. 2023 Jun 1;239:124291.

[1960] Li L, Guo WL, Zhang W et al. Grifola frondosa polysaccharides ameliorate lipid metabolic disorders and gut microbiota dysbiosis in high-fat diet fed rats. *Food Funct*. 2019 May 22;10(5):2560-2572.

[1961] Pan Y, Wan X, Zeng F, et al. Regulatory effect of Grifola frondosa extract rich in polysaccharides and organic acids on glycolipid metabolism and gut microbiota in rats. *Int J Biol Macromol*. 2020 Jul 15;155:1030-1039.

[1962] Li N, Gao X, Pan Y, et al. Effects of alkaloid-rich extracts obtained from Grifola frondosa on gut microbiota and glucose homeostasis in rats. *Food Funct*. 2022 Mar 7;13(5):2729-2742.

[1963] Li X, Zeng F, Huang Y, et al. The Positive Effects of Grifola frondosa Heteropolysaccharide on NAFLD and Regulation of the Gut Microbiota. *Int J Mol Sci*. 2019 Oct 24;20(21):5302.

[1964] Liu J, Wu Y, Cai Y, et al. Long-term consumption of different doses of Grifola frondosa affects immunity and metabolism: correlation with intestinal mucosal microbiota and blood lipids. *3 Biotech*. 2023 Jun;13(6):189.

[1965] Pan YY, Zeng F, Guo WL, et al. Effect of Grifola frondosa 95% ethanol extract on lipid metabolism and gut microbiota composition in high-fat diet-fed rats. *Food Funct*. 2018 Dec 13;9(12):6268-6278.

[1966] Chen Y, Liu D, Wang D, Lai S, et al. Hypoglycemic activity and gut microbiota regulation of a novel polysaccharide from Grifola frondosa in type 2 diabetic mice. *Food Chem Toxicol*. 2019 Apr;126:295-302.

[1967] De Giani A, Bovio F, Forcella ME, et al. Prebiotic Effect of Maitake Extract on a Probiotic Consortium and Its Action after Microbial Fermentation on Colorectal Cell Lines. *Foods*. 2021 Oct 21;10(11):2536.

[1968] Kawai J, Mori K, Hirasawa N. et al. Grifola frondosa extract and ergosterol reduce allergic reactions in an allergy mouse model by suppressing the degranulation of mast cells. *Biosci Biotechnol Biochem*. 2019 Dec;83(12):2280-2287.

[1969] Kawai J, Higuchi Y, Hirota M, et al. Ergosterol and its derivatives from Grifola frondosa inhibit antigen-induced degranulation of RBL-2H3 cells by suppressing the aggregation of high affinity IgE receptors. *Biosci Biotechnol Biochem*. 2018 Oct;82(10):1803-1811.

[1970] Han C, Cui B. Pharmacological and pharmacokinetic studies with agaricoglycerides, extracted from Grifola frondosa, in animal models of pain and inflammation. *Inflammation*. 2012 Aug;35(4):1269-75.

[1971] Cui H, Zhu X, Huo Z, et al. A β-glucan from Grifola frondosa effectively delivers therapeutic oligonucleotide into cells via dectin-1 receptor and attenuates TNFα gene expression. *Int J Biol Macromol.* 2020 Apr 15;149:801-808.

[1972] Tomas-Hernandez S, Blanco J, Garcia-Vallvé S, et al. Anti-Inflammatory and Immunomodulatory Effects of the Grifola frondosa Natural Compound o-Orsellinaldehyde on LPS-Challenged Murine Primary Glial Cells. Roles of NF-κβ and MAPK. *Pharmaceutics.* 2021 May 28;13(6):806.

[1973] Su CH, Lu MK, Lu TJ, et al. A (1→6)-Branched (1→4)-β-d-Glucan from Grifola frondosa Inhibits Lipopolysaccharide-Induced Cytokine Production in RAW264.7 Macrophages by Binding to TLR2 Rather than Dectin-1 or CR3 Receptors. *J Nat Prod.* 2020 Feb 28;83(2):231-242.

[1974] Han C, Cui B. Pharmacological and pharmacokinetic studies with agaricoglycerides, extracted from Grifola frondosa, in animal models of pain and inflammation. *Inflammation.* 2012 Aug;35(4):1269-75.

[1975] Zhang Y, Mills GL, Nair MG. Cyclooxygenase inhibitory and antioxidant compounds from the mycelia of the edible mushroom Grifola frondosa. *J Agric Food Chem.* 2002 Dec 18;50(26):7581-5.

[1976] Tomas-Hernandez S, Garcia-Vallvé S, Pujadas G, et al. Anti-inflammatory and Proapoptotic Properties of the Natural Compound o-Orsellinaldehyde. *J Agric Food Chem.* 2018 Oct 24;66(42):10952-10963.

[1977] Chien RC, Lin LM, Chang YH, et al. Anti-Inflammation Properties of Fruiting Bodies and Submerged Cultured Mycelia of Culinary-Medicinal Higher Basidiomycetes Mushrooms. *Int J Med Mushrooms.* 2016;18(11):999-1009.

[1978] Su CH, Tseng YT, Lo KY, et al. Differences in anti-inflammatory properties of water soluble and insoluble bioactive polysaccharides in lipopolysaccharide-stimulated RAW264.7 macrophages. *Glycoconj J.* 2020 Oct;37(5):565-576.

[1979] Shigesue K, Kodama N, Nanba H. Effects of maitake (Grifola frondosa) polysaccharide on collagen-induced arthritis in mice. *Jpn J Pharmacol.* 2000 Nov;84(3):293-300.

[1980] Aranaz P, Peña A, Vettorazzi A, et al. Grifola frondosa (Maitake) Extract Reduces Fat Accumulation and Improves Health Span in C. elegans through the DAF-16/FOXO and SKN-1/NRF2 Signalling Pathways. *Nutrients.* 2021 Nov 7;13(11):3968.

[1981] Shevchuk Y, Kuypers K, Janssens GE. Fungi as a source of bioactive molecules for the development of longevity medicines. *Ageing Res Rev.* 2023 Jun;87:101929.

[1982] Kim JH, Lim SR, Jung DH, et al. Grifola frondosa Extract Containing Bioactive Components Blocks Skin Fibroblastic Inflammation and Cytotoxicity Caused by Endocrine Disrupting Chemical, Bisphenol A. *Nutrients.* 2022 Sep 15;14(18):3812.

[1983] Meng M, Zhang R, Han R, et al. The polysaccharides from the Grifola frondosa fruiting body prevent lipopolysaccharide/D-galactosamine-induced acute liver injury via the miR-122-Nrf2/ARE pathways. *Food Funct.* 2021 Mar 15;12(5):1973-1982.

[1984] Lee EW, He P, Kawagishi H, et al. Suppression of D-galactosamine-induced liver injury by mushrooms in rats. *Biosci Biotechnol Biochem.* 2000 Sep;64(9):2001-4.

[1985] Li X, Zeng F, Huang Y, et al. The Positive Effects of Grifola frondosa Heteropolysaccharide on NAFLD and Regulation of the Gut Microbiota. *Int J Mol Sci.* 2019 Oct 24;20(21):5302.

[1986] Li C, Meng M, Guo M, et al. The polysaccharides from Grifola frondosa attenuate CCl4-induced hepatic fibrosis in rats via the TGF-β/Smad signaling pathway. *RSC Adv.* 2019 Oct 21;9(58):33684-33692.

[1987] Dai XW, Chen ZY, Yan MX, et al. [Experimental study on intervention effect of Grifola frondosa on nonalcoholic steatohepatitis]. *Zhongguo Zhong Yao Za Zhi.* 2015 May;40(9):1808-11.

[1988] Martin KR. Both common and specialty mushrooms inhibit adhesion molecule expression and in vitro binding of monocytes to human aortic endothelial cells in a pro-inflammatory environment. *Nutr J.* 2010 Jul 16;9:29.

[1989] Park HS, Hwang YH, Kim MK, et al. Functional polysaccharides from Grifola frondosa aqueous extract inhibit atopic dermatitis-like skin lesions in NC/Nga mice. *Biosci Biotechnol Biochem.* 2015;79(1):147-54.

[1990] Nagao M, Sato T, Akimoto N, et al. Augmentation of sebaceous lipogenesis by an ethanol extract of Grifola frondosa (Maitake mushroom) in hamsters in vivo and in vitro. *Exp Dermatol.* 2009 Aug;18(8):730-3.

[1991] Bae JT, Sim GS, Lee DH, et al. Production of exopolysaccharide from mycelial culture of Grifola frondosa and its inhibitory effect on matrix metalloproteinase-1 expression in UV-irradiated human dermal fibroblasts. *FEMS Microbiol Lett.* 2005 Oct 15;251(2):347-54.

[1992] Jung K, Kim IH, Han D. Effect of medicinal plant extracts on forced swimming capacity in mice. *J Ethnopharmacol.* 2004 Jul;93(1):75-81.

[1993] Zhang W, Jiang X, Zhao S, et al. A polysaccharide-peptide with mercury clearance activity from dried fruiting bodies of maitake mushroom Grifola frondosa. *Sci Rep.* 2018 Dec 4;8(1):17630.

[1994] Wu WT, Hsu TH, Chen WL, et al. Polysaccharides of Grifola frondosa ameliorate oxidative stress and hypercholesterolaemia in hamsters fed a high-fat, high-cholesterol diet. *J Pharm Pharmacol.* 2022 Sep 1;74(9):1296-1306.

[1995] Kou L, Du M, Liu P, et al. Anti-Diabetic and Anti-Nephritic Activities of Grifola frondosa Mycelium Polysaccharides in Diet-Streptozotocin-Induced Diabetic Rats Via Modulation on Oxidative Stress. *Appl Biochem Biotechnol.* 2019 Jan;187(1):310-322.

[1996] Ting Z, Yina F, Guanghua M, et al. Purification, Characterization and Antioxidant Activities of Enzymolysis Polysaccharide from Grifola frondosa. *Iran J Pharm Res.* 2017 Winter;16(1):347-356.

[1997] Xu X, Liu Y, Pan C, et al. Antioxidant and Immunomodulatory Activities of Polysaccharides from Fermented Wheat Products of Grifola frondosa: In Vitro Methods. *Int J Food Sci.* 2023 Aug 9;2023:3820276.

[1998] Yeh JY, Hsieh LH, Wu KT, et al. Antioxidant properties and antioxidant compounds of various extracts from the edible basidiomycete Grifola frondosa (Maitake). *Molecules.* 2011 Apr 15;16(4):3197-211.

[1999] Chen GT, Ma XM, Liu ST, et al. Isolation, purification and antioxidant activities of polysaccharides from Grifola frondosa. *Carbohydr Polym.* 2012 Jun 5;89(1):61-6.

[2000] Zhang Y, Chen Z, Huang Z, et al. A comparative study on the structures of Grifola frondosa polysaccharides obtained by different decolourization methods and their in vitro antioxidant activities. *Food Funct.* 2019 Oct 16;10(10):6720-6731.

[2001] Fan Y, Wu X, Zhang M, et al. Physical characteristics and antioxidant effect of polysaccharides extracted by boiling water and enzymolysis from Grifola frondosa. *Int J Biol Macromol.* 2011 Jun 1;48(5):798-803.

[2002] Postemsky PD, Curvetto NR. Submerged Culture of Grifola gargal and G. sordulenta (Higher Basidiomycetes) from Argentina as a Source of Mycelia with Antioxidant Activity. *Int J Med Mushrooms.* 2015;17(1):65-76.

[2003] Smith H, Doyle S, Murphy R. Filamentous fungi as a source of natural antioxidants. *Food Chem.* 2015 Oct 15;185:389-97.

[2004] Kido S, Chosa E, Tanaka R. The effect of six dried and UV-C-irradiated mushrooms powder on lipid oxidation and vitamin D contents of fish meat. *Food Chem.* 2023 Jan 1;398:133917.

[2005] Zhao C, Gao L, Wang C, et al. Structural characterization and antiviral activity of a novel heteropolysaccharide isolated from Grifola frondosa against enterovirus 71. *Carbohydr Polym.* 2016 Jun 25;144:382-9.

[2006] Gu CQ, Li J, Chao FH. Inhibition of hepatitis B virus by D-fraction from Grifola frondosa: synergistic effect of combination with interferon-alpha in HepG2 2.2.15. *Antiviral Res.* 2006 Nov;72(2):162-5.

[2007] Gu CQ, Li JW, Chao F, et al. Isolation, identification and function of a novel anti-HSV-1 protein from Grifola frondosa. *Antiviral Res.* 2007 Sep;75(3):250-7.

[2008] Obi N, Hayashi K, Miyahara T, et al. Inhibitory Effect of TNF-alpha Produced by Macrophages Stimulated with Grifola frondosa Extract (ME) on the Growth of Influenza A/Aichi/2/68 Virus in MDCK Cells. *Am J Chin Med.* 2008;36(6):1171-83.

[2009] Sultana SS, Ghosh J, Chakraborty S, et al. Selective in vitro inhibition of Leishmania donovani by a semi-purified fraction of wild mushroom Grifola frondosa. *Exp Parasitol.* 2018 Sep;192:73-84.

[2010] Fasciana T, Gargano ML, Serra N, et al. Potential Activity of Albino Grifola frondosa Mushroom Extract against Biofilm of Meticillin-Resistant Staphylococcus aureus. *J Fungi (Basel).* 2021 Jul 10;7(7):551.

[2011] He X, Du X, Zang X, et al. Extraction, identification and antimicrobial activity of a new furanone, grifolaone A, from Grifola frondosa. *Nat Prod Res.* 2016;30(8):941-7.

[2012] Deng G, Lin H, Seidman A, et al. A phase I/II trial of a polysaccharide extract from Grifola frondosa (Maitake mushroom) in breast cancer patients: immunological effects. *J Cancer Res Clin Oncol.* 2009 Sep;135(9):1215-21.

[2013] Rajamahanty S, Louie B, O'Neill C, et al. Possible disease remission in patient with invasive bladder cancer with D-fraction regimen. *Int J Gen Med.* 2009 Jul 30;2:15-7.

[2014] Kodama N, Komuta K, Nanba H. Effect of Maitake (Grifola frondosa) D-Fraction on the activation of NK cells in cancer patients. *J Med Food.* 2003 Winter;6(4):371-7.

[2015] Hu Q, Xie B. Effect of Maitake D-fraction in advanced laryngeal and pharyngeal cancers during concurrent chemoradiotherapy: A randomized clinical trial. *Acta Biochim Pol.* 2022 Sep 7;69(3):625-632.

[2016] Chen JT, Tominaga K, Sato Y, et al. Maitake mushroom (Grifola frondosa) extract induces ovulation in patients with polycystic ovary syndrome: a possible monotherapy and a combination therapy after failure with first-line clomiphene citrate. *J Altern Complement Med.* 2010;16:1295-9.

[2017] Tsuji T, Du W, Nishioka T, et al. Phellinus linteus extract sensitizes advanced prostate cancer cells to apoptosis in athymic nude mice. *PLoS One.* 2010 Mar 31;5(3):e9885.

[2018] Zhu T, Guo J, Collins L, et al. Phellinus linteus activates different pathways to induce apoptosis in prostate cancer cells. *Br J Cancer.* 2007 Feb 26;96(4):583-90.

[2019] Collins L, Zhu T, Guo J, et al. Phellinus linteus sensitises apoptosis induced by doxorubicin in prostate cancer. *Br J Cancer.* 2006 Aug 7;95(3):282-8.

[2020] Yu K, Tan Z, Xin Y. Systematic evaluation of the anti-tumor effect of Phellinus linteus polysaccharide in thyroid carcinoma in vitro. *Mol Biol Rep.* 2022 Apr;49(4):2785-2793.

[2021] Sliva D, Jedinak A, Kawasaki J, et al. Phellinus linteus suppresses growth, angiogenesis and invasive behaviour of breast cancer cells through the inhibition of AKT signaling. *Br J Cancer.* 2008 Apr 22;98(8):1348-56.

[2022] Lu TL, Huang GJ, Lu TJ, et al. Hispolon from Phellinus linteus has antiproliferative effects via MDM2-recruited ERK1/2 activity in breast and bladder cancer cells. *Food Chem Toxicol.* 2009 Aug;47(8):2013-21.

[2023] Konno S, Chu K, Feuer N, et al. Potent Anticancer Effects of Bioactive Mushroom Extracts (Phellinus linteus) on a Variety of Human Cancer Cells. *J Clin Med Res.* 2015 Feb;7(2):76-82.

[2024] Jang EH, Jang SY, Cho IH, et al. Hispolon inhibits the growth of estrogen receptor positive human breast cancer cells through modulation of estrogen receptor alpha. *Biochem Biophys Res Commun.* 2015 Aug 7;463(4):917-22.

[2025] Lee WY, Hsu KF, Chiang TA, et al. In vitro antioxidant and anticancer activities of Smilax corbularia extract combined with Phellinus linteus extract against breast cancer cell lines. *Biomed Rep.* 2023 Aug 7;19(3):63.

[2026] Lee WY, Hsu KF, Chiang TA, et al. Phellinus linteus extract induces autophagy and synergizes with 5-fluorouracil to inhibit breast cancer cell growth. *Nutr Cancer.* 2015;67(2):275-84.

[2027] Jia X, Gao M, Li M, et al. Molecular Characterization of Two Polysaccharides from Phellinus vaninii Ljup and their Cytotoxicity to Cancer Cell Lines. *Anticancer Agents Med Chem.* 2018;18(9):1356-1363.

[2028] Lu TL, Huang GJ, Lu TJ, et al. Hispolon from Phellinus linteus has antiproliferative effects via MDM2-recruited ERK1/2 activity in breast and bladder cancer cells. *Food Chem Toxicol.* 2009 Aug;47(8):2013-21.

[2029] Konno S, Chu K, Feuer N, et al. Potent Anticancer Effects of Bioactive Mushroom Extracts (Phellinus linteus) on a Variety of Human Cancer Cells. *J Clin Med Res.* 2015 Feb;7(2):76-82.

[2030] Kuo MY, Yang WT, Ho YJ, et al. Hispolon Methyl Ether, a Hispolon Analog, Suppresses the SRC/STAT3/Survivin Signaling Axis to Induce Cytotoxicity in Human Urinary Bladder Transitional Carcinoma Cell Lines. *Int J Mol Sci.* 2022 Dec 21;24(1):138.

[2031] Masood M, Rasul A, Sarfraz I, et al. Hispolon induces apoptosis against prostate DU145 cancer cells via modulation of mitochondrial and STAT3 pathways. *Pak J Pharm Sci.* 2019 Sep;32(5(Supplementary)):2237-2243.

[2032] Chen YC, Chang HY, Deng JS, et al. Hispolon from Phellinus linteus induces G0/G1 cell cycle arrest and apoptosis in NB4 human leukaemia cells. *Am J Chin Med.* 2013;41(6):1439-57.

[2033] Hsieh MJ, Chien SY, Chou YE, et al. Hispolon from Phellinus linteus possesses mediate caspases activation and induces human nasopharyngeal carcinomas cells apoptosis through ERK1/2, JNK1/2 and p38 MAPK pathway Phytomedicine 21 (2014) 1746-1752. *Phytomedicine.* 2018 Jun 1;45:121.

[2034] Hsieh MJ, Chien SY, Chou YE, et al. Hispolon from Phellinus linteus possesses mediate caspases activation and induces human nasopharyngeal carcinomas cells apoptosis through ERK1/2, JNK1/2 and p38 MAPK pathway. *Phytomedicine.* 2014 Oct 15;21(12):1746-52.

[2035] Chen W, He FY, Li YQ. The apoptosis effect of hispolon from Phellinus linteus (Berkeley & Curtis) Teng on human epidermoid KB cells. *J Ethnopharmacol.* 2006 Apr 21;105(1-2):280-5.

[2036] Park HJ, Choi SY, Hong SM, et al. The ethyl acetate extract of Phellinus linteus grown on germinated brown rice induces G0/G1 cell cycle arrest and apoptosis in human colon carcinoma HT29 cells. *Phytother Res*. 2010 Jul;24(7):1019-26.

[2037] Bae IY, Shin JY, Lee HG. Preparation of Black Hoof medicinal mushroom Phellinus linteus (Berk. et M.A. Curt.) Teng (Aphyllophoromycetideae) beta-glucan sulfate and in vitro tumor cell growth inhibitory activity. *Int J Med Mushrooms*. 2011;13(2):115-20.

[2038] Jeon TI, Jung CH, Cho JY, et al. Identification of an anticancer compound against HT-29 cells from Phellinus linteus grown on germinated brown rice. *Asian Pac J Trop Biomed*. 2013 Oct;3(10):785-9.

[2039] Li YG, Ji DF, Zhong S, et al. Anti-tumor effects of proteoglycan from Phellinus linteus by immunomodulating and inhibiting Reg IV/EGFR/Akt signaling pathway in colorectal carcinoma. *Int J Biol Macromol*. 2011 Apr 1;48(3):511-7.

[2040] Song KS, Li G, Kim JS, et al. Protein-bound polysaccharide from Phellinus linteus inhibits tumor growth, invasion, and angiogenesis and alters Wnt/β-catenin in SW480 human colon cancer cells. *BMC Cancer*. 2011 Jul 22;11:307.

[2041] Zhong S, Ji DF, Li YG, et al. Activation of P27kip1-cyclin D1/E-CDK2 pathway by polysaccharide from Phellinus linteus leads to S-phase arrest in HT-29 cells. *Chem Biol Interact*. 2013 Nov 25;206(2):222-9.

[2042] Li G, Kim DH, Kim TD, et al. Protein-bound polysaccharide from Phellinus linteus induces G2/M phase arrest and apoptosis in SW480 human colon cancer cells. *Cancer Lett*. 2004 Dec 28;216(2):175-81.

[2043] Lim JH, Lee YM, Park SR, et al. Anticancer activity of hispidin via reactive oxygen species-mediated apoptosis in colon cancer cells. *Anticancer Res*. 2014 Aug;34(8):4087-93.

[2044] Yu T, Ganapathy S, Shen L, et al. A lethal synergy induced by phellinus linteus and camptothecin11 in colon cancer cells. *Oncotarget*. 2018 Jan 4;9(5):6308-6319.

[2045] Shin JY, Lee S, Bae IY, et al. Structural and biological study of carboxymethylated Phellinus linteus polysaccharides. *J Agric Food Chem*. 2007 May 2;55(9):3368-72.

[2046] Kim GY, Oh WK, Shin BC, et al. Proteoglycan isolated from Phellinus linteus inhibits tumor growth through mechanisms leading to an activation of CD11c+CD8+ DC and type I helper T cell-dominant immune state. *FEBS Lett*. 2004 Oct 22;576(3):391-400.

[2047] Li YG, Ji DF, Zhong S, et al. Polysaccharide from Phellinus linteus induces S-phase arrest in HepG2 cells by decreasing calreticulin expression and activating the P27kip1-cyclin A/D1/E-CDK2 pathway. *J Ethnopharmacol*. 2013 Oct 28;150(1):187-95.

[2048] Pei JJ, Wang ZB, Ma HL, et al. Structural features and antitumor activity of a novel polysaccharide from alkaline extract of Phellinus linteus mycelia. *Carbohydr Polym*. 2015 Jan 22;115:472-7.

[2049] Konno S, Chu K, Feuer N, et al. Potent Anticancer Effects of Bioactive Mushroom Extracts (Phellinus linteus) on a Variety of Human Cancer Cells. *J Clin Med Res*. 2015 Feb;7(2):76-82.

[2050] Jia X, Gao M, Li M, et al. Molecular Characterization of Two Polysaccharides from Phellinus vaninii Ljup and their Cytotoxicity to Cancer Cell Lines. *Anticancer Agents Med Chem*. 2018;18(9):1356-1363.

[2051] Jeong YK, Oh JY, Yoo JK, et al. The Biofunctional Effects of Mesima as a Radiosensitizer for Hepatocellular Carcinoma. *Int J Mol Sci*. 2020 Jan 29;21(3):871.

[2052] Yang CH, Chang HY, Chen YC, et al. Ethanol extract of Phellinus merrillii protects against diethylnitrosamine- and 2-acetylaminofluorene-induced hepatocarcinogenesis in rats. *Chin J Integr Med*. 2017 Feb;23(2):117-124.

[2053] Konno S, Chu K, Feuer N, et al. Potent Anticancer Effects of Bioactive Mushroom Extracts (Phellinus linteus) on a Variety of Human Cancer Cells. *J Clin Med Res*. 2015 Feb;7(2):76-82.

[2054] Lee JJ, Kwon HK, Lee DS, et al. Mycelial Extract of Phellinus linteus Induces Cell Death in A549 Lung Cancer Cells and Elevation of Nitric Oxide in Raw 264.7 Macrophage Cells. *Mycobiology*. 2006 Sep;34(3):143-7.

[2055] Guo J, Zhu T, Collins L, et al. Modulation of lung cancer growth arrest and apoptosis by Phellinus Linteus. *Mol Carcinog*. 2007 Feb;46(2):144-54.

[2056] Chao W, Deng JS, Li PY, et al. 3,4-Dihydroxybenzalactone Suppresses Human Non-Small Cell Lung Carcinoma Cells Metastasis via Suppression of Epithelial to Mesenchymal Transition, ROS-Mediated PI3K/AKT/MAPK/MMP and NFκB Signaling Pathways. *Molecules*. 2017 Mar 28;22(4):537.

[2057] Konno S, Chu K, Feuer N, et al. Potent Anticancer Effects of Bioactive Mushroom Extracts (Phellinus linteus) on a Variety of Human Cancer Cells. *J Clin Med Res*. 2015 Feb;7(2):76-82.

[2058] Arcella A, Oliva MA, Sanchez M, et al. Effects of hispolon on glioblastoma cell growth. *Environ Toxicol*. 2017 Sep;32(9):2113-2123.

[2059] Liao KF, Chiu TL, Chang SF, et al. Hispolon Induces Apoptosis, Suppresses Migration and Invasion of Glioblastoma Cells and Inhibits GBM Xenograft Tumor Growth In Vivo. *Molecules*. 2021 Jul 26;26(15):4497.

[2060] Choi YH, Huh MK, Ryu CH, et al. Induction of apoptotic cell death by mycelium extracts of Phellinus linteus in human neuroblastoma cells. *Int J Mol Med*. 2004 Aug;14(2):227-32.

[2061] Chandimali N, Huynh DL, Jin WY, et al. Combination Effects of Hispidin and Gemcitabine via Inhibition of Stemness in Pancreatic Cancer Stem Cells. *Anticancer Res*. 2018 Jul;38(7):3967-3975.

[2062] Kim JH, Kim YC, Park B. Hispolon from Phellinus linteus induces apoptosis and sensitizes human cancer cells to the tumor necrosis factor-related apoptosis-inducing ligand through upregulation of death receptors. *Oncol Rep*. 2016 Feb;35(2):1020-6.

[2063] Song YS, Kim SH, Sa JH, et al. Anti-angiogenic, antioxidant and xanthine oxidase inhibition activities of the mushroom Phellinus linteus. *J Ethnopharmacol*. 2003 Sep;88(1):113-6.

[2064] Yoon SK, Sung SK, Lee DH, et al. Tissue Inhibitor of Metalloproteinase-1 (TIMP-1) and IL-23 Induced by Polysaccharide of the Black Hoof Medicinal Mushroom, Phellinus linteus (Agaricomycetes). *Int J Med Mushrooms*. 2017;19(3):213-223.

[2065] Hong D, Park MJ, Jang EH, et al. Hispolon as an inhibitor of TGF-β-induced epithelial-mesenchymal transition in human epithelial cancer cells by co-regulation of TGF-β-Snail/Twist axis. *Oncol Lett*. 2017 Oct;14(4):4866-4872.

[2066] Huang GJ, Yang CM, Chang YS, et al. Hispolon suppresses SK-Hep1 human hepatoma cell metastasis by inhibiting matrix metalloproteinase-2/9 and urokinase-plasminogen activator through the PI3K/Akt and ERK signaling pathways. *J Agric Food Chem*. 2010 Sep 8;58(17):9468-75.

[2067] Huang SM, Chen JY, Chen CC, et al. Black Hoof Medicinal Mushroom Phellinus linteus (Agaricomycetes) Extracts Protect Against Radiation-Induced Hematopoietic Abnormality in Mice. *Int J Med Mushrooms*. 2016;18(5):425-31.

[2068] Mei Y, Zhu H, Hu Q, et al. A novel polysaccharide from mycelia of cultured Phellinus linteus displays antitumor activity through apoptosis. *Carbohydr Polym*. 2015 Jun 25;124:90-7.

[2069] Nakamura T, Matsugo S, Uzuka Y, et al. Fractionation and anti-tumor activity of the mycelia of liquid-cultured Phellinus linteus. *Biosci Biotechnol Biochem*. 2004 Apr;68(4):868-72.

[2070] Lee JW, Baek SJ, Bae WC, et al. Antitumor and Antioxidant Activities of the Extracts from Fruiting Body of Phellinus linteus. *Mycobiology*. 2006 Dec;34(4):230-5.

[2071] Lee HJ, Lee HJ, Lim ES, et al. Cambodian Phellinus linteus inhibits experimental metastasis of melanoma cells in mice via regulation of urokinase type plasminogen activator. *Biol Pharm Bull*. 2005 Jan;28(1):27-31.

[2072] Park HJ, Han ES, Park DK. The ethyl acetate extract of PGP (Phellinus linteus grown on Panax ginseng) suppresses B16F10 melanoma cell proliferation through inducing cellular differentiation and apoptosis. *J Ethnopharmacol*. 2010 Oct 28;132(1):115-21.

[2073] Han SB, Lee CW, Kang JS, et al. Acidic polysaccharide from Phellinus linteus inhibits melanoma cell metastasis by blocking cell adhesion and invasion. *Int Immunopharmacol*. 2006 Apr;6(4):697-702.

[2074] Han SB, Lee CW, Jeon YJ, et al. The inhibitory effect of polysaccharides isolated from Phellinus linteus on tumor growth and metastasis. *Immunopharmacology*. 1999 Feb;41(2):157-64.

[2075] Kim GY, Oh YH, Park YM. Acidic polysaccharide isolated from Phellinus linteus induces nitric oxide-mediated tumoricidal activity of macrophages through protein tyrosine kinase and protein kinase C. *Biochem Biophys Res Commun*. 2003 Sep 19;309(2):399-407.

[2076] Kim GY, Choi GS, Lee SH, et al. Acidic polysaccharide isolated from Phellinus linteus enhances through the up-regulation of nitric oxide and tumor necrosis factor-alpha from peritoneal macrophages. *J Ethnopharmacol*. 2004 Nov;95(1):69-76.

[2077] Al Saqr A, Majrashi M, Alrbyawi H, et al. Elucidating the anti-melanoma effect and mechanisms of Hispolon. *Life Sci*. 2020 Sep 1;256:117702.

[2078] Poudel I, Annaji M, Wibowo FS, et al. Hispolon Cyclodextrin Complexes and Their Inclusion in Liposomes for Enhanced Delivery in Melanoma Cell Lines. *Int J Mol Sci*. 2022 Nov 21;23(22):14487.

[2079] Chen YS, Lee SM, Lin CC, et al. Hispolon decreases melanin production and induces apoptosis in melanoma cells through the downregulation of tyrosinase and microphthalmia-associated transcription factor (MITF) expressions and the activation of caspase-3, -8 and -9. *Int J Mol Sci*. 2014 Jan 17;15(1):1201-15.

[2080] Huang HY, Chieh SY, Tso TK, et al. Orally administered mycelial culture of Phellinus linteus exhibits antitumor effects in hepatoma cell-bearing mice. *J Ethnopharmacol*. 2011 Jan 27;133(2):460-6.

[2081] Yang BK, Hwang SL, Yun IJ, et al. Antitumor Effects and Immunomodulating Activities of Phellinus linteus Extract in a CT-26 Cell-Injected Colon Cancer Mouse Model. *Mycobiology*. 2009 Jun;37(2):128-32.

[2082] Park HJ, Park JB, Lee SJ, et al. Phellinus linteus Grown on Germinated Brown Rice Increases Cetuximab Sensitivity of KRAS-Mutated Colon Cancer. *Int J Mol Sci*. 2017 Aug 11;18(8):1746.

[2083] Liu Y, Wang C, Li J, et al. Phellinus linteus polysaccharide extract improves insulin resistance by regulating gut microbiota composition. *FASEB J*. 2020 Jan;34(1):1065-1078.

[2084] Feng H, Zhang S, Wan JM, et al. Polysaccharides extracted from Phellinus linteus ameliorate high-fat high-fructose diet induced insulin resistance in mice. *Carbohydr Polym*. 2018 Nov 15;200:144-153.

[2085] Jang JS, Lee JS, Lee JH, et al. Hispidin produced from Phellinus linteus protects pancreatic beta-cells from damage by hydrogen peroxide. *Arch Pharm Res*. 2010 Jun;33(6):853-61.

[2086] Zhao C, Liao Z, Wu X, et al. Isolation, purification, and structural features of a polysaccharide from Phellinus linteus and its hypoglycemic effect in alloxan-induced diabetic mice. *J Food Sci*. 2014 May;79(5):H1002-10.

[2087] Liu Y, Wang C, Li J, et al. Hypoglycemic and Hypolipidemic Effects of Phellinus Linteus Mycelial Extract from Solid-State Culture in A Rat Model of Type 2 Diabetes. *Nutrients*. 2019 Jan 30;11(2):296.

[2088] Yamac M, Zeytinoglu M, Senturk H, et al. Effects of Black Hoof Medicinal Mushroom, Phellinus linteus (Agaricomycetes), Polysaccharide Extract in Streptozotocin-Induced Diabetic Rats. *Int J Med Mushrooms*. 2016;18(4):301-11.

[2089] Lee YS, Kang YH, Jung JY, et al. Inhibitory constituents of aldose reductase in the fruiting body of Phellinus linteus. *Biol Pharm Bull*. 2008 Apr;31(4):765-8.

[2090] Kim HM, Kang JS, Kim JY, et al. Evaluation of antidiabetic activity of polysaccharide isolated from Phellinus linteus in non-obese diabetic mouse. *Int Immunopharmacol*. 2010 Jan;10(1):72-8.

[2091] Lee YS, Kang IJ, Won MH, et al. Inhibition of protein tyrosine phosphatase 1beta by hispidin derivatives isolated from the fruiting body of Phellinus linteus. *Nat Prod Commun*. 2010 Dec;5(12):1927-30.

[2092] Wu F, Shang C, Jin T, et al. Hispidin Inhibits Ferroptosis Induced by High Glucose via the miR-15b-5p/GLS2 Axis in Pancreatic Beta Cells. *Evid Based Complement Alternat Med*. 2023 Feb 21;2023:9428241.

[2093] Song TY, Yang NC, Chen CL, et al. Protective Effects and Possible Mechanisms of Ergothioneine and Hispidin against Methylglyoxal-Induced Injuries in Rat Pheochromocytoma Cells. *Oxid Med Cell Longev*. 2017;2017:4824371.

[2094] Liu Y, Wang C, Li J, et al. Hypoglycemic and Hypolipidemic Effects of Phellinus Linteus Mycelial Extract from Solid-State Culture in A Rat Model of Type 2 Diabetes. *Nutrients*. 2019 Jan 30;11(2):296.

[2095] Li XH, Li Y, Cheng ZY, Cai XG, et al. The Effects of Phellinus linteus Polysaccharide Extracts on Cholesterol Efflux in Oxidized Low-Density Lipoprotein-Loaded THP-1 Macrophages. *J Investig Med*. 2015 Jun;63(5):752-7.

[2096] Zou X, Guo X, Sun M. pH control strategy in a shaken minibioreactor for polysaccharide production by medicinal mushroom Phellinus linteus and its anti-hyperlipemia activity. *Bioprocess Biosyst Eng*. 2009 Feb;32(2):277-81.

[2097] Liu Y, Wang C, Li J, et al. Phellinus linteus polysaccharide extract improves insulin resistance by regulating gut microbiota composition. *FASEB J*. 2020 Jan;34(1):1065-1078.

[2098] Liu T, Zhao M, Zhang Y, et al. Integrated microbiota and metabolite profiling analysis of prebiotic characteristics of Phellinus linteus polysaccharide in vitro fermentation. *Int J Biol Macromol*. 2023 Jul 1;242(Pt 2):124854.

[2099] Suh MG, Shin HY, Jeong EJ, et al. Identification of galacturonic acid-rich polysaccharide with intestinal immune system modulating activity via Peyer's patch from postbiotics of Phellinus linteus mycelial submerged culture. *Int J Biol Macromol.* 2023 Apr 15;234:123685.

[2100] Choi DJ, Cho S, Seo JY, et al. Neuroprotective effects of the Phellinus linteus ethyl acetate extract against H2O2-induced apoptotic cell death of SK-N-MC cells. *Nutr Res.* 2016 Jan;36(1):31-43.

[2101] Suzuki S, Kawamata T, Okada Y, et al. Filtrate of Phellinus linteus Broth Culture Reduces Infarct Size Significantly in a Rat Model of Permanent Focal Cerebral Ischemia. *Evid Based Complement Alternat Med.* 2011;2011:326319.

[2102] Peng S, Hou Y, Chen Z. Hispolon alleviates oxidative damage by stimulating the Nrf2 signaling pathway in PC12 cells. *Arch Biochem Biophys.* 2022 Sep 30;727:109303.

[2103] Wu MS, Chien CC, Cheng KT, et al. Hispolon Suppresses LPS- or LTA-Induced iNOS/NO Production and Apoptosis in BV-2 Microglial Cells. *Am J Chin Med.* 2017;45(8):1649-1666.

[2104] Jin MH, Chen DQ, Jin YH, et al. Hispidin inhibits LPS-induced nitric oxide production in BV-2 microglial cells via ROS-dependent MAPK signaling. *Exp Ther Med.* 2021 Sep;22(3):970.

[2105] Park IH, Jeon SY, Lee HJ, et al. A beta-secretase (BACE1) inhibitor hispidin from the mycelial cultures of Phellinus linteus. *Planta Med.* 2004 Feb;70(2):143-6.

[2106] Kwon Y, Haam CE, Byeon S, et al. Vasodilatory Effect of Phellinus linteus Extract in Rat Mesenteric Arteries. *Molecules.* 2020 Jul 10;25(14):3160.

[2107] Lee SJ, Lee DH, Kim HW. Novel Antihypertension Mechanism of β-Glucan by Corin and ANP-Mediated Natriuresis in Mice. *Mycobiology.* 2020 Sep 8;48(5):399-409.

[2108] Su HH, Chu YC, Liao JM, et al. Phellinus linteus Mycelium Alleviates Myocardial Ischemia-Reperfusion Injury through Autophagic Regulation. *Front Pharmacol.* 2017 Apr 4;8:175.

[2109] Kim DE, Kim B, Shin HS, et al. The protective effect of hispidin against hydrogen peroxide-induced apoptosis in H9c2 cardiomyoblast cells through Akt/GSK-3β and ERK1/2 signaling pathway. *Exp Cell Res.* 2014 Oct 1;327(2):264-75.

[2110] Zhao L, Zheng L, Li Z, et al. Phellinus linteus polysaccharides mediates acetaminophen-induced hepatotoxicity via activating AMPK/Nrf2 signaling pathways. *Aging (Albany NY).* 2022 Sep 1;14(17):6993-7002.

[2111] Chen C, Liu X, Qi S, et al. Hepatoprotective effect of Phellinus linteus mycelia polysaccharide (PL-N1) against acetaminophen-induced liver injury in mouse. *Int J Biol Macromol.* 2020 Jul 1;154:1276-1284.

[2112] Gao C, Zhong L, Jiang L, et al. Phellinus linteus mushroom protects against tacrine-induced mitochondrial impairment and oxidative stress in HepG2 cells. *Phytomedicine.* 2013 Jun 15;20(8-9):705-9.

[2113] Huang SC, Wang PW, Kuo PC, et al. Hepatoprotective Principles and Other Chemical Constituents from the Mycelium of Phellinus linteus. *Molecules.* 2018 Jul 12;23(7):1705.

[2114] Kim SH, Lee HS, Lee S, et al. Mycelial culture of Phellinus linteus protects primary cultured rat hepatocytes against hepatotoxins. *J Ethnopharmacol.* 2004 Dec;95(2-3):367-72.

[2115] Jeon TI, Hwang SG, Lim BO, et al. Extracts of Phellinus linteus grown on germinated brown rice suppress liver damage induced by carbon tetrachloride in rats. *Biotechnol Lett.* 2003 Dec;25(24):2093-6.

[2116] Chiu CH, Chang CC, Lin JJ, et al. Styrylpyrones from Phellinus linteus Mycelia Alleviate Non-Alcoholic Fatty Liver by Modulating Lipid and Glucose Metabolic Homeostasis in High-Fat and High-Fructose Diet-Fed Mice. *Antioxidants (Basel).* 2022 Apr 30;11(5):898.

[2117] Chiu CH, Chen MY, Lieu JJ, et al. Inhibitory Effect of Styrylpyrone Extract of Phellinus linteus on Hepatic Steatosis in HepG2 Cells. *Int J Mol Sci.* 2023 Feb 12;24(4):3672.

[2118] Huang SC, Kuo PC, Hung HY, et al. Ionone Derivatives from the Mycelium of Phellinus linteus and the Inhibitory Effect on Activated Rat Hepatic Stellate Cells. *Int J Mol Sci.* 2016 May 6;17(5):681.

[2119] Wang H, Wu G, Park HJ, et al. Protective effect of Phellinus linteus polysaccharide extracts against thioacetamide-induced liver fibrosis in rats: a proteomics analysis. *Chin Med.* 2012 Oct 18;7(1):23.

[2120] Wan F, Yang RC, Shi YP, et al. The protective effect of Phellinus linteus decoction on podocyte injury in the kidney of FSGS rats. *BMC Complement Altern Med.* 2019 Oct 21;19(1):272.

[2121] Feng W, Ruchun Y, Yuewen T. Uncovering pharmacological mechanisms of Phellinus linteus on focal segmental glomeruloscleosis rats through tandem mass tag-based quantitative proteomic analysis, network pharmacology analysis and experimental validation. *J Tradit Chin Med.* 2023 Aug;43(4):744-750.

[2122] Su X, Liu K, Xie Y, et al. Protective effect of a polyphenols-rich extract from Inonotus Sanghuang on bleomycin-induced acute lung injury in mice. *Life Sci.* 2019 Aug 1;230:208-217.

[2123] Chao W, Deng JS, Huang SS, et al. 3, 4-dihydroxybenzalacetone attenuates lipopolysaccharide-induced inflammation in acute lung injury via down-regulation of MMP-2 and MMP-9 activities through suppressing ROS-mediated MAPK and PI3K/AKT signaling pathways. *Int Immunopharmacol.* 2017 Sep;50:77-86.

[2124] Kim JH, Kwon HJ, Kim BW. Protective Effect of 4-(3,4-Dihydroxyphenyl)-3-Buten-2-One from Phellinus linteus on Naproxen-Induced Gastric Antral Ulcers in Rats. *J Microbiol Biotechnol.* 2016 May 28;26(5):823-8.

[2125] Lee JH, Lee SJ, Choi YH, et al. Effects of mycelial culture of Phellinus linteus on ethanol-induced gastric ulcer in rats. *Phytother Res.* 2006 May;20(5):396-402.

[2126] Min BS, Yun BS, Lee HK, et al. Two novel furan derivatives from Phellinus linteus with anti-complement activity. *Bioorg Med Chem Lett.* 2006 Jun 15;16(12):3255-7.

[2127] Yan GH, Choi YH. Phellinus linteus Extract Exerts Anti-asthmatic Effects by Suppressing NF-κB and p38 MAPK Activity in an OVA-induced Mouse Model of Asthma. *Immune Netw.* 2014 Apr;14(2):107-15.

[2128] Kwon HK, Park HJ. Phellinus linteus Grown on Germinated Brown Rice Inhibits IgE-Mediated Allergic Activity through the Suppression of FcεRI-Dependent Signaling Pathway In Vitro and In Vivo. *Evid Based Complement Alternat Med.* 2019 Nov 29;2019:1485015.

[2129] Park HJ. Anti-allergic and anti-inflammatory activity of Phellinus linteus grown on Panax ginseng. *Food Sci Biotechnol.* 2017 Apr 30;26(2):467-472.

[2130] Lim BO, Yamada K, Cho BG, et al. Comparative study on the modulation of IgE and cytokine production by Phellinus linteus grown on germinated brown Rice, Phellinus Linteus and germinated brown rice in murine splenocytes. *Biosci Biotechnol Biochem*. 2004 Nov;68(11):2391-4.

[2131] Lim BO, Jeon TI, Hwang SG, et al. Phellinus linteus grown on germinated brown rice suppresses IgE production by the modulation of Th1/Th2 balance in murine mesenteric lymph node lymphocytes. *Biotechnol Lett*. 2005 May;27(9):613-7.

[2132] Choi YH, Yan GH, Chai OH, et al. Inhibition of anaphylaxis-like reaction and mast cell activation by water extract from the fruiting body of Phellinus linteus. *Biol Pharm Bull*. 2006 Jul;29(7):1360-5.

[2133] Inagaki N, Shibata T, Itoh T, et al. Inhibition of IgE-dependent mouse triphasic cutaneous reaction by a boiling water fraction separated from mycelium of Phellinus linteus. *Evid Based Complement Alternat Med*. 2005 Sep;2(3):369-74.

[2134] Shin MR, Lee JH, Lee JA, et al. Immunomodulatory and anti-inflammatory effects of Phellinus linteus mycelium. *BMC Complement Med Ther*. 2021 Oct 26;21(1):269.

[2135] Matsuba S, Matsuno H, Sakuma M, et al. Phellinus linteus Extract Augments the Immune Response in Mitomycin C-Induced Immunodeficient Mice. *Evid Based Complement Alternat Med*. 2008 Mar;5(1):85-90.

[2136] Song KS, Cho SM, Lee JH, et al. B-lymphocyte-stimulating polysaccharide from mushroom Phellinus linteus. *Chem Pharm Bull (Tokyo)*. 1995 Dec;43(12):2105-8.

[2137] Harikrishnan R, Balasundaram C, Heo MS. Diet enriched with mushroom Phellinus linteus extract enhances the growth, innate immune response, and disease resistance of kelp grouper, Epinephelus bruneus against vibriosis. *Fish Shellfish Immunol*. 2011 Jan;30(1):128-34.

[2138] Oh GS, Lee MS, Pae HO, et al. Effects of oral administration of Phellinus linteus on the production of Th1- and Th2-type cytokines in mice. *Immunopharmacol Immunotoxicol*. 2006;28(2):281-93.

[2139] Kim GY, Park SK, Lee MK, et al. Proteoglycan isolated from Phellinus linteus activates murine B lymphocytes via protein kinase C and protein tyrosine kinase. *Int Immunopharmacol*. 2003 Sep;3(9):1281-92.

[2140] Kim GY, Han MG, Song YS, et al. Proteoglycan isolated from Phellinus linteus induces toll-like receptors 2- and 4-mediated maturation of murine dendritic cells via activation of ERK, p38, and NF-kappaB. *Biol Pharm Bull*. 2004 Oct;27(10):1656-62.

[2141] Park SK, Kim GY, Lim JY, et al. Acidic polysaccharides isolated from Phellinus linteus induce phenotypic and functional maturation of murine dendritic cells. *Biochem Biophys Res Commun*. 2003 Dec 12;312(2):449-58.

[2142] Kim GY, Lee JY, Lee JO, et al. Partial characterization and immunostimulatory effect of a novel polysaccharide-protein complex extracted from Phellinus linteus. *Biosci Biotechnol Biochem*. 2006 May;70(5):1218-26.

[2143] Lee JH, Cho SM, Song KS, et al. Characterization of carbohydrate-peptide linkage of acidic heteroglycopeptide with immuno-stimulating activity from mycelium of Phellinus linteus. *Chem Pharm Bull (Tokyo)*. 1996 May;44(5):1093-5.

[2144] Kim HM, Han SB, Oh GT, et al. Stimulation of humoral and cell mediated immunity by polysaccharide from mushroom Phellinus linteus. *Int J Immunopharmacol*. 1996 May;18(5):295-303.

[2145] Lin CJ, Lien HM, Lin HJ, et al. Modulation of T cell response by Phellinus linteus. *J Biosci Bioeng*. 2016 Jan;121(1):84-88.

[2146] Suabjakyong P, Nishimura K, Toida T, et al. Structural characterization and immunomodulatory effects of polysaccharides from Phellinus linteus and Phellinus igniarius on the IL-6/IL-10 cytokine balance of the mouse macrophage cell lines (RAW 264.7). *Food Funct*. 2015 Aug;6(8):2834-44.

[2147] Lim BO, Yamada K, Cho BG, et al. Comparative study on the modulation of IgE and cytokine production by Phellinus linteus grown on germinated brown Rice, Phellinus Linteus and germinated brown rice in murine splenocytes. *Biosci Biotechnol Biochem*. 2004 Nov;68(11):2391-4.

[2148] Lee EK, Koh EM, Kim YN, et al. Immunomodulatory Effect of Hispolon on LPS-Induced RAW264.7 Cells and Mitogen/Alloantigen-Stimulated Spleen Lymphocytes of Mice. *Pharmaceutics*. 2022 Jul 6;14(7):1423.

[2149] Kim GY, Roh SI, Park SK, et al. Alleviation of experimental septic shock in mice by acidic polysaccharide isolated from the medicinal mushroom Phellinus linteus. *Biol Pharm Bull*. 2003 Oct;26(10):1418-23.

[2150] Bae JS, Jang KH, Jin HK. Comparison of intraperitoneal anti-adhesive polysaccharides derived from Phellinus mushrooms in a rat peritonitis model. *World J Gastroenterol*. 2005 Feb 14;11(6):810-6.

[2151] Bae JS, Ahn SJ, Yim H, et al. Prevention of intraperitoneal adhesions and abscesses by polysaccharides isolated from Phellinus spp in a rat peritonitis model. *Ann Surg*. 2005 Mar;241(3):534-40.

[2152] Chang HY, Sheu MJ, Yang CH, et al. Analgesic effects and the mechanisms of anti-inflammation of hispolon in mice. *Evid Based Complement Alternat Med*. 2011;2011:478246.

[2153] Shin MR, Lee JH, Lee JA, et al. Immunomodulatory and anti-inflammatory effects of Phellinus linteus mycelium. *BMC Complement Med Ther*. 2021 Oct 26;21(1):269.

[2154] Lin CJ, Lien HM, Chang HY, et al. Biological evaluation of Phellinus linteus-fermented broths as anti-inflammatory agents. *J Biosci Bioeng*. 2014 Jul;118(1):88-93.

[2155] Kim HG, Yoon DH, Lee WH, et al. Phellinus linteus inhibits inflammatory mediators by suppressing redox-based NF-kappaB and MAPKs activation in lipopolysaccharide-induced RAW 264.7 macrophage. *J Ethnopharmacol*. 2007 Dec 3;114(3):307-15.

[2156] Song M, Park HJ. Anti-inflammatory effect of Phellinus linteus grown on germinated brown rice on dextran sodium sulfate-induced acute colitis in mice and LPS-activated macrophages. *J Ethnopharmacol*. 2014 Jun 11;154(2):311-8.

[2157] Xie Z, Wang Y, Huang J, et al. Anti-inflammatory activity of polysaccharides from Phellinus linteus by regulating the NF-κB translocation in LPS-stimulated RAW264.7 macrophages. *Int J Biol Macromol*. 2019 May 15;129:61-67.

[2158] Park HJ. Anti-allergic and anti-inflammatory activity of Phellinus linteus grown on Panax ginseng. *Food Sci Biotechnol*. 2017 Apr 30;26(2):467-472.

[2159] Hu T, Lin Q, Guo T, et al. Polysaccharide isolated from Phellinus linteus mycelia exerts anti-inflammatory effects via MAPK and PPAR signaling pathways. *Carbohydr Polym*. 2018 Nov 15;200:487-497.

[2160] Park HJ, Han ES, Park DK, et al. An extract of Phellinus linteus grown on germinated brown rice inhibits inflammation markers in RAW264.7 macrophages by suppressing inflammatory cytokines, chemokines, and mediators and up-regulating antioxidant activity. *J Med Food*. 2010 Dec;13(6):1468-77.

[2161] Huang GJ, Huang SS, Deng JS. Anti-inflammatory activities of inotilone from Phellinus linteus through the inhibition of MMP-9, NF-κB, and MAPK activation in vitro and in vivo. *PLoS One*. 2012;7(5):e35922.

[2162] Kim SH, Song YS, Kim SK, et al. Anti-inflammatory and related pharmacological activities of the n-BuOH subfraction of mushroom Phellinus linteus. *J Ethnopharmacol.* 2004 Jul;93(1):141-6.

[2163] Kim BC, Jeon WK, Hong HY, et al. The anti-inflammatory activity of Phellinus linteus (Berk. & M.A. Curt.) is mediated through the PKCdelta/Nrf2/ARE signaling to up-regulation of heme oxygenase-1. *J Ethnopharmacol.* 2007 Sep 5;113(2):240-7.

[2164] Kim BC, Choi JW, Hong HY, et al. Heme oxygenase-1 mediates the anti-inflammatory effect of mushroom Phellinus linteus in LPS-stimulated RAW264.7 macrophages. *J Ethnopharmacol.* 2006 Jul 19;106(3):364-71.

[2165] Chang HY, Sheu MJ, Yang CH, et al. Analgesic effects and the mechanisms of anti-inflammation of hispolon in mice. *Evid Based Complement Alternat Med.* 2011;2011:478246.

[2166] Yang LY, Shen SC, Cheng KT, et al. Hispolon inhibition of inflammatory apoptosis through reduction of iNOS/NO production via HO-1 induction in macrophages. *J Ethnopharmacol.* 2014 Oct 28;156:61-72.

[2167] Kim GY, Kim SH, Hwang SY, et al. Oral administration of proteoglycan isolated from Phellinus linteus in the prevention and treatment of collagen-induced arthritis in mice. *Biol Pharm Bull.* 2003 Jun;26(6):823-31.

[2168] Shin MR, Lee JA, Kim MJ, et al. Protective Effects of Phellinus linteus Mycelium on the Development of Osteoarthritis after Monosodium Iodoacetate Injection. *Evid Based Complement Alternat Med.* 2020 Aug 15;2020:7240858.

[2169] Kim IH, Chung MY, Shin JY, et al. Protective Effects of Black Hoof Medicinal Mushroom from Korea, Phellinus linteus (Higher Basidiomycetes), on Osteoporosis In Vitro and In Vivo. *Int J Med Mushrooms.* 2016;18(1):39-47.

[2170] Kim YN, Kim MS, Chun SS, et al. Effect of Phellius linteus water extract on benign prostatic hyperplasia. *Nutr Res Pract.* 2013 Jun;7(3):172-7.

[2171] Shibata Y, Kashiwagi B, Arai S, et al. Administration of extract of mushroom Phellinus linteus induces prostate enlargement with increase in stromal component in experimentally developed rat model of benign prostatic hyperplasia. *Urology.* 2005 Aug;66(2):455-60.

[2172] Seo JH, Sung YH, Kim KJ, et al. Effects of Phellinus linteus administration on serotonin synthesis in the brain and expression of monocarboxylate transporters in the muscle during exhaustive exercise in rats. *J Nutr Sci Vitaminol (Tokyo).* 2011;57(1):95-103.

[2173] Lin CH, Shih CC. Potential Protective Activities of Extracts of Phellinus linteus and the Altered Expressions of GSTM3 on Age-Related Cataract. *Evid Based Complement Alternat Med.* 2021 Jan 21;2021:4313805.

[2174] Lee JK, Jang JH, Lee JT, et al. Extraction and Characteristics of Anti-obesity Lipase Inhibitor from Phellinus linteus. *Mycobiology.* 2010 Mar;38(1):52-7.

[2175] Lee JK, Song JH, Lee JS. Optimal Extraction Conditions of Anti-obesity Lipase Inhibitor from Phellinus linteus and Nutritional Characteristics of the Extracts. *Mycobiology.* 2010 Mar;38(1):58-61.

[2176] Hwang BS, Lee MS, Lee SW, et al. Neuraminidase Inhibitors from the Fermentation Broth of Phellinus linteus. *Mycobiology.* 2014 Jun;42(2):189-92.

[2177] Yeom JH, Lee IK, Ki DW, et al. Neuraminidase Inhibitors from the Culture Broth of Phellinus linteus. *Mycobiology.* 2012 Jun;40(2):142-4.

[2178] Gao N, Zhang W, Hu D, et al. Study on Extraction, Physicochemical Properties, and Bacterio-Static Activity of Polysaccharides from Phellinus linteus. *Molecules.* 2023 Jun 29;28(13):5102.

[2179] Contato AG, de Araújo CAV, Zanzarin DM, et al. Biological Characterization and Antimicrobial Bioactives of Mycelium Extracts from Medicinal Mushrooms Phellinus linteus and Pleurotus albidus (Agaricomycetes). *Int J Med Mushrooms.* 2022;24(6):47-55.

[2180] Hur JM, Yang CH, Han SH, et al. Antibacterial effect of Phellinus linteus against methicillin-resistant Staphylococcus aureus. *Fitoterapia.* 2004 Sep;75(6):603-5.

[2181] Shirahata T, Ino C, Mizuno F, et al. γ-Ionylidene-type sesquiterpenoids possessing antimicrobial activity against Porphyromonas gingivalis from Phellinus linteus and their absolute structure determination. *J Antibiot (Tokyo).* 2017 May;70(5):695-698.

[2182] Cho JY, Kwon YJ, Sohn MJ, et al. Phellinstatin, a new inhibitor of enoyl-ACP reductase produced by the medicinal fungus Phellinus linteus. *Bioorg Med Chem Lett.* 2011 Mar 15;21(6):1716-8.

[2183] Hwang JS, Kwon HK, Kim JE, et al. Immunomodulatory effect of water soluble extract separated from mycelium of Phellinus linteus on experimental atopic dermatitis. *BMC Complement Altern Med.* 2012 Sep 18;12:159.

[2184] Han J, Wu T, Jin J, et al. Exosome-like nanovesicles derived from Phellinus linteus inhibit Mical2 expression through cross-kingdom regulation and inhibit ultraviolet-induced skin aging. *J Nanobiotechnology.* 2022 Oct 21;20(1):455.

[2185] Ahn HY, Choo YM, Cho YS. Anti-Pigmentation Effects of Eight Phellinus linteus-Fermented Traditional Crude Herbal Extracts on Brown Guinea Pigs of Ultraviolet B-Induced Hyperpigmentation. *J Microbiol Biotechnol.* 2018 Mar 28;28(3):375-380.

[2186] Kang HS, Choi JH, Cho WK, et al. A sphingolipid and tyrosinase inhibitors from the fruiting body of Phellinus linteus. *Arch Pharm Res.* 2004 Jul;27(7):742-50.

[2187] Lee IS, Bae K, Kuk Yoo J, et al. Inhibition of human neutrophil elastase by ergosterol derivatives from the mycelium of Phellinus linteus. *J Antibiot (Tokyo).* 2012 Aug;65(8):437-40.

[2188] Mukai M, Kasai A, Hiramatsu N, et al. Blockade of the aryl hydrocarbon receptor pathway triggered by dioxin, polycyclic aromatic hydrocarbons and cigarette smoke by Phellinus linteus. *Biol Pharm Bull.* 2008 Oct;31(10):1888-93.

[2189] Lee YS, Kang YH, Jung JY, et al. Protein glycation inhibitors from the fruiting body of Phellinus linteus. *Biol Pharm Bull.* 2008 Oct;31(10):1968-72.

[2190] Chen W, Shen Y, Su H, et al. Hispidin derived from Phellinus linteus affords protection against acrylamide-induced oxidative stress in Caco-2 cells. *Chem Biol Interact.* 2014 Aug 5;219:83-9.

[2191] Chen W, Feng L, Huang Z, et al. Hispidin produced from Phellinus linteus protects against peroxynitrite-mediated DNA damage and hydroxyl radical generation. *Chem Biol Interact.* 2012 Sep 30;199(3):137-42.

[2192] Lee JH, Lee JS, Kim YR, et al. Hispidin isolated from Phellinus linteus protects against hydrogen peroxide-induced oxidative stress in pancreatic MIN6N β-cells. *J Med Food.* 2011 Nov;14(11):1431-8.

2193 Ye SF, Hou ZQ, Zhang QQ. Protective effects of Phellinus linteus extract against iron overload-mediated oxidative stress in cultured rat hepatocytes. *Phytother Res.* 2007 Oct;21(10):948-53.

2194 Park JM, Lee JS, Song JE, et al. Cytoprotective effect of hispidin against palmitate-induced lipotoxicity in C2C12 myotubes. *Molecules.* 2015 Mar 27;20(4):5456-67.

2195 Shon YH, Nam KS. Antimutagenicity and induction of anticarcinogenic phase II enzymes by basidiomycetes. *J Ethnopharmacol.* 2001 Sep;77(1):103-9.

2196 Wu Y, Liu H, Li Z, et al. Purification of polysaccharides from Phellinus linteus by using an aqueous two-phase system and evaluation of the physicochemical and antioxidant properties of polysaccharides in vitro. *Prep Biochem Biotechnol.* 2022;52(1):89-98.

2197 Lee MS, Hwang BS, Lee IK, et al. Chemical Constituents of the Culture Broth of Phellinus linteus and Their Antioxidant Activity. *Mycobiology.* 2015 Mar;43(1):43-8.

2198 Yan JK, Wang YY, Wang ZB, et al. Structure and antioxidative property of a polysaccharide from an ammonium oxalate extract of Phellinus linteus. *Int J Biol Macromol.* 2016 Oct;91:92-9.

2199 Song YS, Kim SH, Sa JH, et al. Anti-angiogenic, antioxidant and xanthine oxidase inhibition activities of the mushroom Phellinus linteus. *J Ethnopharmacol.* 2003 Sep;88(1):113-6.

2200 Wang ZB, Pei JJ, Ma HL, et al. Effect of extraction media on preliminary characterizations and antioxidant activities of Phellinus linteus polysaccharides. *Carbohydr Polym.* 2014 Aug 30;109:49-55.

2201 Yan JK, Wang YY, Ma HL, et al. Ultrasonic effects on the degradation kinetics, preliminary characterization and antioxidant activities of polysaccharides from Phellinus linteus mycelia. *Ultrason Sonochem.* 2016 Mar;29:251-7.

2202 Park IH, Chung SK, Lee KB, et al. An antioxidant hispidin from the mycelial cultures of Phellinus linteus. *Arch Pharm Res.* 2004 Jun;27(6):615-8.

2203 El Hassane A, Shah SA, Hassan NB, et al. Antioxidant activity of hispidin oligomers from medicinal fungi: a DFT study. *Molecules.* 2014 Mar 21;19(3):3489-507.

2204 Ku YH, Kang JH, Lee H. Effects of Phellinus linteus extract on immunity improvement: A CONSORT-randomized, double-blinded, placebo-controlled trial. *Medicine (Baltimore).* 2022 Aug 26;101(34):e30226.

2205 Ryu HY, Lee H, Kang J. A Pilot Clinical Study of the Efficacy and Safety of Phellinus Linteus (Sanghuang) Extract Treatment for Knee Osteoarthritis. *J Acupuncture Res.* 2022 May;39(2):115-121.

2206 Shibata Y, Kurita S, Okugi H, et al. Dramatic remission of hormone refractory prostate cancer achieved with extract of the mushroom, Phellinus linteus. *Urol Int.* 2004;73(2):188-90.

2207 Kojima H, Tanigawa N, Kariya S, et al. A case of spontaneous regression of hepatocellular carcinoma with multiple lung metastases. *Radiat Med.* 2006 Feb;24(2):139-42.

2208 Lee SH, Hwang HK, Kang CM, et al. Potential Impact of Phellinus linteus on Adherence to Adjuvant Treatment After Curative Resection of Pancreatic Ductal Adenocarcinoma: Outcomes of a Propensity Score-Matched Analysis. *Integr Cancer Ther.* 2019 Jan-Dec;18:1534735418816825.

2209 Hamad D, El-Sayed H, Ahmed W, et al. GC-MS Analysis of Potentially Volatile Compounds of Pleurotus ostreatus Polar Extract: In vitro Antimicrobial, Cytotoxic, Immunomodulatory, and Antioxidant Activities. *Front Microbiol.* 2022 Feb 18;13:834525.

2210 Bakir T, Karadeniz M, Unal S. Investigation of antioxidant activities of Pleurotus ostreatus stored at different temperatures. *Food Sci Nutr.* 2018 Apr 16;6(4):1040-1044.

2211 Jedinak A, Sliva D. Pleurotus ostreatus inhibits proliferation of human breast and colon cancer cells through p53-dependent as well as p53-independent pathway. *Int J Oncol.* 2008 Dec;33(6):1307-13.

2212 Khan AA, Gani A, Ahmad M, et al. Mushroom varieties found in the Himalayan regions of India: Antioxidant, antimicrobial, and antiproliferative activities. *Food Sci Biotechnol.* 2016 Aug 31;25(4):1095-1100.

2213 Arora S, Goyal S, Balani J, et al. Enhanced antiproliferative effects of aqueous extracts of some medicinal mushrooms on colon cancer cells. *Int J Med Mushrooms.* 2013;15(3):301-14.

2214 Elbatrawy EN, Ghonimy EA, Alassar MM, et al. Medicinal Mushroom Extracts Possess Differential Antioxidant Activity and Cytotoxicity to Cancer Cells. *Int J Med Mushrooms.* 2015;17(5):471-9.

2215 Elhusseiny SM, El-Mahdy TS, Awad MF, et al. Proteome Analysis and In Vitro Antiviral, Anticancer and Antioxidant Capacities of the Aqueous Extracts of Lentinula edodes and Pleurotus ostreatus Edible Mushrooms. *Molecules.* 2021 Jul 30;26(15):4623.

2216 Gu YH, Sivam G. Cytotoxic effect of oyster mushroom Pleurotus ostreatus on human androgen-independent prostate cancer PC-3 cells. *J Med Food.* 2006 Summer;9(2):196-204.

2217 Silva S, Martins S, Karmali A, et al. Production, purification and characterisation of polysaccharides from Pleurotus ostreatus with antitumour activity. *J Sci Food Agric.* 2012 Jul;92(9):1826-32.

2218 Elhusseiny SM, El-Mahdy TS, Awad MF, et al. Proteome Analysis and In Vitro Antiviral, Anticancer and Antioxidant Capacities of the Aqueous Extracts of Lentinula edodes and Pleurotus ostreatus Edible Mushrooms. *Molecules.* 2021 Jul 30;26(15):4623.

2219 Arora S, Goyal S, Balani J, et al. Enhanced antiproliferative effects of aqueous extracts of some medicinal mushrooms on colon cancer cells. *Int J Med Mushrooms.* 2013;15(3):301-14.

2220 Elhusseiny SM, El-Mahdy TS, Awad MF, et al. Proteome Analysis and In Vitro Antiviral, Anticancer and Antioxidant Capacities of the Aqueous Extracts of Lentinula edodes and Pleurotus ostreatus Edible Mushrooms. *Molecules.* 2021 Jul 30;26(15):4623.

2221 Wu JY, Chen CH, Chang WH, et al. Anti-Cancer Effects of Protein Extracts from Calvatia lilacina, Pleurotus ostreatus and Volvariella volvacea. *Evid Based Complement Alternat Med.* 2011;2011:982368.

2222 Lavi I, Friesem D, Geresh S, et al. An aqueous polysaccharide extract from the edible mushroom Pleurotus ostreatus induces anti-proliferative and pro-apoptotic effects on HT-29 colon cancer cells. *Cancer Lett.* 2006 Nov 28;244(1):61-70.

2223 Jedinak A, Sliva D. Pleurotus ostreatus inhibits proliferation of human breast and colon cancer cells through p53-dependent as well as p53-independent pathway. *Int J Oncol.* 2008 Dec;33(6):1307-13.

[2224] Zusman I, Reifen R, Livni O, et al. Role of apoptosis, proliferating cell nuclear antigen and p53 protein in chemically induced colon cancer in rats fed corncob fiber treated with the fungus Pleurotus ostreatus. *Anticancer Res*. 1997 May-Jun;17(3C):2105-13.

[2225] Khan AA, Gani A, Ahmad M, et al. Mushroom varieties found in the Himalayan regions of India: Antioxidant, antimicrobial, and antiproliferative activities. *Food Sci Biotechnol*. 2016 Aug 31;25(4):1095-1100.

[2226] Arora S, Goyal S, Balani J, et al. Enhanced antiproliferative effects of aqueous extracts of some medicinal mushrooms on colon cancer cells. *Int J Med Mushrooms*. 2013;15(3):301-14.

[2227] Garmanchuk LV, Vedenicheva NP, Al-Maali GA, et al. ANTIPROLIFERATIVE ACTIVITIES Of EXTRACTS FROM MYCELIAL BIOMASS OF SOME MEDICINAL BASIDIOMYCETES IN HUMAN COLON CANCER CELLS COLO 205. *Exp Oncol*. 2022 Nov;44(3):213-216.

[2228] Arora S, Tandon S. Mushroom Extracts Induce Human Colon Cancer Cell (COLO-205) Death by Triggering the Mitochondrial Apoptosis Pathway and Go/G1-Phase Cell Cycle Arrest. *Arch Iran Med*. 2015 May;18(5):284-95.

[2229] Bobek P, Galbavy S. Effect of pleuran (beta-glucan from Pleurotus ostreatus) on the antioxidant status of the organism and on dimethylhydrazine-induced precancerous lesions in rat colon. *Br J Biomed Sci*. 2001;58(3):164-8.

[2230] Jedinak A, Dudhgaonkar S, Jiang J, et al. Pleurotus ostreatus inhibits colitis-related colon carcinogenesis in mice. *Int J Mol Med*. 2010 Nov;26(5):643-50.

[2231] Elhusseiny SM, El-Mahdy TS, Awad MF, et al. Proteome Analysis and In Vitro Antiviral, Anticancer and Antioxidant Capacities of the Aqueous Extracts of Lentinula edodes and Pleurotus ostreatus Edible Mushrooms. *Molecules*. 2021 Jul 30;26(15):4623.

[2232] Deo GS, Khatra J, Buttar S, et al. Antiproliferative, Immunostimulatory, and Anti-Inflammatory Activities of Extracts Derived from Mushrooms Collected in Haida Gwaii, British Columbia (Canada). *Int J Med Mushrooms*. 2019;21(7):629-643.

[2233] Contreras-Ochoa CO, Maza-Lopez J, Mendoza de Gives P, et al. Cell death induction by mycelium extracts from Pleurotus spp. on cervical cancer cell lines. *Nat Prod Res*. 2022 Dec;36(23):6091-6095.

[2234] Meza-Menchaca T, Poblete-Naredo I, Albores-Medina A, et al. Ergosterol Peroxide Isolated from Oyster Medicinal Mushroom, Pleurotus ostreatus (Agaricomycetes), Potentially Induces Radiosensitivity in Cervical Cancer. *Int J Med Mushrooms*. 2020;22(11):1109-1119.

[2235] Cao XY, Liu JL, Yang W, et al. Antitumor activity of polysaccharide extracted from Pleurotus ostreatus mycelia against gastric cancer in vitro and in vivo. *Mol Med Rep*. 2015 Aug;12(2):2383-9.

[2236] Elbatrawy EN, Ghonimy EA, Alassar MM, et al. Medicinal Mushroom Extracts Possess Differential Antioxidant Activity and Cytotoxicity to Cancer Cells. *Int J Med Mushrooms*. 2015;17(5):471-9.

[2237] Kobayashi H, Motoyoshi N, Itagaki T, et al. The inhibition of human tumor cell proliferation by RNase Pol, a member of the RNase T1 family, from Pleurotus ostreatus. *Biosci Biotechnol Biochem*. 2013;77(7):1486-91.

[2238] Kobayashi H, Motoyoshi N, Itagaki T, et al. The inhibition of human tumor cell proliferation by RNase Pol, a member of the RNase T1 family, from Pleurotus ostreatus. *Biosci Biotechnol Biochem*. 2013;77(7):1486-91.

[2239] Ebrahimi A, Atashi A, Soleimani M, et al. Comparison of anticancer effect of Pleurotus ostreatus extract with doxorubicin hydrochloride alone and plus thermotherapy on erythroleukemia cell line. *J Complement Integr Med*. 2017 Dec 19;15(2):/j/jcim.2018.15.issue-2/jcim-2016-0136/jcim-2016-0136.xml.

[2240] Ebrahimi A, Atashi A, Soleimani M, et al. Anti-invasive and antiproliferative effects of Pleurotus ostreatus extract on acute leukemia cell lines. *J Basic Clin Physiol Pharmacol*. 2018 Jan 26;29(1):95-102.

[2241] Wu JY, Chen CH, Chang WH, et al. Anti-Cancer Effects of Protein Extracts from Calvatia lilacina, Pleurotus ostreatus and Volvariella volvacea. *Evid Based Complement Alternat Med*. 2011;2011:982368.

[2242] Olufemi AE, Terry AO, Kola OJ. Anti-leukemic and immunomodulatory effects of fungal metabolites of Pleurotus pulmonarius and Pleurotus ostreatus on benzene-induced leukemia in Wister rats. *Korean J Hematol*. 2012 Mar;47(1):67-73.

[2243] Xu B, Li C, Sung C. Telomerase inhibitory effects of medicinal mushrooms and lichens, and their anticancer activity. *Int J Med Mushrooms*. 2014;16(1):17-28.

[2244] Perduca M, Destefanis L, Bovi M, et al. Structure and properties of the oyster mushroom (Pleurotus ostreatus) lectin. *Glycobiology*. 2020 Jul 16;30(8):550-562.

[2245] Khinsar KH, Abdul S, Hussain A, et al. Anti-tumor effect of polysaccharide from Pleurotus ostreatus on H22 mouse Hepatoma ascites in-vivo and hepatocellular carcinoma in-vitro model. *AMB Express*. 2021 Dec 2;11(1):160.

[2246] Perduca M, Destefanis L, Bovi M, et al. Structure and properties of the oyster mushroom (Pleurotus ostreatus) lectin. *Glycobiology*. 2020 Jul 16;30(8):550-562.

[2247] Kong F, Li FE, He Z, et al. Anti-tumor and macrophage activation induced by alkali-extracted polysaccharide from Pleurotus ostreatus. *Int J Biol Macromol*. 2014 Aug;69:561-6.

[2248] Facchini JM, Alves EP, Aguilera C, et al. Antitumor activity of Pleurotus ostreatus polysaccharide fractions on Ehrlich tumor and Sarcoma 180. *Int J Biol Macromol*. 2014 Jul;68:72-7.

[2249] Maiti S, Mallick SK, Bhutia SK, et al. Antitumor effect of culinary-medicinal oyster mushroom, Pleurotus ostreatus (Jacq.: Fr.) P. Kumm., derived protein fraction on tumor-bearing mice models. *Int J Med Mushrooms*. 2011;13(5):427-40.

[2250] Wang H, Gao J, Ng TB. A new lectin with highly potent antihepatoma and antisarcoma activities from the oyster mushroom Pleurotus ostreatus. *Biochem Biophys Res Commun*. 2000 Sep 7;275(3):810-6.

[2251] Sarangi I, Ghosh D, Bhutia SK, et al. Anti-tumor and immunomodulating effects of Pleurotus ostreatus mycelia-derived proteoglycans. *Int Immunopharmacol*. 2006 Aug;6(8):1287-97.

[2252] Wisbeck E, Facchini JM, Alves EP, et al. A polysaccharide fraction extracted from Pleurotus ostreatus mycelial biomass inhibit Sarcoma 180 tumor. *An Acad Bras Cienc*. 2017;89(3 Suppl):2013-2020.

[2253] Uddin Pk MM, Islam MS, Pervin R, et al. Optimization of extraction of antioxidant polysaccharide from Pleurotus ostreatus (Jacq.) P. Kumm and its cytotoxic activity against murine lymphoid cancer cell line. *PLoS One*. 2019 Jan 3;14(1):e0209371.

[2254] Maiti S, Mallick SK, Bhutia SK, et al. Antitumor effect of culinary-medicinal oyster mushroom, Pleurotus ostreatus (Jacq.: Fr.) P. Kumm., derived protein fraction on tumor-bearing mice models. *Int J Med Mushrooms*. 2011;13(5):427-40.

[2255] Devi KS, Behera B, Mishra D, et al. Immune augmentation and Dalton's Lymphoma tumor inhibition by glucans/glycans isolated from the mycelia and fruit body of Pleurotus ostreatus. *Int Immunopharmacol*. 2015 Mar;25(1):207-17.

[2256] Wolff ER, Wisbeck E, Silveira ML, et al. Antimicrobial and antineoplasic activity of Pleurotus ostreatus. *Appl Biochem Biotechnol*. 2008 Dec;151(2-3):402-12.

[2257] Wang H, Gao J, Ng TB. A new lectin with highly potent antihepatoma and antisarcoma activities from the oyster mushroom Pleurotus ostreatus. *Biochem Biophys Res Commun*. 2000 Sep 7;275(3):810-6.

[2258] Kurashige S, Akuzawa Y, Endo F. Effects of Lentinus edodes, Grifola frondosa and Pleurotus ostreatus administration on cancer outbreak, and activities of macrophages and lymphocytes in mice treated with a carcinogen, N-butyl-N-butanolnitrosoamine. *Immunopharmacol Immunotoxicol*. 1997 May;19(2):175-83.

[2259] Maiti S, Mallick SK, Bhutia SK, et al. Antitumor effect of culinary-medicinal oyster mushroom, Pleurotus ostreatus (Jacq.: Fr.) P. Kumm., derived protein fraction on tumor-bearing mice models. *Int J Med Mushrooms*. 2011;13(5):427-40.

[2260] Zhang Y, Yang X, Jin G, et al. Polysaccharides from Pleurotus ostreatus alleviate cognitive impairment in a rat model of Alzheimer's disease. *Int J Biol Macromol*. 2016 Nov;92:935-941.

[2261] Ćilerdžić J, Galić M, Vukojević J, et al. Pleurotus ostreatus and Laetiporus sulphureus (Agaricomycetes): Possible Agents against Alzheimer and Parkinson Diseases. *Int J Med Mushrooms*. 2019;21(3):275-289.

[2262] Agunloye OM, Oboh G, Falade AO. Pleurotus ostreatus and Lentinus subnudus supplemented diets restore altered acetylcholinesterase and butyrylcholinesterase activities and improve antioxidant status in transgenic Drosophila melanogaster model. *J Diet Suppl*. 2021;18(4):372-386.

[2263] Wang L, Li K, Cui Y, et al. Preparation, structural characterization and neuroprotective effects to against H2O2-induced oxidative damage in PC12 cells of polysaccharides from Pleurotus ostreatus. *Food Res Int*. 2023 Jan;163:112146.

[2264] J B, Das A, Sakthivel KM. Anthraquinone from Edible Fungi Pleurotus ostreatus Protects Human SH-SY5Y Neuroblastoma Cells Against 6-Hydroxydopamine-Induced Cell Death-Preclinical Validation of Gene Knockout Possibilities of PARK7, PINK1, and SNCA1 Using CRISPR SpCas9. *Appl Biochem Biotechnol*. 2020 Jun;191(2):555-566.

[2265] Llauradó G, Morris HJ, Tamayo V, et al. Haematopoiesis radioprotection in Balb/c mice by an aqueous mycelium extract from the Basidiomycete Pleurotus ostreatus mushroom. *Nat Prod Res*. 2015;29(16):1557-61.

[2266] Törős G, El-Ramady H, Prokisch J, et al. Modulation of the Gut Microbiota with Prebiotics and Antimicrobial Agents from Pleurotus ostreatus Mushroom. *Foods*. 2023 May 16;12(10):2010.

[2267] Hu Y, Xu J, Sheng Y, et al. Pleurotus Ostreatus Ameliorates Obesity by Modulating the Gut Microbiota in Obese Mice Induced by High-Fat Diet. *Nutrients*. 2022 Apr 29;14(9):1868.

[2268] Mitsou EK, Saxami G, Stamoulou E, et al. Effects of Rich in B-Glucans Edible Mushrooms on Aging Gut Microbiota Characteristics: An In Vitro Study. *Molecules*. 2020 Jun 18;25(12):2806.

[2269] Adams S, Che D, Hailong J, et al. Effects of pulverized oyster mushroom (Pleurotus ostreatus) on diarrhea incidence, growth performance, immunity, and microbial composition in piglets. *J Sci Food Agric*. 2019 May;99(7):3616-3627.

[2270] Saxami G, Mitsou EK, Kerezoudi EN, et al. In Vitro Fermentation of Edible Mushrooms: Effects on Faecal Microbiota Characteristics of Autistic and Neurotypical Children. *Microorganisms*. 2023 Feb 6;11(2):414.

[2271] Robinson J, Anike FN, Willis W, et al. Medicinal Mushrooms Supplements Alter Chicken Intestinal Microbiome. *Int J Med Mushrooms*. 2018;20(7):685-693.

[2272] Zhang Y, Hu T, Zhou H, et al. Antidiabetic effect of polysaccharides from Pleurotus ostreatus in streptozotocin-induced diabetic rats. *Int J Biol Macromol*. 2016 Feb;83:126-32.

[2273] Xiong M, Huang Y, Liu Y, et al. Antidiabetic Activity of Ergosterol from Pleurotus Ostreatus in KK-Ay Mice with Spontaneous Type 2 Diabetes Mellitus. *Mol Nutr Food Res*. 2018 Feb;62(3).

[2274] Jayasuriya WJ, Suresh TS, Abeytunga D, et al. Oral hypoglycemic activity of culinary-medicinal mushrooms Pleurotus ostreatus and P. cystidiosus (higher basidiomycetes) in normal and alloxan-induced diabetic Wistar rats. *Int J Med Mushrooms*. 2012;14(4):347-55.

[2275] Ravi B, Renitta RE, Prabha ML, et al. Evaluation of antidiabetic potential of oyster mushroom (Pleurotus ostreatus) in alloxan-induced diabetic mice. *Immunopharmacol Immunotoxicol*. 2013 Feb;35(1):101-9.

[2276] Singh V, Bedi GK, Shri R. In Vitro and In Vivo Antidiabetic Evaluation of Selected Culinary-Medicinal Mushrooms (Agaricomycetes). *Int J Med Mushrooms*. 2017;19(1):17-25.

[2277] Llauradó Maury G, Morris-Quevedo HJ, Heykers A, et al. Differential Induction Pattern Towards Classically Activated Macrophages in Response to an Immunomodulatory Extract from Pleurotus ostreatus Mycelium. *J Fungi (Basel)*. 2021 Mar 11;7(3):206.

[2278] Kong F, Li FE, He Z, et al. Anti-tumor and macrophage activation induced by alkali-extracted polysaccharide from Pleurotus ostreatus. *Int J Biol Macromol*. 2014 Aug;69:561-6.

[2279] El-Deeb NM, El-Adawi HI, El-Wahab AEA, et al. Modulation of NKG2D, KIR2DL and Cytokine Production by Pleurotus ostreatus Glucan Enhances Natural Killer Cell Cytotoxicity Toward Cancer Cells. *Front Cell Dev Biol*. 2019 Aug 13;7:165.

[2280] Sun Y, Liu J. Purification, structure and immunobiological activity of a water-soluble polysaccharide from the fruiting body of Pleurotus ostreatus. *Bioresour Technol*. 2009 Jan;100(2):983-6.

[2281] Paulík S, Svrcek S, Mojzisová J, et al. The immunomodulatory effect of the soluble fungal glucan (Pleurotus ostreatus) on delayed hypersensitivity and phagocytic ability of blood leucocytes in mice. *Zentralbl Veterinarmed B*. 1996 May;43(3):129-35.

[2282] Devi KS, Roy B, Patra P, et al. Characterization and lectin microarray of an immunomodulatory heteroglucan from Pleurotus ostreatus mycelia. *Carbohydr Polym*. 2013 May 15;94(2):857-65.

[2283] Seong SK, Kim HW. Potentiation of Innate Immunity by β-Glucans. *Mycobiology*. 2010 Jun;38(2):144-8.

[2284] Xu J, Xu D, Hu Q, et al. Immune regulatory functions of biologically active proteins from edible fungi. *Front Immunol*. 2023 Jan 12;13:1034545.

[2285] Deo GS, Khatra J, Buttar S, et al. Antiproliferative, Immunostimulatory, and Anti-Inflammatory Activities of Extracts Derived from Mushrooms Collected in Haida Gwaii, British Columbia (Canada). *Int J Med Mushrooms*. 2019;21(7):629-643.

[2286] Jeurink PV, Noguera CL, Savelkoul HF, et al. Immunomodulatory capacity of fungal proteins on the cytokine production of human peripheral blood mononuclear cells. *Int Immunopharmacol*. 2008 Aug;8(8):1124-33.

[2287] Elhusseiny SM, El-Mahdy TS, Elleboudy NS, et al. Immunomodulatory activity of extracts from five edible basidiomycetes mushrooms in Wistar albino rats. *Sci Rep*. 2022 Jul 20;12(1):12423.

2288 Paulík S, Svrcek S, Húska M, et al. [The effect of fungal and yeast glucan and levamisole on the level of the cellular immune response in vivo and leukocyte phagocytic activity in mice]. *Vet Med (Praha)*. 1992 Dec;37(12):675-85.

2289 Llauradó G, Morris HJ, Lebeque Y, et al. Oral administration of an aqueous extract from the oyster mushroom Pleurotus ostreatus enhances the immunonutritional recovery of malnourished mice. *Biomed Pharmacother*. 2016 Oct;83:1456-1463.

2290 Abdel-Monem NM, El-Saadani MA, Daba AS, et al. Exopolysaccharide-peptide complex from oyster mushroom (Pleurotus ostreatus) protects against hepatotoxicity in rats. *Biochem Biophys Rep*. 2020 Nov 12;24:100852.

2291 Zhu B, Li Y, Hu T, et al. The hepatoprotective effect of polysaccharides from Pleurotus ostreatus on carbon tetrachloride-induced acute liver injury rats. *Int J Biol Macromol*. 2019 Jun 15;131:1-9.

2292 Jayakumar T, Ramesh E, Geraldine P. Antioxidant activity of the oyster mushroom, Pleurotus ostreatus, on CCl(4)-induced liver injury in rats. *Food Chem Toxicol*. 2006 Dec;44(12):1989-96.

2293 Naguib YM, Azmy RM, Samaka RM, et al. Pleurotus ostreatus opposes mitochondrial dysfunction and oxidative stress in acetaminophen-induced hepato-renal injury. *BMC Complement Altern Med*. 2014 Dec 15;14:494.

2294 Bobek P, Ginter E, Jurcovicová M, et al. Effect of oyster fungus (Pleurotus ostreatus) on serum and liver lipids of Syrian hamsters with a chronic alcohol intake. *Physiol Res*. 1991;40(3):327-32.

2295 Bobek P, Ginter E, Kuniak L, et al. Effect of mushroom Pleurotus ostreatus and isolated fungal polysaccharide on serum and liver lipids in Syrian hamsters with hyperlipoproteinemia. *Nutrition*. 1991 Mar-Apr;7(2):105-8.

2296 Ahmed OM, Ebaid H, El-Nahass ES, et al. Nephroprotective Effect of Pleurotus ostreatus and Agaricus bisporus Extracts and Carvedilol on Ethylene Glycol-Induced Urolithiasis: Roles of NF-κB, p53, Bcl-2, Bax and Bak. *Biomolecules*. 2020 Sep 14;10(9):1317.

2297 Dkhil MA, Diab MSM, Lokman MS, et al. Nephroprotective effect of Pleurotus ostreatus extract against cadmium chloride toxicity in rats. *An Acad Bras Cienc*. 2020;92(1):e20191121.

2298 Bobek P, Nosálová V, Cerná S. Effect of pleuran (beta-glucan from Pleurotus ostreatus) in diet or drinking fluid on colitis in rats. *Nahrung*. 2001 Oct;45(5):360-3.

2299 Bobek P, Galbavy S, Ozdin L. Effect of oyster mushroom (Pleurotus ostreatus) on pathological changes in dimethylhydrazine-induced rat colon cancer. *Oncol Rep*. 1998 May-Jun;5(3):727-30.

2300 Yang Q, Huang B, Li H, et al. Gastroprotective activities of a polysaccharide from the fruiting bodies of Pleurotus ostreatus in rats. *Int J Biol Macromol*. 2012 Jun 1;50(5):1224-8.

2301 Reguła J, Krejpcio Z, Staniek H. Iron bioavailability from cereal products enriched with Pleurotus ostreatus mushrooms in rats with induced anaemia. *Ann Agric Environ Med*. 2016 Jun 2;23(2):310-4.

2302 Martin KR. Both common and specialty mushrooms inhibit adhesion molecule expression and in vitro binding of monocytes to human aortic endothelial cells in a pro-inflammatory environment. *Nutr J*. 2010 Jul 16;9:29.

2303 Agunloye OM. Effect of aqueous extracts of Pleurotus ostreatus and Lentinus subnudus on activity of adenosine deaminase, arginase, cholinergic enzyme, and angiotensin-1-converting enzyme. *J Food Biochem*. 2021 Mar;45(3):e13490.

2304 Piskov S, Timchenko L, Grimm WD, et al. Effects of Various Drying Methods on Some Physico-Chemical Properties and the Antioxidant Profile and ACE Inhibition Activity of Oyster Mushrooms (Pleurotus Ostreatus). *Foods*. 2020 Feb 7;9(2):160.

2305 Zhang Y, Wang Z, Jin G, et al. Regulating dyslipidemia effect of polysaccharides from Pleurotus ostreatus on fat-emulsion-induced hyperlipidemia rats. *Int J Biol Macromol*. 2017 Aug;101:107-116.

2306 Dong Y, Zhang J, Gao Z, et al. Characterization and anti-hyperlipidemia effects of enzymatic residue polysaccharides from Pleurotus ostreatus. *Int J Biol Macromol*. 2019 May 15;129:316-325.

2307 Alam N, Yoon KN, Lee TS, et al. Hypolipidemic Activities of Dietary Pleurotus ostreatus in Hypercholesterolemic Rats. *Mycobiology*. 2011 Mar;39(1):45-51.

2308 Bobek P, Hromadová M, Ozdín L. Oyster mushroom (Pleurotus ostreatus) reduces the activity of 3-hydroxy-3-methylglutaryl CoA reductase in rat liver microsomes. *Experientia*. 1995 Jun 14;51(6):589-91.

2309 Bobek P, Ginter E, Jurcovicová M, et al. Cholesterol-lowering effect of the mushroom Pleurotus ostreatus in hereditary hypercholesterolemic rats. *Ann Nutr Metab*. 1991;35(4):191-5.

2310 Bobek P, Ozdín L, Kajaba I. Dose-dependent hypocholesterolaemic effect of oyster mushroom (Pleurotus ostreatus) in rats. *Physiol Res*. 1997;46(4):327-9.

2311 Bobek P, Ozdin L, Kuniak L. The effect of oyster mushroom (Pleurotus ostreatus), its ethanolic extract and extraction residues on cholesterol levels in serum, lipoproteins and liver of rat. *Nahrung*. 1995;39(1):98-9.

2312 Bobek P, Ozdin L. Oyster mushroom (Pleurotus ostreatus) reduces the production and secretion of very low density lipoproteins in hypercholesterolemic rats. *Z Ernahrungswiss*. 1996 Sep;35(3):249-52.

2313 Bobek P, Kuniak L, Ozdín L. The mushroom Pleurotus ostreatus reduces secretion and accelerates the fractional turnover rate of very-low-density lipoproteins in the rat. *Ann Nutr Metab*. 1993;37(3):142-5.

2314 Opletal L, Jahodár L, Chobot V, et al. Evidence for the anti-hyperlipidaemic activity of the edible fungus Pleurotus ostreatus. *Br J Biomed Sci*. 1997 Dec;54(4):240-3.

2315 Bobek P, Ozdín O, Mikus M. Dietary oyster mushroom (Pleurotus ostreatus) accelerates plasma cholesterol turnover in hypercholesterolaemic rat. *Physiol Res*. 1995;44(5):287-91.

2316 Gil-Ramirez A, Smiderle FR, Morales D, et al. Water-Soluble Polysaccharide Extracts from the Oyster Culinary-Medicinal Mushroom Pleurotus ostreatus (Agaricomycetes) with HMGCR Inhibitory Activity. *Int J Med Mushrooms*. 2017;19(10):879-892.

2317 Bobek P, Ozdín L, Kuniak L. Effect of oyster mushroom (Pleurotus Ostreatus) and its ethanolic extract in diet on absorption and turnover of cholesterol in hypercholesterolemic rat. *Nahrung*. 1996 Aug;40(4):222-4.

2318 Bobek P, Ozdín L. The mushroom Pleurotus ostreatus accelerates plasma very-low-density lipoprotein clearance in hypercholesterolemic rat. *Physiol Res*. 1994;43(3):205-6.

2319 Bobek P, Ozdín L, Kuniak L, et al. [Regulation of cholesterol metabolism with dietary addition of oyster mushrooms (Pleurotus ostreatus) in rats with hypercholesterolemia]. *Cas Lek Cesk*. 1997 Mar 19;136(6):186-90.

2320 Anandhi R, Annadurai T, Anitha TS, et al. Antihypercholesterolemic and antioxidative effects of an extract of the oyster mushroom, Pleurotus ostreatus, and its major constituent, chrysin, in Triton WR-1339-induced hypercholesterolemic rats. *J Physiol Biochem*. 2013 Jun;69(2):313-23.

265

[2321] Chorváthová V, Bobek P, Ginter E, et al. Effect of the oyster fungus on glycaemia and cholesterolaemia in rats with insulin-dependent diabetes. *Physiol Res*. 1993;42(6):175-9.

[2322] Alam N, Amin R, Khan A, et al. Comparative effects of oyster mushrooms on lipid profile, liver and kidney function in hypercholesterolemic rats. *Mycobiology*. 2009 Mar;37(1):37-42.

[2323] Bobek P, Ozdin L, Kuniak L. Mechanism of hypocholesterolemic effect of oyster mushroom (Pleurotus ostreatus) in rats: reduction of cholesterol absorption and increase of plasma cholesterol removal. *Z Ernahrungswiss*. 1994 Mar;33(1):44-50.

[2324] Bobek P, Ozdin L, Kuniak L. Influence of water and ethanol extracts of the oyster mushroom (Pleurotus ostreatus) on serum and liver lipids of the Syrian hamsters. *Nahrung*. 1993;37(6):571-5.

[2325] Piskov SI, Timchenko LD, Rzhepakovsky IV, et al. [The influence of the drying method for food properties and hypolidemic potential of oyster mushrooms (Pleurotus ostreatus)]. *Vopr Pitan*. 2018;87(2):65-76.

[2326] Chowdhury HH, Rebolj K, Kreft M, et al. Lysophospholipids prevent binding of a cytolytic protein ostreolysin to cholesterol-enriched membrane domains. *Toxicon*. 2008 Jun 15;51(8):1345-56.

[2327] Sato M, Tokuji Y, Yoneyama S, et al. Profiling of hepatic gene expression of mice fed with edible japanese mushrooms by DNA microarray analysis: comparison among Pleurotus ostreatus, Grifola frondosa, and Hypsizigus marmoreus. *J Agric Food Chem*. 2011 Oct 12;59(19):10723-31.

[2328] Caz V, Gil-Ramírez A, Largo C, Tabernero M, et al. Modulation of Cholesterol-Related Gene Expression by Dietary Fiber Fractions from Edible Mushrooms. *J Agric Food Chem*. 2015 Aug 26;63(33):7371-80.

[2329] Bobek P, Galbavý S. [The oyster mushroom (Pleurotus ostreatus) effectively prevents the development of atherosclerosis in rabbits]. *Ceska Slov Farm*. 1999 Sep;48(5):226-30.

[2330] Hossain S, Hashimoto M, Choudhury EK, et al. Dietary mushroom (Pleurotus ostreatus) ameliorates atherogenic lipid in hypercholesterolaemic rats. *Clin Exp Pharmacol Physiol*. 2003 Jul;30(7):470-5.

[2331] Bobek P, Galbavý S. Hypocholesterolemic and antiatherogenic effect of oyster mushroom (Pleurotus ostreatus) in rabbits. *Nahrung*. 1999 Oct;43(5):339-42.

[2332] Pang L, Wang T, Liao Q, et al. Protective role of ergothioneine isolated from Pleurotus ostreatus against dextran sulfate sodium-induced ulcerative colitis in rat model. *J Food Sci*. 2022 Jan;87(1):415-426.

[2333] Nosál'ová V, Bobek P, Cerná S, et al. Effects of pleuran (beta-glucan isolated from Pleurotus ostreatus) on experimental colitis in rats. *Physiol Res*. 2001;50(6):575-81.

[2334] Hu Y, Xu J, Sheng Y, et al. Pleurotus Ostreatus Ameliorates Obesity by Modulating the Gut Microbiota in Obese Mice Induced by High-Fat Diet. *Nutrients*. 2022 Apr 29;14(9):1868.

[2335] J B, Das A. An edible fungi Pleurotus ostreatus inhibits adipogenesis via suppressing expression of PPAR γ and C/EBP α in 3T3-L1 cells: In vitro validation of gene knock out of RNAs in PPAR γ using CRISPR spcas9. *Biomed Pharmacother*. 2019 Aug;116:109030.

[2336] Kawagishi H, Suzuki H, Watanabe H, et al. A lectin from an edible mushroom Pleurotus ostreatus as a food intake-suppressing substance. *Biochim Biophys Acta*. 2000 May 1;1474(3):299-308.

[2337] González-Ibáñez L, Meneses ME, Sánchez-Tapia M, et al. Edible and medicinal mushrooms (Pleurotus ostreatus, Ustilago maydis, Ganoderma lucidum) reduce endoplasmic reticulum stress and inflammation in adipose tissue of obese Wistar rats fed with a high fat plus saccharose diet. *Food Funct*. 2023 Jun 6;14(11):5048-5061.

[2338] Rivero-Pérez N, Ayala-Martínez M, Zepeda-Bastida A, et al. Anti-inflammatory effect of aqueous extracts of spent Pleurotus ostreatus substrates in mouse ears treated with 12-O-tetradecanoylphorbol-13-acetate. *Indian J Pharmacol*. 2016 Mar-Apr;48(2):141-4.

[2339] Jayasuriya WJABN, Handunnetti SM, Wanigatunge CA, et al. Anti-Inflammatory Activity of Pleurotus ostreatus, a Culinary Medicinal Mushroom, in Wistar Rats. *Evid Based Complement Alternat Med*. 2020 Mar 5;2020:6845383.

[2340] Deo GS, Khatra J, Buttar S, et al. Antiproliferative, Immunostimulatory, and Anti-Inflammatory Activities of Extracts Derived from Mushrooms Collected in Haida Gwaii, British Columbia (Canada). *Int J Med Mushrooms*. 2019;21(7):629-643.

[2341] Gunawardena D, Bennett L, Shanmugam K, et al. Anti-inflammatory effects of five commercially available mushroom species determined in lipopolysaccharide and interferon-γ activated murine macrophages. *Food Chem*. 2014 Apr 1;148:92-6.

[2342] Jedinak A, Dudhgaonkar S, Wu QL, et al. Anti-inflammatory activity of edible oyster mushroom is mediated through the inhibition of NF-κB and AP-1 signaling. *Nutr J*. 2011 May 16;10:52.

[2343] Stastny J, Marsik P, Tauchen J, et al. Antioxidant and Anti-Inflammatory Activity of Five Medicinal Mushrooms of the Genus Pleurotus. *Antioxidants (Basel)*. 2022 Aug 13;11(8):1569.

[2344] Jang IT, Hyun SH, Shin JW, et al. Characterization of an Anti-gout Xanthine Oxidase Inhibitor from Pleurotus ostreatus. *Mycobiology*. 2014 Sep;42(3):296-300.

[2345] Chourasia A, Tiwari A, Ganeshpurkar A, et al. Evaluation of Antiarthritic Effect of Culinary-Medicinal Oyster Mushroom Pleurotus ostreatus cv. Florida (Agaricomycetes) on Complete Freund's Adjuvant Induced Arthritis in Rats. *Int J Med Mushrooms*. 2019;21(11):1123-1136.

[2346] Bauerová K, Paulovicová E, Mihalová D, et al. Study of new ways of supplementary and combinatory therapy of rheumatoid arthritis with immunomodulators. Glucomannan and Imunoglukán in adjuvant arthritis. *Toxicol Ind Health*. 2009 May-Jun;25(4-5):329-35.

[2347] Rovenský J, Stančíkova M, Svík K, et al. The effects of β-glucan isolated from Pleurotus ostreatus on methotrexate treatment in rats with adjuvant arthritis. *Rheumatol Int*. 2011 Apr;31(4):507-11.

[2348] Isai M, Elanchezhian R, Sakthivel M, et al. Anticataractogenic effect of an extract of the oyster mushroom, Pleurotus ostreatus, in an experimental animal model. *Curr Eye Res*. 2009 Apr;34(4):264-73.

[2349] Ebigwai JK, Edu EA, Itam EH, et al. Activity of crude cold-water extract of the culinary-medicinal oyster mushroom, Pleurotus ostreatus (Jacq.:Fr.) P.Kumm. (higher Basidiomycetes), and timolol. *Int J Med Mushrooms*. 2012;14(5):467-70.

[2350] Ruggeri M, Miele D, Contardi M, et al. Mycelium-based biomaterials as smart devices for skin wound healing. *Front Bioeng Biotechnol*. 2023 Aug 15;11:1225722.

[2351] Majtán J, Kumar P, Koller J, et al. Induction of metalloproteinase 9 secretion from human keratinocytes by pleuran (beta-glucan from Pleurotus ostreatus). *Z Naturforsch C J Biosci*. 2009 Jul-Aug;64(7-8):597-600.

[2352] Hsiao Y, Shao Y, Wu Y, et al. Physicochemical properties and protective effects on UVA-induced photoaging in Hs68 cells of Pleurotus ostreatus polysaccharides by fractional precipitation. *Int J Biol Macromol*. 2023 Feb 15;228:537-547.

[2353] Choi J, Song E, Gwon H, et al. Aqueous Extracts of Pleurotus ostreatus and Hericium erinaceus Protect against Ultraviolet A-Induced Damage in Human Dermal Fibroblasts. *Int J Med Mushrooms*. 2022;24(2):63-74.

[2354] Alam N, Yoon KN, Lee KR, et al. Antioxidant Activities and Tyrosinase Inhibitory Effects of Different Extracts from Pleurotus ostreatus Fruiting Bodies. *Mycobiology*. 2010 Dec;38(4):295-301.

[2355] Sharif S, Atta A, Huma T, et al. Anticancer, antithrombotic, antityrosinase, and anti-α-glucosidase activities of selected wild and commercial mushrooms from Pakistan. *Food Sci Nutr*. 2018 Sep 14;6(8):2170-2176.

[2356] Espinosa-Páez E, Alanis-Guzmán MG, Hernández-Luna CE, et al. Increasing Antioxidant Activity and Protein Digestibility in Phaseolus vulgaris and Avena sativa by Fermentation with the Pleurotus ostreatus Fungus. *Molecules*. 2017 Dec 20;22(12):2275.

[2357] Solomko EF, Eliseeva GS. [Biosynthesis of vitamins B by the fungus Pleurotus ostreatus in a submerged culture]. *Prikl Biokhim Mikrobiol*. 1988 Mar-Apr;24(2):164-9.

[2358] Aguilar Uscanga BR, Cavazos Garduño A, et al. In-vivo assessment of the protection of β-glucans of Pleurotus ostreatus against oxidative stress caused by acrylamide intake (part II). *Nutr Hosp*. 2020 Oct 21;37(5):1028-1032.

[2359] Jayakumar T, Sakthivel M, Thomas PA, et al. Pleurotus ostreatus, an oyster mushroom, decreases the oxidative stress induced by carbon tetrachloride in rat kidneys, heart and brain. *Chem Biol Interact*. 2008 Nov 25;176(2-3):108-20.

[2360] Kylyc A, Yesilada E. Preliminary results on antigenotoxic effects of dried mycelia of two medicinal mushrooms in Drosophila melanogaster somatic mutation and recombination test. *Int J Med Mushrooms*. 2013;15(4):415-21.

[2361] Agunloye OM. Effect of aqueous extracts of Pleurotus ostreatus and Lentinus subnudus on activity of adenosine deaminase, arginase, cholinergic enzyme, and angiotensin-1-converting enzyme. *J Food Biochem*. 2021 Mar;45(3):e13490.

[2362] Bakir T, Karadeniz M, Unal S. Investigation of antioxidant activities of Pleurotus ostreatus stored at different temperatures. *Food Sci Nutr*. 2018 Apr 16;6(4):1040-1044.

[2363] Rahimah SB, Djunaedi DD, Soeroto AY, et al. The Phytochemical Screening, Total Phenolic Contents and Antioxidant Activities in Vitro of White Oyster Mushroom (Pleurotus Ostreatus) Preparations. *Open Access Maced J Med Sci*. 2019 Jun 30;7(15):2404-2412.

[2364] Jin Z, Li Y, Ren J, Qin N. Yield, Nutritional Content, and Antioxidant Activity of Pleurotus ostreatus on Corncobs Supplemented with Herb Residues. *Mycobiology*. 2018 Mar 29;46(1):24-32.

[2365] Vamanu E. Antioxidant properties of polysaccharides obtained by batch cultivation of Pleurotus ostreatus mycelium. *Nat Prod Res*. 2013;27(12):1115-8.

[2366] González-Palma I, Escalona-Buendía HB, Ponce-Alquicira E, et al. Evaluation of the Antioxidant Activity of Aqueous and Methanol Extracts of Pleurotus ostreatus in Different Growth Stages. *Front Microbiol*. 2016 Jul 12;7:1099.

[2367] Alam N, Yoon KN, Lee KR, et al. Antioxidant Activities and Tyrosinase Inhibitory Effects of Different Extracts from Pleurotus ostreatus Fruiting Bodies. *Mycobiology*. 2010 Dec;38(4):295-301.

[2368] Li H, Zhang Z, Li M, et al. Yield, size, nutritional value, and antioxidant activity of oyster mushrooms grown on perilla stalks. *Saudi J Biol Sci*. 2017 Feb;24(2):347-354.

[2369] Bobek P, Ozdin L, Kuniak L. Antioxidative effect of oyster mushroom (Pleurotus ostreatus) in hypercholesterolemic rat. *Pharmazie*. 1995 Jun;50(6):441-2.

[2370] Patra S, Patra P, Maity KK, et al. A heteroglycan from the mycelia of Pleurotus ostreatus: structure determination and study of antioxidant properties. *Carbohydr Res*. 2013 Mar 7;368:16-21.

[2371] Zhang Y, Dai L, Kong X, et al. Characterization and in vitro antioxidant activities of polysaccharides from Pleurotus ostreatus. *Int J Biol Macromol*. 2012 Oct;51(3):259-65.

[2372] Krishnamoorthy D, Sankaran M. Modulatory effect of Pleurotus ostreatus on oxidant/antioxidant status in 7, 12-dimethylbenz (a) anthracene induced mammary carcinoma in experimental rats--A dose-response study. *J Cancer Res Ther*. 2016 Jan-Mar;12(1):386-94.

[2373] Vamanu E. In vitro antimicrobial and antioxidant activities of ethanolic extract of lyophilized mycelium of Pleurotus ostreatus PQMZ91109. *Molecules*. 2012 Mar 26;17(4):3653-71.

[2374] Vamanu E. Biological activities of the polysaccharides produced in submerged culture of two edible Pleurotus ostreatus mushrooms. *J Biomed Biotechnol*. 2012;2012:565974.

[2375] Ćilerdžić J, Stajić M, Vukojević J, et al. Antioxidant and antifungal potential of Pleurotus ostreatus and Agrocybe cylindracea basidiocarps and mycelia. *Curr Pharm Biotechnol*. 2015;16(2):179-86.

[2376] Yim HS Jr, Chye FY, Tan CT, et al. Antioxidant Activities and Total Phenolic Content of Aqueous Extract of Pleurotus ostreatus (Cultivated Oyster Mushroom). *Malays J Nutr*. 2010 Aug;16(2):281-91.

[2377] Lam YS, Okello EJ. Determination of Lovastatin, β-glucan, Total Polyphenols, and Antioxidant Activity in Raw and Processed Oyster Culinary-Medicinal Mushroom, Pleurotus ostreatus (Higher Basidiomycetes). *Int J Med Mushrooms*. 2015;17(2):117-28.

[2378] Ahmad N, Mahmood F, Khalil SA, et al. Antioxidant activity via DPPH, gram-positive and gram-negative antimicrobial potential in edible mushrooms. *Toxicol Ind Health*. 2014 Oct;30(9):826-34.

[2379] Vamanu E. In vitro antioxidant and antimicrobial activities of two edible mushroom mycelia obtained in the presence of different nitrogen sources. *J Med Food*. 2013 Feb;16(2):155-66.

[2380] Emsen B, Guven B, Uzun Y, et al. Antioxidant and Genotoxic Effects of Aqueous and Methanol Extracts from Two Edible Mushrooms from Turkey in Human Peripheral Lymphocytes. *Int J Med Mushrooms*. 2020;22(2):161-170.

[2381] Reis FS, Martins A, Barros L, et al. Antioxidant properties and phenolic profile of the most widely appreciated cultivated mushrooms: a comparative study between in vivo and in vitro samples. *Food Chem Toxicol*. 2012 May;50(5):1201-7.

[2382] Udeh AS, Ezebialu CU, Eze EA, et al. Antibacterial and Antioxidant Activity of Different Extracts of Some Wild Medicinal Mushrooms from Nigeria. *Int J Med Mushrooms*. 2021;23(10):83-95.

[2383] Piljac-Zegarac J, Samec D, et al. Antioxidant properties of extracts of wild medicinal mushroom species from Croatia. *Int J Med Mushrooms*. 2011;13(3):257-63.

[2384] Obodai M, Ferreira IC, Fernandes A, et al. Evaluation of the chemical and antioxidant properties of wild and cultivated mushrooms of Ghana. *Molecules*. 2014 Nov 26;19(12):19532-48.

[2385] Elbatrawy EN, Ghonimy EA, Alassar MM, et al. Medicinal Mushroom Extracts Possess Differential Antioxidant Activity and Cytotoxicity to Cancer Cells. *Int J Med Mushrooms*. 2015;17(5):471-9.

[2386] Lin S, Ching LT, Ke X, et al. Comparison of the Composition and Antioxidant Activities of Phenolics from the Fruiting Bodies of Cultivated Asian Culinary-Medicinal Mushrooms. *Int J Med Mushrooms*. 2016;18(10):871-881.

[2387] Jayakumar T, Thomas PA, Geraldine P. Protective effect of an extract of the oyster mushroom, Pleurotus ostreatus, on antioxidants of major organs of aged rats. *Exp Gerontol*. 2007 Mar;42(3):183-91.

[2388] Jayakumar T, Thomas PA, Ramesh E, et al. An extract of the pleurotus ostreatus mushroom bolsters the glutathione redox system in various organs of aged rats. *J Med Food*. 2010 Aug;13(4):771-8.

[2389] Jayakumar T, Thomas PA, Isai M, et al. An extract of the oyster mushroom, Pleurotus ostreatus, increases catalase gene expression and reduces protein oxidation during aging in rats. *Zhong Xi Yi Jie He Xue Bao*. 2010 Aug;8(8):774-80.

[2390] Thomas PA, Geraldine P, Jayakumar T. Pleurotus ostreatus, an edible mushroom, enhances glucose 6-phosphate dehydrogenase, ascorbate peroxidase and reduces xanthine dehydrogenase in major organs of aged rats. *Pharm Biol*. 2014 May;52(5):646-54.

[2391] Elhusseiny SM, El-Mahdy TS, Elleboudy NS, et al. In vitro Anti SARS-CoV-2 Activity and Docking Analysis of Pleurotus ostreatus, Lentinula edodes and Agaricus bisporus Edible Mushrooms. *Infect Drug Resist*. 2022 Jul 2;15:3459-3475.

[2392] He M, Su D, Liu Q, et al. Mushroom lectin overcomes hepatitis B virus tolerance via TLR6 signaling. *Sci Rep*. 2017 Jul 19;7(1):5814.

[2393] El-Fakharany EM, Haroun BM, Ng TB, et al. Oyster mushroom laccase inhibits hepatitis C virus entry into peripheral blood cells and hepatoma cells. *Protein Pept Lett*. 2010 Aug;17(8):1031-9.

[2394] Elhusseiny SM, El-Mahdy TS, Awad MF, et al. Proteome Analysis and In Vitro Antiviral, Anticancer and Antioxidant Capacities of the Aqueous Extracts of Lentinula edodes and Pleurotus ostreatus Edible Mushrooms. *Molecules*. 2021 Jul 30;26(15):4623.

[2395] Razumov IA, Kazachinskaia EI, Puchkova LI, et al. [Protective activity of aqueous extracts from higher mushrooms against Herpes simplex virus type-2 on albino mice model]. *Antibiot Khimioter*. 2013;58(9-10):8-12.

[2396] Wang HX, Ng TB. Isolation of a novel ubiquitin-like protein from Pleurotus ostreatus mushroom with anti-human immunodeficiency virus, translation-inhibitory, and ribonuclease activities. *Biochem Biophys Res Commun*. 2000 Sep 24;276(2):587-93.

[2397] Krupodorova T, Rybalko S, Barshteyn V. Antiviral activity of Basidiomycete mycelia against influenza type A (serotype H1N1) and herpes simplex virus type 2 in cell culture. *Virol Sin*. 2014 Oct;29(5):284-90.

[2398] Hamad D, El-Sayed H, Ahmed W, et al. GC-MS Analysis of Potentially Volatile Compounds of Pleurotus ostreatus Polar Extract: In vitro Antimicrobial, Cytotoxic, Immunomodulatory, and Antioxidant Activities. *Front Microbiol*. 2022 Feb 18;13:834525.

[2399] Mishra V, Tomar S, Yadav P, et al. Elemental Analysis, Phytochemical Screening and Evaluation of Antioxidant, Antibacterial and Anticancer Activity of Pleurotus ostreatus through In Vitro and In Silico Approaches. *Metabolites*. 2022 Aug 31;12(9):821.

[2400] Ganeshpurkar A, Bhadoriya SS, Pardhi P, et al. Study of Antimicrobial and Cytotoxic Potential of the Oyster Mushroom Pleurotus ostreatus cv. Florida (Agaricomycetes). *Int J Med Mushrooms*. 2016;18(4):321-5.

[2401] Vamanu E. In vitro antimicrobial and antioxidant activities of ethanolic extract of lyophilized mycelium of Pleurotus ostreatus PQMZ91109. *Molecules*. 2012 Mar 26;17(4):3653-71.

[2402] Wolff ER, Wisbeck E, Silveira ML, et al. Antimicrobial and antineoplasic activity of Pleurotus ostreatus. *Appl Biochem Biotechnol*. 2008 Dec;151(2-3):402-12.

[2403] Skariyachan S, Prasanna A, Manjunath SP, et al. Exploring the Medicinal Potential of the Fruit Bodies of Oyster Mushroom, Pleurotus ostreatus (Agaricomycetes), against Multidrug-Resistant Bacterial Isolates. *Int J Med Mushrooms*. 2016;18(3):245-52.

[2404] Younis AM, Wu FS, El Shikh HH. Antimicrobial Activity of Extracts of the Oyster Culinary Medicinal Mushroom Pleurotus ostreatus (Higher Basidiomycetes) and Identification of a New Antimicrobial Compound. *Int J Med Mushrooms*. 2015;17(6):579-90.

[2405] Baraza LD, Neser W, Jackson KC, et al. Antimicrobial Coumarins from the Oyster Culinary-Medicinal Mushroom, Pleurotus ostreatus (Agaricomycetes), from Kenya. *Int J Med Mushrooms*. 2016;18(10):905-913.

[2406] Yakobi SH, Mkhize S, Pooe OJ. Screening of Antimicrobial Properties and Bioactive Compounds of Pleurotus Ostreatus Extracts against Staphylococcus Aureus, Escherichia coli, and Neisseria Gonorrhoeae. *Biochem Res Int*. 2023 Apr 17;2023:1777039.

[2407] Kunjadia PD, Nagee A, Pandya PY, et al. Medicinal and antimicrobial role of the oyster culinary-medicinal mushroom Pleurotus ostreatus (higher Basidiomycetes) cultivated on banana agrowastes in India. *Int J Med Mushrooms*. 2014;16(3):227-38.

[2408] Ahmad N, Mahmood F, Khalil SA, et al. Antioxidant activity via DPPH, gram-positive and gram-negative antimicrobial potential in edible mushrooms. *Toxicol Ind Health*. 2014 Oct;30(9):826-34.

[2409] Chowdhury M, Kubra K, Ahmed S. Screening of antimicrobial, antioxidant properties and bioactive compounds of some edible mushrooms cultivated in Bangladesh. *Ann Clin Microbiol Antimicrob*. 2015 Feb 7;14:8.

[2410] Klančnik A, Megušar P, Sterniša M, et al. Aqueous Extracts of Wild Mushrooms Show Antimicrobial and Antiadhesion Activities against Bacteria and Fungi. *Phytother Res*. 2017 Dec;31(12):1971-1976.

[2411] Kalyoncu F, Oskay M, Sağlam H, et al. Antimicrobial and antioxidant activities of mycelia of 10 wild mushroom species. *J Med Food*. 2010 Apr;13(2):415-9.

[2412] Castillo TA, Lemos RA, Pereira JRG, et al. Mycelial Growth and Antimicrobial Activity of Pleurotus Species (Agaricomycetes). *Int J Med Mushrooms*. 2018;20(2):191-200.

[2413] Hearst R, Nelson D, McCollum G, et al. An examination of antibacterial and antifungal properties of constituents of Shiitake (Lentinula edodes) and oyster (Pleurotus ostreatus) mushrooms. *Complement Ther Clin Pract*. 2009 Feb;15(1):5-7.

[2414] Udeh AS, Ezebialu CU, Eze EA, et al. Antibacterial and Antioxidant Activity of Different Extracts of Some Wild Medicinal Mushrooms from Nigeria. *Int J Med Mushrooms*. 2021;23(10):83-95.

[2415] Ramos-Ligonio A, López-Monteon A, et al. Trypanocidal activity of ergosterol peroxide from Pleurotus ostreatus. *Biotechnol Biofuels*. 2015 Apr 11;8:63.

[2416] Alotaibi BS, Malak N, Khan A, et al. Acaricidal assessment of the fungal extract of Pleurotus ostreatus against Rhipicephalus microplus: Role of in vitro and in silico analysis. *Heliyon*. 2023 Aug 29;9(9):e19600.

[2417] Meza-Menchaca T, Suárez-Medellín J, Del Ángel-Piña C, et al. The Amoebicidal Effect of Ergosterol Peroxide Isolated from Pleurotus ostreatus. *Phytother Res*. 2015 Dec;29(12):1982-6.

[2418] Satou T, Kaneko K, Li W, et al. The toxin produced by pleurotus ostreatus reduces the head size of nematodes. *Biol Pharm Bull*. 2008 Apr;31(4):574-6.

[2419] de Matos AFIM, Greesler LT, Giacometi M, et al. Nematocidal Effect of Oyster Culinary-Medicinal Mushroom Pleurotus ostreatus (Agaricomycetes) against Haemonchus contortus. *Int J Med Mushrooms*. 2020;22(11):1089-1098.

[2420] Afieroho OE, Noundou XS, Onyia CP, et al. Antiplasmodial Activity of the n-Hexane Extract from Pleurotus ostreatus (Jacq. ex. Fr) P. Kumm. *Turk J Pharm Sci*. 2019 Mar;16(1):37-42.

[2421] Ullah MI, Akhtar M, Iqbal Z, et al. Immunomodulating and Antiprotozoal Effects of Different Extracts of the Oyster Culinary-Medicinal Mushroom Pleurotus ostreatus (Higher Basidiomycetes) Against Coccidiosis in Broiler. *Int J Med Mushrooms*. 2015;17(3):309-17.

[2422] Annang F, Pérez-Victoria I, Appiah T, et al. Antiprotozoan sesterterpenes and triterpenes isolated from two Ghanaian mushrooms. *Fitoterapia*. 2018 Jun;127:341-348.

[2423] Nobre C, González A, Losoya C, et al. Detoxification of ochratoxin A and zearalenone by Pleurotus ostreatus during in vitro gastrointestinal digestion. *Food Chem*. 2022 Aug 1;384:132525.

[2424] Das A, Bhattacharya S, Palaniswamy M, et al. Biodegradation of aflatoxin B1 in contaminated rice straw by Pleurotus ostreatus MTCC 142 and Pleurotus ostreatus GHBBF10 in the presence of metal salts and surfactants. *World J Microbiol Biotechnol*. 2014 Aug;30(8):2315-24.

[2425] Aguilar Uscanga BR, Cavazos Garduño A, Solís Pacheco JR, et al. In vivo assessment of the protection conferred by β-glucans from Pleurotus ostreatus against the harmful effects of acrylamide intake (Part I). *Nutr Hosp*. 2020 Aug 27;37(4):850-854.

[2426] Jackson LW 3rd, Pryor BM. Degradation of aflatoxin B1 from naturally contaminated maize using the edible fungus Pleurotus ostreatus. *AMB Express*. 2017 Dec;7(1):110.

[2427] Das A, Bhattacharya S, Palaniswamy M, et al. Aflatoxin B1 degradation during co-cultivation of Aspergillus flavus and Pleurotus ostreatus strains on rice straw. *3 Biotech*. 2015 Jun;5(3):279-284.

[2428] Wang L, Huang W, Shen Y, et al. Enhancing the degradation of Aflatoxin B1 by co-cultivation of two fungi strains with the improved production of detoxifying enzymes. *Food Chem*. 2022 Mar 1;371:131092.

[2429] Singh SK, Khajuria R, Kaur L. Biodegradation of ciprofloxacin by white rot fungus Pleurotus ostreatus. *3 Biotech*. 2017 May;7(1):69.

[2430] Kózka B, Nałęcz-Jawecki G, Turło J, et al. Application of Pleurotus ostreatus to efficient removal of selected antidepressants and immunosuppressant. *J Environ Manage*. 2020 Nov 1;273:111131.

[2431] Golovko O, Kaczmarek M, Asp H, et al. Uptake of perfluoroalkyl substances, pharmaceuticals, and parabens by oyster mushrooms (Pleurotus ostreatus) and exposure risk in human consumption. *Chemosphere*. 2022 Mar;291(Pt 2):132898.

[2432] Křesinová Z, Linhartová L, Filipová A, et al. Biodegradation of endocrine disruptors in urban wastewater using Pleurotus ostreatus bioreactor. *N Biotechnol*. 2018 Jul 25;43:53-61.

[2433] Bhattacharya S, Das A, Prashanthi K, et al. Mycoremediation of Benzo[a]pyrene by Pleurotus ostreatus in the presence of heavy metals and mediators. *3 Biotech*. 2014 Apr;4(2):205-211.

[2434] Migliore L, Fiori M, Spadoni A, et al. Biodegradation of oxytetracycline by Pleurotus ostreatus mycelium: a mycoremediation technique. *J Hazard Mater*. 2012 May 15;215-216:227-32.

[2435] Dickson UJ, Coffey M, George Mortimer RJ, et al. Investigating the potential of sunflower species, fermented palm wine and Pleurotus ostreatus for treatment of petroleum-contaminated soil. *Chemosphere*. 2020 Feb;240:124881.

[2436] Hultberg M, Ahrens L, Golovko O. Use of lignocellulosic substrate colonized by oyster mushroom (Pleurotus ostreatus) for removal of organic micropollutants from water. *J Environ Manage*. 2020 Oct 15;272:111087.

[2437] Liu X, Deng W, Yang Y. Characterization of a Novel Laccase LAC-Yang1 from White-Rot Fungus Pleurotus ostreatus Strain Yang1 with a Strong Ability to Degrade and Detoxify Chlorophenols. *Molecules*. 2021 Jan 18;26(2):473.

[2438] Ahuactzin-Pérez M, Tlecuitl-Beristain S, García-Dávila J, et al. A novel biodegradation pathway of the endocrine-disruptor di(2-ethyl hexyl) phthalate by Pleurotus ostreatus based on quantum chemical investigation. *Ecotoxicol Environ Saf*. 2018 Jan;147:494-499.

[2439] Hwang SS, Kim HY, Ka JO, et al. Changes in the activities of enzymes involved in the degradation of butylbenzyl phthalate by Pleurotus ostreatus. *J Microbiol Biotechnol*. 2012 Feb;22(2):239-43.

[2440] Patel H, Gupte A, Gupte S. Biodegradation of fluoranthene by basidiomycetes fungal isolate Pleurotus ostreatus HP-1. *Appl Biochem Biotechnol*. 2009 Jun;157(3):367-76.

[2441] Pozdnyakova N, Dubrovskaya E, Chernyshova M, et al. The degradation of three-ringed polycyclic aromatic hydrocarbons by wood-inhabiting fungus Pleurotus ostreatus and soil-inhabiting fungus Agaricus bisporus. *Fungal Biol*. 2018 May;122(5):363-372.

[2442] Skariyachan S, Prasanna A, Manjunath SP, et al. Environmental assessment of the degradation potential of mushroom fruit bodies of Pleurotus ostreatus (Jacq.: Fr.) P. Kumm. towards synthetic azo dyes and contaminating effluents collected from textile industries in Karnataka, India. *Environ Monit Assess*. 2016 Feb;188(2):121.

[2443] Hirano T, Honda Y, Watanabe T, et al. Degradation of bisphenol A by the lignin-degrading enzyme, manganese peroxidase, produced by the white-rot basidiomycete, Pleurotus ostreatus. *Biosci Biotechnol Biochem*. 2000 Sep;64(9):1958-62.

[2444] Pozdnyakova NN, Chernyshova MP, Grinev VS, et al. [Degradation of fluorene and fluoranthene by the basidiomycete Pleurotus ostreatus]. *Prikl Biokhim Mikrobiol*. 2016 Nov-Dec;52(6):590-8.

[2445] Economou CN, Philippoussis AN, Diamantopoulou PA. Spent mushroom substrate for a second cultivation cycle of Pleurotus mushrooms and dephenolization of agro-industrial wastewaters. *FEMS Microbiol Lett*. 2020 Apr 1;367(8):fnaa060.

[2446] Jiang GX, Niu JF, Zhang SP, et al. Prediction of biodegradation rate constants of hydroxylated polychlorinated biphenyls by fungal laccases from Trametes versicolor and Pleurotus ostreatus. *Bull Environ Contam Toxicol*. 2008 Jul;81(1):1-6.

[2447] Kubátová A, Erbanová P, Eichlerová I, et al. PCB congener selective biodegradation by the white rot fungus Pleurotus ostreatus in contaminated soil. *Chemosphere*. 2001 Apr;43(2):207-15.

[2448] Šrédlová K, Šírová K, Stella T, et al. Degradation Products of Polychlorinated Biphenyls and Their In Vitro Transformation by Ligninolytic Fungi. *Toxics*. 2021 Apr 8;9(4):81.

[2449] Purnomo AS, Putra SR, Shimizu K, et al. Biodegradation of heptachlor and heptachlor epoxide-contaminated soils by white-rot fungal inocula. *Environ Sci Pollut Res Int*. 2014 Oct;21(19):11305-12.

[2450] Bezalel L, Hadar Y, Fu PP, et al. Initial Oxidation Products in the Metabolism of Pyrene, Anthracene, Fluorene, and Dibenzothiophene by the White Rot Fungus Pleurotus ostreatus. *Appl Environ Microbiol*. 1996 Jul;62(7):2554-9.

[2451] Faraco V, Pezzella C, Miele A, et al. Bio-remediation of colored industrial wastewaters by the white-rot fungi Phanerochaete chrysosporium and Pleurotus ostreatus and their enzymes. *Biodegradation*. 2009 Apr;20(2):209-20.

[2452] Ghasemi R, Golbabaei F, Rezaei S, et al. A comparison of biofiltration performance based on bacteria and fungi for treating toluene vapors from airflow. *AMB Express*. 2020 Jan 14;10(1):8.

[2453] Siracusa G, Becarelli S, Lorenzi R, et al. PCB in the environment: bio-based processes for soil decontamination and management of waste from the industrial production of Pleurotus ostreatus. *N Biotechnol*. 2017 Oct 25;39(Pt B):232-239.

[2454] da Rocha Ferreira GL, Vendruscolo F, et al. Biosorption of hexavalent chromium by Pleurotus ostreatus. *Heliyon*. 2019 Mar 29;5(3):e01450.

[2455] Purnomo AS, Nawfa R, Martak F, et al. Biodegradation of Aldrin and Dieldrin by the White-Rot Fungus Pleurotus ostreatus. *Curr Microbiol*. 2017 Mar;74(3):320-324.

[2456] Gayosso-Canales M, Rodríguez-Vázquez R, et al. PCBs stimulate laccase production and activity in Pleurotus ostreatus thus promoting their removal. *Folia Microbiol (Praha)*. 2012 Mar;57(2):149-58.

[2457] Dementyev DV, Zotina TA, Manukovsky NS, et al. Biosorption of (241)Am from aqueous solutions and its biochemical fractionation in Pleurotus ostreatus mycelium. *Dokl Biochem Biophys*. 2015;460:34-6.

[2458] Šrédlová K, Škrob Z, Filipová A, et al. Biodegradation of PCBs in contaminated water using spent oyster mushroom substrate and a trickle-bed bioreactor. *Water Res*. 2020 Mar 1;170:115274.

[2459] Espinosa-Valdemar RM, Turpin-Marion S, et al. Disposable diapers biodegradation by the fungus Pleurotus ostreatus. *Waste Manag*. 2011 Aug;31(8):1683-8.

[2460] da Luz JM, Paes SA, Bazzolli DM, et al. Abiotic and biotic degradation of oxo-biodegradable plastic bags by Pleurotus ostreatus. *PLoS One*. 2014 Nov 24;9(11):e107438.

[2461] Hwang SS, Choi HT, Song HG. Biodegradation of endocrine-disrupting phthalates by Pleurotus ostreatus. *J Microbiol Biotechnol*. 2008 Apr;18(4):767-72.

[2462] Moeder M, Cajthaml T, Koeller G, et al. Structure selectivity in degradation and translocation of polychlorinated biphenyls (Delor 103) with a Pleurotus ostreatus (oyster mushroom) culture. *Chemosphere*. 2005 Dec;61(9):1370-8.

[2463] Mayans B, Camacho-Arévalo R, García-Delgado C, et al. An assessment of Pleurotus ostreatus to remove sulfonamides, and its role as a biofilter based on its own spent mushroom substrate. *Environ Sci Pollut Res Int*. 2021 Feb;28(6):7032-7042.

[2464] Ahuactzin-Pérez M, Tlécuitl-Beristain S, García-Dávila J, et al. Kinetics and pathway of biodegradation of dibutyl phthalate by Pleurotus ostreatus. *Fungal Biol*. 2018 Oct;122(10):991-997.

[2465] Vaseem H, Singh VK, Singh MP. Heavy metal pollution due to coal washery effluent and its decontamination using a macrofungus, Pleurotus ostreatus. *Ecotoxicol Environ Saf*. 2017 Nov;145:42-49.

[2466] Stella T, Covino S, Čvančarová M, et al. Bioremediation of long-term PCB-contaminated soil by white-rot fungi. *J Hazard Mater*. 2017 Feb 15;324(Pt B):701-710.

[2467] Silva ADM, Sousa J, Hultberg M, et al. Fluoxetine Removal from Aqueous Solutions Using a Lignocellulosic Substrate Colonized by the White-Rot Fungus Pleurotus ostreatus. *Int J Environ Res Public Health*. 2022 Feb 25;19(5):2672.

[2468] Palli L, Castellet-Rovira F, Pérez-Trujillo M, et al. Preliminary evaluation of Pleurotus ostreatus for the removal of selected pharmaceuticals from hospital wastewater. *Biotechnol Prog*. 2017 Nov;33(6):1529-1537.

[2469] Karas PA, Makri S, Papadopoulou ES, et al. The potential of organic substrates based on mushroom substrate and straw to dissipate fungicides contained in effluents from the fruit-packaging industry - Is there a role for Pleurotus ostreatus? *Ecotoxicol Environ Saf*. 2016 Feb;124:447-454.

[2470] George J, Rajendran DS, Senthil Kumar P, et al. Efficient decolorization and detoxification of triarylmethane and azo dyes by porous-cross-linked enzyme aggregates of Pleurotus ostreatus laccase. *Chemosphere*. 2023 Feb;313:137612.

[2471] Byss M, Elhottová D, Tříska J, et al. Fungal bioremediation of the creosote-contaminated soil: influence of Pleurotus ostreatus and Irpex lacteus on polycyclic aromatic hydrocarbons removal and soil microbial community composition in the laboratory-scale study. *Chemosphere*. 2008 Nov;73(9):1518-24.

[2472] Novotný C, Vyas BR, Erbanová P, et al. Removal of PCBs by various white rot fungi in liquid cultures. *Folia Microbiol (Praha)*. 1997;42(2):136-40.

[2473] Rodríguez S, Fernández M, Bermúdez RC, et al. [Treatment of coloured industrial effluents with Pleurotus spp]. *Rev Iberoam Micol*. 2003 Dec;20(4):164-8.

[2474] Blanco-Orta MF, García-de la Cruz RF, Paz-Maldonado LMT, et al. Assessing three industrially produced fungi for the bioremediation of diclofenac. *J Environ Sci Health A Tox Hazard Subst Environ Eng*. 2023;58(7):661-670.

[2475] Muzikář M, Křesinová Z, Svobodová K, et al. Biodegradation of chlorobenzoic acids by ligninolytic fungi. *J Hazard Mater*. 2011 Nov 30;196:386-94.

[2476] Mai C, Schormann W, Majcherczyk A, et al. Degradation of acrylic copolymers by white-rot fungi. *Appl Microbiol Biotechnol*. 2004 Sep;65(4):479-87.

[2477] Linhartová L, Michalíková K, Šrédlová K, et al. Biodegradability of Dental Care Antimicrobial Agents Chlorhexidine and Octenidine by Ligninolytic Fungi. *Molecules*. 2020 Jan 18;25(2):400.

[2478] Wang S, Li W, Liu L, et al. Biodegradation of decabromodiphenyl ethane (DBDPE) by white-rot fungus Pleurotus ostreatus: Characteristics, mechanisms, and toxicological response. *J Hazard Mater*. 2022 Feb 15;424(Pt D):127716.

[2479] Zhao X, Lu Y, Phillips DR, et al. Study of biodegradation products from azo dyes in fungal degradation by capillary electrophoresis/electrospray mass spectrometry. *J Chromatogr A*. 2007 Aug 3;1159(1-2):217-24.

[2480] Loffredo E, Castellana G, Senesi N. Decontamination of a municipal landfill leachate from endocrine disruptors using a combined sorption/bioremoval approach. *Environ Sci Pollut Res Int*. 2014 Feb;21(4):2654-62.

[2481] Kajaba I, Simoncic R, Frecerova K, et al. Clinical studies on the hypolipidemic and antioxidant effects of selected natural substances. *Bratisl Lek Listy*. 2008;109(6):267-72.

[2482] Schneider I, Kressel G, Meyer A, et al. Lipid lowering effects of oyster mushroom (Pleurotus ostreatus) in humans. *J Funct Foods*. 2011;3:17–24.

[2483] Jayasuriya WJ, Wanigatunge CA, Fernando GH, et al. Hypoglycaemic activity of culinary Pleurotus ostreatus and P. cystidiosus mushrooms in healthy volunteers and type 2 diabetic patients on diet control and the possible mechanisms of action. *Phytother Res*. 2015 Feb;29(2):303-9.

[2484] Dicks L, Jakobs L, Sari M, et al. Fortifying a meal with oyster mushroom powder beneficially affects postprandial glucagon-like peptide-1, non-esterified free fatty acids and hunger sensation in adults with impaired glucose tolerance: a double-blind randomized controlled crossover trial. *Eur J Nutr*. 2022 Mar;61(2):687-701.

[2485] Khatun K, Mahtab H, Khanam PA, et al. Oyster mushroom reduced blood glucose and cholesterol in diabetic subjects. *Mymensingh Med J*. 2007;16:94–99.

[2486] Choudhury BK, Rahman T, Kakon A, et al. Effects of Pleurotus ostreatus on Blood Pressure and Glycemic Status of Hypertensive Diabetic Male Volunteers. *J Med Biochem*. 2013 Jan;6(1):5-10.

[2487] Choudhury MBK. Pleurotus ostreatus improves lipid profile of obese hypertensive nondiabetic males. *Bangladesh J Med Biochem*. 2013;7:37–44.

[2488] Sayeed MA, Banu A, Khatun K, et al. Effect of Edible Mushroom (Pleurotus ostreatus) on Type-2 Diabetics. *Ibrahim Med College J*. 2015 Apr;8(1):6-11.

[2489] Jesenak M, Hrubisko M, Majtan J, et al. Anti-allergic effect of Pleuran (β-glucan from Pleurotus ostreatus) in children with recurrent respiratory tract infections. *Phytother Res*. 2014 Mar;28(3):471-4.

[2490] Jesenak M, Majtan J, Rennerova Z, et al. Immunomodulatory effect of pleuran (β-glucan from Pleurotus ostreatus) in children with recurrent respiratory tract infections. *Int Immunopharmacol*. 2013 Feb;15(2):395-9.

[2491] Rennerova Z, Picó Sirvent L, Carvajal Roca E, et al. Beta-(1,3/1,6)-D-glucan from Pleurotus ostreatus in the prevention of recurrent respiratory tract infections: An international, multicentre, open-label, prospective study. *Front Pediatr*. 2022 Oct 14;10:999701.

[2492] Minov J, Bislimovska-Karadzhinska J, Petrova T, et al. Effects of Pleuran (B-Glucan from Pleurotus Ostreatus) Supplementation on Incidence and Duration of COPD Exacerbations. *Open Access Maced J Med Sci*. 2017 Nov 16;5(7):893-898.

[2493] Urbancikova I, Hudackova D, Majtan J, et al. Efficacy of Pleuran (β-Glucan from Pleurotus ostreatus) in the Management of Herpes Simplex Virus Type 1 Infection. *Evid Based Complement Alternat Med*. 2020 Apr 13;2020:8562309.

[2494] González-Bonilla A, Meneses ME, Pérez-Herrera A, et al. Dietary Supplementation with Oyster Culinary-Medicinal Mushroom, Pleurotus ostreatus (Agaricomycetes), Reduces Visceral Fat and Hyperlipidemia in Inhabitants of a Rural Community in Mexico. *Int J Med Mushrooms*. 2022;24(9):49-61.

[2495] Majtan J. Pleuran (β-glucan from Pleurotus ostreatus): an effective nutritional supplement against upper respiratory tract infections? *Med Sport Sci*. 2012;59:57-61.

[2496] Bobovčák M, Kuniaková R, Gabriž J, et al. Effect of Pleuran (β-glucan from Pleurotus ostreatus) supplementation on cellular immune response after intensive exercise in elite athletes. *Appl Physiol Nutr Metab*. 2010 Dec;35(6):755-62.

[2497] Spacek J, Vocka M, Zavadova E, et al. Immunomodulation with β-glucan from Pleurotus ostreatus in patients with endocrine-dependent breast cancer. *Immunotherapy*. 2022 Jan;14(1):31-40.

[2498] Jesenak M, Urbancek S, Majtan J, et al. β-Glucan-based cream (containing pleuran isolated from pleurotus ostreatus) in supportive treatment of mild-to-moderate atopic dermatitis. *J Dermatolog Treat*. 2016 Aug;27(4):351-4.

[2499] Schiano I, Raco S, Cestone E, et al. Pleuran-β-Glucan from Oyster Culinary-Medicinal Mushroom, Pleurotus ostreatus (Agaricomycetes), Soothes and Improves Skin Parameters. *Int J Med Mushrooms*. 2021;23(12):75-83.

[2500] Jagadeesh R, Babu G, Lakshmanan H, et al. Bioactive Sterol Derivatives Isolated from the Pleurotus djamor var. Roseus Induced Apoptosis in Cancer Cell Lines. *Cardiovasc Hematol Agents Med Chem*. 2020;18(2):124-134.

[2501] Inci Ş, Akyüz M, Kirbag S. Antimicrobial, Antioxidant, Cytotoxicity and DNA Protective Properties of the Pink Oyster Mushroom, Pleurotus djamor (Agaricomycetes). *Int J Med Mushrooms*. 2023;25(2):55-66.

[2502] Maity GN, Maity P, Choudhuri I, et al. Structural studies of a water insoluble β-glucan from Pleurotus djamor and its cytotoxic effect against PA1, ovarian carcinoma cells. *Carbohydr Polym*. 2019 Oct 15;222:114990.

[2503] Jagadeesh R, Babu G, Lakshmanan H, et al. Bioactive Sterol Derivatives Isolated from the Pleurotus djamor var. Roseus Induced Apoptosis in Cancer Cell Lines. *Cardiovasc Hematol Agents Med Chem*. 2020;18(2):124-134.

[2504] Borges GM, De Barba FF, Schiebelbein AP, et al. Extracellular polysaccharide production by a strain of Pleurotus djamor isolated in the south of Brazil and antitumor activity on Sarcoma 180. *Braz J Microbiol*. 2014 Mar 10;44(4):1059-65.

[2505] Nayak H, Kushwaha A, Behera PC, et al. The Pink Oyster Mushroom, Pleurotus djamor (Agaricomycetes): A Potent Antioxidant and Hypoglycemic Agent. *Int J Med Mushrooms*. 2021;23(12):29-36.

[2506] Zhang J, Meng G, Zhang C, et al. The antioxidative effects of acidic-, alkalic-, and enzymatic-extractable mycelium zinc polysaccharides by Pleurotus djamor on liver and kidney of streptozocin-induced diabetic mice. *BMC Complement Altern Med*. 2015 Dec 18;15:440.

[2507] Li H, Feng Y, Sun W, Kong Y, et al. Antioxidation, anti-inflammation and anti-fibrosis effect of phosphorylated polysaccharides from Pleurotus djamor mycelia on adenine-induced chronic renal failure mice. *Int J Biol Macromol*. 2021 Feb 15;170:652-663.

[2508] Zhang J, Liu M, Yang Y, et al. Purification, characterization and hepatoprotective activities of mycelia zinc polysaccharides by Pleurotus djamor. *Carbohydr Polym*. 2016 Jan 20;136:588-97.

[2509] Sánchez JE, Jiménez-Pérez G, Liedo P. Can consumption of antioxidant rich mushrooms extend longevity?: antioxidant activity of Pleurotus spp. and its effects on Mexican fruit flies' (Anastrepha ludens) longevity. *Age (Dordr)*. 2015 Dec;37(6):107.

[2510] Li H, Zhao H, Gao Z, et al. The Antioxidant and Anti-Aging Effects of Acetylated Mycelia Polysaccharides from Pleurotus djamor. *Molecules*. 2019 Jul 24;24(15):2698.

[2511] Nayak H, Kushwaha A, Behera PC, et al. The Pink Oyster Mushroom, Pleurotus djamor (Agaricomycetes): A Potent Antioxidant and Hypoglycemic Agent. *Int J Med Mushrooms*. 2021;23(12):29-36.

[2512] Jiao F, Wang X, Song X, et al. Processing optimization and anti-oxidative activity of enzymatic extractable polysaccharides from Pleurotus djamor. *Int J Biol Macromol*. 2017 May;98:469-478.

[2513] Maity GN, Maity P, Khatua S, et al. Structural features and antioxidant activity of a new galactoglucan from edible mushroom Pleurotus djamor. *Int J Biol Macromol*. 2021 Jan 31;168:743-749.

[2514] Sudha G, Janardhanan A, Moorthy A, et al. Comparative study on the antioxidant activity of methanolic and aqueous extracts from the fruiting bodies of an edible mushroom Pleurotus djamor. *Food Sci Biotechnol*. 2016 Apr 30;25(2):371-377.

[2515] Inci Ş, Akyüz M, Kirbag S. Antimicrobial, Antioxidant, Cytotoxicity and DNA Protective Properties of the Pink Oyster Mushroom, Pleurotus djamor (Agaricomycetes). *Int J Med Mushrooms*. 2023;25(2):55-66.

[2516] Oropeza-Guerrero MP, Santos-Sánchez NF, Salas-Coronado R, et al. Productivity and Antioxidant Activity of Wild, Reconstituted, and Hybrid Strains of the Pink Oyster Mushroom, Pleurotus djamor (Agaricomycetes), from Mexico. *Int J Med Mushrooms*. 2018;20(7):607-621.

[2517] Babu DR, Pandey M, Rao GN. Antioxidant and electrochemical properties of cultivated Pleurotus spp. and their sporeless/low sporing mutants. *J Food Sci Technol*. 2014 Nov;51(11):3317-24.

[2518] Inci Ş, Akyüz M, Kirbag S. Antimicrobial, Antioxidant, Cytotoxicity and DNA Protective Properties of the Pink Oyster Mushroom, Pleurotus djamor (Agaricomycetes). *Int J Med Mushrooms*. 2023;25(2):55-66.

[2519] Illuri R, M E, M K, et al. Bio-prospective potential of Pleurotus djamor and Pleurotus florida mycelial extracts towards Gram positive and Gram negative microbial pathogens causing infectious disease. *J Infect Public Health*. 2022 Feb;15(2):297-306.

[2520] Inci Ş, Akyüz M, Kirbag S. Antimicrobial, Antioxidant, Cytotoxicity and DNA Protective Properties of the Pink Oyster Mushroom, Pleurotus djamor (Agaricomycetes). *Int J Med Mushrooms*. 2023;25(2):55-66.

[2521] Pineda-Alegría JA, Sánchez-Vázquez JE, González-Cortazar M, et al. The Edible Mushroom Pleurotus djamor Produces Metabolites with Lethal Activity Against the Parasitic Nematode Haemonchus contortus. *J Med Food*. 2017 Dec;20(12):1184-1192.

[2522] González-Cortázar M, Sánchez JE, Huicochea-Medina M, et al. In Vitro and In Vivo Nematicide Effect of Extract Fractions of Pleurotus djamor Against Haemonchus contortus. *J Med Food*. 2021 Mar;24(3):310-318.

[2523] Colmenares-Cruz S, González-Cortazar M, Castañeda-Ramírez GS, et al. Nematocidal activity of hydroalcoholic extracts of spent substrate of Pleurotus djamor on L3 larvae of Haemonchus contortus. *Vet Parasitol*. 2021 Dec;300:109608.

[2524] Cruz-Ornelas R, Sánchez-Vázquez JE, Amaya-Delgado L, et al. Biodegradation of NSAIDs and their effect on the activity of ligninolytic enzymes from Pleurotus djamor. *3 Biotech*. 2019 Oct;9(10):373.

[2525] Wu F, Li SJ, Dong CH, Dai YC, et al. The Genus Pachyma (Syn. Wolfiporia) Reinstated and Species Clarification of the Cultivated Medicinal Mushroom "Fuling" in China. *Front Microbiol*. 2020 Dec 15;11:590788.

[2526] Cheng S, Castillo V, Silva D. CDC20 associated with cancer metastasis and novel mushroom-derived CDC20 inhibitors with antimetastatic activity. *Int J Oncol*. 2019 Jun;54(6):2250-56.

[2527] Jiang Y, Fan L. The effect of Poria cocos ethanol extract on the intestinal barrier function and intestinal microbiota in mice with breast cancer. *J Ethnopharmacol*. 2021 Feb 10;266:113456.

[2528] Jiang TT, Ding LF, Nie W, et al. Tetranorlanostane and Lanostane Triterpenoids with Cytotoxic Activity from the Epidermis of Poria cocos. *Chem Biodivers*. 2021 May;18(5):e2100196.

[2529] Ma X, Wu J, Liu C, et al. Deciphering of Key Pharmacological Pathways of Poria Cocos Intervention in Breast Cancer Based on Integrated Pharmacological Method. *Evid Based Complement Alternat Med*. 2020 Oct 9;2020:4931531.

[2530] Jiang Y, Fan L. Evaluation of anticancer activities of Poria cocos ethanol extract in breast cancer: In vivo and in vitro, identification and mechanism. *J Ethnopharmacol*. 2020 Jul 15;257:112851.

[2531] Liu X, Wang X, Xu X, et al. Purification, antitumor and anti-inflammation activities of an alkali-soluble and carboxymethyl polysaccharide CMP33 from Poria cocos. *Int J Biol Macromol*. 2019 Apr 15;127:39-47.

[2532] Hu K, Luo Q, Zhu XF, et al. [Isolation of homogeneous polysaccharide from Poria cocos and effect of its sulfated derivatives on migration of human breast cancer MDA-MB-231 cells]. *Zhongguo Zhong Yao Za Zhi*. 2019 Jul;44(13):2835-2840.

[2533] Zhang M, Chiu LC, Cheung PC, et al. Growth-inhibitory effects of a beta-glucan from the mycelium of Poria cocos on human breast carcinoma MCF-7 cells: cell-cycle arrest and apoptosis induction. *Oncol Rep*. 2006 Mar;15(3):637-43.

[2534] Miao G, Han J, Zhang J, et al. Targeting Pyruvate Kinase M2 and Hexokinase II, Pachymic Acid Impairs Glucose Metabolism and Induces Mitochondrial Apoptosis. *Biol Pharm Bull*. 2019 Jan 1;42(1):123-129.

[2535] Ling H, Zhang Y, Ng KY, et al. Pachymic acid impairs breast cancer cell invasion by suppressing nuclear factor-κB-dependent matrix metalloproteinase-9 expression. *Breast Cancer Res Treat*. 2011 Apr;126(3):609-20.

[2536] Li Y, Li X, Lu Y, et al. Co-delivery of Poria cocos extract and doxorubicin as an 'all-in-one' nanocarrier to combat breast cancer multidrug resistance during chemotherapy. *Nanomedicine*. 2020 Jan;23:102095.

[2537] Wang N, Liu D, Guo J, et al. Molecular mechanism of Poria cocos combined with oxaliplatin on the inhibition of epithelial-mesenchymal transition in gastric cancer cells. *Biomed Pharmacother*. 2018 Jun:102:865-873.

[2538] Liu X, Wang X, Xu X, et al. Purification, antitumor and anti-inflammation activities of an alkali-soluble and carboxymethyl polysaccharide CMP33 from Poria cocos. *Int J Biol Macromol*. 2019 Apr 15;127:39-47.

[2539] Wang Y, Zhang L, Li Y, et al. Correlation of structure to antitumor activities of five derivatives of a beta-glucan from Poria cocos sclerotium. *Carbohydr Res*. 2004 Oct 20;339(15):2567-74.

[2540] Wang H, Luo Y, Chu Z, et al. Poria Acid, Triterpenoids Extracted from Poria cocos, Inhibits the Invasion and Metastasis of Gastric Cancer Cells. *Molecules*. 2022 Jun 6;27(11):3629.

[2541] Xu H, Wang Y, Zhao J, et al. Triterpenes from Poria cocos are revealed as potential retinoid X receptor selective agonists based on cell and in silico evidence. *Chem Biol Drug Des*. 2020 May;95(5):493-502.

[2542] Lee S, Lee S, Roh HS, et al. Cytotoxic constituents from the sclerotia of Poria cocos against human lung adenocarcinoma cells by inducing mitochondrial apoptosis. *Cells*. 2018;7(9):116.

[2543] Jiang TT, Ding LF, Nie W, et al. Tetranorlanostane and Lanostane Triterpenoids with Cytotoxic Activity from the Epidermis of Poria cocos. *Chem Biodivers*. 2021 May;18(5):e2100196.

[2544] Lee S, Lee S, Roh HS, et al. Cytotoxic Constituents from the Sclerotia of Poria cocos against Human Lung Adenocarcinoma Cells by Inducing Mitochondrial Apoptosis. *Cells*. 2018 Aug 24;7(9):116.

[2545] Liu X, Wang X, Xu X, et al. Purification, antitumor and anti-inflammation activities of an alkali-soluble and carboxymethyl polysaccharide CMP33 from Poria cocos. *Int J Biol Macromol*. 2019 Apr 15;127:39-47.

[2546] Kikuchi T, Uchiyama E, Ukiya M, et al. Cytotoxic and apoptosis-inducing activities of triterpene acids from Poria cocos. *J Nat Prod*. 2011 Feb 25;74(2):137-44.

[2547] Zhou L, Zhang Y, Gapter LA, et al. Cytotoxic and anti-oxidant activities of lanostane-type triterpenes isolated from Poria cocos. *Chem Pharm Bull (Tokyo)*. 2008 Oct;56(10):1459-62.

[2548] Ma J, Liu J, Lu C, et al. Pachymic acid induces apoptosis via activating ROS-dependent JNK and ER stress pathways in lung cancer cells. *Cancer Cell Int*. 2015 Aug 5;15:78.

[2549] Ling H, Zhou L, Jia X, et al. Polyporenic acid C induces caspase-8-mediated apoptosis in human lung cancer A549 cells. *Mol Carcinog*. 2009 Jun;48(6):498-507.

[2550] Lin TY, Lu MK, Chang CC. Structural identification of a fucose-containing 1,3-β-mannoglucan from Poria cocos and its anti-lung cancer CL1-5 cells migration via inhibition of TGFβR-mediated signaling. *Int J Biol Macromol*. 2020 Aug 15;157:311-318.

[2551] Qin L, Huang D, Huang J, et al. Integrated Analysis and Finding Reveal Anti-Liver Cancer Targets and Mechanisms of Pachyman (Poria cocos Polysaccharides). *Front Pharmacol*. 2021 Sep 17;12:742349.

[2552] Jiang TT, Ding LF, Nie W, et al. Tetranorlanostane and Lanostane Triterpenoids with Cytotoxic Activity from the Epidermis of Poria cocos. *Chem Biodivers*. 2021 May;18(5):e2100196.

[2553] Liu X, Wang X, Xu X, et al. Purification, antitumor and anti-inflammation activities of an alkali-soluble and carboxymethyl polysaccharide CMP33 from Poria cocos. *Int J Biol Macromol*. 2019 Apr 15;127:39-47.

[2554] Wang H, Sun X, Wei C, et al. Synthesis and bioactivity evaluation of pachymic acid derivatives as potential cytotoxic agents. *Med Chem Res*. 2023;32(2):342-354.

[2555] Lai KH, Lu MC, Du YC, et al. Cytotoxic Lanostanoids from Poria cocos. *J Nat Prod*. 2016 Nov 23;79(11):2805-2813.

[2556] Kikuchi T, Uchiyama E, Ukiya M, et al. Cytotoxic and apoptosis-inducing activities of triterpene acids from Poria cocos. *J Nat Prod*. 2011 Feb 25;74(2):137-44.

[2557] Choi YH. Induction of apoptosis by an ethanol extract of Poria cocos Wolf. in human leukemia U937 cells. *Oncol Rep*. 2015 Nov;34(5):2533-40.

[2558] Ukiya M, Akihisa T, Tokuda H, et al. Inhibition of tumor-promoting effects by poricoic acids G and H and other lanostane-type triterpenes and cytotoxic activity of poricoic acids A and G from Poria cocos. *J Nat Prod*. 2002 Apr;65(4):462-5.

[2559] Chen YY, Chang HM. Antiproliferative and differentiating effects of polysaccharide fraction from fu-ling (Poria cocos) on human leukemic U937 and HL-60 cells. *Food Chem Toxicol*. 2004 May;42(5):759-69.

[2560] Chen L, Fang W, Liu J, et al. Poricoic acid A (PAA) inhibits T-cell acute lymphoblastic leukemia through inducing autophagic cell death and ferroptosis. *Biochem Biophys Res Commun*. 2022 Jun 11;608:108-115.

[2561] Jiang TT, Ding LF, Nie W, et al. Tetranorlanostane and Lanostane Triterpenoids with Cytotoxic Activity from the Epidermis of Poria cocos. *Chem Biodivers*. 2021 May;18(5):e2100196.

[2562] Li G, Xu ML, Lee CS, et al. Cytotoxicity and DNA topoisomerases inhibitory activity of constituents from the sclerotium of Poria cocos. *Arch Pharm Res*. 2004 Aug;27(8):829-33.

[2563] Cheng S, Eliaz I, Lin J, et al. Triterpenes from Poria cocos suppress growth and invasiveness of pancreatic cancer cells through the downregulation of MMP-7. *Int J Oncol*. 2013 Jun;42(6):1869-74.

[2564] Cheng S, Swanson K, Eliaz I, et al. Pachymic acid inhibits growth and induces apoptosis of pancreatic cancer in vitro and in vivo by targeting ER stress. *PLoS One*. 2015 Apr 27;10(4):e0122270.

[2565] Zhou L, Zhang Y, Gapter LA, et al. Cytotoxic and anti-oxidant activities of lanostane-type triterpenes isolated from Poria cocos. *Chem Pharm Bull (Tokyo)*. 2008 Oct;56(10):1459-62.

[2566] Gapter L, Wang Z, Glinski J, et al. Induction of apoptosis in prostate cancer cells by pachymic acid from Poria cocos. *Biochem Biophys Res Commun*. 2005 Jul 15;332(4):1153-61.

[2567] Ma R, Zhang Z, Xu J, et al. Poricoic acid A induces apoptosis and autophagy in ovarian cancer via modulating the mTOR/p70s6k signaling axis. *Braz J Med Biol Res*. 2021 Oct 18;54(12):e11183.

[2568] Wen H, Wu Z, Hu H, et al. The anti-tumor effect of pachymic acid on osteosarcoma cells by inducing PTEN and Caspase 3/7-dependent apoptosis. *J Nat Med*. 2018 Jan;72(1):57-63.

[2569] Jeong JW, Lee WS, Go SI, et al. Pachymic Acid Induces Apoptosis of EJ Bladder Cancer Cells by DR5 Up-Regulation, ROS Generation, Modulation of Bcl-2 and IAP Family Members. *Phytother Res*. 2015 Oct;29(10):1516-24.

[2570] Akihisa T, Nakamura Y, Tokuda H, et al. Triterpene acids from Poria cocos and their anti-tumor-promoting effects. *J Nat Prod*. 2007 Jun;70(6):948-53.

[2571] Akihisa T, Uchiyama E, Kikuchi T, et al. Anti-tumor-promoting effects of 25-methoxyporicoic acid A and other triterpene acids from Poria cocos. *J Nat Prod*. 2009 Oct;72(10):1786-92.

[2572] Kaminaga T, Yasukawa K, Kanno H, et al. Inhibitory effects of lanostane-type triterpene acids, the components of Poria cocos, on tumor promotion by 12-O-tetradecanoylphorbol-13-acetate in two-stage carcinogenesis in mouse skin. *Oncology*. 1996 Sep-Oct;53(5):382-5.

[2573] Cheng S, Castillo V, Sliva D. CDC20 associated with cancer metastasis and novel mushroom-derived CDC20 inhibitors with antimetastatic activity. *Int J Oncol*. 2019 Jun;54(6):2250-2256.

[2574] Kang HM, Lee SK, Shin DS, et al. Dehydrotrametenolic acid selectively inhibits the growth of H-ras transformed rat2 cells and induces apoptosis through caspase-3 pathway. *Life Sci*. 2006 Jan 2;78(6):607-13.

[2575] Yin L, Huang G, Khan I, et al. Poria cocos polysaccharides exert prebiotic function to attenuate the adverse effects and improve the therapeutic outcome of 5-FU in ApcMin/+ mice. *Chin Med.* 2022 Oct 3;17(1):116.

[2576] Lee D, Lee S, Shim SH, et al. Protective effect of lanostane triterpenoids from the sclerotia of Poria cocos Wolf against cisplatin-induced apoptosis in LLC-PK1 cells. *Bioorg Med Chem Lett.* 2017 Jul 1;27(13):2881-2885.

[2577] Wang C, Yang S, Gao L, et al. Carboxymethyl pachyman (CMP) reduces intestinal mucositis and regulates the intestinal microflora in 5-fluorouracil-treated CT26 tumour-bearing mice. *Food Funct.* 2018 May 23;9(5):2695-2704.

[2578] Jin Y, Zhang L, Zhang M, et al. Antitumor activities of heteropolysaccharides of Poria cocos mycelia from different strains and culture media. *Carbohydr Res.* 2003 Jul 4;338(14):1517-21.

[2579] Chen X, Zhang L, Cheung PC. Immunopotentiation and anti-tumor activity of carboxymethylated-sulfated beta-(1-->3)-d-glucan from Poria cocos. *Int Immunopharmacol.* 2010 Apr;10(4):398-405.

[2580] Zhang L, Chen L, Xu X, et al. Effect of molecular mass on antitumor activity of heteropolysaccharide from Poria cocos. *Biosci Biotechnol Biochem.* 2005 Mar;69(3):631-4.

[2581] Lin Y, Zhang L, Chen L, et al. Molecular mass and antitumor activities of sulfated derivatives of alpha-glucan from Poria cocos mycelia. *Int J Biol Macromol.* 2004 Oct;34(5):289-94.

[2582] Wang Y, Zhang L, Li Y, et al. Correlation of structure to antitumor activities of five derivatives of a beta-glucan from Poria cocos sclerotium. *Carbohydr Res.* 2004 Oct 20;339(15):2567-74.

[2583] Sun Y, Liu Z, Pi Z, et al. Poria cocos could ameliorate cognitive dysfunction in APP/PS1 mice by restoring imbalance of Aβ production and clearance and gut microbiota dysbiosis. *Phytother Res.* 2021 May;35(5):2768-90.

[2584] Jiang Y, Fan L. The effect of Poria cocos ethanol extract on the intestinal barrier function and intestinal microbiota in mice with breast cancer. *J Ethnopharmacol.* 2021 Feb 10;266:113456.

[2585] Zou YT, Zhou J, Wu CY, et al. Protective effects of Poria cocos and its components against cisplatin-induced intestinal injury. *J Ethnopharmacol.* 2021;269:113722.

[2586] Yin L, Huang G, Khan I, et al. Poria cocos polysaccharides exert prebiotic function to attenuate the adverse effects and improve the therapeutic outcome of 5-FU in ApcMin/+ mice. *Chin Med.* 2022 Oct 3;17(1):116.

[2587] Zhu L, Ye C, Hu B, et al. Regulation of gut microbiota and intestinal metabolites by Poria cocos oligosaccharides improves glycolipid metabolism disturbance in high-fat diet-fed mice. *J Nutr Biochem.* 2022 Sep;107:109019.

[2588] Xu H, Wang Y, Jurutka PW, et al. 16α-Hydroxytrametenolic Acid from Poria cocos Improves Intestinal Barrier Function Through the Glucocorticoid Receptor-Mediated PI3K/Akt/NF-κB Pathway. *J Agric Food Chem.* 2019 Oct 2;67(39):10871-10879.

[2589] Sun SS, Wang K, Ma K, et al. An insoluble polysaccharide from the sclerotium of Poria cocos improves hyperglycemia, hyperlipidemia and hepatic steatosis in ob/ob mice via modulation of gut microbiota. *Chin J Nat Med.* 2019 Jan;17(1):3-14.

[2590] Lai Y, Yu H, Deng H, et al. Three main metabolites from Wolfiporia cocos (F. A. Wolf) Ryvarden & Gilb regulate the gut microbiota in mice: A comparative study using microbiome-metabolomics. *Front Pharmacol.* 2022 Aug 3;13:911140.

[2591] Wang C, Yang S, Gao L, et al. Carboxymethyl pachyman (CMP) reduces intestinal mucositis and regulates the intestinal microflora in 5-fluorouracil-treated CT26 tumour-bearing mice. *Food Funct.* 2018 May 23;9(5):2695-2704.

[2592] Jiang Y, Fan L. The effect of Poria cocos ethanol extract on the intestinal barrier function and intestinal microbiota in mice with breast cancer. *J Ethnopharmacol.* 2021 Feb 10;266:113456.

[2593] Xu H, Wang Y, Jurutka PW, et al. 16α-hydroxytrametenolic acid from Poria cocos improves intestinal barrier function through the glucocorticoid receptor-mediated PI3K/Akt/NF-κB pathway. *J Agric Food Chem.* 2019;67(39):10871-10879.

[2594] Zou YT, Zhou J, Wu CY, et al. Protective effects of Poria cocos and its components against cisplatin-induced intestinal injury. *J Ethnopharmacol.* 2021;269:113722.

[2595] Ye H, Ma S, Qiu Z, et al. Poria cocos polysaccharides rescue pyroptosis-driven gut vascular barrier disruption in order to alleviates non-alcoholic steatohepatitis. *J Ethnopharmacol.* 2022 Oct 5;296:115457.

[2596] Duan Y, Huang J, Sun M, et al. Poria cocos polysaccharide improves intestinal barrier function and maintains intestinal homeostasis in mice. *Int J Biol Macromol.* 2023 Sep 30;249:125953.

[2597] Jiang YH, Wang L, Chen WD, et al. Poria cocos polysaccharide prevents alcohol-induced hepatic injury and inflammation by repressing oxidative stress and gut leakiness. *Front Nutr.* 2022 Aug 17;9:963598.

[2598] Yin L, Huang G, Khan I, et al. Poria cocos polysaccharides exert prebiotic function to attenuate the adverse effects and improve the therapeutic outcome of 5-FU in ApcMin/+ mice. *Chin Med.* 2022 Oct 3;17(1):116.

[2599] Lan K, Yang H, Zheng J, et al. Poria cocos oligosaccharides ameliorate dextran sodium sulfate-induced colitis mice by regulating gut microbiota dysbiosis. *Food Funct.* 2023 Jan 23;14(2):857-873.

[2600] Tan Z, Zhang Q, Zhao R, et al. A Comparative Study on the Effects of Different Sources of Carboxymethyl Poria Polysaccharides on the Repair of DSS-Induced Colitis in Mice. *Int J Mol Sci.* 2023 May 20;24(10):9034.

[2601] Liu X, Yu X, Xu X, et al. The protective effects of Poria cocos-derived polysaccharide CMP33 against IBD in mice and its molecular mechanism. *Food Funct.* 2018 Nov 14;9(11):5936-5949.

[2602] Xu H, Wang S, Jiang Y, et al. Poria cocos Polysaccharide Ameliorated Antibiotic-Associated Diarrhea in Mice via Regulating the Homeostasis of the Gut Microbiota and Intestinal Mucosal Barrier. *Int J Mol Sci.* 2023 Jan 11;24(2):1423.

[2603] Lai Y, Deng H, Fang Q, et al. Water-Insoluble Polysaccharide Extracted from Poria cocos Alleviates Antibiotic-Associated Diarrhea Based on Regulating the Gut Microbiota in Mice. *Foods.* 2023 Aug 16;12(16):3080.

[2604] Tu Y, Luo X, Liu D, et al. Extracts of Poria cocos improve functional dyspepsia via regulating brain-gut peptides, immunity and repairing of gastrointestinal mucosa. *Phytomedicine.* 2022 Jan;95:153875.

[2605] Sun Y, Liu Z, Pi Z, et al. Poria cocos could ameliorate cognitive dysfunction in APP/PS1 mice by restoring imbalance of Aβ production and clearance and gut microbiota dysbiosis. *Phytother Res.* 2021 May;35(5):2768-90.

[2606] Zhou X, Zhang Y, Jiang Y, et al. Poria cocos polysaccharide attenuates damage of nervus in Alzheimer's disease rat model induced by D-galactose and aluminum trichloride. *Neuroreport.* 2021 May 19;32(8):727-737.

[2607] Sun Y, Liu Z, Pi Z, et al. Poria cocos could ameliorate cognitive dysfunction in APP/PS1 mice by restoring imbalance of Aβ production and clearance and gut microbiota dysbiosis. *Phytother Res.* 2021 Jan 11. Online ahead of print.

[2608] Lv Q, Di X, Bian B, Li K, et al. Neuroprotective Effects of Poria cocos (Agaricomycetes) Essential Oil on Aβ1-40-Induced Learning and Memory Deficit in Rats. *Int J Med Mushrooms*. 2022;24(10):73-82.

[2609] Wu T, Hou W, Liu C, et al. Efficient Combination of Complex Chromatography, Molecular Docking and Enzyme Kinetics for Exploration of Acetylcholinesterase Inhibitors from Poria cocos. *Molecules*. 2023 Jan 27;28(3):1228.

[2610] Yu M, Xu X, Jiang N, et al. Dehydropachymic acid decreases bafilomycin A1 induced β-Amyloid accumulation in PC12 cells. *J Ethnopharmacol*. 2017 Feb 23;198:167-173.

[2611] Chen W, An W, Chu J. [Effect of water extract of Poria on cytosolic free calcium concentration in brain nerve cells of neonatal rats]. *Zhongguo Zhong Xi Yi Jie He Za Zhi*. 1998 May;18(5):293-5.

[2612] Pang Y, Zhu S, Pei H. Pachymic acid protects against cerebral ischemia/reperfusion injury by the PI3K/Akt signaling pathway. *Metab Brain Dis*. 2020 Apr;35(4):673-680.

[2613] Li TH, Hou CC, Chang CL, et al. Anti-hyperglycemic properties of crude extract and triterpenes from Poria cocos. *Evid Based Complement Alternat Med*. 2011;2011:128402.

[2614] Dai B, Wu Q, Zeng C, et al. The effect of Liuwei Dihuang decoction on PI3K/Akt signaling pathway in liver of type 2 diabetes mellitus (T2DM) rats with insulin resistance. *J Ethnopharmacol*. 2016;192:382-389.

[2615] Li TH, Hou CC, Chang CL, et al. Anti-Hyperglycemic Properties of Crude Extract and Triterpenes from Poria cocos. *Evid Based Complement Alternat Med*. 2011;2011:128402.

[2616] Ma C, Lu J, Ren M, et al. Rapid identification of α-glucosidase inhibitors from Poria using spectrum-effect, component knock-out, and molecular docking technique. *Front Nutr*. 2023 Aug 10;10:1089829.

[2617] Huang YC, Chang WL, Huang SF, et al. Pachymic acid stimulates glucose uptake through enhanced GLUT4 expression and translocation. *Eur J Pharmacol*. 2010 Dec 1;648(1-3):39-49.

[2618] Sato M, Tai T, Nunoura Y, et al. Dehydrotrametenolic acid induces preadipocyte differentiation and sensitizes animal models of noninsulin-dependent diabetes mellitus to insulin. *Biol Pharm Bull*. 2002 Jan;25(1):81-6.

[2619] Yoon JJ, Lee YJ, Lee SM, et al. Poria cocos inhibits high glucose-induced proliferation of rat mesangial cells. *Am J Chin Med*. 2013;41(1):71-83.

[2620] Wu Y, Deng H, Sun J, et al. Poricoic acid A induces mitophagy to ameliorate podocyte injury in diabetic kidney disease via downregulating FUNDC1. *J Biochem Mol Toxicol*. 2023 Sep 14:e23503.

[2621] Huang YJ, Hsu NY, Lu KH, et al. Poria cocos water extract ameliorates the behavioral deficits induced by unpredictable chronic mild stress in rats by down-regulating inflammation. *J Ethnopharmacol*. 2020;258:112566.

[2622] Lee CY, Lee CT, Tzeng IS, et al. Poria cocos Regulates Cell Migration and Actin Filament Aggregation in B35 and C6 Cells by Modulating the RhoA, CDC42, and Rho Signaling Pathways. *Evid Based Complement Alternat Med*. 2021 Sep 1;2021:6854860.

[2623] Chen YC, Lee CT, Tsai FM, et al. The Effects of Poria cocos on Rho Signaling-Induced Regulation of Mobility and F-Actin Aggregation in MK-801-Treated B35 and C6 Cells. *Behav Neurol*. 2022 Jul 12;2022:8225499.

[2624] Zhang W, Chen L, Li P, et al. Antidepressant and immunosuppressive activities of two polysaccharides from Poria cocos (Schw.) Wolf. *Int J Biol Macromol*. 2018 Dec;120(Pt B):1696-1704.

[2625] Zhang DD, Li HJ, Zhang HR, et al. Poria cocos water-soluble polysaccharide modulates anxiety-like behavior induced by sleep deprivation by regulating the gut dysbiosis, metabolic disorders and TNF-α/NF-κB signaling pathway. *Food Funct*. 2022 Jun 20;13(12):6648-6664.

[2626] Zhang D, Li H, Luo X, et al. Integrated 16S rDNA, metabolomics, and TNF-α/NF-κB signaling pathway analyses to explain the modulatory effect of Poria cocos aqueous extract on anxiety-like behavior. *Phytomedicine*. 2022 Sep;104:154300.

[2627] Shah VK, Choi JJ, Han JY, et al. Pachymic acid enhances pentobarbital-induced sleeping behaviors via GABAA-ergic systems in mice. *Biomol Ther (Seoul)*. 2014;22(4):314-320.

[2628] Kim H, Park I, Park K, et al. The Positive Effects of Poria cocos Extract on Quality of Sleep in Insomnia Rat Models. *Int J Environ Res Public Health*. 2022 May 29;19(11):6629.

[2629] Shah VK, Choi JJ, Han JY, et al. Pachymic Acid Enhances Pentobarbital-Induced Sleeping Behaviors via GABAA-ergic Systems in Mice. *Biomol Ther (Seoul)*. 2014 Jul;22(4):314-20.

[2630] Li W, Yu J, Zhao J, et al. Poria cocos polysaccharides reduces high-fat diet-induced arteriosclerosis in ApoE-/- mice by inhibiting inflammation. *Phytother Res*. 2021;35(4):2220-2229.

[2631] Zhao J, Niu X, Yu J, et al. Poria cocos polysaccharides attenuated ox-LDL-induced inflammation and oxidative stress via ERK activated Nrf2/HO-1 signaling pathway and inhibited foam cell formation in VSMCs. *Int Immunopharmacol*. 2020;80:106173.

[2632] Son TH, Kim SH, Shin HL, et al. Inhibition of Osteoclast Differentiation and Promotion of Osteogenic Formation by Wolfiporia extensa Mycelium. *J Microbiol Biotechnol*. 2023 Sep 28;33(9):1197-1205.

[2633] Hwang YH, Jang SA, Lee A, et al. Poria cocos ameliorates bone loss in ovariectomized mice and inhibits osteoclastogenesis in vitro. *Nutrients*. 2020;12(5):1383.

[2634] Song D, Cao Z, Tickner J, et al. Poria cocos polysaccharide attenuates RANKL-induced osteoclastogenesis by suppressing NFATc1 activity and phosphorylation of ERK and STAT3. *Arch Biochem Biophys*. 2018 Jun 1;647:76-83.

[2635] Liu J, Yu J, Peng X. Poria cocos Polysaccharides alleviates chronic nonbacterial prostatitis by preventing oxidative stress, regulating hormone production, modifying gut microbiota, and remodeling the DNA methylome. *J Agric Food Chem*. 2020;68(45):12661-12670.

[2636] Yu J, Hu Q, Liu J, et al. Metabolites of gut microbiota fermenting Poria cocos polysaccharide alleviates chronic nonbacterial prostatitis in rats. *Int J Biol Macromol*. 2022 Jun 1;209(Pt B):1593-1604.

[2637] Jin J, Chowdhury MHU, Hafizur Rahman M, et al. Bioactive Compounds and Signaling Pathways of Wolfiporia extensa in Suppressing Inflammatory Response by Network Pharmacology. *Life (Basel)*. 2023 Mar 27;13(4):893.

[2638] Lu MK, Chao CH, Hsu YC. Effect of carbohydrate-feeding strategy on the production, physiochemical changes, anti-inflammation activities of polysaccharides of Poria cocos. *Int J Biol Macromol*. 2021 Dec 1;192:435-443.

[2639] Liu X, Wang X, Xu X, et al. Purification, antitumor and anti-inflammation activities of an alkali-soluble and carboxymethyl polysaccharide CMP33 from Poria cocos. *Int J Biol Macromol*. 2019 Apr 15:127:39-47.

[2640] Lee SR, Lee S, Moon E, et al. Bioactivity-guided isolation of anti-inflammatory triterpenoids from the sclerotia of Poria cocos using LPS-stimulated Raw264.7 cells. *Bioorg Chem.* 2017 Feb;70:94-99.

[2641] Cai TG, Cai Y. Triterpenes from the fungus Poria cocos and their inhibitory activity on nitric oxide production in mouse macrophages via blockade of activating protein-1 pathway. *Chem Biodivers.* 2011 Nov;8(11):2135-43.

[2642] Jeong JW, Lee HH, Han MH, et al. Ethanol extract of Poria cocos reduces the production of inflammatory mediators by suppressing the NF-kappaB signaling pathway in lipopolysaccharide-stimulated RAW 264.7 macrophages. *BMC Complement Altern Med.* 2014 Mar 15;14:101.

[2643] Cuellar MJ, Giner RM, Recio MC, et al. Effect of the basidiomycete Poria cocos on experimental dermatitis and other inflammatory conditions. *Chem Pharm Bull (Tokyo).* 1997 Mar;45(3):492-4.

[2644] Yasukawa K, Kaminaga T, Kitanaka S, et al. 3 beta-p-hydroxybenzoyldehydrotumulosic acid from Poria cocos, and its anti-inflammatory effect. *Phytochemistry.* 1998 Aug;48(8):1357-60.

[2645] Nukaya H, Yamashiro H, Fukazawa H, et al. Isolation of inhibitors of TPA-induced mouse ear edema from Hoelen, Poria cocos. *Chem Pharm Bull (Tokyo).* 1996 Apr;44(4):847-9.

[2646] Tseng J, Chang JG. Suppression of tumor necrosis factor-alpha, interleukin-1 beta, interleukin-6 and granulocyte-monocyte colony stimulating factor secretion from human monocytes by an extract of Poria cocos. *Zhonghua Min Guo Wei Sheng Wu Ji Mian Yi Xue Za Zhi.* 1992 Feb;25(1):1-11.

[2647] Cuélla MJ, Giner RM, Recio MC, et al. Two fungal lanostane derivatives as phospholipase A2 inhibitors. *J Nat Prod.* 1996 Oct;59(10):977-9.

[2648] Giner-Larza EM, Máñez S, Giner-Pons RM, et al. On the anti-inflammatory and anti-phospholipase A(2) activity of extracts from lanostane-rich species. *J Ethnopharmacol.* 2000 Nov;73(1-2):61-9.

[2649] Yu SJ, Tseng J. Fu-Ling, a Chinese herbal drug, modulates cytokine secretion by human peripheral blood monocytes. *Int J Immunopharmacol.* 1996 Jan;18(1):37-44.

[2650] Wu Y, Ying J, Zhu X, et al. Pachymic acid suppresses the inflammatory response of chondrocytes and alleviates the progression of osteoarthritis via regulating the Sirtuin 6/NF-κB signal axis. *Int Immunopharmacol.* 2023 Aug 30;124(Pt A):110854.

[2651] Liang D, Yong T, Diao X, et al. Hypouricaemic and nephroprotective effects of Poria cocos in hyperuricemic mice by up-regulating ATP-binding cassette super-family G member 2. *Pharm Biol.* 2021 Dec;59(1):275-286.

[2652] Gai W, Zheng X, Wang C, et al. Marburg virus-like particles by co-expression of glycoprotein and matrix protein in insect cells induces immune responses in mice. *Virol J.* 2017;14(1):204.

[2653] Tian H, Liu Z, Pu Y, et al. Immunomodulatory effects exerted by Poria Cocos polysaccharides via TLR4/TRAF6/NF-κB signaling in vitro and in vivo. *Biomed Pharmacother.* 2019 Apr;112:108709.

[2654] Hu X, Hong B, Shan X, et al. The Effect of Poria cocos Polysaccharide PCP-1C on M1 Macrophage Polarization via the Notch Signaling Pathway. *Molecules.* 2023 Feb 24;28(5):2140.

[2655] Li YR, Liu ST, Gan Q, et al. Four polysaccharides isolated from Poria cocos mycelium and fermentation broth supernatant possess different activities on regulating immune response. *Int J Biol Macromol.* 2023 Jan 31;226:935-945.

[2656] Pu Y, Liu Z, Tian H, et al. The immunomodulatory effect of Poria cocos polysaccharides is mediated by the Ca2+/PKC/p38/NF-κB signaling pathway in macrophages. *Int Immunopharmacol.* 2019 Jul;72:252-257.

[2657] Liang J, Zhao M, Xie S, et al. Effect of steam explosion pretreatment on polysaccharide isolated from Poria cocos: Structure and immunostimulatory activity. *J Food Biochem.* 2022 Oct;46(10):e14355.

[2658] Liu J, Hong W, Li M, et al. Transcriptome analysis reveals immune and metabolic regulation effects of Poria cocos polysaccharides on Bombyx mori larvae. *Front Immunol.* 2022 Oct 28;13:1014985.

[2659] Wang H, Mukerabigwi JF, Zhang Y, et al. In vivo immunological activity of carboxymethylated-sulfated (1→3)-β-D-glucan from sclerotium of Poria cocos. *Int J Biol Macromol.* 2015 Aug;79:511-7.

[2660] Chang HH, Yeh CH, Sheu F. A novel immunomodulatory protein from Poria cocos induces Toll-like receptor 4-dependent activation within mouse peritoneal macrophages. *J Agric Food Chem.* 2009 Jul 22;57(14):6129-39.

[2661] Chen X, Zhang L, Cheung PC. Immunopotentiation and anti-tumor activity of carboxymethylated-sulfated beta-(1-->3)-d-glucan from Poria cocos. *Int Immunopharmacol.* 2010 Apr;10(4):398-405.

[2662] Lee KY, Jeon YJ. Polysaccharide isolated from Poria cocos sclerotium induces NF-kappaB/Rel activation and iNOS expression in murine macrophages. *Int Immunopharmacol.* 2003 Oct;3(10-11):1353-62.

[2663] Lee KY, You HJ, Jeong HG, et al. Polysaccharide isolated from Poria cocos sclerotium induces NF-kappaB/Rel activation and iNOS expression through the activation of p38 kinase in murine macrophages. *Int Immunopharmacol.* 2004 Aug;4(8):1029-38.

[2664] Liu F, Zhang L, Feng X, et al. Immunomodulatory Activity of Carboxymethyl Pachymaran on Immunosuppressed Mice Induced by Cyclophosphamide. *Molecules.* 2021 Sep 22;26(19):5733.

[2665] Chao CL, Huang HW, Su MH, et al. The Lanostane Triterpenoids in Poria cocos Play Beneficial Roles in Immunoregulatory Activity. *Life (Basel).* 2021 Feb 1;11(2):111.

[2666] Li YR, Liu ST, Gan Q, et al. Four polysaccharides isolated from Poria cocos mycelium and fermentation broth supernatant possess different activities on regulating immune response. *Int J Biol Macromol.* 2023 Jan 31;226:935-945.

[2667] Zhang W, Chen L, Li P, et al. Antidepressant and immunosuppressive activities of two polysaccharides from Poria cocos (Schw.) Wolf. *Int J Biol Macromol.* 2018 Dec;120(Pt B):1696-1704.

[2668] Jang TR, Kao MF, Chen CH, et al. Alleviating effects of dehydration under no hyperthermia on the immunomodulatory response to the polysaccharide fraction from fu-ling (Poria cocos) in male collegiate wrestlers. *Chin Med J (Engl).* 2011 Feb;124(4):530-6.

[2669] Kakegawa T, Yoshida LS, Takada M, et al. Comparison of the effects of pachymic acid, moronic acid and hydrocortisone on the polysome loading of RNAs in lipopolysaccharide-treated THP-1 macrophages. *J Nat Med.* 2019 Jan;73(1):190-201.

[2670] Zhang GW, Liu HY, Xia QM, et al. Anti-rejection effect of ethanol extract of Poria cocos wolf in rats after cardiac allograft implantation. *Chin Med J (Engl).* 2004 Jun;117(6):932-5.

[2671] Ding CG, Tian PX, Xue WJ. [Preventive effect of poria cocos on acute rejection of renal transplantation in rats]. *Zhongguo Zhong Xi Yi Jie He Za Zhi.* 2010 Mar;30(3):308-11.

[2672] Chao CL, Wang CJ, Huang HW, et al. Poria cocos Modulates Th1/Th2 Response and Attenuates Airway Inflammation in an Ovalbumin-Sensitized Mouse Allergic Asthma Model. *Life (Basel)*. 2021 Apr 21;11(5):372.

[2673] Bae MJ, See HJ, Choi G, et al. Regulatory T Cell Induced by Poria cocos Bark Exert Therapeutic Effects in Murine Models of Atopic Dermatitis and Food Allergy. *Mediators Inflamm*. 2016;2016:3472608.

[2674] Jiang GP, Liao YJ, Huang LL, et al. Effects and molecular mechanism of pachymic acid on ferroptosis in renal ischemia reperfusion injury. *Mol Med Rep*. 2021;23(1):63.

[2675] Liang D, Yong T, Diao X, et al. Hypouricaemic and nephroprotective effects of Poria cocos in hyperuricemic mice by up-regulating ATP-binding cassette super-family G member 2. *Pharm Biol*. 2021 Dec;59(1):275-286.

[2676] Zan JF, Shen CJ, Zhang LP, et al. Effect of Poria cocos hydroethanolic extract on treating adriamycin-induced rat model of nephrotic syndrome. *Chin J Integr Med*. 2017 Dec;23(12):916-922.

[2677] Jiang GP, Liao YJ, Huang LL, et al. Effects and molecular mechanism of pachymic acid on ferroptosis in renal ischemia reperfusion injury. *Mol Med Rep*. 2021 Jan;23(1):63.

[2678] Lee SM, Lee YJ, Yoon JJ, et al. Effect of Poria cocos on Puromycin Aminonucleoside-Induced Nephrotic Syndrome in Rats. *Evid Based Complement Alternat Med*. 2014;2014:570420.

[2679] Lee SM, Lee YJ, Yoon JJ, et al. Effect of Poria cocos on hypertonic stress-induced water channel expression and apoptosis in renal collecting duct cells. *J Ethnopharmacol*. 2012 May 7;141(1):368-76.

[2680] Chen DQ, Chen L, Guo Y, et al. Poricoic acid A suppresses renal fibroblast activation and interstitial fibrosis in UUO rats via upregulating Sirt3 and promoting β-catenin K49 deacetylation. *Acta Pharmacol Sin*. 2023 May;44(5):1038-1050.

[2681] Zhao YY, Lei P, Chen DQ, et al. Renal metabolic profiling of early renal injury and renoprotective effects of Poria cocos epidermis using UPLC Q-TOF/HSMS/MSE. *J Pharm Biomed Anal*. 2013 Jul-Aug;81-82:202-9.

[2682] Hattori T, Hayashi K, Nagao T, et al. Studies on antinephritic effects of plant components (3): Effect of pachyman, a main component of Poria cocos Wolf on original-type anti-GBM nephritis in rats and its mechanisms. *Jpn J Pharmacol*. 1992 May;59(1):89-96.

[2683] Wang M, Hu HH, Chen YY, et al. Novel poricoic acids attenuate renal fibrosis through regulating redox signalling and aryl hydrocarbon receptor activation. *Phytomedicine*. 2020 Dec;79:153323.

[2684] Chen L, Cao G, Wang M, et al. The Matrix Metalloproteinase-13 Inhibitor Poricoic Acid ZI Ameliorates Renal Fibrosis by Mitigating Epithelial-Mesenchymal Transition. *Mol Nutr Food Res*. 2019 Jul;63(13):e1900132.

[2685] Li Q, Ming Y, Jia H, et al. Poricoic acid A suppresses TGF-β1-induced renal fibrosis and proliferation via the PDGF-C, Smad3 and MAPK pathways. *Exp Ther Med*. 2021 Apr;21(4):289.

[2686] Wang M, Chen DQ, Wang MC, et al. Poricoic acid ZA, a novel RAS inhibitor, attenuates tubulo-interstitial fibrosis and podocyte injury by inhibiting TGF-β/Smad signaling pathway. *Phytomedicine*. 2017 Dec 1;36:243-253.

[2687] Wang M, Chen DQ, Chen L, et al. Novel RAS Inhibitors Poricoic Acid ZG and Poricoic Acid ZH Attenuate Renal Fibrosis via a Wnt/β-Catenin Pathway and Targeted Phosphorylation of smad3 Signaling. *J Agric Food Chem*. 2018 Feb 28;66(8):1828-1842.

[2688] Wang M, Chen DQ, Chen L, et al. Novel inhibitors of the cellular renin-angiotensin system components, poricoic acids, target Smad3 phosphorylation and Wnt/β-catenin pathway against renal fibrosis. *Br J Pharmacol*. 2018 Jul;175(13):2689-2708.

[2689] Chen DQ, Wang YN, Vaziri ND, et al. Poricoic acid A activates AMPK to attenuate fibroblast activation and abnormal extracellular matrix remodelling in renal fibrosis. *Phytomedicine*. 2020 Jul;72:153232.

[2690] Zhao YY, Feng YL, Bai X, et al. Ultra performance liquid chromatography-based metabonomic study of therapeutic effect of the surface layer of Poria cocos on adenine-induced chronic kidney disease provides new insight into anti-fibrosis mechanism. *PLoS One*. 2013;8(3):e59617.

[2691] Zhao YY, Li HT, Feng YL, et al. Urinary metabonomic study of the surface layer of Poria cocos as an effective treatment for chronic renal injury in rats. *J Ethnopharmacol*. 2013 Jul 9;148(2):403-10.

[2692] Chen DQ, Feng YL, Chen L, et al. Poricoic acid A enhances melatonin inhibition of AKI-to-CKD transition by regulating Gas6/AxlNFκB/Nrf2 axis. *Free Radic Biol Med*. 2019 Apr;134:484-497.

[2693] Yi XL, Hu J, Wu QT, et al. Effect of Different-Volume Fluid Resuscitation on Organ Functions in Severe Acute Pancreatitis and Therapeutic Effect of Poria cocos. *Evid Based Complement Alternat Med*. 2020 Oct 14;2020:6408202.

[2694] Li CY, Liu L, Zhao YW, et al. Inhibition of Calcium Oxalate Formation and Antioxidant Activity of Carboxymethylated Poria cocos Polysaccharides. *Oxid Med Cell Longev*. 2021 Mar 1;2021:6653593.

[2695] Xiong P, Cheng XY, Sun XY, et al. Interaction between nanometer calcium oxalate and renal epithelial cells repaired with carboxymethylated polysaccharides. *Biomater Adv*. 2022 Jun;137:212854.

[2696] Feng Z, Shi H, Liang B, et al. Bioinformatics and experimental findings reveal the therapeutic actions and targets of pachymic acid against cystitis glandularis. *Biofactors*. 2021 Jul;47(4):665-673.

[2697] Wu K, Guo C, Yang B, et al. Antihepatotoxic benefits of Poria cocos polysaccharides on acetaminophen-lesioned livers in vivo and in vitro. *J Cell Biochem*. 2019;120(5):7482-7488.

[2698] Cheng Y, Xie Y, Ge JC, et al. Structural characterization and hepatoprotective activity of a galactoglucan from Poria cocos. *Carbohydr Polym*. 2021 Jul 1;263:117979.

[2699] Wu K, Qin J, Liu M, et al. Bioinformatics approach and experimental validation reveal the hepatoprotective effect of pachyman against acetaminophen-associated liver injury. *Aging (Albany NY)*. 2023 Sep 6;15(17):8800-8811.

[2700] Jiang YH, Wang L, Chen WD, et al. Poria cocos polysaccharide prevents alcohol-induced hepatic injury and inflammation by repressing oxidative stress and gut leakiness. *Front Nutr*. 2022 Aug 17;9:963598.

[2701] Wu K, Fan J, Huang X, et al. Hepatoprotective effects exerted by Poria Cocos polysaccharides against acetaminophen-induced liver injury in mice. *Int J Biol Macromol*. 2018 Jul 15;114:137-142.

[2702] Wu K, Guo C, Yang B, et al. Antihepatotoxic benefits of Poria cocos polysaccharides on acetaminophen-lesioned livers in vivo and in vitro. *J Cell Biochem*. 2019 May;120(5):7482-7488.

[2703] Kim JH, Sim HA, Jung DY, et al. Poria cocus Wolf extract ameliorates hepatic steatosis through regulation of lipid metabolism, inhibition of ER stress, and activation of autophagy via AMPK activation. *Int J Mol Sci*. 2019;20(19):4801.

2704 Ye H, Ma S, Qiu Z, et al. Poria cocos polysaccharides rescue pyroptosis-driven gut vascular barrier disruption in order to alleviates non-alcoholic steatohepatitis. *J Ethnopharmacol*. 2022 Oct 5;296:115457.

2705 He J, Yang Y, Zhang F, et al. Effects of Poria cocos extract on metabolic dysfunction-associated fatty liver disease via the FXR/PPARα-SREBPs pathway. *Front Pharmacol*. 2022 Oct 5;13:1007274.

2706 Wang J, Zheng D, Huang F, et al. Theabrownin and Poria cocos Polysaccharide Improve Lipid Metabolism via Modulation of Bile Acid and Fatty Acid Metabolism. *Front Pharmacol*. 2022 Jun 27;13:875549.

2707 Tan YY, Yue SR, Lu AP, et al. The improvement of nonalcoholic steatohepatitis by Poria cocos polysaccharides associated with gut microbiota and NF-κB/CCL3/CCR1 axis. *Phytomedicine*. 2022 Aug;103:154208.

2708 Li W, Yu J, Zhao J, et al. Poria cocos polysaccharides reduces high-fat diet-induced arteriosclerosis in ApoE-/- mice by inhibiting inflammation. *Phytother Res*. 2021 Apr;35(4):2220-2229.

2709 Kim JH, Sim HA, Jung DY, et al. Poria cocus Wolf Extract Ameliorates Hepatic Steatosis through Regulation of Lipid Metabolism, Inhibition of ER Stress, and Activation of Autophagy via AMPK Activation. *Int J Mol Sci*. 2019 Sep 27;20(19):4801.

2710 Sun SS, Wang K, Ma K, et al. An insoluble polysaccharide from the sclerotium of Poria cocos improves hyperglycemia, hyperlipidemia and hepatic steatosis in ob/ob mice via modulation of gut microbiota. *Chin J Nat Med*. 2019 Jan;17(1):3-14.

2711 Jiang YH, Zhang Y, Wang YY, et al. [Extracts of Poria cocos polysaccharides improves alcoholic liver disease in mice via CYP2E1 and NF-κB inflammatory pathways]. *Zhongguo Zhong Yao Za Zhi*. 2022 Jan;47(1):134-140.

2712 Li FF, Yuan Y, Liu Y, et al. Pachymic acid protects H9c2 cardiomyocytes from lipopolysaccharide-induced inflammation and apoptosis by inhibiting the extracellular signal-regulated kinase 1/2 and p38 pathways. *Mol Med Rep*. 2015 Aug;12(2):2807-13.

2713 Sekiya N, Goto H, Shimada Y, et al. Inhibitory effects of triterpenes isolated from Hoelen on free radical-induced lysis of red blood cells. *Phytother Res*. 2003 Feb;17(2):160-2.

2714 Wu ZL, Ren H, Lai WY, et al. Scleroderma of Poria cocos exerts its diuretic effect via suppression of renal aquaporin-2 expression in rats with chronic heart failure. *J Ethnopharmacol*. 2014 Aug 8;155(1):563-71.

2715 Feng YL, Lei P, Tian T, et al. Diuretic activity of some fractions of the epidermis of Poria cocos. *J Ethnopharmacol*. 2013 Dec 12;150(3):1114-8.

2716 Hu GS, Huang CG, Zhang Y, et al. Accumulation of biomass and four triterpenoids in two-stage cultured Poria cocos mycelia and diuretic activity in rats. *Chin J Nat Med*. 2017 Apr;15(4):265-270.

2717 Zhao YY, Feng YL, Du X, et al. Diuretic activity of the ethanol and aqueous extracts of the surface layer of Poria cocos in rat. *J Ethnopharmacol*. 2012 Dec 18;144(3):775-8.

2718 Zhu L, Chen G, Guo Y, et al. Structural characterization of Poria cocos oligosaccharides and their effects on the hepatic metabolome in high-fat diet-fed mice. *Food Funct*. 2022 Jun 20;13(12):6813-6829.

2719 Cai H, Cheng Y, Zhu Q, et al. Identification of Triterpene Acids in Poria cocos Extract as Bile Acid Uptake Transporter Inhibitors. *Drug Metab Dispos*. 2021 May;49(5):353-360.

2720 Miao H, Zhao YH, Vaziri ND, et al. Lipidomics Biomarkers of Diet-Induced Hyperlipidemia and Its Treatment with Poria cocos. *J Agric Food Chem*. 2016 Feb 3;64(4):969-79.

2721 Sun SS, Wang K, Ma K, et al. An insoluble polysaccharide from the sclerotium of Poria cocos improves hyperglycemia, hyperlipidemia and hepatic steatosis in ob/ob mice via modulation of gut microbiota. *Chin J Nat Med*. 2019 Jan;17(1):3-14.

2722 Pan ZS, Chen YL, Tang KJ, et al. Pachymic acid modulates sirtuin 6 activity to alleviate lipid metabolism disorders. *Exp Ther Med*. 2023 May 15;26(1):320.

2723 Kim TH, Yu GR, Kim H, et al. Network Pharmacological Analysis of a New Herbal Combination Targeting Hyperlipidemia and Efficacy Validation In Vitro. *Curr Issues Mol Biol*. 2023 Feb 4;45(2):1314-1332.

2724 Zhu L, Ye C, Hu B, et al. Regulation of gut microbiota and intestinal metabolites by Poria cocos oligosaccharides improves glycolipid metabolism disturbance in high-fat diet-fed mice. *J Nutr Biochem*. 2022 Sep;107:109019.

2725 Xie Q, Jia X, Zhang W, et al. Effects of Poria cocos extract and protein powder mixture on glucolipid metabolism and rhythm changes in obese mice. *Food Sci Nutr*. 2023 Mar 9;11(5):2356-2371.

2726 Wong AR, Hung A, Yang AWH, et al. Poria cocos compounds targeting neuropeptide Y1 receptor (Y1R) for weight management: A computational ligand- and structure-based study with molecular dynamics simulations identified beta-amyrin acetate as a putative Y1R inhibitor. *PLoS One*. 2023 Jun 30;18(6):e0277873.

2727 Wu Y, Li D, Wang H, et al. Protective Effect of Poria Cocos Polysaccharides on Fecal Peritonitis-Induced Sepsis in Mice Through Inhibition of Oxidative Stress, Inflammation, Apoptosis, and Reduction of Treg Cells. *Front Microbiol*. 2022 May 27;13:887949.

2728 Zhang Y, Huang J, Sun M, et al. Preparation, characterization, antioxidant and antianemia activities of Poria cocos polysaccharide iron (III) complex. *Heliyon*. 2023 Jan 7;9(1):e12819.

2729 Wang S, Tan W, Zhang L, et al. Pachymic Acid Protects Against Bleomycin-Induced Pulmonary Fibrosis by Suppressing Fibrotic, Inflammatory, and Oxidative Stress Pathways in Mice. *Appl Biochem Biotechnol*. 2023 Aug 31. Online ahead of print.

2730 Ye C, Gao ZH, Chen KQ, et al. Research on Pachymaran to Ameliorate CsA-Induced Immunosuppressive Lung Injury by Regulating Microflora Metabolism. *Microorganisms*. 2023 Sep 7;11(9):2249.

2731 Gui Y, Sun L, Liu R, et al. Pachymic acid inhibits inflammation and cell apoptosis in lipopolysaccharide (LPS)-induced rat model with pneumonia by regulating NF-κB and MAPK pathways. *Allergol Immunopathol (Madr)*. 2021 Sep 1;49(5):87-93.

2732 Liu YC, Liu GY, Liu RL. [Effects of poria cocos on ototoxicity induced by kanamycin in guinea-pigs]. *Zhongguo Zhong Xi Yi Jie He Za Zhi*. 1995 Jul;15(7):422-3.

2733 Lee SG, Kim MM. Pachymic acid promotes induction of autophagy related to IGF-1 signaling pathway in WI-38 cells. *Phytomedicine*. 2017 Dec 1;36:82-87.

2734 Gao Y, Yan H, Jin R, et al. Antiepileptic activity of total triterpenes isolated from Poria cocos is mediated by suppression of aspartic and glutamic acids in the brain. *Pharm Biol*. 2016 Nov;54(11):2528-2535.

2735 Wu Z, Chen X, Ni W, et al. The inhibition of Mpro, the primary protease of COVID-19, by Poria cocos and its active compounds: a network pharmacology and molecular docking study. *RSC Adv*. 2021 Mar 25;11(20):11821-11843.

[2736] Akihisa T, Nakamura Y, Tokuda H, et al. Triterpene acids from Poria cocos and their anti-tumor-promoting effects. *J Nat Prod*. 2007 Jun;70(6):948-53.

[2737] Ukiya M, Akihisa T, Tokuda H, et al. Inhibition of tumor-promoting effects by poricoic acids G and H and other lanostane-type triterpenes and cytotoxic activity of poricoic acids A and G from Poria cocos. *J Nat Prod*. 2002 Apr;65(4):462-5.

[2738] Shan H, Qinglin Z, Fengjun X, et al. Reversal of multidrug resistance of KBV200 cells by triterpenoids isolated from Poria cocos. *Planta Med*. 2012 Mar;78(5):428-33.

[2739] Wang J, Yu Z, Wu W, et al. Molecular mechanism of epicatechin gallate binding with carboxymethyl β-glucan and its effect on antibacterial activity. *Carbohydr Polym*. 2022 Dec 15;298:120105.

[2740] Zhang L, Ravipati AS, Koyyalamudi SR, et al. Anti-fungal and anti-bacterial activities of ethanol extracts of selected traditional Chinese medicinal herbs. *Asian Pac J Trop Med*. 2013 Sep;6(9):673-81.

[2741] Park YH. Son IH, Kim B, et al. Poria cocos water extract (PCW) protects PC12 neuronal cells from beta-amyloid-induced cell death through antioxidant and antiapoptotic functions. *Pharmazie*. 2009 Nov;64(11):760-4.

[2742] Zhai X, Zhang W, Pei H, et al. Structure and physicochemical properties of polysaccharides from Poria cocos extracted by deep eutectic solvent. *Glycoconj J*. 2022 Aug;39(4):475-486.

[2743] Yi Y, Hua H, Sun X, et al. Rapid determination of polysaccharides and antioxidant activity of Poria cocos using near-infrared spectroscopy combined with chemometrics. *Spectrochim Acta A Mol Biomol Spectrosc*. 2020 Oct 15;240:118623.

[2744] Tang J, Nie J, Li D, et al. Characterization and antioxidant activities of degraded polysaccharides from Poria cocos sclerotium. *Carbohydr Polym*. 2014 May 25;105:121-6.

[2745] Wang Y, Yu Y, Mao J. Carboxymethylated beta-glucan derived from Poria cocos with biological activities. *J Agric Food Chem*. 2009 Nov 25;57(22):10913-5.

[2746] Chen S, Zhang H, Yang L, et al. Optimization of Ultrasonic-Assisted Extraction Conditions for Bioactive Components and Antioxidant Activity of Poria cocos (Schw.) Wolf by an RSM-ANN-GA Hybrid Approach. *Foods*. 2023 Feb 1;12(3):619.

[2747] Wang N, Zhang Y, Wang X, et al. Antioxidant property of water-soluble polysaccharides from Poria cocos Wolf using different extraction methods. *Int J Biol Macromol*. 2016 Feb;83:103-10.

[2748] Kang KY, Hwang YH, Lee SJ, et al. Verification of the Functional Antioxidant Activity and Antimelanogenic Properties of Extracts of Poria cocos Mycelium Fermented with Freeze-Dried Plum Powder. *Int J Biomater*. 2019 Jun 2;2019:9283207.

[2749] Wang Q, Chen S, Han L, et al. Antioxidant activity of carboxymethyl (1→3)-β-d-glucan (from the sclerotium of Poria cocos) sulfate (in vitro). *Int J Biol Macromol*. 2014 Aug;69:229-35.

[2750] Zhou L, Zhang Y, Gapter LA, et al. Cytotoxic and anti-oxidant activities of lanostane-type triterpenes isolated from Poria cocos. *Chem Pharm Bull (Tokyo)*. 2008 Oct;56(10):1459-62.

[2751] Wu SJ, Ng LT, Lin CC. Antioxidant activities of some common ingredients of traditional chinese medicine, Angelica sinensis, Lycium barbarum and Poria cocos. *Phytother Res*. 2004 Dec;18(12):1008-12.

[2752] Schinella GR, Tournier HA, Prieto JM, et al. Antioxidant activity of anti-inflammatory plant extracts. *Life Sci*. 2002 Jan 18;70(9):1023-33.

[2753] Bae MJ, See HJ, Choi G, et al. Regulatory T Cell Induced by Poria cocos Bark Exert Therapeutic Effects in Murine Models of Atopic Dermatitis and Food Allergy. *Mediators Inflamm*. 2016;2016:3472608.

[2754] Cuellar MJ, Giner RM, Recio MC, et al. Effect of the basidiomycete Poria cocos on experimental dermatitis and other inflammatory conditions. *Chem Pharm Bull (Tokyo)*. 1997 Mar;45(3):492-4.

[2755] Fuchs SM, Heinemann C, Schliemann-Willers S, et al. Assessment of anti-inflammatory activity of Poria cocos in sodium lauryl sulphate-induced irritant contact dermatitis. *Skin Res Technol*. 2006 Nov;12(4):223-7.

[2756] Lee H, Cha HJ. Poria cocos Wolf extracts represses pigmentation in vitro and in vivo. *Cell Mol Biol (Noisy-le-grand)*. 2018;64(5):80-84.

[2757] Shah FH, Eom YS, Kim SJ. Evaluation of phytochemicals of Poria cocos against tyrosinase protein: a virtual screening, pharmacoinformatics and molecular dynamics study. *3 Biotech*. 2023 Jun;13(6):199.

[2758] Kang KY, Hwang YH, Lee SJ, et al. Verification of the Functional Antioxidant Activity and Antimelanogenic Properties of Extracts of Poria cocos Mycelium Fermented with Freeze-Dried Plum Powder. *Int J Biomater*. 2019 Jun 2;2019:9283207.

[2759] Park SG, Jo IJ, Park SA, et al. Poria cocos Extract from Mushrooms Stimulates Aquaporin-3 via the PI3K/Akt/mTOR Signaling Pathway. *Clin Cosmet Investig Dermatol*. 2022 Sep 15;15:1919-1931.

[2760] Choi E, Kang YG, Hwang SH, et al. In Vitro Effects of Dehydrotrametenolic Acid on Skin Barrier Function. *Molecules*. 2019 Dec 14;24(24):4583.

[2761] Fang CL, Paul CR, Day CH, et al. Poria cocos (Fuling) targets TGFβ/Smad7 associated collagen accumulation and enhances Nrf2-antioxidant mechanism to exert anti-skin aging effects in human dermal fibroblasts. *Environ Toxicol*. 2021;36(5):729-736.

[2762] Zhang T, Huang S, Qiu J, et al. Beneficial Effect of Gastrodia elata Blume and Poria cocos Wolf Administration on Acute UVB Irradiation by Alleviating Inflammation through Promoting the Gut-Skin Axis. *Int J Mol Sci*. 2022 Sep 16;23(18):10833.

[2763] Prieto JM, Recio MC, Giner RM, et al. Influence of traditional Chinese anti-inflammatory medicinal plants on leukocyte and platelet functions. *J Pharm Pharmacol*. 2003 Sep;55(9):1275-82.

[2764] Zhou J, Zhang K, Gao J, et al. Effect of Poria cocos Mushroom Polysaccharides (PCPs) on the Quality and DNA Methylation of Cryopreserved Shanghai White Pig Spermatozoa. *Cells*. 2023 May 24;12(11):1456.

[2765] Tai T, Akita Y, Kinoshita K, Koyama K, et al. Anti-emetic principles of Poria cocos. *Planta Med*. 1995 Dec;61(6):527-30.

[2766] Li GH, Shen YM, Zhang KQ. Nematicidal activity and chemical component of Poria cocos. *J Microbiol*. 2005 Feb;43(1):17-20.

[2767] Schinella GR, Tournier HA, Prieto JM, et al. Inhibition of Trypanosoma cruzi growth by medical plant extracts. *Fitoterapia*. 2002 Dec;73(7-8):569-75.

[2768] Peng X, Jia C, Chi H, et al. Efficacy and Pharmacological Mechanism of Poria cocos-Based Formulas Combined With Chemotherapy for Ovarian Cancer: A Integrated Systems Pharmacology Study. *Front Pharmacol*. 2022 Mar 21;13:788810.

[2769] Di YM, Sun L, Lu C, et al. Benefits of herbal formulae containing Poria cocos (Fuling) for type 2 diabetes mellitus: A systematic review and meta-analysis. *PLoS One*. 2022 Dec 1;17(12):e0278536.

[2770] Prochazkova L, Lipperlt DP, Colxzato LS, et al. Exploring the effect of microdosing psychedelics on creativity in an open-label natural setting. *Psychopharmacology (Berl)*. 2018; 235(12): 3401–3413.

[2771] Kopra EI, Ferris JA, Winstock AR, et al. Adverse experiences resulting in emergency medical treatment seeking following the use of magic mushrooms. *J Psychopharmacol*. 2022 Aug;36(8):965-973.

[2772] Mahmood ZA. Chapter 18, Bioactive Alkaloids from Fungi: Psilocybin. *Natural products*. pp. 535-552.

[2773] Musshoff F, Madea B, Beike J. Hallucinogenic mushrooms on the German market - simple instructions for examination and identification. *Forensic Sci Int*. 2000 Sep 11;113(1-3):389-95.

[2774] Gotvaldova K, Borovicka J, Hajkova K, et al. Extensive Collection of Psychotropic Mushrooms with Determination of Their Tryptamine Alkaloids. *Int J Mol Sci*. 2022 Nov; 23(22): 14068.

[2775] Christiansen AL, Rasmussen KE, Hoiland K. The content of Psilocybin in Norwegian Psilocybe semilanceata. *Planta Med*. 1981 Jul;42(7):229-35.

[2776] Gartz J. Extraction and analysis of indole derivatives from fungal biomass. *J Basic Microbiol*. 1994;34(1):17-22.

[2777] Gartz J, Allen JW, Merlin MD. Ethnomycology, biochemistry, and cultivation of Psilocybe samuiensis Guzmán, Bandala and Allen, a new psychoactive fungus from Koh Samui, Thailand. *J Ethnopharmacol*. 1994 Jul 8;43(2):73-80.

[2778] Perkal M. Analysis of hallucinogens in psilocybe-type mushrooms [microform]. Monash University.

[2779] Erowid.org. The psilometric scale of comparative potency of selected Psilocybe mushrooms. Available at: https://www.erowid.org/plants/mushrooms/mushrooms_info4.shtml. Accessed November 6, 2023.

[2780] Koike Y, Wada K, Kusano G, et al. Isolation of psilocybin from Psilocybe argentipes and its determination in specimens of some mushrooms. *HIGEO NOZOE Institute of Pharmaceutical Sciences*. 1981 May-Hun:362-365.

[2781] Gümüştaş M, Kılıç CS, Kaya A, et al. Psilocin and psilocybin contents of some Panaeolis spp. growing in Turkey. *Ankara University Faculty of Pharmacy*. 2012 Sep.

[2782] Musshoff F, Madea B, Beike J. Hallucinogenic mushrooms on the German market - simple instructions for examination and identification. *Forensic Sci Int*. 2000 Sep 11;113(1-3):389-95.

[2783] Christiansen AL, Rasmussen KE, Hoiland K. Detection of psilocybin and psilocin in norwegian species of pluteus and conocybe. *Planta Med*. 1984 Aug;50(4):341-3.

[2784] Gartz J. Extraction and analysis of indole derivatives from fungal biomass. *J Basic Microbiol*. 1994;34(1):17-22.

[2785] Ling S, Ceban F, Lui LMW, et al. Molecular Mechanisms of Psilocybin and Implications for the Treatment of Depression. *CNS Drugs*. 2022 Jan;36(1):17-30.

[2786] Hakami Zanjani AA, Nguyen TQT, et al. The molecular basis of the antidepressant action of the magic mushroom extract, psilocin. *Biochim Biophys Acta Proteins Proteom*. 2023 Jul 1;1871(4):140914.

[2787] Hesselgrave N, Troppoli TA, Wulff AB, et al. Harnessing psilocybin: antidepressant-like behavioral and synaptic actions of psilocybin are independent of 5-HT2R activation in mice. *Proc Natl Acad Sci U S A*. 2021 Apr 27;118(17):e2022489118.

[2788] Ling S, Ceban F, Lui LMW, et al. Molecular Mechanisms of Psilocybin and Implications for the Treatment of Depression. *CNS Drugs*. 2022 Jan;36(1):17-30.

[2789] Hibicke M, Landry AN, Kramer HM, et al. Psychedelics, but Not Ketamine, Produce Persistent Antidepressant-like Effects in a Rodent Experimental System for the Study of Depression. *ACS Chem Neurosci*. 2020 Mar 18;11(6):864-871.

[2790] Malikowska-Racia N, Koniewski M, Golebiowska J, et al. Acute but not long-lasting antidepressant-like effect of psilocybin in differential reinforcement of low-rate 72 schedule in rats. *J Psychopharmacol*. 2023 Oct 16:2698811231205692.

[2791] Hibicke M, Nichols CD. Validation of the forced swim test in Drosophila, and its use to demonstrate psilocybin has long-lasting antidepressant-like effects in flies. *Sci Rep*. 2022 Jun 15;12(1):10019.

[2792] Higgins GA, Carroll NK, Brown M, et al. Low Doses of Psilocybin and Ketamine Enhance Motivation and Attention in Poor Performing Rats: Evidence for an Antidepressant Property. *Front Pharmacol*. 2021 Feb 26;12:640241.

[2793] Thomas CW, Blanco-Duque C, Bréant BJ, et al. Psilocin acutely alters sleep-wake architecture and cortical brain activity in laboratory mice. *Transl Psychiatry*. 2022 Feb 23;12(1):77.

[2794] Matsushima Y, Shirota O, Kikura-Hanajiri R, et al. Effects of Psilocybe argentipes on marble-burying behavior in mice. *Biosci Biotechnol Biochem*. 2009 Aug;73(8):1866-8.

[2795] Odland AU, Kristensen JL, Andreasen JT. Investigating the role of 5-HT2A and 5-HT2C receptor activation in the effects of psilocybin, DOI, and citalopram on marble burying in mice. *Behav Brain Res*. 2021 Mar 5;401:113093.

[2796] Singh S, Botvinnik A, Shahar O, et al. Effect of psilocybin on marble burying in ICR mice: role of 5-HT1A receptors and implications for the treatment of obsessive-compulsive disorder. *Transl Psychiatry*. 2023 May 10;13(1):164.

[2797] Kiilerich KF, Lorenz J, Scharff MB, et al. Repeated low doses of psilocybin increase resilience to stress, lower compulsive actions, and strengthen cortical connections to the paraventricular thalamic nucleus in rats. *Mol Psychiatry*. 2023 Oct 2. Online ahead of print.

[2798] Jones NT, Zahid Z, Grady SM, et al. Transient Elevation of Plasma Glucocorticoids Supports Psilocybin-Induced Anxiolysis in Mice. *ACS Pharmacol Transl Sci*. 2023 Aug 2;6(8):1221-1231.

[2799] Moldavan MG, Grodzinskaya AA, Solomko EF, et al. The effect of Psilocybe cubensis extract on hippocampal neurons in vitro. *Fiziol Zh (1994)*. 2001;47(6):15-23.

[2800] Jastrzebski M, Bala A. [The impact of psilocybin on visual perception and spatial orientation--neuropsychological approach]. *Psychiatr Pol*. 2013 Nov-Dec;47(6):1157-67.

[2801] Jefsen OH, Elfving B, Wegener G, et al. Transcriptional regulation in the rat prefrontal cortex and hippocampus after a single administration of psilocybin. *J Psychopharmacol*. 2021 Apr;35(4):483-493.

[2802] Erkizia-Santamaría I, Alles-Pascual R, Horrillo I, et al. Serotonin 5-HT2A, 5-HT2c and 5-HT1A receptor involvement in the acute effects of psilocybin in mice. In vitro pharmacological profile and modulation of thermoregulation and head-twich response. *Biomed Pharmacother*. 2022 Oct;154:113612.

[2803] Liu J, Wang Y, Xia K, et al. Acute psilocybin increased cortical activities in rats. *Front Neurosci*. 2023 May 23;17:1168911.

[2804] Golden CT, Chadderton P. Psilocybin reduces low frequency oscillatory power and neuronal phase-locking in the anterior cingulate cortex of awake rodents. *Sci Rep*. 2022 Jul 26;12(1):12702.

[2805] Madsen MK, Stenbæk DS, Arvidsson A, et al. Psilocybin-induced changes in brain network integrity and segregation correlate with plasma psilocin level and psychedelic experience. *Eur Neuropsychopharmacol.* 2021 Sep;50:121-132.

[2806] Winter JC, Rice KC, Amorosi DJ, et al. Psilocybin-induced stimulus control in the rat. *Pharmacol Biochem Behav.* 2007 Oct;87(4):472-80.

[2807] Raval NR, Johansen A, Donovan LL, et al. A Single Dose of Psilocybin Increases Synaptic Density and Decreases 5-HT2A Receptor Density in the Pig Brain. *Int J Mol Sci.* 2021 Jan 15;22(2):835.

[2808] Gilmour LP, O'Brien RD. Psilocybin: reaction with a fraction of rat brain. *Science.* 1967 Jan 13;155(3759):207-8.

[2809] Davoudian PA, Shao LX, Kwan AC. Shared and Distinct Brain Regions Targeted for Immediate Early Gene Expression by Ketamine and Psilocybin. *ACS Chem Neurosci.* 2023 Feb 1;14(3):468-480.

[2810] Rijsketic DR, Casey AB, Barbosa DAN, et al. UNRAVELing the synergistic effects of psilocybin and environment on brain-wide immediate early gene expression in mice. *Neuropsychopharmacology.* 2023 Nov;48(12):1798-1807.

[2811] Popik P, Hogendorf A, Bugno R, et al. Effects of ketamine optical isomers, psilocybin, psilocin and norpsilocin on time estimation and cognition in rats. *Psychopharmacology (Berl).* 2022 Jun;239(6):1689-1703.

[2812] Rijsketic DR, Casey AB, Barbosa DAN, et al. UNRAVELing the synergistic effects of psilocybin and environment on brain-wide immediate early gene expression in mice. *bioRxiv.* 2023 Feb 21:2023.02.19.528997.

[2813] Moldavan MG, Grodzinskaya AA, Solomko EF, et al. The effect of Psilocybe cubensis extract on hippocampal neurons in vitro. *Fiziol Zh (1994).* 2001;47(6):15-23.

[2814] Spain A, Howarth C, Khrapitchev AA, et al. Neurovascular and neuroimaging effects of the hallucinogenic serotonin receptor agonist psilocin in the rat brain. *Neuropharmacology.* 2015 Dec;99:210-20.

[2815] Tylš F, Vejmola Č, Koudelka V, Piorecká V, et al. Underlying pharmacological mechanisms of psilocin-induced broadband desynchronization and disconnection of EEG in rats. *Front Neurosci.* 2023 Jun 22;17:1152578.

[2816] Moliner R, Girych M, Brunello CA, et al. Psychedelics promote plasticity by directly binding to BDNF receptor TrkB. *Nat Neurosci.* 2023 Jun;26(6):1032-1041.

[2817] Effinger DP, Quadir SG, Ramage MC, et al. Sex-specific effects of psychedelic drug exposure on central amygdala reactivity and behavioral responding. *Transl Psychiatry.* 2023 Apr 8;13(1):119.

[2818] Vohra HZ, Saunders JM, Jaster AM, et al. Sex-specific effects of psychedelics on prepulse inhibition of startle in 129S6/SvEv mice. *Psychopharmacology (Berl).* 2022 Jun;239(6):1649-1664.

[2819] Sakashita Y, Abe K, Katagiri N, et al. Effect of psilocin on extracellular dopamine and serotonin levels in the mesoaccumbens and mesocortical pathway in awake rats. *Biol Pharm Bull.* 2015;38(1):134-8.

[2820] Zhuk O, Jasicka-Misiak I, Poliwoda A, et al. Research on acute toxicity and the behavioral effects of methanolic extract from psilocybin mushrooms and psilocin in mice. *Toxins (Basel).* 2015 Mar 27;7(4):1018-29.

[2821] Wojtas A, Bysiek A, Wawrzczak-Bargiela A, Szych Z, et al. Effect of Psilocybin and Ketamine on Brain Neurotransmitters, Glutamate Receptors, DNA and Rat Behavior. *Int J Mol Sci.* 2022 Jun 16;23(12):6713.

[2822] Grandjean J, Buehlmann D, Buerge M, et al. Psilocybin exerts distinct effects on resting state networks associated with serotonin and dopamine in mice. *Neuroimage.* 2021 Jan 15;225:117456.

[2823] Shao LX, Liao C, Gregg I, et al. Psilocybin induces rapid and persistent growth of dendritic spines in frontal cortex in vivo. *Neuron.* 2021 Aug 18;109(16):2535-2544.e4.

[2824] Torrado Pacheco A, Olson RJ, Garza G, et al. Acute psilocybin enhances cognitive flexibility in rats. *bioRxiv.* 2023 Jan 9:2023.01.09.523291.

[2825] Buzzelli V, Carbone E, Manduca A, et al. Psilocybin mitigates the cognitive deficits observed in a rat model of Fragile X syndrome. *Psychopharmacology (Berl).* 2023 Jan;240(1):137-147.

[2826] Roberts BF, Zylko AL, Waters CE, et al. Effect of psilocybin on decision-making and motivation in the healthy rat. *Behav Brain Res.* 2023 Feb 25;440:114262.

[2827] Du Y, Li Y, Zhao X, et al. Psilocybin facilitates fear extinction in mice by promoting hippocampal neuroplasticity. *Chin Med J (Engl).* 2023 Mar 30. Online ahead of print.

[2828] Catlow BJ, Song S, Paredes DA, et al. Effects of psilocybin on hippocampal neurogenesis and extinction of trace fear conditioning. *Exp Brain Res.* 2013 Aug;228(4):481-91.

[2829] Davis M, Walters JK. Psilocybin: biphasic dose-response effects on the acoustic startle reflex in the rat. *Pharmacol Biochem Behav.* 1977 Apr;6(4):427-31.

[2830] Wang J, Liang M, Shang Q, et al. Psilocin suppresses methamphetamine-induced hyperlocomotion and acquisition of conditioned place preference via D2R-mediated ERK signaling. *CNS Neurosci Ther.* 2023 Mar;29(3):831-841.

[2831] Nguyen TQT, Lund FW, Zanjani AAH, et al. Magic mushroom extracts in lipid membranes. *Biochim Biophys Acta Biomembr.* 2022 Sep 1;1864(9):183957.

[2832] Alper K, Cange J, Sah R, et al. Psilocybin sex-dependently reduces alcohol consumption in C57BL/6J mice. *Front Pharmacol.* 2023 Jan 4;13:1074633.

[2833] Benvenuti F, Colombo D, Soverchia L, et al. Psilocybin prevents reinstatement of alcohol seeking by disrupting the reconsolidation of alcohol-related memories. *Psychopharmacology (Berl).* 2023 Jul;240(7):1521-1530.

[2834] Meinhardt MW, Pfarr S, Fouquet G, et al. Psilocybin targets a common molecular mechanism for cognitive impairment and increased craving in alcoholism. *Sci Adv.* 2021 Nov 19;7(47):eabh2399.

[2835] Huang J, Pham M, Panenka WJ, et al. Chronic Treatment With Psilocybin Decreases Changes in Body Weight in a Rodent Model of Obesity. *Front Psychiatry.* 2022 May 18;13:891512.

[2836] Fadahunsi N, Lund J, Breum AW, et al. Acute and long-term effects of psilocybin on energy balance and feeding behavior in mice. *Transl Psychiatry.* 2022 Aug 11;12(1):330.

[2837] Nkadimeng SM, Nabatanzi A, Steinmann CML, et al. Phytochemical, Cytotoxicity, Antioxidant and Anti-Inflammatory Effects of Psilocybe Natalensis Magic Mushroom. *Plants (Basel).* 2020 Aug 31;9(9):1127.

[2838] Nkadimeng SM, Steinmann CML, Eloff JN. Anti-Inflammatory Effects of Four Psilocybin-Containing Magic Mushroom Water Extracts in vitro on 15-Lipoxygenase Activity and on Lipopolysaccharide-Induced Cyclooxygenase-2 and Inflammatory Cytokines in Human U937 Macrophage Cells. *J Inflamm Res.* 2021 Aug 5;14:3729-3738.

281

[2839] Robinson GI, Li D, Wang B, et al. Anti-Inflammatory Effects of Serotonin Receptor and Transient Receptor Potential Channel Ligands in Human Small Intestinal Epithelial Cells. *Curr Issues Mol Biol*. 2023 Aug 15;45(8):6743-6774.

[2840] Flanagan TW, Nichols CD. Psychedelics and Anti-inflammatory Activity in Animal Models. *Curr Top Behav Neurosci*. 2022;56:229-245.

[2841] Zanikov T, Gerasymchuk M, Ghasemi Gojani E, et al. The Effect of Combined Treatment of Psilocybin and Eugenol on Lipopolysaccharide-Induced Brain Inflammation in Mice. *Molecules*. 2023 Mar 14;28(6):2624.

[2842] Meldrum BS, Naquet R. Effects of psilocybin, dimethyltryptamine, mescaline and various lysergic acid derivatives on the EEG and on photically induced epilepsy in the baboon (Papio papio). *Electroencephalogr Clin Neurophysiol*. 1971 Dec;31(6):563-72.

[2843] Donovan LL, Johansen JV, Ros NF, et al. Effects of a single dose of psilocybin on behaviour, brain 5-HT2A receptor occupancy and gene expression in the pig. *Eur Neuropsychopharmacol*. 2021 Jan;42:1-11.

[2844] Meltzer HY, Fessler RG, Simonovic M, et al. Stimulation of rat prolactin secretion by indolealkylamine hallucinogens. *Psychopharmacology (Berl)*. 1978 Apr 11;56(3):255-9.

[2845] Nkadimeng SM, Nabatanzi A, Steinmann CML, et al. Phytochemical, Cytotoxicity, Antioxidant and Anti-Inflammatory Effects of Psilocybe Natalensis Magic Mushroom. *Plants (Basel)*. 2020 Aug 31;9(9):1127.

[2846] Khan FI, Hassan F, Lai D. In Silico Studies on Psilocybin Drug Derivatives Against SARS-CoV-2 and Cytokine Storm of Human Interleukin-6 Receptor. *Front Immunol*. 2022 Jan 14;12:794780.

[2847] Dhanasekaran D, Latha S, Suganya P, et al. Taxonomic identification and bioactive compounds characterization of Psilocybe cubensis DPT1 to probe its antibacterial and mosquito larvicidal competency. *Microb Pathog*. 2020 Jun;143:104138.

[2848] Bianco Coletto MA. [Basidiomycetes in relation to antibiosis. II. Antibiotic activity of mycelia and culture liquids]. *G Batteriol Virol Immunol*. 1981 Jul-Dec;74(7-12):267-74.

[2849] Dhanasekaran D, Latha S, Suganya P, et al. Taxonomic identification and bioactive compounds characterization of Psilocybe cubensis DPT1 to probe its antibacterial and mosquito larvicidal competency. *Microb Pathog*. 2020 Jun;143:104138.

[2850] Carhart-Harris R, Giribaldi B, Watts R, et al. Trial of Psilocybin versus Escitalopram for Depression. *N Engl J Med*. 2021 Apr 15;384(15):1402-1411.

[2851] Gukasyan N, Davis AK, Barrett FS, Cosimano MP, et al. Efficacy and safety of psilocybin-assisted treatment for major depressive disorder: Prospective 12-month follow-up. *J Psychopharmacol*. 2022 Feb;36(2):151-158.

[2852] Griffiths RR, Johnson MW, Carducci MA, et al. Psilocybin produces substantial and sustained decreases in depression and anxiety in patients with life-threatening cancer: A randomized double-blind trial. *J Psychopharmacol*. 2016 Dec;30(12):1181-1197.

[2853] Ross S, Bossis A, Guss J, et al. Rapid and sustained symptom reduction following psilocybin treatment for anxiety and depression in patients with life-threatening cancer: a randomized controlled trial. *J Psychopharmacol*. 2016 Dec;30(12):1165-1180.

[2854] Sloshower J, Skosnik PD, Safi-Aghdam H, et al. Psilocybin-assisted therapy for major depressive disorder: An exploratory placebo-controlled, fixed-order trial. *J Psychopharmacol*. 2023 Jul;37(7):698-706.

[2855] Lewis BR, Garland EL, Byrne K, et al. HOPE: A Pilot Study of Psilocybin Enhanced Group Psychotherapy in Patients With Cancer. *J Pain Symptom Manage*. 2023 Sep;66(3):258-269.

[2856] Grob CS, Danforth AL, Chopra GS, et al. Pilot study of psilocybin treatment for anxiety in patients with advanced-stage cancer. *Arch Gen Psychiatry*. 2011 Jan;68(1):71-8.

[2857] Daws RE, Timmermann C, Giribaldi B, et al. Increased global integration in the brain after psilocybin therapy for depression. *Nat Med*. 2022 Apr;28(4):844-851.

[2858] Carhart-Harris RL, Bolstridge M, Day CMJ, et al. Psilocybin with psychological support for treatment-resistant depression: six-month follow-up. *Psychopharmacology (Berl)*. 2018 Feb;235(2):399-408.

[2859] Roseman L, Demetriou L, Wall MB, et al. Increased amygdala responses to emotional faces after psilocybin for treatment-resistant depression. *Neuropharmacology*. 2018 Nov;142:263-269.

[2860] Skosnik PD, Sloshower J, Safi-Aghdam H, et al. Sub-acute effects of psilocybin on EEG correlates of neural plasticity in major depression: Relationship to symptoms. *J Psychopharmacol*. 2023 Jul;37(7):687-697.

[2861] Davis AK, Barrett FS, May DG, et al. Effects of Psilocybin-Assisted Therapy on Major Depressive Disorder: A Randomized Clinical Trial. *JAMA Psychiatry*. 2021 May 1;78(5):481-489.

[2862] Siegel JS, Subramanian S, Perry D, et al. Psilocybin desynchronizes brain networks. *medRxiv*. 2023 Aug 24:2023.08.22.23294131.

[2863] Goodwin GM, Aaronson ST, Alvarez O, et al. Single-Dose Psilocybin for a Treatment-Resistant Episode of Major Depression. *N Engl J Med*. 2022 Nov 3;387(18):1637-1648.

[2864] Erritzoe D, Roseman L, Nour MM, et al. Effects of psilocybin therapy on personality structure. *Acta Psychiatr Scand*. 2018 Nov;138(5):368-378.

[2865] Stroud JB, Freeman TP, Leech R, et al. Psilocybin with psychological support improves emotional face recognition in treatment-resistant depression. *Psychopharmacology (Berl)*. 2018 Feb;235(2):459-466.

[2866] Carhart-Harris RL, Roseman L, Bolstridge M, et al. Psilocybin for treatment-resistant depression: fMRI-measured brain mechanisms. *Sci Rep*. 2017 Oct 13;7(1):13187.

[2867] Goodwin GM, Aaronson ST, Alvarez O, et al. Single-dose psilocybin for a treatment-resistant episode of major depression: Impact on patient-reported depression severity, anxiety, function, and quality of life. *J Affect Disord*. 2023 Apr 14;327:120-127.

[2868] Raison CL, Sanacora G, Woolley J, et al. Single-Dose Psilocybin Treatment for Major Depressive Disorder: A Randomized Clinical Trial. *JAMA*. 2023 Sep 5;330(9):843-853.

[2869] Wall MB, Lam C, Ertl N, et al. Increased low-frequency brain responses to music after psilocybin therapy for depression. *J Affect Disord*. 2023 Jul 15;333:321-330.

[2870] Shukuroglou M, Roseman L, Wall M, et al. Changes in music-evoked emotion and ventral striatal functional connectivity after psilocybin therapy for depression. *J Psychopharmacol*. 2023 Jan;37(1):70-79.

[2871] Kometer M, Schmidt A, Bachmann R, et al. Psilocybin biases facial recognition, goal-directed behavior, and mood state toward positive relative to negative emotions through different serotonergic subreceptors. *Biol Psychiatry*. 2012 Dec 1;72(11):898-906.

[2872] Preller KH, Duerler P, Burt JB, et al. Psilocybin Induces Time-Dependent Changes in Global Functional Connectivity. *Biol Psychiatry*. 2020 Jul 15;88(2):197-207.

[2873] Kinderlehrer DA. The Effectiveness of Microdosed Psilocybin in the Treatment of Neuropsychiatric Lyme Disease: A Case Study. *Int Med Case Rep J*. 2023 Mar 3;16:109-115.

[2874] Doss MK, Považan M, Rosenberg MD, et al. Psilocybin therapy increases cognitive and neural flexibility in patients with major depressive disorder. *Transl Psychiatry*. 2021 Nov 8;11(1):574.

[2875] Krediet E, Bostoen T, Breeksema J, et al. Reviewing the Potential of Psychedelics for the Treatment of PTSD. *Int J Neuropsychopharmacol*. 2020 Jun;23(6):385–400.

[2876] Lyons T, Carhart-Harris RL. Increased nature relatedness and decreased authoritarian political views after psilocybin for treatment-resistant depression. *J Psychopharmacol*. 2018 Jul;32(7):811-819.

[2877] Lawrence DW. Self-administration of Psilocybin for the Acute Treatment of Migraine: A Case Report. *Innov Clin Neurosci*. 2023 Sep 1;20(7-9):37-39.

[2878] Schindler EAD, Sewell RA, Gottschalk CH, et al. Exploratory Controlled Study of the Migraine-Suppressing Effects of Psilocybin. *Neurotherapeutics*. 2021 Jan;18(1):534-543.

[2879] Schindler EAD, Sewell RA, Gottschalk CH, et al. Exploratory investigation of a patient-informed low-dose psilocybin pulse regimen in the suppression of cluster headache: Results from a randomized, double-blind, placebo-controlled trial. *Headache*. 2022 Nov;62(10):1383-1394.

[2880] Mason NL, Szabo A, Kuypers KPC, et al. Psilocybin induces acute and persisting alterations in immune status in healthy volunteers: An experimental, placebo-controlled study. *Brain Behav Immun*. 2023 Nov;114:299-310.

[2881] Lyes M, Yang KH, Castellanos J, et al. Microdosing psilocybin for chronic pain: a case series. *Pain*. 2023 Apr 1;164(4):698-702.

[2882] Meikle SE, Liknaitzky P, Rossell SL, et al. Psilocybin-assisted therapy for depression: How do we advance the field? *Aust N Z J Psychiatry*. 2020 Mar;54(3):225-231.

[2883] Bogenschutz MP, Forcehimes AA, Pommy JA, et al. Psilocybin-assisted treatment for alcohol dependence: a proof-of-concept study. *J Psychopharmacol*. 2015 Mar;29(3):289-99.

[2884] Heinzerling KG, Sergi K, Linton M, et al. Nature-themed video intervention may improve cardiovascular safety of psilocybin-assisted therapy for alcohol use disorder. *Front Psychiatry*. 2023 Sep 18;14:1215972.

[2885] Bogenschutz MP, Ross S, Bhatt S, et al. Percentage of Heavy Drinking Days Following Psilocybin-Assisted Psychotherapy vs Placebo in the Treatment of Adult Patients With Alcohol Use Disorder: A Randomized Clinical Trial. *JAMA Psychiatry*. 2022 Oct 1;79(10):953-962.

[2886] Barrett SP, Archambault J, Engelberg MJ, et al. Hallucinogenic drugs attenuate the subjective response to alcohol in humans. *Hum Psychopharmacol*. 2000 Oct;15(7):559-565.

[2887] Johnson MW, Garcia-Romeu A, Griffiths RR. Long-term follow-up of psilocybin-facilitated smoking cessation. *Am J Drug Alcohol Abuse*. 2017 Jan;43(1):55-60.

[2888] Garcia-Romeu A, Griffiths RR, Johnson MW. Psilocybin-occasioned mystical experiences in the treatment of tobacco addiction. *Curr Drug Abuse Rev*. 2014;7(3):157-64.

[2889] Johnson MW, Garcia-Romeu A, Cosimano MP, et al. Pilot study of the 5-HT2AR agonist psilocybin in the treatment of tobacco addiction. *J Psychopharmacol*. 2014 Nov;28(11):983-92.

[2890] Garcia-Romeu A, Davis AK, Erowid E, et al. Persisting Reductions in Cannabis, Opioid, and Stimulant Misuse After Naturalistic Psychedelic Use: An Online Survey. *Front Psychiatry*. 2020 Jan 22;10:955.

[2891] Barrett FS, Doss MK, Sepeda ND, et al. Emotions and brain function are altered up to one month after a single high dose of psilocybin. *Sci Rep*. 2020 Feb 10;10(1):2214.

[2892] Pokorny T, Preller KH, Kometer M, et al. Effect of Psilocybin on Empathy and Moral Decision-Making. *Int J Neuropsychopharmacol*. 2017 Sep 1;20(9):747-757.

[2893] Nicholas CR, Henriquez KM, Gassman MC, et al. High dose psilocybin is associated with positive subjective effects in healthy volunteers. *J Psychopharmacol*. 2018 Jul;32(7):770-778.

[2894] Nayak SM, Jackson H, Sepeda ND, et al. Naturalistic psilocybin use is associated with persisting improvements in mental health and wellbeing: results from a prospective, longitudinal survey. *Front Psychiatry*. 2023 Sep 19;14:1199642.

[2895] Stauffer CS, Anderson BT, Ortigo KM, et al. Psilocybin-Assisted Group Therapy and Attachment: Observed Reduction in Attachment Anxiety and Influences of Attachment Insecurity on the Psilocybin Experience. *ACS Pharmacol Transl Sci*. 2020 Dec 9;4(2):526-532.

[2896] Anderson BT, Danforth A, Daroff PR, et al. Psilocybin-assisted group therapy for demoralized older long-term AIDS survivor men: An open-label safety and feasibility pilot study. *EClinicalMedicine*. 2020 Sep 24;27:100538.

[2897] Kraehenmann R, Preller KH, Scheidegger M, et al. Psilocybin-Induced Decrease in Amygdala Reactivity Correlates with Enhanced Positive Mood in Healthy Volunteers. *Biol Psychiatry*. 2015 Oct 15;78(8):572-81.

[2898] Moreno FA, Weigand CB, Taitano EK, et al. Safety, tolerability, and efficacy of psilocybin in 9 patients with obsessive-compulsive disorder. *J clin Psychiatry*. 2006 Nov;67(11):1735-40.

[2899] Schneier FR, Feusner J, Wheaton MG, et al. Pilot study of single-dose psilocybin for serotonin reuptake inhibitor-resistant body dysmorphic disorder. *J Psychiatr Res*. 2023 May;161:364-370.

[2900] Kiraga MK, Kuypers KPC, Uthaug MV, et al. Decreases in State and Trait Anxiety Post-psilocybin: A Naturalistic, Observational Study Among Retreat Attendees. *Front Psychiatry*. 2022 Jul 7;13:883869.

[2901] McCulloch DE, Madsen MK, Stenbæk DS, et al. Lasting effects of a single psilocybin dose on resting-state functional connectivity in healthy individuals. *J Psychopharmacol*. 2022 Jan;36(1):74-84.

[2902] Søndergaard A, Madsen MK, Ozenne B, et al. Lasting increases in trait mindfulness after psilocybin correlate positively with the mystical-type experience in healthy individuals. *Front Psychol*. 2022 Oct 5;13:948729.

[2903] Madsen MK, Fisher PM, Stenbæk DS, et al. A single psilocybin dose is associated with long-term increased mindfulness, preceded by a proportional change in neocortical 5-HT2A receptor binding. *Eur Neuropsychopharmacol*. 2020 Apr;33:71-80.

[2904] Smigielski L, Scheidegger M, Kometer M, et al. Psilocybin-assisted mindfulness training modulates self-consciousness and brain default mode network connectivity with lasting effects. *Neuroimage*. 2019 Aug 1;196:207-215.

[2905] Mason NL, Mischler E, Uthaug MV, et al. Sub-Acute Effects of Psilocybin on Empathy, Creative Thinking, and Subjective Well-Being. *J Psychoactive Drugs*. 2019 Apr-Jun;51(2):123-134.

[2906] Mason NL, Kuypers KPC, Reckweg JT, et al. Spontaneous and deliberate creative cognition during and after psilocybin exposure. *Transl Psychiatry*. 2021 Apr 8;11(1):209.

[2907] Barrett FS, Carbonaro TM, Hurwitz E, et al. Double-blind comparison of the two hallucinogens psilocybin and dextromethorphan: effects on cognition. *Psychopharmacology (Berl)*. 2018 Oct;235(10):2915-2927.

[2908] Carter OL, Hasler F, Pettigrew JD, et al. Psilocybin links binocular rivalry switch rate to attention and subjective arousal levels in humans. *Psychopharmacology (Berl)*. 2007 Dec;195(3):415-24.

[2909] MacLean KA, Johnson MW, Griffiths RR. Mystical experiences occasioned by the hallucinogen psilocybin lead to increases in the personality domain of openness. *J Psychopharmacol*. 2011 Nov;25(11):1453-61.

[2910] van Elk M, Fejer G, Lempe P, et al. Effects of psilocybin microdosing on awe and aesthetic experiences: a preregistered field and lab-based study. *Psychopharmacology (Berl)*. 2022 Jun;239(6):1705-1720.

[2911] Kometer M, Pokorny T, Seifritz E, et al. Psilocybin-induced spiritual experiences and insightfulness are associated with synchronization of neuronal oscillations. *Psychopharmacology (Berl)*. 2015 Oct;232(19):3663-76.

[2912] Nikolič M, Viktorin V, Zach P, et al. Psilocybin intoxication did not affect daytime or sleep-related declarative memory consolidation in a small sample exploratory analysis. *Eur Neuropsychopharmacol*. 2023 Sep;74:78-88.

[2913] Rucker JJ, Marwood L, Ajantaival RJ, et al. The effects of psilocybin on cognitive and emotional functions in healthy participants: Results from a phase 1, randomised, placebo-controlled trial involving simultaneous psilocybin administration and preparation. *J Psychopharmacol*. 2022 Jan;36(1):114-125.

[2914] Rootman JM, Kryskow P, Harvey K, et al. Adults who microdose psychedelics report health related motivations and lower levels of anxiety and depression compared to non-microdosers. *Sci Rep*. 2021 Nov 18;11(1):22479.

[2915] Perez N, Langlest F, Mallet L, et al. Psilocybin-assisted therapy for depression: A systematic review and dose-response meta-analysis of human studies. *Eur Neuropsychopharmacol*. 2023 Nov:76:61-76.

[2916] Cavarra M, Mason NL, Kuypers KPC, et al. Potential analgesic effects of psychedelics on select chronic pain conditions: A survey study. *Eur J Pain*. 2023 Aug 20. Online ahead of print.

[2917] Simonsson O, Osika W, Carhart-Harris R, et al. Associations between lifetime classic psychedelic use and cardiometabolic diseases. *Sci Rep*. 2021 Jul 13;11(1):14427.

[2918] Jones GM, Nock MK. MDMA/ecstasy use and psilocybin use are associated with lowered odds of psychological distress and suicidal thoughts in a sample of US adults. *J Psychopharmacol*. 2022 Jan;36(1):46-56.

[2919] Jones G, Arias D, Nock M. Associations between MDMA/ecstasy, classic psychedelics, and suicidal thoughts and behaviors in a sample of U.S. adolescents. *Sci Rep*. 2022 Dec 19;12(1):21927.

[2920] Johnson MW, Garcia-Romeu A, Johnson PS, et al. An online survey of tobacco smoking cessation associated with naturalistic psychedelic use. *J Psychopharmacol*. 2017 Jul;31(7):841-850.

[2921] Jones GM, Nock MK. Psilocybin use is associated with lowered odds of crime arrests in US adults: A replication and extension. *J Psychopharmacol*. 2022 Jan;36(1):66-73.

[2922] Barrett FS, Doss MK, Sepeda ND, et al. Emotions and brain function are altered up to one month after a single high dose of psilocybin. *Sci Reports*. 2020;10(2214).

[2923] Cao L, Jin H, Liang Q, et al. A new anti-tumor cytotoxic triterpene from Ganoderma lucidum. *Nat Prod Res*. 2022 Aug;36(16):4125-4131.

[2924] Chen S, Yong T, Zhang Y, et al. Anti-tumor and Anti-angiogenic Ergosterols from Ganoderma lucidum. *Front Chem*. 2017 Oct 30;5:85.

[2925] Tang C, Zhao R, Ni H, et al. Molecule mechanisms of Ganoderma lucidum treated hepatocellular carcinoma based on the transcriptional profiles and miRNA-target network. *Biomed Pharmacother*. 2020 May;125:110028.

[2926] Huang XR, Cai F, Chen J, et al. Cytotoxic lanostane-type triterpenes from the fruiting bodies of Ganoderma lucidum. *Nat Prod Res*. 2023 Aug-Sep;37(18):3042-3047.

[2927] Fang L, Zhao Q, Guo C, et al. Removing the sporoderm from the sporoderm-broken spores of Ganoderma lucidum improves the anticancer and immune-regulatory activity of the water-soluble polysaccharide. *Front Nutr*. 2022 Sep 16;9:1006127.

[2928] Chen S, Li X, Yong T, et al. Cytotoxic lanostane-type triterpenoids from the fruiting bodies of Ganoderma lucidum and their structure-activity relationships. *Oncotarget*. 2017 Feb 7;8(6):10071-10084.

[2929] Shen J, Park HS, Xia YM, et al. The polysaccharides from fermented Ganoderma lucidum mycelia induced miRNAs regulation in suppressed HepG2 cells. *Carbohydr Polym*. 2014 Mar 15;103:319-24.

[2930] Ruan W, Lim AH, Huang LG, et al. Extraction optimisation and isolation of triterpenoids from Ganoderma lucidum and their effect on human carcinoma cell growth. *Nat Prod Res*. 2014;28(24):2264-72.

[2931] Yang HL. Ganoderic acid produced from submerged culture of Ganoderma lucidum induces cell cycle arrest and cytotoxicity in human hepatoma cell line BEL7402. *Biotechnol Lett*. 2005 Jun;27(12):835-8.

[2932] Zhu L, Wu M, Li P, et al. High-Pressure Supercritical CO_2 Extracts of Ganoderma lucidum Fruiting Body and Their Anti-hepatoma Effect Associated With the Ras/Raf/MEK/ERK Signaling Pathway. *Front Pharmacol*. 2020 Dec 14;11:602702.

[2933] Lu H, Song J, Jia XB, et al. Antihepatoma activity of the acid and neutral components from Ganoderma lucidum. *Phytother Res*. 2012 Sep;26(9):1294-300.

[2934] Ren F, Cao KY, Gong RZ, et al. The role of post-transcriptional modification on a new tRNAIle(GAU) identified from Ganoderma lucidum in its fragments' cytotoxicity on cancer cells. *Int J Biol Macromol*. 2023 Feb 28;229:885-895.

[2935] Li GL, Tang JF, Tan WL, et al. The anti-hepatocellular carcinoma effects of polysaccharides from Ganoderma lucidum by regulating macrophage polarization via the MAPK/NF-κB signaling pathway. *Food Funct*. 2023 Apr 3;14(7):3155-3168.

[2936] Wu TS, Shi LS, Kuo SC. Cytotoxicity of Ganoderma lucidum triterpenes. *J Nat Prod*. 2001 Aug;64(8):1121-2.

[2937] Li N, Hu YL, He CX, et al. Preparation, characterisation and anti-tumour activity of Ganoderma lucidum polysaccharide nanoparticles. *J Pharm Pharmacol*. 2010 Jan;62(1):139-44.

[2938] Li L, Li T, Wang XJ, et al. [Effects of Ganoderma lucidum spores on HepG2 cells proliferation and growth cycle]. *Zhong Yao Cai*. 2008 Oct;31(10):1514-8.

[2939] Weng CJ, Chau CF, Chen KD, et al. The anti-invasive effect of lucidenic acids isolated from a new Ganoderma lucidum strain. *Mol Nutr Food Res*. 2007 Dec;51(12):1472-7.

[2940] Chen YK, Kuo YH, Chiang BH, et al. Cytotoxic activities of 9,11-dehydroergosterol peroxide and ergosterol peroxide from the fermentation mycelia of ganoderma lucidum cultivated in the medium containing leguminous plants on Hep 3B cells. *J Agric Food Chem*. 2009 Jul 8;57(13):5713-9.

[2941] Lin CN, Tome WP, Won SJ. Novel cytotoxic principles of Formosan Ganoderma lucidum. *J Nat Prod*. 1991 Jul-Aug;54(4):998-1002.

[2942] Aslaminabad R, Rahimianshahreza N, Hosseini SA, et al. Regulation of Nrf2 and Nrf2-related proteins by ganoderma lucidum in hepatocellular carcinoma. *Mol Biol Rep*. 2022 Oct;49(10):9605-9612.

[2943] Lin SB, Li CH, Lee SS, et al. Triterpene-enriched extracts from Ganoderma lucidum inhibit growth of hepatoma cells via suppressing protein kinase C, activating mitogen-activated protein kinases and G2-phase cell cycle arrest. *Life Sci*. 2003 Apr 11;72(21):2381-90.

[2944] Weng CJ, Chau CF, Yen GC, et al. Inhibitory effects of ganoderma lucidum on tumorigenesis and metastasis of human hepatoma cells in cells and animal models. *J Agric Food Chem*. 2009 Jun 10;57(11):5049-57.

[2945] Ding Z, Zhou Z, Cheng X, et al. Inhibitory effects of Ganoderma lucidum triterpenoid on the growth and metastasis of hepatocellular carcinoma. *Am J Transl Res*. 2023 May 15;15(5):3410-3423.

[2946] Song M, Li ZH, Gu HS, et al. Ganoderma lucidum Spore Polysaccharide Inhibits the Growth of Hepatocellular Carcinoma Cells by Altering Macrophage Polarity and Induction of Apoptosis. *J Immunol Res*. 2021 Mar 5;2021:6696606.

[2947] Li A, Shuai X, Jia Z, et al. Ganoderma lucidum polysaccharide extract inhibits hepatocellular carcinoma growth by downregulating regulatory T cells accumulation and function by inducing microRNA-125b. *J Transl Med*. 2015 Mar 26;13:100.

[2948] Huang D, Fan Q, Liu Z, et al. An Epitope on EGFR Loading Catastrophic Internalization Serve as a Novel Oncotarget for Hepatocellular Carcinoma Therapy. *Cancers (Basel)*. 2020 Feb 16;12(2):456.

[2949] Weng CJ, Chau CF, Hsieh YS, et al. Lucidenic acid inhibits PMA-induced invasion of human hepatoma cells through inactivating MAPK/ERK signal transduction pathway and reducing binding activities of NF-kappaB and AP-1. *Carcinogenesis*. 2008 Jan;29(1):147-56.

[2950] Wang XL, Ding ZY, Zhao Y, et al. Efficient Accumulation and In Vitro Antitumor Activities of Triterpene Acids from Submerged Batch--Cultured Lingzhi or Reishi Medicinal Mushroom, Ganoderma lucidum (Agaricomycetes). *Int J Med Mushrooms*. 2017;19(5):419-431.

[2951] Wu JR, Hu CT, You RI, et al. Preclinical trials for prevention of tumor progression of hepatocellular carcinoma by LZ-8 targeting c-Met dependent and independent pathways. *PLoS One*. 2015 Jan 21;10(1):e0114495.

[2952] Gill BS, Kumar S, Navgeet. Ganoderic acid targeting nuclear factor erythroid 2-related factor 2 in lung cancer. *Tumour Biol*. 2017 Mar;39(3):1010428317695530.

[2953] Gao Y, Gao H, Chan E, et al. Antitumor activity and underlying mechanisms of ganopoly, the refined polysaccharides extracted from Ganoderma lucidum, in mice. *Immunol Invest*. 2005;34(2):171-98.

[2954] Cao L, Jin H, Liang Q, et al. A new anti-tumor cytotoxic triterpene from Ganoderma lucidum. *Nat Prod Res*. 2022 Aug;36(16):4125-4131.

[2955] Shi YJ, Zheng HX, Hong ZP, et al. Antitumor effects of different Ganoderma lucidum spore powder in cell- and zebrafish-based bioassays. *J Integr Med*. 2021 Mar;19(2):177-184.

[2956] Cilerdžić J, Vukojević J, Stajić M, et al. Biological activity of Ganoderma lucidum basidiocarps cultivated on alternative and commercial substrate. *J Ethnopharmacol*. 2014 Aug 8;155(1):312-9.

[2957] Fang L, Zhao Q, Guo C, et al. Removing the sporoderm from the sporoderm-broken spores of Ganoderma lucidum improves the anticancer and immune-regulatory activity of the water-soluble polysaccharide. *Front Nutr*. 2022 Sep 16;9:1006127.

[2958] Hsu WH, Qiu WL, Tsao SM, et al. Effects of WSG, a polysaccharide from Ganoderma lucidum, on suppressing cell growth and mobility of lung cancer. *Int J Biol Macromol*. 2020 Dec 15;165(Pt A):1604-1613.

[2959] Guo J, Yuan C, Huang M, et al. Ganoderma lucidum-derived polysaccharide enhances coix oil-based microemulsion on stability and lung cancer-targeted therapy. *Drug Deliv*. 2018 Nov;25(1):1802-1810.

[2960] Wang PY, Zhu XL, Lin ZB. Antitumor and Immunomodulatory Effects of Polysaccharides from Broken-Spore of Ganoderma lucidum. *Front Pharmacol*. 2012 Jul 13;3:135.

[2961] Chen SN, Chang CS, Hung MH, et al. The Effect of Mushroom Beta-Glucans from Solid Culture of Ganoderma lucidum on Inhibition of the Primary Tumor Metastasis. *Evid Based Complement Alternat Med*. 2014;2014:252171.

[2962] Cao QZ, Lin SQ, Wang SZ. [Effect of Ganoderma lucidum polysaccharides peptide on invasion of human lung carcinoma cells in vitro]. *Beijing Da Xue Xue Bao Yi Xue Ban*. 2007 Dec 18;39(6):653-6.

[2963] Li N, Hu YL, He CX, et al. Preparation, characterisation and anti-tumour activity of Ganoderma lucidum polysaccharide nanoparticles. *J Pharm Pharmacol*. 2010 Jan;62(1):139-44.

[2964] Gao JJ, Min BS, Ahn EM, et al. New triterpene aldehydes, lucialdehydes A-C, from Ganoderma lucidum and their cytotoxicity against murine and human tumor cells. *Chem Pharm Bull (Tokyo)*. 2002 Jun;50(6):837-40.

[2965] Cao QZ, Lin ZB. Ganoderma lucidum polysaccharides peptide inhibits the growth of vascular endothelial cell and the induction of VEGF in human lung cancer cell. *Life Sci*. 2006 Feb 23;78(13):1457-63.

[2966] Zolj S, Smith MP, Goines JC, et al. Antiproliferative Effects of a Triterpene-Enriched Extract from Lingzhi or Reishi Medicinal Mushroom, Ganoderma lucidum (Agaricomycetes), on Human Lung Cancer Cells. *Int J Med Mushrooms*. 2018;20(12):1173-1183.

[2967] Min BS, Gao JJ, Nakamura N, et al. Triterpenes from the spores of Ganoderma lucidum and their cytotoxicity against meth-A and LLC tumor cells. *Chem Pharm Bull (Tokyo)*. 2000 Jul;48(7):1026-33.

[2968] Kimura Y, Taniguchi M, Baba K. Antitumor and antimetastatic effects on liver of triterpenoid fractions of Ganoderma lucidum: mechanism of action and isolation of an active substance. *Anticancer Res*. 2002 Nov-Dec;22(6A):3309-18.

2969 Wang W, Gou X, Xue H, et al. Ganoderan (GDN) Regulates The Growth, Motility And Apoptosis Of Non-Small Cell Lung Cancer Cells Through ERK Signaling Pathway In Vitro And In Vivo. *Onco Targets Ther*. 2019 Oct 25;12:8821-8832.

2970 Wu CT, Lin TY, Hsu HY, et al. Ling Zhi-8 mediates p53-dependent growth arrest of lung cancer cells proliferation via the ribosomal protein S7-MDM2-p53 pathway. *Carcinogenesis*. 2011 Dec;32(12):1890-6.

2971 Lin TY, Hsu HY, Sun WH, et al. Induction of Cbl-dependent epidermal growth factor receptor degradation in Ling Zhi-8 suppressed lung cancer. *Int J Cancer*. 2017 Jun 1;140(11):2596-2607.

2972 Tang W, Liu JW, Zhao WM, et al. Ganoderic acid T from Ganoderma lucidum mycelia induces mitochondria mediated apoptosis in lung cancer cells. *Life Sci*. 2006 Dec 23;80(3):205-11.

2973 Lin TY, Hsu HY. Ling Zhi-8 reduces lung cancer mobility and metastasis through disruption of focal adhesion and induction of MDM2-mediated Slug degradation. *Cancer Lett*. 2016 Jun 1;375(2):340-348.

2974 Vetchinkina E, Shirokov A, Bucharskaya A, et al. Antitumor Activity of Extracts from Medicinal Basidiomycetes Mushrooms. *Int J Med Mushrooms*. 2016;18(11):955-964.

2975 Wang WJ, Wu YS, Chen S, et al. Mushroom β-Glucan May Immunomodulate the Tumor-Associated Macrophages in the Lewis Lung Carcinoma. *Biomed Res Int*. 2015;2015:604385.

2976 Chen Y, Lv J, Li K, et al. Sporoderm-Broken Spores of Ganoderma lucidum Inhibit the Growth of Lung Cancer: Involvement of the Akt/mTOR Signaling Pathway. *Nutr Cancer*. 2016 Oct;68(7):1151-60.

2977 Sharif S, Atta A, Huma T, et al. Anticancer, antithrombotic, antityrosinase, and anti-α-glucosidase activities of selected wild and commercial mushrooms from Pakistan. *Food Sci Nutr*. 2018 Sep 14;6(8):2170-2176.

2978 Sohretoglu D, Zhang C, Luo J, et al. ReishiMax inhibits mTORC1/2 by activating AMPK and inhibiting IGFR/PI3K/Rheb in tumor cells. *Signal Transduct Target Ther*. 2019 Jun 28;4:21.

2979 Liu W, Yuan R, Hou A, et al. Ganoderma triterpenoids attenuate tumour angiogenesis in lung cancer tumour-bearing nude mice. *Pharm Biol*. 2020 Dec;58(1):1061-1068.

2980 Chen NH, Liu JW, Zhong JJ. Ganoderic acid Me inhibits tumor invasion through down-regulating matrix metalloproteinases 2/9 gene expression. *J Pharmacol Sci*. 2008 Oct;108(2):212-6.

2981 Sadava D, Still DW, Mudry RR, et al. Effect of Ganoderma on drug-sensitive and multidrug-resistant small-cell lung carcinoma cells. *Cancer Lett*. 2009 May 18;277(2):182-9.

2982 Chung WT, Lee SH, Kim JD, et al. Effect of mycelial culture broth of Ganoderma lucidum on the growth characteristics of human cell lines. *J Biosci Bioeng*. 2001;92(6):550-5.

2983 Sun LX, Li WD, Lin ZB, et al. Protection against lung cancer patient plasma-induced lymphocyte suppression by Ganoderma lucidum polysaccharides. *Cell Physiol Biochem*. 2014;33(2):289-99.

2984 Shahid A, Chen M, Yeung S, et al. The medicinal mushroom Ganoderma lucidum prevents lung tumorigenesis induced by tobacco smoke carcinogens. *Front Pharmacol*. 2023 Sep 6;14:1244150.

2985 Kashimoto N, Hayama M, Kamiya K, et al. Inhibitory effect of a water-soluble extract from the culture medium of Ganoderma lucidum (Rei-shi) mycelia on the development of pulmonary adenocarcinoma induced by N-nitrosobis (2-hydroxypropyl) amine in Wistar rats. *Oncol Rep*. 2006 Dec;16(6):1181-7.

2986 Wang X, Wang B, Zhou L, et al. Ganoderma lucidum put forth anti-tumor activity against PC-3 prostate cancer cells via inhibition of Jak-1/STAT-3 activity. *Saudi J Biol Sci*. 2020 Oct;27(10):2632-2637.

2987 Jiang J, Slivova V, Valachovicova T, et al. Ganoderma lucidum inhibits proliferation and induces apoptosis in human prostate cancer cells PC-3. *Int J Oncol*. 2004 May;24(5):1093-9.

2988 Qu L, Li S, Zhuo Y, Chen J, et al. Anticancer effect of triterpenes from Ganoderma lucidum in human prostate cancer cells. *Oncol Lett*. 2017 Dec;14(6):7467-7472.

2989 Kao CH, Bishop KS, Xu Y, et al. Identification of Potential Anticancer Activities of Novel Ganoderma lucidum Extracts Using Gene Expression and Pathway Network Analysis. *Genomics Insights*. 2016 Feb 16;9:1-16.

2990 Sliva D, Sedlak M, Slivova V, et al. Biologic activity of spores and dried powder from Ganoderma lucidum for the inhibition of highly invasive human breast and prostate cancer cells. *J Altern Complement Med*. 2003 Aug;9(4):491-7.

2991 Liu J, Shimizu K, Kondo R. The effects of ganoderma alcohols isolated from Ganoderma lucidum on the androgen receptor binding and the growth of LNCaP cells. *Fitoterapia*. 2010 Dec;81(8):1067-72.

2992 Wang T, Xie ZP, Huang ZS, et al. Total triterpenoids from Ganoderma Lucidum suppresses prostate cancer cell growth by inducing growth arrest and apoptosis. *J Huazhong Univ Sci Technolog Med Sci*. 2015 Oct;35(5):736-741.

2993 Zaidman BZ, Wasser SP, Nevo E, et al. Coprinus comatus and Ganoderma lucidum interfere with androgen receptor function in LNCaP prostate cancer cells. *Mol Biol Rep*. 2008 Jun;35(2):107-17.

2994 Sliva D, Labarrere C, Slivova V, et al. Ganoderma lucidum suppresses motility of highly invasive breast and prostate cancer cells. *Biochem Biophys Res Commun*. 2002 Nov 8;298(4):603-12.

2995 Stanley G, Harvey K, Slivova V, et al. Ganoderma lucidum suppresses angiogenesis through the inhibition of secretion of VEGF and TGF-beta1 from prostate cancer cells. *Biochem Biophys Res Commun*. 2005 Apr 29;330(1):46-52.

2996 Zaidman BZ, Wasser SP, Nevo E, et al. Androgen receptor-dependent and -independent mechanisms mediate Ganoderma lucidum activities in LNCaP prostate cancer cells. *Int J Oncol*. 2007 Oct;31(4):959-67.

2997 Zhao X, Zhou D, Liu Y, et al. Ganoderma lucidum polysaccharide inhibits prostate cancer cell migration via the protein arginine methyltransferase 6 signaling pathway. *Mol Med Rep*. 2018 Jan;17(1):147-157.

2998 Wu K, Na K, Chen D, et al. Effects of non-steroidal anti-inflammatory drug-activated gene-1 on Ganoderma lucidum polysaccharides-induced apoptosis of human prostate cancer PC-3 cells. *Int J Oncol*. 2018 Dec;53(6):2356-2368.

2999 Zhao S, Ye G, Fu G, et al. Ganoderma lucidum exerts anti-tumor effects on ovarian cancer cells and enhances their sensitivity to cisplatin. *Int J Oncol*. 2011 May;38(5):1319-27.

3000 Hsieh TC, Wu JM. Suppression of proliferation and oxidative stress by extracts of Ganoderma lucidum in the ovarian cancer cell line OVCAR-3. *Int J Mol Med*. 2011 Dec;28(6):1065-9.

3001 Dai S, Liu J, Sun X, et al. Ganoderma lucidum inhibits proliferation of human ovarian cancer cells by suppressing VEGF expression and up-regulating the expression of connexin 43. *BMC Complement Altern Med*. 2014 Nov 5;14:434.

3002 Jin H, Song C, Zhao Z, et al. Ganoderma Lucidum Polysaccharide, an Extract from Ganoderma Lucidum, Exerts Suppressive Effect on Cervical Cancer Cell Malignancy through Mitigating Epithelial-Mesenchymal and JAK/STAT5 Signaling Pathway. *Pharmacology*. 2020;105(7-8):461-470.

3003 Huang XR, Cai F, Chen J, et al. Cytotoxic lanostane-type triterpenes from the fruiting bodies of Ganoderma lucidum. *Nat Prod Res*. 2023 Aug-Sep;37(18):3042-3047.

3004 Cheng CR, Yue QX, Wu ZY, et al. Cytotoxic triterpenoids from Ganoderma lucidum. *Phytochemistry*. 2010 Sep;71(13):1579-85.

3005 Cilerdžić J, Vukojević J, Stajić M, et al. Biological activity of Ganoderma lucidum basidiocarps cultivated on alternative and commercial substrate. *J Ethnopharmacol*. 2014 Aug 8;155(1):312-9.

3006 Ruan W, Wei Y, Popovich DG. Distinct Responses of Cytotoxic Ganoderma lucidum Triterpenoids in Human Carcinoma Cells. *Phytother Res*. 2015 Nov;29(11):1744-52.

3007 Veljović S, Veljović M, Nikićević N, et al. Chemical composition, antiproliferative and antioxidant activity of differently processed Ganoderma lucidum ethanol extracts. *J Food Sci Technol*. 2017 Apr;54(5):1312-1320.

3008 Ruan W, Lim AH, Huang LG, et al. Extraction optimisation and isolation of triterpenoids from Ganoderma lucidum and their effect on human carcinoma cell growth. *Nat Prod Res*. 2014;28(24):2264-72.

3009 Cui YJ, Guan SH, Feng LX, et al. Cytotoxicity of 9,11-dehydroergosterol peroxide isolated from Ganoderma lucidum and its target-related proteins. *Nat Prod Commun*. 2010 Aug;5(8):1183-6.

3010 Zhu HS, Yang XL, Wang LB, et al. Effects of extracts from sporoderm-broken spores of Ganoderma lucidum on HeLa cells. *Cell Biol Toxicol*. 2000;16(3):201-6.

3011 Li N, Hu YL, He CX, et al. Preparation, characterisation and anti-tumour activity of Ganoderma lucidum polysaccharide nanoparticles. *J Pharm Pharmacol*. 2010 Jan;62(1):139-44.

3012 Liu RM, Li YB, Liang XF, et al. Structurally related ganoderic acids induce apoptosis in human cervical cancer HeLa cells: Involvement of oxidative stress and antioxidant protective system. *Chem Biol Interact*. 2015 Oct 5;240:134-44.

3013 Liu RM, Zhong JJ. Ganoderic acid Mf and S induce mitochondria mediated apoptosis in human cervical carcinoma HeLa cells. *Phytomedicine*. 2011 Mar 15;18(5):349-55.

3014 Yue QX, Song XY, Ma C, et al. Effects of triterpenes from Ganoderma lucidum on protein expression profile of HeLa cells. *Phytomedicine*. 2010 Jul;17(8-9):606-13.

3015 Lu J, Zhang A, Zhang F, et al. Ganoderenic acid D-loaded functionalized graphene oxide-based carrier for active targeting therapy of cervical carcinoma. *Biomed Pharmacother*. 2023 Aug;164:114947.

3016 Liu RM, Li YB, Zhong JJ. Cytotoxic and pro-apoptotic effects of novel ganoderic acid derivatives on human cervical cancer cells in vitro. *Eur J Pharmacol*. 2012 Apr 15;681(1-3):23-33.

3017 Gao Y, Gao H, Chan E, et al. Antitumor activity and underlying mechanisms of ganopoly, the refined polysaccharides extracted from Ganoderma lucidum, in mice. *Immunol Invest*. 2005;34(2):171-98.

3018 Zhang JJ, Wang DW, Cai D, et al. Meroterpenoids From Ganoderma lucidum Mushrooms and Their Biological Roles in Insulin Resistance and Triple-Negative Breast Cancer. *Front Chem*. 2021 Nov 3;9:772740.

3019 Jiang J, Slivova V, Harvey K, et al. Ganoderma lucidum suppresses growth of breast cancer cells through the inhibition of Akt/NF-kappaB signaling. *Nutr Cancer*. 2004;49(2):209-16.

3020 Chen S, Yong T, Zhang Y, et al. Anti-tumor and Anti-angiogenic Ergosterols from Ganoderma lucidum. *Front Chem*. 2017 Oct 30;5:85.

3021 Barbieri A, Quagliariello V, Del Vecchio V, et al. Anticancer and Anti-Inflammatory Properties of Ganoderma lucidum Extract Effects on Melanoma and Triple-Negative Breast Cancer Treatment. *Nutrients*. 2017 Feb 28;9(3):210.

3022 Lu QY, Sartippour MR, Brooks MN, et al. Ganoderma lucidum spore extract inhibits endothelial and breast cancer cells in vitro. *Oncol Rep*. 2004 Sep;12(3):659-62.

3023 Hu H, Ahn NS, Yang X, et al. Ganoderma lucidum extract induces cell cycle arrest and apoptosis in MCF-7 human breast cancer cell. *Int J Cancer*. 2002 Nov 20;102(3):250-3.

3024 Fang L, Zhao Q, Guo C, et al. Removing the sporoderm from the sporoderm-broken spores of Ganoderma lucidum improves the anticancer and immune-regulatory activity of the water-soluble polysaccharide. *Front Nutr*. 2022 Sep 16;9:1006127.

3025 Martínez-Montemayor MM, Ling T, Suárez-Arroyo IJ, et al. Identification of Biologically Active Ganoderma lucidum Compounds and Synthesis of Improved Derivatives That Confer Anti-cancer Activities in vitro. *Front Pharmacol*. 2019 Feb 19;10:115.

3026 Ai-Lati A, Liu S, Ji Z, et al. Structure and bioactivities of a polysaccharide isolated from Ganoderma lucidum in submerged fermentation. *Bioengineered*. 2017 Sep 3;8(5):565-571.

3027 Chen S, Li X, Yong T, et al. Cytotoxic lanostane-type triterpenoids from the fruiting bodies of Ganoderma lucidum and their structure-activity relationships. *Oncotarget*. 2017 Feb 7;8(6):10071-10084.

3028 Chen Y, Lan P. Total Syntheses and Biological Evaluation of the Ganoderma lucidum Alkaloids Lucidimines B and C. *ACS Omega*. 2018 Mar 31;3(3):3471-3481.

3029 Sliva D, Sedlak M, Slivova V, et al. Biologic activity of spores and dried powder from Ganoderma lucidum for the inhibition of highly invasive human breast and prostate cancer cells. *J Altern Complement Med*. 2003 Aug;9(4):491-7.

3030 Larypoor M. Investigation of HER-3 gene expression under the influence of carbohydrate biopolymers extract of shiitake and reishi in MCF-7 cell line. *Mol Biol Rep*. 2022 Jul;49(7):6563-6572.

3031 Zhang Y. Ganoderma lucidum (Reishi) suppresses proliferation and migration of breast cancer cells via inhibiting Wnt/β-catenin signaling. *Biochem Biophys Res Commun*. 2017 Jul 8;488(4):679-684.

3032 Zhong C, Li Y, Li W, et al. Ganoderma lucidum extract promotes tumor cell pyroptosis and inhibits metastasis in breast cancer. *Food Chem Toxicol*. 2023 Apr;174:113654.

3033 Kolniak-Ostek J, Oszmiański J, Szyjka A, et al. Anticancer and Antioxidant Activities in Ganoderma lucidum Wild Mushrooms in Poland, as Well as Their Phenolic and Triterpenoid Compounds. *Int J Mol Sci*. 2022 Aug 19;23(16):9359.

3034 Acevedo-Díaz A, Ortiz-Soto G, Suárez-Arroyo IJ, et al. Ganoderma lucidum Extract Reduces the Motility of Breast Cancer Cells Mediated by the RAC⁻Lamellipodin Axis. *Nutrients*. 2019 May 19;11(5):1116.

[3035] Smina TP, Nitha B, Devasagayam TP, et al. Ganoderma lucidum total triterpenes induce apoptosis in MCF-7 cells and attenuate DMBA induced mammary and skin carcinomas in experimental animals. *Mutat Res Genet Toxicol Environ Mutagen.* 2017 Jan;813:45-51.

[3036] Gonul O, Aydin HH, Kalmis E, et al. Effects of Ganoderma lucidum (Higher Basidiomycetes) Extracts on the miRNA Profile and Telomerase Activity of the MCF-7 Breast Cancer Cell Line. *Int J Med Mushrooms.* 2015;17(3):231-9.

[3037] Sliva D, Labarrere C, Slivova V, et al. Ganoderma lucidum suppresses motility of highly invasive breast and prostate cancer cells. *Biochem Biophys Res Commun.* 2002 Nov 8;298(4):603-12.

[3038] Wu G, Qian Z, Guo J, et al. Ganoderma lucidum extract induces G1 cell cycle arrest, and apoptosis in human breast cancer cells. *Am J Chin Med.* 2012;40(3):631-42.

[3039] Jiao C, Chen W, Tan X, et al. Ganoderma lucidum spore oil induces apoptosis of breast cancer cells in vitro and in vivo by activating caspase-3 and caspase-9. *J Ethnopharmacol.* 2020 Jan 30;247:112256.

[3040] Qin FY, Chen YY, Zhang JJ, et al. Meroterpenoid Dimers from Ganoderma Mushrooms and Their Biological Activities Against Triple Negative Breast Cancer Cells. *Front Chem.* 2022 May 3;10:888371.

[3041] Mousavi SM, Hashemi SA, Gholami A, et al. Ganoderma lucidum methanolic extract as a potent phytoconstituent: characterization, in-vitro antimicrobial and cytotoxic activity. *Sci Rep.* 2023 Oct 13;13(1):17326.

[3042] Jiang J, Slivova V, Sliva D. Ganoderma lucidum inhibits proliferation of human breast cancer cells by down-regulation of estrogen receptor and NF-kappaB signaling. *Int J Oncol.* 2006 Sep;29(3):695-703.

[3043] Thyagarajan A, Jiang J, Hopf A, et al. Inhibition of oxidative stress-induced invasiveness of cancer cells by Ganoderma lucidum is mediated through the suppression of interleukin-8 secretion. *Int J Mol Med.* 2006 Oct;18(4):657-64.

[3044] Yue GG, Fung KP, Tse GM, et al. Comparative studies of various ganoderma species and their different parts with regard to their antitumor and immunomodulating activities in vitro. *J Altern Complement Med.* 2006 Oct;12(8):777-89.

[3045] Jiang J, Jedinak A, Sliva D. Ganodermanontriol (GDNT) exerts its effect on growth and invasiveness of breast cancer cells through the down-regulation of CDC20 and uPA. *Biochem Biophys Res Commun.* 2011 Nov 18;415(2):325-9.

[3046] Wu GS, Song YL, Yin ZQ, et al. Ganoderiol A-enriched extract suppresses migration and adhesion of MDA-MB-231 cells by inhibiting FAK-SRC-paxillin cascade pathway. *PLoS One.* 2013 Oct 29;8(10):e76620.

[3047] Chen P, Yong Y, Gu Y, et al. Comparison of antioxidant and antiproliferation activities of polysaccharides from eight species of medicinal mushrooms. *Int J Med Mushrooms.* 2015;17(3):287-95.

[3048] Jia Y, Li Y, Shang H, et al. Ganoderic Acid A and Its Amide Derivatives as Potential Anti-Cancer Agents by Regulating the p53-MDM2 Pathway: Synthesis and Biological Evaluation. *Molecules.* 2023 Mar 4;28(5):2374.

[3049] Wu GS, Lu JJ, Guo JJ, et al. Ganoderic acid DM, a natural triterpenoid, induces DNA damage, G1 cell cycle arrest and apoptosis in human breast cancer cells. *Fitoterapia.* 2012 Mar;83(2):408-14.

[3050] Jiang J, Grieb B, Thyagarajan A, et al. Ganoderic acids suppress growth and invasive behavior of breast cancer cells by modulating AP-1 and NF-kappaB signaling. *Int J Mol Med.* 2008 May;21(5):577-84.

[3051] Gao Y, Gao H, Chan E, et al. Antitumor activity and underlying mechanisms of ganopoly, the refined polysaccharides extracted from Ganoderma lucidum, in mice. *Immunol Invest.* 2005;34(2):171-98.

[3052] Suárez-Arroyo IJ, Acevedo-Díaz A, Ríos-Fuller TJ, et al. Ganoderma lucidum enhances carboplatin chemotherapy effect by inhibiting the DNA damage response pathway and stemness. *Am J Cancer Res.* 2022 Mar 15;12(3):1282-1294.

[3053] Martínez-Montemayor MM, Ling T, Suárez-Arroyo IJ, et al. Identification of Biologically Active Ganoderma lucidum Compounds and Synthesis of Improved Derivatives That Confer Anti-cancer Activities in vitro. *Front Pharmacol.* 2019 Feb 19:10:115.

[3054] Martínez-Montemayor MM, Acevedo RR, Otero-Franqui E, et al. Ganoderma lucidum (Reishi) inhibits cancer cell growth and expression of key molecules in inflammatory breast cancer. *Nutr Cancer.* 2011;63(7):1085-94.

[3055] Suarez-Arroyo IJ, Rosario-Acevedo R, Aguilar-Perez A, et al. Anti-tumor effects of Ganoderma lucidum (reishi) in inflammatory breast cancer in in vivo and in vitro models. *PLoS One.* 2013;8(2):e57431.

[3056] Rios-Fuller TJ, Ortiz-Soto G, Lacourt-Ventura M, et al. Ganoderma lucidum extract (GLE) impairs breast cancer stem cells by targeting the STAT3 pathway. *Oncotarget.* 2018 Nov 13;9(89):35907-35921.

[3057] Deepalakshmi K, Mirunalini S. Modulatory effect of Ganoderma lucidum on expression of xenobiotic enzymes, oxidant-antioxidant and hormonal status in 7,12-dimethylbenz(a)anthracene-induced mammary carcinoma in rats. *Pharmacogn Mag.* 2013 Apr;9(34):167-75.

[3058] Loganathan J, Jiang J, Smith A, et al. The mushroom Ganoderma lucidum suppresses breast-to-lung cancer metastasis through the inhibition of pro-invasive genes. *Int J Oncol.* 2014 Jun;44(6):2009-15.

[3059] Jiang J, Thyagarajan-Sahu A, Loganathan J, et al. BreastDefend™ prevents breast-to-lung cancer metastases in an orthotopic animal model of triple-negative human breast cancer. *Oncol Rep.* 2012 Oct;28(4):1139-45.

[3060] Liu G, Zeng T. Sporoderm-Removed Ganoderma lucidum Spore Powder May Suppress the Proliferation, Migration, and Invasion of Esophageal Squamous Cell Carcinoma Cells Through PI3K/AKT/mTOR and Erk Pathway. *Integr Cancer Ther.* 2021 Jan-Dec;20:15347354211062157.

[3061] Shao CS, Zhou XH, Zheng XX, et al. Ganoderic acid D induces synergistic autophagic cell death except for apoptosis in ESCC cells. *J Ethnopharmacol.* 2020 Nov 15;262:113213.

[3062] Shi YJ, Zheng HX, Hong ZP, et al. Antitumor effects of different Ganoderma lucidum spore powder in cell- and zebrafish-based bioassays. *J Integr Med.* 2021 Mar;19(2):177-184.

[3063] Li P, Deng YP, Wei XX, et al. Triterpenoids from Ganoderma lucidum and their cytotoxic activities. *Nat Prod Res.* 2013;27(1):17-22.

[3064] Cheuk W, Chan JK, Nuovo G, et al. Regression of gastric large B-Cell lymphoma accompanied by a florid lymphoma-like T-cell reaction: immunomodulatory effect of Ganoderma lucidum (Lingzhi)? *Int J Surg Pathol.* 2007 Apr;15(2):180-6.

[3065] Calviño E, Pajuelo L, Casas JA, et al. Cytotoxic action of Ganoderma lucidum on interleukin-3 dependent lymphoma DA-1 cells: involvement of apoptosis proteins. *Phytother Res.* 2011 Jan;25(1):25-32.

[3066] Müller CI, Kumagai T, O'Kelly J, et al. Ganoderma lucidum causes apoptosis in leukemia, lymphoma and multiple myeloma cells. *Leuk Res.* 2006 Jul;30(7):841-8.

288

[3067] Saltarelli R, Ceccaroli P, Buffalini M, et al. Biochemical characterization and antioxidant and antiproliferative activities of different Ganoderma collections. *J Mol Microbiol Biotechnol*. 2015;25(1):16-25.

[3068] Wang SY, Hsu ML, Hsu HC, et al. The anti-tumor effect of Ganoderma lucidum is mediated by cytokines released from activated macrophages and T lymphocytes. *Int J Cancer*. 1997 Mar 17;70(6):699-705.

[3069] Yang G, Yang L, Zhuang Y, et al. Ganoderma lucidum polysaccharide exerts anti-tumor activity via MAPK pathways in HL-60 acute leukemia cells. *J Recept Signal Transduct Res*. 2016;36(1):6-13.

[3070] Calviño E, Manjón JL, Sancho P, et al. Ganoderma lucidum induced apoptosis in NB4 human leukemia cells: involvement of Akt and Erk. *J Ethnopharmacol*. 2010 Mar 2;128(1):71-8.

[3071] Wang JH, Zhou YJ, Zhang M, et al. Active lipids of Ganoderma lucidum spores-induced apoptosis in human leukemia THP-1 cells via MAPK and PI3K pathways. *J Ethnopharmacol*. 2012 Jan 31;139(2):582-9.

[3072] Cheng KC, Huang HC, Chen JH, et al. Ganoderma lucidum polysaccharides in human monocytic leukemia cells: from gene expression to network construction. *BMC Genomics*. 2007 Nov 9;8:411. doi: 10.1186/1471-2164-8-411.

[3073] Zhong L, Jiang D, Wang Q. [Effects of Ganoderma lucidum (Leyss ex Fr) Karst compound on the proliferation and differentiation of K562 leukemic cells]. *Hunan Yi Ke Da Xue Xue Bao*. 1999;24(6):521-4.

[3074] Lee MK, Hung TM, Cuong TD, et al. Ergosta-7,22-diene-2β,3α,9α-triol from the fruit bodies of Ganoderma lucidum induces apoptosis in human myelocytic HL-60 cells. *Phytother Res*. 2011 Nov;25(11):1579-85.

[3075] Wu TS, Shi LS, Kuo SC. Cytotoxicity of Ganoderma lucidum triterpenes. *J Nat Prod*. 2001 Aug;64(8):1121-2.

[3076] Zhong M, Huang J, Mao P, et al. Ganoderma lucidum polysaccharide inhibits the proliferation of leukemic cells through apoptosis. *Acta Biochim Pol*. 2022 Jun 28;69(3):639-645.

[3077] Müller CI, Kumagai T, O'Kelly J, et al. Ganoderma lucidum causes apoptosis in leukemia, lymphoma and multiple myeloma cells. *Leuk Res*. 2006 Jul;30(7):841-8.

[3078] Mousavi SM, Hashemi SA, Gholami A, et al. Ganoderma lucidum methanolic extract as a potent phytoconstituent: characterization, in-vitro antimicrobial and cytotoxic activity. *Sci Rep*. 2023 Oct 13;13(1):17326.

[3079] Lieu CW, Lee SS, Wang SY. The effect of Ganoderma lucidum on induction of differentiation in leukemic U937 cells. *Anticancer Res*. 1992 Jul-Aug;12(4):1211-5.

[3080] Hsu CL, Yu YS, Yen GC. Lucidenic acid B induces apoptosis in human leukemia cells via a mitochondria-mediated pathway. *J Agric Food Chem*. 2008 Jun 11;56(11):3973-80.

[3081] Chen C, Li P, Li Y, et al. Antitumor effects and mechanisms of Ganoderma extracts and spores oil. *Oncol Lett*. 2016 Nov;12(5):3571-3578.

[3082] Wang SY, Hsu ML, Hsu HC, et al. The anti-tumor effect of Ganoderma lucidum is mediated by cytokines released from activated macrophages and T lymphocytes. *Int J Cancer*. 1997 Mar 17;70(6):699-705.

[3083] Müller CI, Kumagai T, O'Kelly J, et al. Ganoderma lucidum causes apoptosis in leukemia, lymphoma and multiple myeloma cells. *Leuk Res*. 2006 Jul;30(7):841-8.

[3084] Wu X, Jiang L, Zhang Z, et al. Pancreatic cancer cell apoptosis is induced by a proteoglycan extracted from Ganoderma lucidum. *Oncol Lett*. 2021 Jan;21(1):34.

[3085] Gill BS, Kumar S, Navgeet. Ganoderic Acid A Targeting β-Catenin in Wnt Signaling Pathway: In Silico and In Vitro Study. *Interdiscip Sci*. 2018 Jun;10(2):233-243.

[3086] Zhang W, Lei Z, Meng J, et al. Water Extract of Sporoderm-Broken Spores of Ganoderma lucidum Induces Osteosarcoma Apoptosis and Restricts Autophagic Flux. *Onco Targets Ther*. 2019 Dec 31;12:11651-11665.

[3087] Zhang QH, Hu QX, et al. Ganoderma lucidum Exerts an Anticancer Effect on Human Osteosarcoma Cells via Suppressing the Wnt/β-Catenin Signaling Pathway. *Integr Cancer Ther*. 2019 Jan-Dec;18:1534735419890917.

[3088] Sun Z, Huang K, Fu X, et al. A chemically sulfated polysaccharide derived from Ganoderma lucidum induces mitochondrial-mediated apoptosis in human osteosarcoma MG63 cells. *Tumour Biol*. 2014 Oct;35(10):9919-26.

[3089] He J, Zhang W, Di T, et al. Water extract of sporoderm-broken spores of Ganoderma lucidum enhanced pd-l1 antibody efficiency through downregulation and relieved complications of pd-l1 monoclonal antibody. *Biomed Pharmacother*. 2020 Nov;131:110541.

[3090] Min BS, Gao JJ, Nakamura N, et al. Triterpenes from the spores of Ganoderma lucidum and their cytotoxicity against meth-A and LLC tumor cells. *Chem Pharm Bull (Tokyo)*. 2000 Jul;48(7):1026-33.

[3091] Dulay RMR, Valdez BC, Chakrabarti S, et al. Cytotoxicity of Medicinal Mushrooms Oudemansiella canarii and Ganoderma lucidum (Agaricomycetes) Against Hematologic Malignant Cells via Activation of Apoptosis-Related Markers. *Int J Med Mushrooms*. 2022;24(11):83-95.

[3092] da Silva Milhorini S, de Lima Bellan D, Zavadinack M, et al. Antimelanoma effect of a fucoxylomannan isolated from Ganoderma lucidum fruiting bodies. *Carbohydr Polym*. 2022 Oct 15;294:119823.

[3093] Barbieri A, Quagliariello V, Del Vecchio V, et al. Anticancer and Anti-Inflammatory Properties of Ganoderma lucidum Extract Effects on Melanoma and Triple-Negative Breast Cancer Treatment. *Nutrients*. 2017 Feb 28;9(3):210.

[3094] Zheng S, Jia Y, Zhao J, et al. Ganoderma lucidum polysaccharides eradicates the blocking effect of fibrinogen on NK cytotoxicity against melanoma cells. *Oncol Lett*. 2012 Mar;3(3):613-616.

[3095] Zheng L, Wong YS, Shao M, et al. Apoptosis induced by 9,11-dehydroergosterol peroxide from Ganoderma Lucidum mycelium in human malignant melanoma cells is Mcl-1 dependent. *Mol Med Rep*. 2018 Jul;18(1):938-944.

[3096] Xian H, Li J, Zhang Y, et al. Antimetastatic Effects of Ganoderma lucidum Polysaccharide Peptide on B16-F10-luc-G5 Melanoma Mice With Sleep Fragmentation. *Front Pharmacol*. 2021 Jul 8;12:650216.

[3097] Ai-Lati A, Liu S, Ji Z, et al. Structure and bioactivities of a polysaccharide isolated from Ganoderma lucidum in submerged fermentation. *Bioengineered*. 2017 Sep 3;8(5):565-571.

[3098] Shahid A, Huang M, Liu M, et al. The medicinal mushroom Ganoderma lucidum attenuates UV-induced skin carcinogenesis and immunosuppression. *PLoS One*. 2022 Mar 21;17(3):e0265615.

[3099] Zheng DS, Chen LS. Triterpenoids from Ganoderma lucidum inhibit the activation of EBV antigens as telomerase inhibitors. *Exp Ther Med*. 2017 Oct;14(4):3273-3278.

3100 Liu L, Yu Z, Chen J, et al. Lucialdehyde B suppresses proliferation and induces mitochondria-dependent apoptosis in nasopharyngeal carcinoma CNE2 cells. *Pharm Biol.* 2023 Dec;61(1):918-926.

3101 Vetchinkina E, Shirokov A, Bucharskaya A, et al. Antitumor Activity of Extracts from Medicinal Basidiomycetes Mushrooms. *Int J Med Mushrooms.* 2016;18(11):955-964.

3102 Cai D, Zhang JJ, Wu ZH, et al. Lucidumones B-H, racemic meroterpenoids that inhibit tumor cell migration from Ganoderma lucidum. *Bioorg Chem.* 2021 May;110:104774.

3103 Abdullah NR, Sharif F, Azizan NH, et al. Pellet diameter of Ganoderma lucidum in a repeated-batch fermentation for the trio total production of biomass-exopolysaccharide-endopolysaccharide and its anti-oral cancer beta-glucan response. *AIMS Microbiol.* 2020 Oct 22;6(4):379-400.

3104 Wu X, Wu Q, Wang Y, et al. Aqueous-soluble components of sporoderm-removed Ganoderma lucidum spore powder promote ferroptosis in oral squamous cell carcinoma. *Chin J Cancer Res.* 2023 Apr 30;35(2):176-190.

3105 Hsu WH, Hua WJ, Qiu WL, et al. WSG, a glucose-enriched polysaccharide from Ganoderma lucidum, suppresses tongue cancer cells via inhibition of EGFR-mediated signaling and potentiates cisplatin-induced apoptosis. *Int J Biol Macromol.* 2021 Dec 15;193(Pt B):1201-1208.

3106 de Camargo MR, Frazon TF, Inacio KK, et al. Ganoderma lucidum polysaccharides inhibit in vitro tumorigenesis, cancer stem cell properties and epithelial-mesenchymal transition in oral squamous cell carcinoma. *J Ethnopharmacol.* 2022 Mar 25;286:114891.

3107 Li L, Guo HJ, Zhu LY, et al. A supercritical-CO2 extract of Ganoderma lucidum spores inhibits cholangiocarcinoma cell migration by reversing the epithelial-mesenchymal transition. *Phytomedicine.* 2016 May 15;23(5):491-7.

3108 Wang C, Lin D, Chen Q, et al. Polysaccharide peptide isolated from grass-cultured Ganoderma lucidum induces anti-proliferative and pro-apoptotic effects in the human U251 glioma cell line. *Oncol Lett.* 2018 Apr;15(4):4330-4336.

3109 Wang C, Shi S, Chen Q, et al. Antitumor and Immunomodulatory Activities of Ganoderma lucidum Polysaccharides in Glioma-Bearing Rats. *Integr Cancer Ther.* 2018 Sep;17(3):674-683.

3110 Cheng AY, Chien YC, Lee HC, et al. Water-Extracted Ganoderma lucidum Induces Apoptosis and S-Phase Arrest via Cyclin-CDK2 Pathway in Glioblastoma Cells. *Molecules.* 2020 Aug 6;25(16):3585.

3111 Li R, Tang X, Xu C, et al. Circular RNA NF1-419 Inhibits Proliferation and Induces Apoptosis by Regulating Lipid Metabolism in Astroglioma Cells. *Recent Pat Anticancer Drug Discov.* 2022;17(2):162-177.

3112 Gill BS, Navgeet, Kumar S. Antioxidant potential of ganoderic acid in Notch-1 protein in neuroblastoma. *Mol Cell Biochem.* 2019 Jun;456(1-2):1-14.

3113 Cheng Y, Xie P. Ganoderic acid A holds promising cytotoxicity on human glioblastoma mediated by incurring apoptosis and autophagy and inactivating PI3K/AKT signaling pathway. *J Biochem Mol Toxicol.* 2019 Nov;33(11):e22392.

3114 Das A, Alshareef M, Henderson F Jr, et al. Ganoderic acid A/DM-induced NDRG2 over-expression suppresses high-grade meningioma growth. *Clin Transl Oncol.* 2020 Jul;22(7):1138-1145.

3115 Lu QY, Jin YS, Zhang Q, et al. Ganoderma lucidum extracts inhibit growth and induce actin polymerization in bladder cancer cells in vitro. *Cancer Lett.* 2004 Dec 8;216(1):9-20.

3116 Shi YJ, Zheng HX, Hong ZP, et al. Antitumor effects of different Ganoderma lucidum spore powder in cell- and zebrafish-based bioassays. *J Integr Med.* 2021 Mar;19(2):177-184.

3117 Zhong J, Fang L, Chen R, et al. Polysaccharides from sporoderm-removed spores of Ganoderma lucidum induce apoptosis in human gastric cancer cells via disruption of autophagic flux. *Oncol Lett.* 2021 May;21(5):425.

3118 Wang DH, Weng XC. [Antitumor activity of extracts of Ganoderma lucidum and their protective effects on damaged HL-7702 cells induced by radiotherapy and chemotherapy]. *Zhongguo Zhong Yao Za Zhi.* 2006 Oct;31(19):1618-22.

3119 Oliveira M, Reis FS, Sousa D, et al. A methanolic extract of Ganoderma lucidum fruiting body inhibits the growth of a gastric cancer cell line and affects cellular autophagy and cell cycle. *Food Funct.* 2014 Jul 25;5(7):1389-94.

3120 Liang C, Li H, Zhou H, et al. Recombinant Lz-8 from Ganoderma lucidum induces endoplasmic reticulum stress-mediated autophagic cell death in SGC-7901 human gastric cancer cells. *Oncol Rep.* 2012 Apr;27(4):1079-89.

3121 Jang KJ, Son IS, Shin DY, et al. Anti-invasive activity of ethanol extracts of Ganoderma lucidum through tightening of tight junctions and inhibition of matrix metalloproteinase activities in human gastric carcinoma cells. *J Acupunct Meridian Stud.* 2011 Dec;4(4):225-35.

3122 Jang KJ, Han MH, Lee BH, et al. Induction of apoptosis by ethanol extracts of Ganoderma lucidum in human gastric carcinoma cells. *J Acupunct Meridian Stud.* 2010 Mar;3(1):24-31.

3123 Kim TH, Kim JS, Kim ZH, et al. Khz-cp (crude polysaccharide extract obtained from the fusion of Ganoderma lucidum and Polyporus umbellatus mycelia) induces apoptosis by increasing intracellular calcium levels and activating P38 and NADPH oxidase-dependent generation of reactive oxygen species in SNU-1 cells. *BMC Complement Altern Med.* 2014 Jul 10;14:236.

3124 Huh S, Lee S, Choi SJ, et al. Quercetin Synergistically Inhibit EBV-Associated Gastric Carcinoma with Ganoderma lucidum Extracts. *Molecules.* 2019 Oct 24;24(21):3834.

3125 Bai JH, Xu J, Zhao J, et al. Ganoderma lucidum Polysaccharide Enzymatic Hydrolysate Suppresses the Growth of Human Colon Cancer Cells via Inducing Apoptosis. *Cell Transplant.* 2020 Jan-Dec;29:963689720931435.

3126 Liu X, Xu Y, Li Y, et al. Ganoderma lucidum fruiting body extracts inhibit colorectal cancer by inducing apoptosis, autophagy, and G0/G1 phase cell cycle arrest in vitro and in vivo. *Am J Transl Res.* 2020 Jun 15;12(6):2675-2684.

3127 Shin MJ, Chae HJ, Lee JW, et al. Lucidumol A, Purified Directly from Ganoderma lucidum, Exhibits Anticancer Effect and Cellular Inflammatory Response in Colorectal Cancer. *Evid Based Complement Alternat Med.* 2022 Nov 8;2022:7404493.

3128 Liu MM, Liu T, Yeung S, et al. Inhibitory activity of medicinal mushroom Ganoderma lucidum on colorectal cancer by attenuating inflammation. *Precis Clin Med.* 2021 Aug 28;4(4):231-245.

3129 Dan X, Liu W, Wong JH, et al. A Ribonuclease Isolated from Wild Ganoderma Lucidum Suppressed Autophagy and Triggered Apoptosis in Colorectal Cancer Cells. *Front Pharmacol.* 2016 Jul 25;7:217.

3130 Fang L, Zhao Q, Guo C, et al. Removing the sporoderm from the sporoderm-broken spores of Ganoderma lucidum improves the anticancer and immune-regulatory activity of the water-soluble polysaccharide. *Front Nutr.* 2022 Sep 16;9:1006127.

3131 Tülüce Y, Keleş AY, Köstekci S. Assessment of redox homeostasis via genotoxicity, cytotoxicity, apoptosis and NRF-2 in colorectal cancer cell lines after treatment with Ganoderma lucidum extract. *Drug Chem Toxicol.* 2023 Sep 13:1-16.

3132 Pan K, Jiang Q, Liu G, et al. Optimization extraction of Ganoderma lucidum polysaccharides and its immunity and antioxidant activities. *Int J Biol Macromol.* 2013 Apr;55:301-6.

3133 Ruan W, Wei Y, Popovich DG. Distinct Responses of Cytotoxic Ganoderma lucidum Triterpenoids in Human Carcinoma Cells. *Phytother Res.* 2015 Nov;29(11):1744-52.

3134 Xie JT, Wang CZ, Wicks S, et al. Ganoderma lucidum extract inhibits proliferation of SW 480 human colorectal cancer cells. *Exp Oncol.* 2006 Mar;28(1):25-9.

3135 Ruan W, Lim AH, Huang LG, et al. Extraction optimisation and isolation of triterpenoids from Ganoderma lucidum and their effect on human carcinoma cell growth. *Nat Prod Res.* 2014;28(24):2264-72.

3136 Kim TH, Kim JS, Kim ZH, et al. Khz (fusion product of Ganoderma lucidum and Polyporus umbellatus mycelia) induces apoptosis in human colon carcinoma HCT116 cells, accompanied by an increase in reactive oxygen species, activation of caspase 3, and increased intracellular Ca^{2+}. *J Med Food.* 2015 Mar;18(3):332-6.

3137 Ren F, Cao KY, Gong RZ, et al. The role of post-transcriptional modification on a new tRNAIle(GAU) identified from Ganoderma lucidum in its fragments' cytotoxicity on cancer cells. *Int J Biol Macromol.* 2023 Feb 28;229:885-895.

3138 Jiang D, Wang L, Zhao T, et al. Restoration of the tumor-suppressor function to mutant p53 by Ganoderma lucidum polysaccharides in colorectal cancer cells. *Oncol Rep.* 2017 Jan;37(1):594-600.

3139 Liang Z, Guo YT, Yi YJ, et al. Ganoderma lucidum polysaccharides target a Fas/caspase dependent pathway to induce apoptosis in human colon cancer cells. *Asian Pac J Cancer Prev.* 2014;15(9):3981-6.

3140 Kolniak-Ostek J, Oszmiański J, Szyjka A, et al. Anticancer and Antioxidant Activities in Ganoderma lucidum Wild Mushrooms in Poland, as Well as Their Phenolic and Triterpenoid Compounds. *Int J Mol Sci.* 2022 Aug 19;23(16):9359.

3141 Li P, Liu L, Huang S, et al. Anti-cancer Effects of a Neutral Triterpene Fraction from Ganoderma lucidum and its Active Constituents on SW620 Human Colorectal Cancer Cells. *Anticancer Agents Med Chem.* 2020;20(2):237-244.

3142 Ji Z, Tang Q, Hao, et al. Induction of apoptosis in the SW620 colon carcinoma cell line by triterpene-enriched extracts from Ganoderma lucidum through activation of caspase-3. *Oncol Lett.* 2011 May;2(3):565-570.

3143 Jedinak A, Thyagarajan-Sahu A, Jiang J, et al. Ganodermanontriol, a lanostanoid triterpene from Ganoderma lucidum, suppresses growth of colon cancer cells through ß-catenin signaling. *Int J Oncol.* 2011 Mar;38(3):761-7.

3144 Thyagarajan A, Jedinak A, Nguyen H, et al. Triterpenes from Ganoderma Lucidum induce autophagy in colon cancer through the inhibition of p38 mitogen-activated kinase (p38 MAPK). *Nutr Cancer.* 2010;62(5):630-40.

3145 Liang ZE, Yi YJ, Guo YT, et al. Inhibition of migration and induction of apoptosis in LoVo human colon cancer cells by polysaccharides from Ganoderma lucidum. *Mol Med Rep.* 2015 Nov;12(5):7629-36.

3146 Li K, Na K, Sang T, Wu K, et al. The ethanol extracts of sporoderm-broken spores of Ganoderma lucidum inhibit colorectal cancer in vitro and in vivo. *Oncol Rep.* 2017 Nov;38(5):2803-2813.

3147 Pan H, Wang Y, Na K, et al. Autophagic flux disruption contributes to Ganoderma lucidum polysaccharide-induced apoptosis in human colorectal cancer cells via MAPK/ERK activation. *Cell Death Dis.* 2019 Jun 11;10(6):456.

3148 Hong KJ, Dunn DM, Shen CL, et al. Effects of Ganoderma lucidum on apoptotic and anti-inflammatory function in HT-29 human colonic carcinoma cells. *Phytother Res.* 2004 Sep;18(9):768-70.

3149 Chen NH, Liu JW, Zhong JJ. Ganoderic acid T inhibits tumor invasion in vitro and in vivo through inhibition of MMP expression. *Pharmacol Rep.* 2010 Jan-Feb;62(1):150-63.

3150 Gao Y, Gao H, Chan E, et al. Antitumor activity and underlying mechanisms of ganopoly, the refined polysaccharides extracted from Ganoderma lucidum, in mice. *Immunol Invest.* 2005;34(2):171-98.

3151 Guo C, Guo D, Fang L, et al. Ganoderma lucidum polysaccharide modulates gut microbiota and immune cell function to inhibit inflammation and tumorigenesis in colon. *Carbohydr Polym.* 2021 Sep 1;267:118231.

3152 Lu H, Uesaka T, Katoh O, et al. Prevention of the development of preneoplastic lesions, aberrant crypt foci, by a water-soluble extract from cultured medium of Ganoderma lucidum (Rei-shi) mycelia in male F344 rats. *Oncol Rep.* 2001 Nov-Dec;8(6):1341-5.

3153 Lu H, Kyo E, Uesaka T, et al. Prevention of development of N,N'-dimethylhydrazine-induced colon tumors by a water-soluble extract from cultured medium of Ganoderma lucidum (Rei-shi) mycelia in male ICR mice. *Int J Mol Med.* 2002 Feb;9(2):113-7.

3154 Watanabe H, Kashimoto N, Ushijima M, et al. Effects of a water-soluble extract of Ganoderma lucidum mycelia on aberrant crypt foci induced by azoxymethane and small-intestinal injury by 5-FU in F344 rats. *Med Mol Morphol.* 2013 Jun;46(2):97-103.

3155 Na K, Li K, Sang T, et al. Anticarcinogenic effects of water extract of sporoderm-broken spores of Ganoderma lucidum on colorectal cancer in vitro and in vivo. *Int J Oncol.* 2017 May;50(5):1541-1554.

3156 Lu H, Kyo E, Uesaka T, et al. A water-soluble extract from cultured medium of Ganoderma lucidum (Rei-shi) mycelia suppresses azoxymethane-induction of colon cancers in male F344 rats. *Oncol Rep.* 2003 Mar-Apr;10(2):375-9.

3157 Yuen JW, Gohel MD, Au DW. Telomerase-associated apoptotic events by mushroom ganoderma lucidum on premalignant human urothelial cells. *Nutr Cancer.* 2008;60(1):109-19.

3158 Yuen JW, Gohel MD, Ng CF. The differential immunological activities of Ganoderma lucidum on human pre-cancerous uroepithelial cells. *J Ethnopharmacol.* 2011 Jun 1;135(3):711-8.

3159 Yuen JW, Gohel MD. The dual roles of Ganoderma antioxidants on urothelial cell DNA under carcinogenic attack. *J Ethnopharmacol.* 2008 Jul 23;118(2):324-30.

3160 Wu QP, Xie YZ, Deng Z, et al. Ergosterol peroxide isolated from Ganoderma lucidum abolishes microRNA miR-378-mediated tumor cells on chemoresistance. *PLoS One.* 2012;7(8):e44579.

3161 Xia QH, Lu CT, Tong MQ, et al. Ganoderma Lucidum Polysaccharides Enhance the Abscopal Effect of Photothermal Therapy in Hepatoma-Bearing Mice Through Immunomodulatory, Anti-Proliferative, Pro-Apoptotic and Anti-Angiogenic. *Front Pharmacol.* 2021 Jul 6;12:648708.

3162 Wu M, Shen CE, Lin QF, et al. Sterols and triterpenoids from Ganoderma lucidum and their reversal activities of tumor multidrug resistance. *Nat Prod Res.* 2022 Mar;36(5):1396-1399.

[3163] Li WD, Zhang BD, Wei R, et al. Reversal effect of Ganoderma lucidum polysaccharide on multidrug resistance in K562/ADM cell line. *Acta Pharmacol Sin.* 2008 May;29(5):620-7.

[3164] Liu DL, Li YJ, Yang DH, et al. Ganoderma lucidum derived ganoderenic acid B reverses ABCB1-mediated multidrug resistance in HepG2/ADM cells. *Int J Oncol.* 2015 May;46(5):2029-38.

[3165] Kim KC, Jun HJ, Kim JS, et al. Enhancement of radiation response with combined Ganoderma lucidum and Duchesnea chrysantha extracts in human leukemia HL-60 cells. *Int J Mol Med.* 2008 Apr;21(4):489-98.

[3166] Zhao S, Ye G, Fu G, et al. Ganoderma lucidum exerts anti-tumor effects on ovarian cancer cells and enhances their sensitivity to cisplatin. *Int J Oncol.* 2011 May;38(5):1319-27.

[3167] Cen K, Chen M, He M, et al. Sporoderm-Broken Spores of Ganoderma lucidum Sensitizes Ovarian Cancer to Cisplatin by ROS/ERK Signaling and Attenuates Chemotherapy-Related Toxicity. *Front Pharmacol.* 2022 Feb 21;13:826716.

[3168] Zhu J, Xu J, Jiang LL, et al. Improved antitumor activity of cisplatin combined with Ganoderma lucidum polysaccharides in U14 cervical carcinoma-bearing mice. *Kaohsiung J Med Sci.* 2019 Apr;35(4):222-229.

[3169] Shao CS, Feng N, Zhou S, et al. Ganoderic acid T improves the radiosensitivity of HeLa cells via converting apoptosis to necroptosis. *Toxicol Res (Camb).* 2021 May 13;10(3):531-541.

[3170] Qiu WL, Hsu WH, Tsao SM, et al. WSG, a Glucose-Rich Polysaccharide from Ganoderma lucidum, Combined with Cisplatin Potentiates Inhibition of Lung Cancer In Vitro and In Vivo. *Polymers (Basel).* 2021 Dec 13;13(24):4353.

[3171] Yu Y, Qian L, Du N, et al. Ganoderma lucidum polysaccharide enhances radiosensitivity of hepatocellular carcinoma cell line HepG2 through Akt signaling pathway. *Exp Ther Med.* 2017 Dec;14(6):5903-5907.

[3172] Yao X, Li G, Xu H, et al. Inhibition of the JAK-STAT3 signaling pathway by ganoderic acid A enhances chemosensitivity of HepG2 cells to cisplatin. *Planta Med.* 2012 Nov;78(16):1740-8.

[3173] Opattova A, Horak J, Vodenkova S, et al. Ganoderma Lucidum induces oxidative DNA damage and enhances the effect of 5-Fluorouracil in colorectal cancer in vitro and in vivo. *Mutat Res Genet Toxicol Environ Mutagen.* 2019 Sep;845:403065.

[3174] Lei X, Zhi C, Huang W, et al. Recombinant Ganoderma lucidum Immunomodulatory Protein Improves the Treatment for Chemotherapy-Induced Neutropenia. *Front Pharmacol.* 2020 Jun 26;11:956.

[3175] Zhou H, Sun F, Li H, et al. Effect of recombinant Ganoderma lucidum immunoregulatory protein on cyclophosphamide-induced leukopenia in mice. *Immunopharmacol Immunotoxicol.* 2013 Jun;35(3):426-33.

[3176] Li Y, Lei Z, Guo Y, et al. Fermentation of Ganoderma lucidum and Raphani Semen with a probiotic mixture attenuates cyclophosphamide-induced immunosuppression through microbiota-dependent or -independent regulation of intestinal mucosal barrier and immune responses. *Phytomedicine.* 2023 Dec;121:155082.

[3177] Xu F, Li X, Xiao X, et al. Effects of Ganoderma lucidum polysaccharides against doxorubicin-induced cardiotoxicity. *Biomed Pharmacother.* 2017 Nov;95:504-512.

[3178] Veena RK, Ajith TA, Janardhanan KK. Lingzhi or Reishi Medicinal Mushroom, Ganoderma lucidum (Agaricomycetes), Prevents Doxorubicin-Induced Cardiotoxicity in Rats. *Int J Med Mushrooms.* 2018;20(8):761-774.

[3179] Fang H, Lin D, Li X, et al. Therapeutic potential of Ganoderma lucidum polysaccharide peptide in Doxorubicin-induced nephropathy: modulation of renin-angiotensin system and proteinuria. *Front Pharmacol.* 2023 Sep 29;14:1287908.

[3180] Veena RK, Janardhanan KK. Polysaccharide-Protein Complex Isolated from Fruiting Bodies and Cultured Mycelia of Lingzhi or Reishi Medicinal Mushroom, Ganoderma lucidum (Agaricomycetes), Attenuates Doxorubicin-Induced Oxidative Stress and Myocardial Injury in Rats. *Int J Med Mushrooms.* 2022;24(2):31-40.

[3181] Wu SY, Ou CC, Lee ML, et al. Polysaccharide of Ganoderma lucidum Ameliorates Cachectic Myopathy Induced by the Combination Cisplatin plus Docetaxel in Mice. *Microbiol Spectr.* 2023 Jun 15;11(3):e0313022.

[3182] Hassan HM, Al-Wahaibi LH, Elmorsy MA, et al. Suppression of Cisplatin-Induced Hepatic Injury in Rats Through Alarmin High-Mobility Group Box-1 Pathway by Ganoderma lucidum: Theoretical and Experimental Study. *Drug Des Devel Ther.* 2020 Jun 11;14:2335-2353.

[3183] Pillai TG, John M, Sara Thomas G. Prevention of cisplatin induced nephrotoxicity by terpenes isolated from Ganoderma lucidum occurring in Southern Parts of India. *Exp Toxicol Pathol.* 2011 Jan;63(1-2):157-60.

[3184] Mahran YF, Hassan HM. Ganoderma lucidum Prevents Cisplatin-Induced Nephrotoxicity through Inhibition of Epidermal Growth Factor Receptor Signaling and Autophagy-Mediated Apoptosis. *Oxid Med Cell Longev.* 2020 Jul 6;2020:4932587.

[3185] Kashimoto N, Ishii S, Myojin Y, et al. A water-soluble extract from cultured medium of Ganoderma lucidum (Reishi) mycelia attenuates the small intestinal injury induced by anti-cancer drugs. *Oncol Lett.* 2010 Jan;1(1):63-68.

[3186] Chen LH, Lin ZB, Li WD. Ganoderma lucidum polysaccharides reduce methotrexate-induced small intestinal damage in mice via induction of epithelial cell proliferation and migration. *Acta Pharmacol Sin.* 2011 Dec;32(12):1505-12.

[3187] Abulizi A, Ran J, Ye Y, et al. Ganoderic acid improves 5-fluorouracil-induced cognitive dysfunction in mice. *Food Funct.* 2021 Dec 13;12(24):12325-12337.

[3188] Li D, Gao L, Li M, et al. Polysaccharide from spore of Ganoderma lucidum ameliorates paclitaxel-induced intestinal barrier injury: Apoptosis inhibition by reversing microtubule polymerization. *Biomed Pharmacother.* 2020 Oct;130:110539.

[3189] Wang CZ, Basila D, Aung HH, et al. Effects of ganoderma lucidum extract on chemotherapy-induced nausea and vomiting in a rat model. *Am J Chin Med.* 2005;33(5):807-15.

[3190] Abulizi A, Hu L, Ma A, et al. Ganoderic acid alleviates chemotherapy-induced fatigue in mice bearing colon tumor. *Acta Pharmacol Sin.* 2021 Oct;42(10):1703-1713.

[3191] Song YS, Kim SH, Sa JH, et al. Anti-angiogenic and inhibitory activity on inducible nitric oxide production of the mushroom Ganoderma lucidum. *J Ethnopharmacol.* 2004 Jan;90(1):17-20.

[3192] Cao QZ, Lin ZB. Antitumor and anti-angiogenic activity of Ganoderma lucidum polysaccharides peptide. *Acta Pharmacol Sin.* 2004 Jun;25(6):833-8.

[3193] Sillapapongwarakorn S, Yanarojana S, Pinthong D, et al. Molecular docking based screening of triterpenoids as potential G-quadruplex stabilizing ligands with anti-cancer activity. *Bioinformation.* 2017 Sep 30;13(9):284-292.

[3194] Wang J, Pu J, Zhang Z, et al. Triterpenoids of Ganoderma lucidum inhibited S180 sarcoma and H22 hepatoma in mice by regulating gut microbiota. *Heliyon.* 2023 Jun 7;9(6):e16682.

[3195] El-Khashab IH. Antiangiogenic and Proapoptotic Activities of Atorvastatin and Ganoderma lucidum in Tumor Mouse Model via VEGF and Caspase-3 Pathways. *Asian Pac J Cancer Prev.* 2021 Apr 1;22(4):1095-1104.

[3196] Fu Y, Shi L, Ding K. Structure elucidation and anti-tumor activity in vivo of a polysaccharide from spores of Ganoderma lucidum (Fr.) Karst. *Int J Biol Macromol.* 2019 Dec 1;141:693-699.

[3197] Jiang Y, Wang H, Lü L, et al. [Chemistry of polysaccharide Lzps-1 from Ganoderma lucidum spore and anti-tumor activity of its total polysaccharides]. *Yao Xue Xue Bao.* 2005 Apr;40(4):347-50.

[3198] Wang PY, Zhu XL, Lin ZB. Antitumor and Immunomodulatory Effects of Polysaccharides from Broken-Spore of Ganoderma lucidum. *Front Pharmacol.* 2012 Jul 13;3:135.

[3199] Liu X, Yuan JP, Chung CK, et al. Antitumor activity of the sporoderm-broken germinating spores of Ganoderma lucidum. *Cancer Lett.* 2002 Aug 28;182(2):155-61.

[3200] Zhang J, Tang Q, Zhou C, et al. GLIS, a bioactive proteoglycan fraction from Ganoderma lucidum, displays anti-tumour activity by increasing both humoral and cellular immune response. *Life Sci.* 2010 Nov 20;87(19-22):628-37.

[3201] Rubel R, Santa HSD, Dos Santos LF, et al. Immunomodulatory and Antitumoral Properties of Ganoderma lucidum and Agaricus brasiliensis (Agaricomycetes) Medicinal Mushrooms. *Int J Med Mushrooms.* 2018;20(4):393-403.

[3202] Joseph S, Sabulal B, George V, et al. Antitumor and anti-inflammatory activities of polysaccharides isolated from Ganoderma lucidum. *Acta Pharm.* 2011 Sep 1;61(3):335-42.

[3203] Gao JJ, Min BS, Ahn EM, et al. New triterpene aldehydes, lucialdehydes A-C, from Ganoderma lucidum and their cytotoxicity against murine and human tumor cells. *Chem Pharm Bull (Tokyo).* 2002 Jun;50(6):837-40.

[3204] Nonaka Y, Shibata H, Nakai M, et al. Anti-tumor activities of the antlered form of Ganoderma lucidum in allogeneic and syngeneic tumor-bearing mice. *Biosci Biotechnol Biochem.* 2006 Sep;70(9):2028-34.

[3205] Li JJ, Lei LS, Yu CL, et al. [Effect of Ganoderma lucidum polysaccharides on tumor cell nucleotide content and cell cycle in S180 ascitic tumor-bearing mice]. *Nan Fang Yi Ke Da Xue Xue Bao.* 2007 Jul;27(7):1003-5.

[3206] Wang J, Zhang L, Yu Y, et al. Enhancement of antitumor activities in sulfated and carboxymethylated polysaccharides of Ganoderma lucidum. *J Agric Food Chem.* 2009 Nov 25;57(22):10565-72.

[3207] Wang J, Pu J, Zhang Z, et al. Triterpenoids of Ganoderma lucidum inhibited S180 sarcoma and H22 hepatoma in mice by regulating gut microbiota. *Heliyon.* 2023 Jun 7;9(6):e16682.

[3208] Liu X, Yuan JP, Chung CK, et al. Antitumor activity of the sporoderm-broken germinating spores of Ganoderma lucidum. *Cancer Lett.* 2002 Aug 28;182(2):155-61.

[3209] Zhao RL, He YM. Network pharmacology analysis of the anti-cancer pharmacological mechanisms of Ganoderma lucidum extract with experimental support using Hepa1-6-bearing C57 BL/6 mice. *J Ethnopharmacol.* 2018 Jan 10;210:287-295.

[3210] Chen Y, Lu H, Song S, et al. [Preparation of Ganoderma lucidum polysaccharides and triterpenes microemulsion and its anticancer effect in mice with transplant Heps tumors]. *Zhongguo Zhong Yao Za Zhi.* 2010 Oct;35(20):2679-83.

[3211] Zhou GQ, Zhao HY, Lu C. [Effect of Ganoderma lucidum polysaccharides on intestinal mucosal immune system in H22 liver cancer bearing mice]. *Zhongguo Zhong Xi Yi Jie He Za Zhi.* 2009 Apr;29(4):335-9.

[3212] Su J, Li D, Chen Q, Li M, et al. Anti-breast Cancer Enhancement of a Polysaccharide From Spore of Ganoderma lucidum With Paclitaxel: Suppression on Tumor Metabolism With Gut Microbiota Reshaping. *Front Microbiol.* 2018 Dec 17;9:3099.

[3213] Su J, Su L, Li D, et al. Antitumor Activity of Extract From the Sporoderm-Breaking Spore of Ganoderma lucidum: Restoration on Exhausted Cytotoxic T Cell With Gut Microbiota Remodeling. *Front Immunol.* 2018 Jul 31;9:1765.

[3214] Roda E, Luca F, Iorio CD, et al. Novel Medicinal Mushroom Blend as a Promising Supplement in Integrative Oncology: A Multi-Tiered Study using 4T1 Triple-Negative Mouse Breast Cancer Model. *Int J Mol Sci.* 2020 May 14;21(10):3479.

[3215] Kong M, Yao Y, Zhang H. Antitumor activity of enzymatically hydrolyzed Ganoderma lucidum polysaccharide on U14 cervical carcinoma-bearing mice. *Int J Immunopathol Pharmacol.* 2019 Jan-Dec;33:2058738419869489.

[3216] Yuen JWM, Mak DSY, Chan ES, et al. Tumor inhibitory effects of intravesical Ganoderma lucidum instillation in the syngeneic orthotopic MB49/C57 bladder cancer mice model. *J Ethnopharmacol.* 2018 Sep 15;223:113-121.

[3217] Tomasi S, Lohézic-Le Dévéhat F, Sauleau P, et al. Cytotoxic activity of methanol extracts from Basidiomycete mushrooms on murine cancer cell lines. *Pharmazie.* 2004 Apr;59(4):290-3.

[3218] Liu X, Yuan JP, Chung CK, et al. Antitumor activity of the sporoderm-broken germinating spores of Ganoderma lucidum. *Cancer Lett.* 2002 Aug 28;182(2):155-61.

[3219] Yue GG, Fung KP, Leung PC, et al. Comparative studies on the immunomodulatory and antitumor activities of the different parts of fruiting body of Ganoderma lucidum and Ganoderma spores. *Phytother Res.* 2008 Oct;22(10):1282-91.

[3220] Krasnopolskaya LM, Yarina MS, Avtonomova AV, et al. [Antitumor Activity of Polysaccharides from Ganoderma lucidum Mycelium: in vivo Comparative Study]. *Antibiot Khimioter.* 2015;60(11-12):29-34.

[3221] Chen J, Yu YH. [Inhibitory effects of sporoderm-broken Ganoderma lucidum spores on growth of lymphoma implanted in nude mouse]. *Zhongguo Shi Yan Xue Ye Xue Za Zhi.* 2012 Apr;20(2):310-4.

[3222] Chang YH, Yang JS, Yang JL, et al. Ganoderma lucidum extracts inhibited leukemia WEHI-3 cells in BALB/c mice and promoted an immune response in vivo. *Biosci Biotechnol Biochem.* 2009 Dec;73(12):2589-94.

[3223] Tomasi S, Lohézic-Le Dévéhat F, Sauleau P, et al. Cytotoxic activity of methanol extracts from Basidiomycete mushrooms on murine cancer cell lines. *Pharmazie.* 2004 Apr;59(4):290-3.

[3224] Sun LX, Lin ZB, Duan XS, et al. Ganoderma lucidum polysaccharides counteract inhibition on CD71 and FasL expression by culture supernatant of B16F10 cells upon lymphocyte activation. *Exp Ther Med.* 2013 Apr;5(4):1117-1122.

[3225] Lu J, Sun LX, Lin ZB, et al. Antagonism by Ganoderma lucidum polysaccharides against the suppression by culture supernatants of B16F10 melanoma cells on macrophage. *Phytother Res.* 2014 Feb;28(2):200-6.

[3226] Xu XY, Luo X, Song Y, et al. [Ganoderma lucidum polysaccharides promote T lymphocyte infiltration into tumor by regulating expression of ICAM-1 in endothelial cells]. *Zhongguo Zhong Yao Za Zhi.* 2021 Oct;46(19):5072-5079.

[3227] Harhaji Trajković LM, Mijatović SA, Maksimović-Ivanić DD, et al. Anticancer properties of Ganoderma lucidum methanol extracts in vitro and in vivo. *Nutr Cancer.* 2009;61(5):696-707.

[3228] Sun LX, Li WD, Lin ZB, et al. Cytokine production suppression by culture supernatant of B16F10 cells and amelioration by Ganoderma lucidum polysaccharides in activated lymphocytes. *Cell Tissue Res.* 2015 May;360(2):379-89.

[3229] Sun LX, Lin ZB, Li XJ, et al. Promoting effects of Ganoderma lucidum polysaccharides on B16F10 cells to activate lymphocytes. *Basic Clin Pharmacol Toxicol.* 2011 Mar;108(3):149-54.

[3230] Sun LX, Lin ZB, Duan XS, et al. Enhanced MHC class I and costimulatory molecules on B16F10 cells by Ganoderma lucidum polysaccharides. *J Drug Target.* 2012 Aug;20(7):582-92.

[3231] Sun LX, Lin ZB, Duan XS, et al. Ganoderma lucidum polysaccharides antagonize the suppression on lymphocytes induced by culture supernatants of B16F10 melanoma cells. *J Pharm Pharmacol.* 2011 May;63(5):725-35.

[3232] Gu YH, Belury MA. Selective induction of apoptosis in murine skin carcinoma cells (CH72) by an ethanol extract of Lentinula edodes. *Cancer Lett.* 2005 Mar 18;220(1):21-8.

[3233] Lin CN, Tome WP, Won SJ. Novel cytotoxic principles of Formosan Ganoderma lucidum. *J Nat Prod.* 1991 Jul-Aug;54(4):998-1002.

[3234] Hernández-Márquez E, Lagunas-Martínez A, Bermudez-Morales VH, et al. Inhibitory activity of Lingzhi or Reishi medicinal mushroom, Ganoderma lucidum (higher Basidiomycetes) on transformed cells by human papillomavirus. *Int J Med Mushrooms.* 2014;16(2):179-87.

[3235] Sun XZ, Liao Y, Li W, et al. Neuroprotective effects of ganoderma lucidum polysaccharides against oxidative stress-induced neuronal apoptosis. *Neural Regen Res.* 2017 Jun;12(6):953-958.

[3236] Zhang W, Zhang Q, Deng W, et al. Neuroprotective effect of pretreatment with ganoderma lucidum in cerebral ischemia/reperfusion injury in rat hippocampus. *Neural Regen Res.* 2014 Aug 1;9(15):1446-52.

[3237] Ćilerdžić JL, Sofrenić IV, Tešević VV, et al. Neuroprotective Potential and Chemical Profile of Alternatively Cultivated Ganoderma lucidum Basidiocarps. *Chem Biodivers.* 2018 May;15(5):e1800036.

[3238] Ahmad F, Singh G, Soni H, et al. Identification of potential neuroprotective compound from Ganoderma lucidum extract targeting microtubule affinity regulation kinase 4 involved in Alzheimer's disease through molecular dynamics simulation and MMGBSA. *Aging Med (Milton).* 2022 Dec 12;6(2):144-154.

[3239] Lu SY, Peng XR, Dong JR, et al. Aromatic constituents from Ganoderma lucidum and their neuroprotective and anti-inflammatory activities. *Fitoterapia.* 2019 Apr;134:58-64.

[3240] Gokce EC, Kahveci R, Atanur OM, et al. Neuroprotective effects of Ganoderma lucidum polysaccharides against traumatic spinal cord injury in rats. *Injury.* 2015 Nov;46(11):2146-55.

[3241] Wang C, Liu X, Lian C, et al. Triterpenes and Aromatic Meroterpenoids with Antioxidant Activity and Neuroprotective Effects from Ganoderma lucidum. *Molecules.* 2019 Nov 28;24(23):4353.

[3242] Aguirre Moreno AC, Campos Peña V, et al. Ganoderma lucidum reduces kainic acid-induced hippocampal neuronal damage via inflammatory cytokines and glial fibrillary acid protein expression. *Proc West Pharmacol Soc.* 2011;54:78-9.

[3243] Kahveci R, Kahveci FO, Gokce EC, et al. Effects of Ganoderma lucidum Polysaccharides on Different Pathways Involved in the Development of Spinal Cord Ischemia Reperfusion Injury: Biochemical, Histopathologic, and Ultrastructural Analysis in a Rat Model. *World Neurosurg.* 2021 Jun;150:e287-e297.

[3244] Zhao HB, Lin SQ, Liu JH, et al. Polysaccharide extract isolated from ganoderma lucidum protects rat cerebral cortical neurons from hypoxia/reoxygenation injury. *J Pharmacol Sci.* 2004 Jun;95(2):294-8.

[3245] Zhou Y, Qu ZQ, Zeng YS, et al. Neuroprotective effect of preadministration with Ganoderma lucidum spore on rat hippocampus. *Exp Toxicol Pathol.* 2012 Nov;64(7-8):673-80.

[3246] Wang SQ, Li XJ, Zhou S, et al. Intervention effects of ganoderma lucidum spores on epileptiform discharge hippocampal neurons and expression of neurotrophin-4 and N-cadherin. *PLoS One.* 2013 Apr 24;8(4):e61687.

[3247] Zhou ZY, Tang YP, Xiang J, et al. Neuroprotective effects of water-soluble Ganoderma lucidum polysaccharides on cerebral ischemic injury in rats. *J Ethnopharmacol.* 2010 Aug 19;131(1):154-64.

[3248] Cheung WM, Hui WS, Chu PW, et al. Ganoderma extract activates MAP kinases and induces the neuronal differentiation of rat pheochromocytoma PC12 cells. *FEBS Lett.* 2000 Dec 15;486(3):291-6.

[3249] Jiang ZM, Qiu HB, Wang SQ, et al. Ganoderic acid A potentiates the antioxidant effect and protection of mitochondrial membranes and reduces the apoptosis rate in primary hippocampal neurons in magnesium free medium. *Pharmazie.* 2018 Feb 1;73(2):87-91.

[3250] Shen B, Truong J, Helliwell R, et al. An in vitro study of neuroprotective properties of traditional Chinese herbal medicines thought to promote healthy ageing and longevity. *BMC Complement Altern Med.* 2013 Dec 27;13:373.

[3251] Cai Q, Li Y, Pei G. Polysaccharides from Ganoderma lucidum attenuate microglia-mediated neuroinflammation and modulate microglial phagocytosis and behavioural response. *J Neuroinflammation.* 2017 Mar 24;14(1):63.

[3252] Li DW, Liu M, Leng YQ, et al. Lanostane triterpenoids from Ganoderma lucidum and their inhibitory effects against FAAH. *Phytochemistry.* 2022 Nov;203:113339.

[3253] Lin YX, Sun JT, Liao ZZ, et al. Triterpenoids from the fruiting bodies of Ganoderma lucidum and their inhibitory activity against FAAH. *Fitoterapia.* 2022 Apr;158:105161.

[3254] Li D, Leng Y, Liao Z, et al. Nor-triterpenoids from the fruiting bodies of Ganoderma lucidum and their inhibitory activity against FAAH. *Nat Prod Res.* 2023 Feb;37(4):579-585.

[3255] Sadiq NB, Ryu DH, Cho JY, et al. Postharvest Drying Techniques Regulate Secondary Metabolites and Anti-Neuroinflammatory Activities of Ganoderma lucidum. *Molecules.* 2021 Jul 25;26(15):4484.

[3256] Yoon HM, Jang KJ, Han MS, et al. Ganoderma lucidum ethanol extract inhibits the inflammatory response by suppressing the NF-κB and toll-like receptor pathways in lipopolysaccharide-stimulated BV2 microglial cells. *Exp Ther Med.* 2013 Mar;5(3):957-963.

[3257] Kou RW, Gao YQ, Xia B, et al. Ganoderterpene A, a New Triterpenoid from Ganoderma lucidum, Attenuates LPS-Induced Inflammation and Apoptosis via Suppressing MAPK and TLR-4/NF-κB Pathways in BV-2 Cells. *J Agric Food Chem.* 2021 Nov 3;69(43):12730-12740.

[3258] Hilliard A, Mendonca P, Soliman KFA. Involvement of NFκB and MAPK signaling pathways in the preventive effects of Ganoderma lucidum on the inflammation of BV-2 microglial cells induced by LPS. *J Neuroimmunol.* 2020 Aug 15;345:577269.

3259 Chi B, Wang S, Bi S, et al. Effects of ganoderic acid A on lipopolysaccharide-induced proinflammatory cytokine release from primary mouse microglia cultures. *Exp Ther Med*. 2018 Jan;15(1):847-853.

3260 Sheng F, Zhang L, Wang S, et al. Deacetyl Ganoderic Acid F Inhibits LPS-Induced Neural Inflammation via NF-κB Pathway Both In Vitro and In Vivo. *Nutrients*. 2019 Dec 27;12(1):85.

3261 Jia Y, Zhang D, Yin H, et al. Ganoderic Acid A Attenuates LPS-Induced Neuroinflammation in BV2 Microglia by Activating Farnesoid X Receptor. *Neurochem Res*. 2021 Jul;46(7):1725-1736.

3262 Zeng M, Qi L, Guo Y, et al. Long-Term Administration of Triterpenoids From Ganoderma lucidum Mitigates Age-Associated Brain Physiological Decline via Regulating Sphingolipid Metabolism and Enhancing Autophagy in Mice. *Front Aging Neurosci*. 2021 May 6;13:628860.

3263 Zhang XQ, Ip FC, Zhang DM, et al. Triterpenoids with neurotrophic activity from Ganoderma lucidum. *Nat Prod Res*. 2011 Oct;25(17):1607-13.

3264 Ling-Sing Seow S, Naidu M, et al. Potentiation of neuritogenic activity of medicinal mushrooms in rat pheochromocytoma cells. *BMC Complement Altern Med*. 2013 Jul 4;13:157.

3265 Phan CW, David P, Naidu M, et al. Neurite outgrowth stimulatory effects of culinary-medicinal mushrooms and their toxicity assessment using differentiating Neuro-2a and embryonic fibroblast BALB/3T3. *BMC Complement Altern Med*. 2013 Oct 11;13:261.

3266 Chen LW, Horng LY, Wu CL, et al. Activating mitochondrial regulator PGC-1α expression by astrocytic NGF is a therapeutic strategy for Huntington's disease. *Neuropharmacology*. 2012 Sep;63(4):719-32.

3267 Yamashina K, Yamamoto S, Matsumoto M, et al. Suppressive Effect of Fruiting Bodies of Medicinal Mushrooms on Demyelination and Motor Dysfunction in a Cuprizone-Induced Multiple Sclerosis Mouse Model. *Int J Med Mushrooms*. 2022;24(9):15-24.

3268 Tel G, Ozturk M, Duru ME, et al. Antioxidant and anticholinesterase activities of five wild mushroom species with total bioactive contents. *Pharm Biol*. 2015 Jun;53(6):824-30.

3269 Wei JC, Wang AH, Wei YL, et al. Chemical characteristics of the fungus Ganoderma lucidum and their inhibitory effects on acetylcholinesterase. *J Asian Nat Prod Res*. 2018 Oct;20(10):992-1001.

3270 Lee I, Ahn B, Choi J, et al. Selective cholinesterase inhibition by lanostane triterpenes from fruiting bodies of Ganoderma lucidum. *Bioorg Med Chem Lett*. 2011 Nov 1;21(21):6603-7.

3271 Hasnat A, Pervin M, Lim BO. Acetylcholinesterase inhibition and in vitro and in vivo antioxidant activities of Ganoderma lucidum grown on germinated brown rice. *Molecules*. 2013 Jun 7;18(6):6663-78.

3272 Lai G, Guo Y, Chen D, et al. Alcohol Extracts From Ganoderma lucidum Delay the Progress of Alzheimer's Disease by Regulating DNA Methylation in Rodents. *Front Pharmacol*. 2019 Mar 26;10:272.

3273 Zhang Y, Li H, Song L, et al. Polysaccharide from Ganoderma lucidum ameliorates cognitive impairment by regulating the inflammation of the brain-liver axis in rats. *Food Funct*. 2021 Aug 2;12(15):6900-6914.

3274 Pinweha S, Wanikiat P, Sanvarinda Y, et al. The signaling cascades of Ganoderma lucidum extracts in stimulating non-amyloidogenic protein secretion in human neuroblastoma SH-SY5Y cell lines. *Neurosci Lett*. 2008 Dec 19;448(1):62-6.

3275 Zhang Y, Song S, Li H, et al. Polysaccharide from Ganoderma lucidum alleviates cognitive impairment in a mouse model of chronic cerebral hypoperfusion by regulating CD4+CD25+Foxp3+ regulatory T cells. *Food Funct*. 2022 Feb 21;13(4):1941-1952.

3276 Ajith TA, Sudheesh NP, Roshny D, et al. Effect of Ganoderma lucidum on the activities of mitochondrial dehydrogenases and complex I and II of electron transport chain in the brain of aged rats. *Exp Gerontol*. 2009 Mar;44(3):219-23.

3277 Qin C, Wu SQ, Chen BS, et al. Pathological Changes in APP/PS-1 Transgenic Mouse Models of Alzheimer's Disease Treated with Ganoderma Lucidum Preparation. *Zhongguo Yi Xue Ke Xue Yuan Xue Bao*. 2017 Aug 20;39(4):552-561.

3278 Qin C, Wu S, Chen B, et al. Effect of Ganoderma Lucidum Preparation on the Behavior, Biochemistry, and Autoimmune Parameters of Mouse Models of APP/PS1 Double Transgenic Alzheimer's Disease. *Zhongguo Yi Xue Ke Xue Yuan Xue Bao*. 2017 Jun 20;39(3):330-335.

3279 Lai CS, Yu MS, Yuen WH, et al. Antagonizing beta-amyloid peptide neurotoxicity of the anti-aging fungus Ganoderma lucidum. *Brain Res*. 2008 Jan 23;1190:215-24.

3280 Huang S, Mao J, Ding K, et al. Polysaccharides from Ganoderma lucidum Promote Cognitive Function and Neural Progenitor Proliferation in Mouse Model of Alzheimer's Disease. *Stem Cell Reports*. 2017 Jan 10;8(1):84-94.

3281 Rahman MA, Hossain S, Abdullah N, et al. Lingzhi or Reishi Medicinal Mushroom, Ganoderma lucidum (Agaricomycetes), Ameliorates Nonspatial Learning and Memory Deficits in Rats with Hypercholesterolemia and Alzheimer's Disease. *Int J Med Mushrooms*. 2020;22(11):1067-1078.

3282 Zhao HL, Cui SY, Qin Y, et al. Prophylactic effects of sporoderm-removed Ganoderma lucidum spores in a rat model of streptozotocin-induced sporadic Alzheimer's disease. *J Ethnopharmacol*. 2021 Apr 6;269:113725.

3283 Yu N, Huang Y, Jiang Y, et al. Ganoderma lucidum Triterpenoids (GLTs) Reduce Neuronal Apoptosis via Inhibition of ROCK Signal Pathway in APP/PS1 Transgenic Alzheimer's Disease Mice. *Oxid Med Cell Longev*. 2020 Jan 28;2020:9894037.

3284 Zhang Y, Wang X, Yang X, et al. Ganoderic Acid A To Alleviate Neuroinflammation of Alzheimer's Disease in Mice by Regulating the Imbalance of the Th17/Tregs Axis. *J Agric Food Chem*. 2021 Dec 1;69(47):14204-14214.

3285 Ahmad F. Ganoderic Acid A targeting leucine-rich repeat kinase 2 involved in Parkinson's disease-A computational study. *Aging Med (Milton)*. 2022 Dec 20;6(3):272-280.

3286 Cheng H, Wang J, Zhang Y, et al. The mechanism of LZ-8-mediated immune response in the mouse model of Parkinson's disease. *J Neuroimmunol*. 2023 Oct 15;383:578144.

3287 Zhang R, Xu S, Cai Y, et al. Ganoderma lucidum Protects Dopaminergic Neuron Degeneration through Inhibition of Microglial Activation. *Evid Based Complement Alternat Med*. 2011;2011:156810.

3288 Rahman MA, Hossain S, Abdullah N, et al. Lingzhi or Reishi Medicinal Mushroom, Ganoderma lucidum (Agaricomycetes) Ameliorates Spatial Learning and Memory Deficits in Rats with Hypercholesterolemia and Alzheimer's Disease. *Int J Med Mushrooms*. 2020;22(1):93-103.

3289 Ren ZL, Wang CD, Wang T, et al. Ganoderma lucidum extract ameliorates MPTP-induced parkinsonism and protects dopaminergic neurons from oxidative stress via regulating mitochondrial function, autophagy, and apoptosis. *Acta Pharmacol Sin*. 2019 Apr;40(4):441-450.

3290 Ding H, Zhou M, Zhang RP, et al. [Ganoderma lucidum extract protects dopaminergic neurons through inhibiting the production of inflammatory mediators by activated microglia]. *Sheng Li Xue Bao*. 2010 Dec 25;62(6):547-54.

3291 Özevren H, İrtegün S, Deveci E, et al. Ganoderma Lucidum Protects Rat Brain Tissue Against Trauma-Induced Oxidative Stress. *Korean J Neurotrauma*. 2017 Oct;13(2):76-84.

3292 Nascimento CP, Luz DA, da Silva CCS, et al. Ganoderma lucidum Ameliorates Neurobehavioral Changes and Oxidative Stress Induced by Ethanol Binge Drinking. *Oxid Med Cell Longev*. 2020 Jul 30;2020:2497845.

3293 Shevelev OB, Akulov AE, Dotsenko AS, et al. Neurometabolic Effect of Altaian Fungus Ganoderma lucidum (Reishi Mushroom) in Rats Under Moderate Alcohol Consumption. *Alcohol Clin Exp Res*. 2015 Jul;39(7):1128-36.

3294 Sharma P, Tulsawani R. Ganoderma lucidum aqueous extract prevents hypobaric hypoxia induced memory deficit by modulating neurotransmission, neuroplasticity and maintaining redox homeostasis. *Sci Rep*. 2020 Jun 2;10(1):8944.

3295 Tello I, Campos-Pena V, Montiel E, et al. Anticonvulsant and neuroprotective effects of oligosaccharides from Lingzhi or Reishi medicinal mushroom, Ganoderma lucidum (Higher Basidiomycetes). *Int J Med Mushrooms*. 2013;15(6):555-68.

3296 Socala K, Nieoczym D, Grzywnowicz K, et al. Evaluation of Anticonvulsant, Antidepressant-, and Anxiolytic-like Effects of an Aqueous Extract from Cultured Mycelia of the Lingzhi or Reishi Medicinal Mushroom Ganoderma lucidum (Higher Basidiomycetes) in Mice. *Int J Med Mushrooms*. 2015;17(3):209-18.

3297 Wang SQ, Li XJ, Qiu HB, et al. Anti-epileptic effect of Ganoderma lucidum polysaccharides by inhibition of intracellular calcium accumulation and stimulation of expression of CaMKII α in epileptic hippocampal neurons. *PLoS One*. 2014 Jul 10;9(7):e102161.

3298 Yang ZW, Wu F, Zhang SL. Effects of ganoderic acids on epileptiform discharge hippocampal neurons: insights from alterations of BDNF,TRPC3 and apoptosis. *Pharmazie*. 2016 Jun;71(6):340-4.

3299 Choi YJ, Yang HS, Jo JH, et al. Anti-Amnesic Effect of Fermented Ganoderma lucidum Water Extracts by Lactic Acid Bacteria on Scopolamine-Induced Memory Impairment in Rats. *Prev Nutr Food Sci*. 2015 Jun;20(2):126-32.

3300 Ezurike PU, Odunola E, Oke TA, et al. Ganoderma lucidum ethanol extract promotes weight loss and improves depressive-like behaviors in male and female Swiss mice. *Physiol Behav*. 2023 Jun 1;265:114155.

3301 Matsuzaki H, Shimizu Y, Iwata N, et al. Antidepressant-like effects of a water-soluble extract from the culture medium of Ganoderma lucidum mycelia in rats. *BMC Complement Altern Med*. 2013 Dec 26;13:370.

3302 Zhao S, Rong C, Gao Y, et al. Antidepressant-like effect of Ganoderma lucidum spore polysaccharide-peptide mediated by upregulation of prefrontal cortex brain-derived neurotrophic factor. *Appl Microbiol Biotechnol*. 2021 Dec;105(23):8675-8688.

3303 Hossen SMM, Yusuf ATM, Emon NU, et al. Biochemical and Pharmacological aspects of Ganoderma lucidum: Exponent from the in vivo and computational investigations. *Biochem Biophys Rep*. 2022 Nov 7;32:101371.

3304 Li H, Xiao Y, Han L, et al. Ganoderma lucidum polysaccharides ameliorated depression-like behaviors in the chronic social defeat stress depression model via modulation of Dectin-1 and the innate immune system. *Brain Res Bull*. 2021 Jun;171:16-24.

3305 Socala K, Nieoczym D, Grzywnowicz K, et al. Evaluation of Anticonvulsant, Antidepressant-, and Anxiolytic-like Effects of an Aqueous Extract from Cultured Mycelia of the Lingzhi or Reishi Medicinal Mushroom Ganoderma lucidum (Higher Basidiomycetes) in Mice. *Int J Med Mushrooms*. 2015;17(3):209-18.

3306 Hossen SMM, Yusuf ATM, Emon NU, et al. Biochemical and Pharmacological aspects of Ganoderma lucidum: Exponent from the in vivo and computational investigations. *Biochem Biophys Rep*. 2022 Nov 7;32:101371.

3307 Socala K, Nieoczym D, Grzywnowicz K, et al. Evaluation of Anticonvulsant, Antidepressant-, and Anxiolytic-like Effects of an Aqueous Extract from Cultured Mycelia of the Lingzhi or Reishi Medicinal Mushroom Ganoderma lucidum (Higher Basidiomycetes) in Mice. *Int J Med Mushrooms*. 2015;17(3):209-18.

3308 Matsuzaki H, Shimizu Y, Iwata N, et al. Antidepressant-like effects of a water-soluble extract from the culture medium of Ganoderma lucidum mycelia in rats. *BMC Complement Altern Med*. 2013 Dec 26;13:370.

3309 Mi X, Zeng GR, Liu JQ, et al. Ganoderma Lucidum Triterpenoids Improve Maternal Separation-Induced Anxiety- and Depression-like Behaviors in Mice by Mitigating Inflammation in the Periphery and Brain. *Nutrients*. 2022 May 28;14(11):2268.

3310 Guo C, Guo D, Fang L, et al. Ganoderma lucidum polysaccharide modulates gut microbiota and immune cell function to inhibit inflammation and tumorigenesis in colon. *Carbohydr Polym*. 2021 Sep 1;267:118231.

3311 Sang T, Guo C, Guo D, et al. Suppression of obesity and inflammation by polysaccharide from sporoderm-broken spore of Ganoderma lucidum via gut microbiota regulation. *Carbohydr Polym*. 2021 Mar 15;256:117594.

3312 Xia Q, Zhao Q, Zhu H, et al. Physicochemical characteristics of Ganoderma lucidum oligosaccharide and its regulatory effect on intestinal flora in vitro fermentation. *Food Chem X*. 2022 Aug 9;15:100421.

3313 Li Y, Liu H, Qi H, et al. Probiotic fermentation of Ganoderma lucidum fruiting body extracts promoted its immunostimulatory activity in mice with dexamethasone-induced immunosuppression. *Biomed Pharmacother*. 2021 Sep;141:111909.

3314 Jin M, Zhang H, Wang J, et al. Response of intestinal metabolome to polysaccharides from mycelia of Ganoderma lucidum. *Int J Biol Macromol*. 2019 Feb 1;122:723-731.

3315 Tong A, Wu W, Chen Z, et al. Modulation of gut microbiota and lipid metabolism in rats fed high-fat diets by Ganoderma lucidum triterpenoids. *Curr Res Food Sci*. 2022 Dec 27;6:100427.

3316 Yang K, Zhang Y, Cai M, et al. In vitro prebiotic activities of oligosaccharides from the by-products in Ganoderma lucidum spore polysaccharide extraction. *RSC Adv*. 2020 Apr 14;10(25):14794-14802.

3317 Su J, Li D, Chen Q, Li M, et al. Anti-breast Cancer Enhancement of a Polysaccharide From Spore of Ganoderma lucidum With Paclitaxel: Suppression on Tumor Metabolism With Gut Microbiota Reshaping. *Front Microbiol*. 2018 Dec 17;9:3099.

3318 Meneses ME, Martínez-Carrera D, Torres N, et al. Hypocholesterolemic Properties and Prebiotic Effects of Mexican Ganoderma lucidum in C57BL/6 Mice. *PLoS One*. 2016 Jul 20;11(7):e0159631.

3319 Su L, Li D, Su J, et al. Polysaccharides of Sporoderm-Broken Spore of Ganoderma lucidum Modulate Adaptive Immune Function via Gut Microbiota Regulation. *Evid Based Complement Alternat Med*. 2021 Mar 23;2021:8842062.

3320 Xiong W, Yang C, Xia J, et al. G. lucidum triterpenes restores intestinal flora balance in non-hepatitis B virus-related hepatocellular carcinoma: evidence of 16S rRNA sequencing and network pharmacology analysis. *Front Pharmacol*. 2023 Sep 18;14:1197418.

[3321] Guo C, Guo D, Fang L, et al. Ganoderma lucidum polysaccharide modulates gut microbiota and immune cell function to inhibit inflammation and tumorigenesis in colon. *Carbohydr Polym*. 2021 Sep 1;267:118231.

[3322] Sang T, Guo C, Guo D, et al. Suppression of obesity and inflammation by polysaccharide from sporoderm-broken spore of Ganoderma lucidum via gut microbiota regulation. *Carbohydr Polym*. 2021 Mar 15;256:117594.

[3323] Li Y, Liu H, Qi H, et al. Probiotic fermentation of Ganoderma lucidum fruiting body extracts promoted its immunostimulatory activity in mice with dexamethasone-induced immunosuppression. *Biomed Pharmacother*. 2021 Sep;141:111909.

[3324] Jin M, Zhu Y, Shao D, et al. Effects of polysaccharide from mycelia of Ganoderma lucidum on intestinal barrier functions of rats. *Int J Biol Macromol*. 2017 Jan;94(Pt A):1-9.

[3325] Sun LX, Chen LH, Lin ZB, et al. Effects of Ganoderma lucidum polysaccharides on IEC-6 cell proliferation, migration and morphology of differentiation benefiting intestinal epithelium healing in vitro. *J Pharm Pharmacol*. 2011 Dec;63(12):1595-603.

[3326] Li K, Zhuo C, Teng C, et al. Effects of Ganoderma lucidum polysaccharides on chronic pancreatitis and intestinal microbiota in mice. *Int J Biol Macromol*. 2016 Dec;93(Pt A):904-912.

[3327] Li K, Yu M, Hu Y, et al. Three kinds of Ganoderma lucidum polysaccharides attenuate DDC-induced chronic pancreatitis in mice. *Chem Biol Interact*. 2016 Mar 5;247:30-8.

[3328] Guo C, Guo D, Fang L, et al. Ganoderma lucidum polysaccharide modulates gut microbiota and immune cell function to inhibit inflammation and tumorigenesis in colon. *Carbohydr Polym*. 2021 Sep 1;267:118231.

[3329] Liu Y, Tang Q, Feng J, et al. Effects of molecular weight on intestinal anti-inflammatory activities of β-D-glucan from Ganoderma lucidum. *Front Nutr*. 2022 Sep 29;9:1028727.

[3330] Hsu HY, Kuan YC, Lin TY, et al. Reishi Protein LZ-8 Induces FOXP3(+) Treg Expansion via a CD45-Dependent Signaling Pathway and Alleviates Acute Intestinal Inflammation in Mice. *Evid Based Complement Alternat Med*. 2013;2013:513542.

[3331] Kubota A, Kobayashi M, Sarashina S, et al. Reishi mushroom Ganoderma lucidum Modulates IgA production and alpha-defensin expression in the rat small intestine. *J Ethnopharmacol*. 2018 Mar 25;214:240-243.

[3332] Koo MH, Chae HJ, Lee JH, et al. Antiinflammatory lanostane triterpenoids from Ganoderma lucidum. *Nat Prod Res*. 2021 Nov;35(22):4295-4302.

[3333] Ren Z, Ding H, Zhou M, et al. Ganoderma lucidum Modulates Inflammatory Responses following 1-Methyl-4-Phenyl-1,2,3,6-Tetrahydropyridine (MPTP) Administration in Mice. *Nutrients*. 2022 Sep 19;14(18):3872.

[3334] Su HG, Peng XR, Shi QQ, et al. Lanostane triterpenoids with anti-inflammatory activities from Ganoderma lucidum. *Phytochemistry*. 2020 May;173:112256.

[3335] Wu YL, Han F, Luan SS, et al. Triterpenoids from Ganoderma lucidum and Their Potential Anti-inflammatory Effects. *J Agric Food Chem*. 2019 May 8;67(18):5147-5158.

[3336] Li S, Hou W, Li Y, et al. Modeling and optimization of the protocol of complex chromatography separation of cyclooxygenase-2 inhibitors from Ganoderma lucidum spore. *Phytochem Anal*. 2023 Jun;34(4):431-442.

[3337] Park M, Kim M. Analysis of Antioxidant and Anti-Inflammatory Activities of Solvent Fractions from Rhynchosia nulubilis Cultivated with Ganoderma lucidum Mycelium. *Prev Nutr Food Sci*. 2017 Dec;22(4):365-371.

[3338] Hasnat MA, Pervin M, Cha KM, et al. Anti-inflammatory activity on mice of extract of Ganoderma lucidum grown on rice via modulation of MAPK and NF-κB pathways. *Phytochemistry*. 2015 Jun;114:125-36.

[3339] Patocka J. Anti-inflammatory triterpenoids from mysterious mushroom Ganoderma lucidum and their potential possibility in modern medicine. *Acta Medica (Hradec Kralove)*. 1999;42(4):123-5.

[3340] Lu SY, Peng XR, Dong JR, et al. Aromatic constituents from Ganoderma lucidum and their neuroprotective and anti-inflammatory activities. *Fitoterapia*. 2019 Apr;134:58-64.

[3341] Feng X, Wang Y. Anti-inflammatory, anti-nociceptive and sedative-hypnotic activities of lucidone D extracted from Ganoderma lucidum. *Cell Mol Biol (Noisy-le-grand)*. 2019 Apr 30;65(4):37-42.

[3342] Liu YJ, Du JL, Cao LP, et al. Anti-inflammatory and hepatoprotective effects of Ganoderma lucidum polysaccharides on carbon tetrachloride-induced hepatocyte damage in common carp (Cyprinus carpio L.). *Int Immunopharmacol*. 2015 Mar;25(1):112-20.

[3343] Xu J, Xiao C, Xu H, et al. Anti-inflammatory effects of Ganoderma lucidum sterols via attenuation of the p38 MAPK and NF-κB pathways in LPS-induced RAW 264.7 macrophages. *Food Chem Toxicol*. 2021 Apr;150:112073.

[3344] Choi S, Nguyen VT, Tae N, et al. Anti-inflammatory and heme oxygenase-1 inducing activities of lanostane triterpenes isolated from mushroom Ganoderma lucidum in RAW264.7 cells. *Toxicol Appl Pharmacol*. 2014 Nov 1;280(3):434-42.

[3345] Wen L, Sheng Z, Wang J, et al. Structure of water-soluble polysaccharides in spore of Ganoderma lucidum and their anti-inflammatory activity. *Food Chem*. 2022 Mar 30;373(Pt A):131374.

[3346] Joseph S, Sabulal B, George V, et al. Antitumor and anti-inflammatory activities of polysaccharides isolated from Ganoderma lucidum. *Acta Pharm*. 2011 Sep 1;61(3):335-42.

[3347] Lin JM, Lin CC, Chiu HF, et al. Evaluation of the anti-inflammatory and liver-protective effects of anoectochilus formosanus, ganoderma lucidum and gynostemma pentaphyllum in rats. *Am J Chin Med*. 1993;21(1):59-69.

[3348] Ryu DH, Cho JY, Sadiq NB, et al. Optimization of antioxidant, anti-diabetic, and anti-inflammatory activities and ganoderic acid content of differentially dried Ganoderma lucidum using response surface methodology. *Food Chem*. 2021 Jan 15;335:127645.

[3349] Li QZ, Chen X, Mao PW, et al. N-Glycosylated Ganoderma lucidum immunomodulatory protein improved anti-inflammatory activity via inhibition of the p38 MAPK pathway. *Food Funct*. 2021 Apr 26;12(8):3393-3404.

[3350] Jia X, Ma B, Xue F, et al. Structure Characterization and Anti-Inflammatory Activity of Polysaccharides from Lingzhi or Reishi Medicinal Mushroom Ganoderma lucidum (Agaricomycetes) by Microwave-Assisted Freeze-Thaw Extraction. *Int J Med Mushrooms*. 2022;24(11):49-61.

[3351] Zhang J, Shi X, Cheng W, et al. Comparison of the Anti-Inflammatory and Antioxidant Activities of Mycelial Polysaccharides from Different Strains of Lingzhi or Reishi Medicinal Mushroom, Ganoderma lucidum (Agaricomycetes). *Int J Med Mushrooms*. 2022;24(7):77-90.

297

3352 Zhang K, Liu Y, Zhao X, et al. Anti-inflammatory properties of GLPss58, a sulfated polysaccharide from Ganoderma lucidum. *Int J Biol Macromol*. 2018 Feb;107(Pt A):486-493.

3353 Lakshmi B, Ajith TA, Sheena N, et al. Antiperoxidative, anti-inflammatory, and antimutagenic activities of ethanol extract of the mycelium of Ganoderma lucidum occurring in South India. *Teratog Carcinog Mutagen*. 2003;Suppl 1:85-97.

3354 Akihisa T, Nakamura Y, Tagata M, et al. Anti-inflammatory and anti-tumor-promoting effects of triterpene acids and sterols from the fungus Ganoderma lucidum. *Chem Biodivers*. 2007 Feb;4(2):224-31.

3355 Ko HH, Hung CF, Wang JP, et al. Antiinflammatory triterpenoids and steroids from Ganoderma lucidum and G. tsugae. *Phytochemistry*. 2008 Jan;69(1):234-9.

3356 Tung NT, Cuong TD, Hung TM, et al. Inhibitory effect on NO production of triterpenes from the fruiting bodies of Ganoderma lucidum. *Bioorg Med Chem Lett*. 2013 Mar 1;23(5):1428-32.

3357 Lin CY, Chen YH, Lin CY, et al. Ganoderma lucidum polysaccharides attenuate endotoxin-induced intercellular cell adhesion molecule-1 expression in cultured smooth muscle cells and in the neointima in mice. *J Agric Food Chem*. 2010 Sep 8;58(17):9563-71.

3358 Dudhgaonkar S, Thyagarajan A, Sliva D. Suppression of the inflammatory response by triterpenes isolated from the mushroom Ganoderma lucidum. *Int Immunopharmacol*. 2009 Oct;9(11):1272-80.

3359 Wu YS, Ho SY, Nan FH, et al. Ganoderma lucidum beta 1,3/1,6 glucan as an immunomodulator in inflammation induced by a high-cholesterol diet. *BMC Complement Altern Med*. 2016 Dec 3;16(1):500.

3360 Liu C, Dunkin D, Lai J, et al. Anti-inflammatory Effects of Ganoderma lucidum Triterpenoid in Human Crohn's Disease Associated with Downregulation of NF-κB Signaling. *Inflamm Bowel Dis*. 2015 Aug;21(8):1918-25.

3361 Cheng J, Zhang G, Liu L, et al. Anti-inflammatory activity of β-glucans from different sources before and after fermentation by fecal bacteria in vitro. *J Sci Food Agric*. 2023 Sep 23. Online ahead of print.

3362 Zheng S, Ma J, Zhao X, et al. Ganoderic Acid A Attenuates IL-1β-Induced Inflammation in Human Nucleus Pulposus Cells Through Inhibiting the NF-κB Pathway. *Inflammation*. 2022 Apr;45(2):851-862.

3363 Aursuwanna T, Noitang S, Sangtanoo P, et al. Investigating the cellular antioxidant and anti-inflammatory effects of the novel peptides in lingzhi mushrooms. *Heliyon*. 2022 Oct 13;8(10):e11067.

3364 Meng M, Yao J, Zhang Y, et al. Potential Anti-Rheumatoid Arthritis Activities and Mechanisms of Ganoderma lucidum Polysaccharides. *Molecules*. 2023 Mar 8;28(6):2483.

3365 Meng M, Wang L, Yao Y, et al. Ganoderma lucidum polysaccharide peptide (GLPP) attenuates rheumatic arthritis in rats through inactivating NF-κB and MAPK signaling pathways. *Phytomedicine*. 2023 Oct;119:155010.

3366 Heo Y, Kim M, Suminda GGD, et al. Inhibitory effects of Ganoderma lucidum spore oil on rheumatoid arthritis in a collagen-induced arthritis mouse model. *Biomed Pharmacother*. 2023 Jan;157:114067.

3367 Ho YW, Yeung JS, Chiu PK, et al. Ganoderma lucidum polysaccharide peptide reduced the production of proinflammatory cytokines in activated rheumatoid synovial fibroblast. *Mol Cell Biochem*. 2007 Jul;301(1-2):173-9.

3368 Chen Z, Qin W, Lin H, et al. Inhibitory effect of polysaccharides extracted from Changbai Mountain Ganoderma lucidum on periodontal inflammation. *Heliyon*. 2023 Jan 28;9(2):e13205.

3369 Lin S, Meng J, Li F, et al. Ganoderma lucidum polysaccharide peptide alleviates hyperuricemia by regulating adenosine deaminase and urate transporters. *Food Funct*. 2022 Dec 13;13(24):12619-12631.

3370 Huang CH, Chen TY, Tsai GJ. Hypouricemic Effect of Submerged Culture of Ganoderma lucidum in Potassium Oxonate-Induced Hyperuricemic Rats. *Metabolites*. 2022 Jun 16;12(6):553.

3371 Koyama K, Imaizumi T, Akiba M, et al. Antinociceptive components of Ganoderma lucidum. *Planta Med*. 1997 Jun;63(3):224-7.

3372 Feng X, Wang Y. Anti-inflammatory, anti-nociceptive and sedative-hypnotic activities of lucidone D extracted from Ganoderma lucidum. *Cell Mol Biol (Noisy-le-grand)*. 2019 Apr 30;65(4):37-42.

3373 Chen X, Veena RK, Ramya H, et al. Gano oil: A novel antinociceptive agent extracted from Ganoderma lucidum inhibits paw oedema and relieves pain by hypnotic and analgesic actions of fatty acid amides. *J Ethnopharmacol*. 2020 Dec 5;263:113144.

3374 Fujita R, Liu J, Shimizu K, et al. Anti-androgenic activities of Ganoderma lucidum. *J Ethnopharmacol*. 2005 Oct 31;102(1):107-12.

3375 Liu J, Kurashiki K, Shimizu K, et al. Structure-activity relationship for inhibition of 5alpha-reductase by triterpenoids isolated from Ganoderma lucidum. *Bioorg Med Chem*. 2006 Dec 15;14(24):8654-60.

3376 Liu J, Kurashiki K, Shimizu K, et al. 5alpha-reductase inhibitory effect of triterpenoids isolated from Ganoderma lucidum. *Biol Pharm Bull*. 2006 Feb;29(2):392-5.

3377 Liu J, Tamura S, Kurashiki K, et al. Anti-androgen effects of extracts and compounds from Ganoderma lucidum. *Chem Biodivers*. 2009 Feb;6(2):231-43.

3378 Liu J, Shimizu K, Konishi F, et al. The anti-androgen effect of ganoderol B isolated from the fruiting body of Ganoderma lucidum. *Bioorg Med Chem*. 2007 Jul 15;15(14):4966-72.

3379 Nahata A, Dixit VK. Ganoderma lucidum is an inhibitor of testosterone-induced prostatic hyperplasia in rats. *Andrologia*. 2012 May;44 Suppl 1:160-74.

3380 Nahata A, Dixit VK. Evaluation of 5α-reductase inhibitory activity of certain herbs useful as antiandrogens. *Andrologia*. 2014 Aug;46(6):592-601.

3381 Hu Y, Lin Z, Fu H, et al. Immunomodulatory effect of Ganoderma lucidum polysaccharide extract on peritoneal macrophage function of BALB/c mice. *Cell Mol Biol (Noisy-le-grand)*. 2022 Apr 30;68(4):31-34.

3382 Kuo MC, Weng CY, Ha CL, et al. Ganoderma lucidum mycelia enhance innate immunity by activating NF-kappaB. *J Ethnopharmacol*. 2006 Jan 16;103(2):217-22.

3383 Xie J, Lin D, Li J, et al. Effects of Ganoderma lucidum polysaccharide peptide ameliorating cyclophosphamide-induced immune dysfunctions based on metabolomics analysis. *Front Nutr*. 2023 May 25;10:1179749.

3384 Li Y, Liu H, Qi H, et al. Probiotic fermentation of Ganoderma lucidum fruiting body extracts promoted its immunostimulatory activity in mice with dexamethasone-induced immunosuppression. *Biomed Pharmacother*. 2021 Sep;141:111909.

3385 Liu Z, Xing J, Zheng S, et al. Ganoderma lucidum polysaccharides encapsulated in liposome as an adjuvant to promote Th1-bias immune response. *Carbohydr Polym*. 2016 May 20;142:141-8.

3386 Liu Z, Xing J, Huang Y, et al. Activation effect of Ganoderma lucidum polysaccharides liposomes on murine peritoneal macrophages. *Int J Biol Macromol*. 2016 Jan;82:973-8.

3387 Wang G, Wang L, Zhou J, et al. The Possible Role of PD-1 Protein in Ganoderma lucidum-Mediated Immunomodulation and Cancer Treatment. *Integr Cancer Ther*. 2019 Jan-Dec;18:1534735419880275.

3388 Liu G, Zhang J, Kan Q, et al. Extraction, Structural Characterization, and Immunomodulatory Activity of a High Molecular Weight Polysaccharide From Ganoderma lucidum. *Front Nutr*. 2022 Mar 25;9:846080.

3389 Wang J, Yuan Y, Yue T. Immunostimulatory activities of β-d-glucan from Ganoderma Lucidum. *Carbohydr Polym*. 2014 Feb 15;102:47-54.

3390 Liu Z, Ma X, Deng B, et al. Development of liposomal Ganoderma lucidum polysaccharide: formulation optimization and evaluation of its immunological activity. *Carbohydr Polym*. 2015 Mar 6;117:510-517.

3391 Pan K, Jiang Q, Liu G, et al. Optimization extraction of Ganoderma lucidum polysaccharides and its immunity and antioxidant activities. *Int J Biol Macromol*. 2013 Apr;55:301-6.

3392 Zhang J, Gao X, Pan Y, et al. Toxicology and immunology of Ganoderma lucidum polysaccharides in Kunming mice and Wistar rats. *Int J Biol Macromol*. 2016 Apr;85:302-10.

3393 Nizhenkovska IV, Pidchenko VT, Bychkova NG, et al. Influence of Ganoderma lucidum (Curt.: Fr.) P. Karst. on T-cell-mediated immunity in normal and immunosuppressed mice line CBA/Ca. *Ceska Slov Farm*. 2015 Sep;64(4):139-43.

3394 Liu J, Zhang J, Feng J, et al. Multiple Fingerprint-Activity Relationship Assessment of Immunomodulatory Polysaccharides from Ganoderma lucidum Based on Chemometric Methods. *Molecules*. 2023 Mar 24;28(7):2913.

3395 Liu T, Zhou J, Li W, et al. Effects of sporoderm-broken spores of Ganoderma lucidum on growth performance, antioxidant function and immune response of broilers. *Anim Nutr*. 2020 Mar;6(1):39-46.

3396 Liu G, Zhang J, Hou T, et al. Extraction kinetics, physicochemical properties and immunomodulatory activity of the novel continuous phase transition extraction of polysaccharides from Ganoderma lucidum. *Food Funct*. 2021 Oct 19;12(20):9708-9718.

3397 Mao PW, Li LD, Wang YL, et al. Optimization of the fermentation parameters for the production of Ganoderma lucidum immunomodulatory protein by Pichia pastoris. *Prep Biochem Biotechnol*. 2020;50(4):357-364.

3398 Ji Z, Tang Q, Zhang J, et al. Immunomodulation of RAW264.7 macrophages by GLIS, a proteopolysaccharide from Ganoderma lucidum. *J Ethnopharmacol*. 2007 Jul 25;112(3):445-50.

3399 Sun LX, Lin ZB, Lu J, et al. The improvement of M1 polarization in macrophages by glycopeptide derived from Ganoderma lucidum. *Immunol Res*. 2017 Jun;65(3):658-665.

3400 Chang CJ, Chen YY, Lu CC, et al. Ganoderma lucidum stimulates NK cell cytotoxicity by inducing NKG2D/NCR activation and secretion of perforin and granulysin. *Innate Immun*. 2014 Apr;20(3):301-11.

3401 Ma C, Guan SH, Yang M, et al. Differential protein expression in mouse splenic mononuclear cells treated with polysaccharides from spores of Ganoderma lucidum. *Phytomedicine*. 2008 Apr;15(4):268-76.

3402 Chen Z, Xiao G. One-Pot Assembly of the Highly Branched Tetradecasaccharide from Ganoderma lucidum Glycan GLSWA-1 with Immune-Enhancing Activities. *Org Lett*. 2023 Oct 13;25(40):7395-7399.

3403 Ahmadi K, Riazipour M. Effect of Ganoderma lucidum on cytokine release by peritoneal macrophages. *Iran J Immunol*. 2007 Dec;4(4):220-6.

3404 Liu YH, Lin YS, Lin KL, et al. Effects of hot-water extracts from Ganoderma lucidum residues and solid-state fermentation residues on prebiotic and immune-stimulatory activities in vitro and the powdered residues used as broiler feed additives in vivo. *Bot Stud*. 2015 Dec;56(1):17.

3405 Wang YY, Khoo KH, Chen ST, et al. Studies on the immuno-modulating and antitumor activities of Ganoderma lucidum (Reishi) polysaccharides: functional and proteomic analyses of a fucose-containing glycoprotein fraction responsible for the activities. *Bioorg Med Chem*. 2002 Apr;10(4):1057-62.

3406 Zhang LX, Mong H, Zhou XB. [Effect of Japanese Ganoderma Lucidum on production of interleukin-2 from murine splenocytes]. *Zhongguo Zhong Xi Yi Jie He Za Zhi*. 1993 Oct;13(10):613-5, 582.

3407 Wang J, Wang Y, Liu X, et al. Free radical scavenging and immunomodulatory activities of Ganoderma lucidum polysaccharides derivatives. *Carbohydr Polym*. 2013 Jan 2;91(1):33-8.

3408 Wang Y, Fan X, Wu X. Ganoderma lucidum polysaccharide (GLP) enhances antitumor immune response by regulating differentiation and inhibition of MDSCs via a CARD9-NF-κB-IDO pathway. *Biosci Rep*. 2020 Jun 26;40(6):BSR20201170.

3409 Tang QJ, Zhang JS, Pan YJ, et al. [Activation of mouse macrophages by the alkali-extracted polysaccharide from spore of Ganoderma lucidum]. *Xi Bao Yu Fen Zi Mian Yi Xue Za Zhi*. 2004 Mar;20(2):142-4.

3410 Yeh CH, Chen HC, Yang JJ, et al. Polysaccharides PS-G and protein LZ-8 from Reishi (Ganoderma lucidum) exhibit diverse functions in regulating murine macrophages and T lymphocytes. *J Agric Food Chem*. 2010 Aug 11;58(15):8535-44.

3411 Zhao H, Luo Y, Lu C, et al. Enteric mucosal immune response might trigger the immunomodulation activity of Ganoderma lucidum polysaccharide in mice. *Planta Med*. 2010 Feb;76(3):223-7.

3412 Cao LZ, Lin ZB. Comparison of the effects of polysaccharides from wood-cultured and bag-cultured Ganoderma lucidum on murine spleen lymphocyte proliferation in vitro. *Yao Xue Xue Bao*. 2003 Feb;38(2):92-7.

3413 Li J, Gu F, Cai C, et al. Purification, structural characterization, and immunomodulatory activity of the polysaccharides from Ganoderma lucidum. *Int J Biol Macromol*. 2020 Jan 15;143:806-813.

3414 Liu Y, Tang Q, Zhang J, et al. Triple helix conformation of β-d-glucan from Ganoderma lucidum and effect of molecular weight on its immunostimulatory activity. *Int J Biol Macromol*. 2018 Jul 15;114:1064-1070.

3415 Huang SQ, Ning ZX. Extraction of polysaccharide from Ganoderma lucidum and its immune enhancement activity. *Int J Biol Macromol*. 2010 Oct 1;47(3):336-41.

3416 Rubel R, Santa HSD, Dos Santos LF, et al. Immunomodulatory and Antitumoral Properties of Ganoderma lucidum and Agaricus brasiliensis (Agaricomycetes) Medicinal Mushrooms. *Int J Med Mushrooms*. 2018;20(4):393-403.

3417 Yi Y, Hu S, Xiong X, et al. [Study the rudimentary immunoregulatory mechanisms of Ganoderma Spore oil on immunocompromized mice]. *Wei Sheng Yan Jiu*. 2012 Sep;41(5):833-9.

3418 Wang Y, Liu Y, Yu H, et al. Structural characterization and immuno-enhancing activity of a highly branched water-soluble β-glucan from the spores of Ganoderma lucidum. *Carbohydr Polym*. 2017 Jul 1;167:337-344.

3419 Sheng Z, Wen L, Yang B. Structure identification of a polysaccharide in mushroom Lingzhi spore and its immunomodulatory activity. *Carbohydr Polym*. 2022 Feb 15;278:118939.

3420 Yoshida H, Suzuki M, Sakaguchi R, et al. Preferential induction of Th17 cells in vitro and in vivo by Fucogalactan from Ganoderma lucidum (Reishi). *Biochem Biophys Res Commun*. 2012 May 25;422(1):174-80.

3421 Bao XF, Zhen Y, Ruan L, et al. Purification, characterization, and modification of T lymphocyte-stimulating polysaccharide from spores of Ganoderma lucidum. *Chem Pharm Bull (Tokyo)*. 2002 May;50(5):623-9.

3422 Liu Y, Tan D, Cui H, et al. Ganoderic acid C2 exerts the pharmacological effects against cyclophosphamide-induced immunosuppression: a study involving molecular docking and experimental validation. *Sci Rep*. 2023 Oct 18;13(1):17745.

3423 Lai CY, Hung JT, Lin HH, et al. Immunomodulatory and adjuvant activities of a polysaccharide extract of Ganoderma lucidum in vivo and in vitro. *Vaccine*. 2010 Jul 12;28(31):4945-54.

3424 Cao LZ, Lin ZB. Regulation on maturation and function of dendritic cells by Ganoderma lucidum polysaccharides. *Immunol Lett*. 2002 Oct 1;83(3):163-9.

3425 Berovic M, Habijanic J, Zore I, et al. Submerged cultivation of Ganoderma lucidum biomass and immunostimulatory effects of fungal polysaccharides. *J Biotechnol*. 2003 Jun 12;103(1):77-86.

3426 Hsu MJ, Lee SS, Lin WW. Polysaccharide purified from Ganoderma lucidum inhibits spontaneous and Fas-mediated apoptosis in human neutrophils through activation of the phosphatidylinositol 3 kinase/Akt signaling pathway. *J Leukoc Biol*. 2002 Jul;72(1):207-16.

3427 Hsu JW, Huang HC, Chen ST, et al. Ganoderma lucidum Polysaccharides Induce Macrophage-Like Differentiation in Human Leukemia THP-1 Cells via Caspase and p53 Activation. *Evid Based Complement Alternat Med*. 2011;2011:358717.

3428 Yuan S, Yang Y, Li J, et al. Ganoderma lucidum Rhodiola compound preparation prevent D-galactose-induced immune impairment and oxidative stress in aging rat model. *Sci Rep*. 2020 Nov 6;10(1):19244.

3429 Tsai CC, Yang FL, Huang ZY, et al. Oligosaccharide and peptidoglycan of Ganoderma lucidum activate the immune response in human mononuclear cells. *J Agric Food Chem*. 2012 Mar 21;60(11):2830-7.

3430 Rubel R, Dalla Santa HS, Bonatto SJ, et al. Medicinal mushroom Ganoderma lucidum (Leyss: Fr) Karst. triggers immunomodulatory effects and reduces nitric oxide synthesis in mice. *J Med Food*. 2010 Feb;13(1):142-8.

3431 Nedeljkovic BB, Ćilerdžić J, Zmijanjac D, et al. Immunomodulatory Effects of Extract of Lingzhi or Reishi Medicinal Mushroom Ganoderma lucidum (Agaricomycetes) Basidiocarps Cultivated on Alternative Substrate. *Int J Med Mushrooms*. 2022;24(8):45-59.

3432 Ahmadi K, Riazipour M. Ganoderma lucidum induces the expression of CD40/CD86 on peripheral blood monocytes. *Iran J Immunol*. 2009 Jun;6(2):87-91.

3433 Chan WK, Cheung CC, Law HK, et al. Ganoderma lucidum polysaccharides can induce human monocytic leukemia cells into dendritic cells with immuno-stimulatory function. *J Hematol Oncol*. 2008 Jul 21;1:9.

3434 Chien CM, Cheng JL, Chang WT, et al. Polysaccharides of Ganoderma lucidum alter cell immunophenotypic expression and enhance CD56+ NK-cell cytotoxicity in cord blood. *Bioorg Med Chem*. 2004 Nov 1;12(21):5603-9.

3435 Bao XF, Wang XS, Dong Q, et al. Structural features of immunologically active polysaccharides from Ganoderma lucidum. *Phytochemistry*. 2002 Jan;59(2):175-81.

3436 Lin YL, Lee SS, Hou SM, et al. Polysaccharide purified from Ganoderma lucidum induces gene expression changes in human dendritic cells and promotes T helper 1 immune response in BALB/c mice. *Mol Pharmacol*. 2006 Aug;70(2):637-44.

3437 Kohguchi M, Kunikata T, Watanabe H, et al. Immuno-potentiating effects of the antler-shaped fruiting body of Ganoderma lucidum (Rokkaku-Reishi). *Biosci Biotechnol Biochem*. 2004 Apr;68(4):881-7.

3438 Hsu PY, Chern JL, Chen HY, et al. Extract of sporoderm-broken germinating spores of ganoderma lucidum activates human polymorphonuclear neutrophils via the P38 mitogen-activated protein kinase pathway. *Chang Gung Med J*. 2012 Mar-Apr;35(2):140-7.

3439 Guo L, Xie J, Ruan Y, et al. Characterization and immunostimulatory activity of a polysaccharide from the spores of Ganoderma lucidum. *Int Immunopharmacol*. 2009 Sep;9(10):1175-82.

3440 Zhao R, Chen Q, He YM. The effect of Ganoderma lucidum extract on immunological function and identify its anti-tumor immunostimulatory activity based on the biological network. *Sci Rep*. 2018 Aug 23;8(1):12680.

3441 Hsu MJ, Lee SS, Lee ST, et al. Signaling mechanisms of enhanced neutrophil phagocytosis and chemotaxis by the polysaccharide purified from Ganoderma lucidum. *Br J Pharmacol*. 2003 May;139(2):289-98.

3442 Cao LZ, Lin ZB. Regulatory effect of Ganoderma lucidum polysaccharides on cytotoxic T-lymphocytes induced by dendritic cells in vitro. *Acta Pharmacol Sin*. 2003 Apr;24(4):321-6.

3443 Hua KF, Hsu HY, Chao LK, et al. Ganoderma lucidum polysaccharides enhance CD14 endocytosis of LPS and promote TLR4 signal transduction of cytokine expression. *J Cell Physiol*. 2007 Aug;212(2):537-50.

3444 Watanabe K, Shuto T, Sato M, et al. Lucidenic acids-rich extract from antlered form of Ganoderma lucidum enhances TNFα induction in THP-1 monocytic cells possibly via its modulation of MAP kinases p38 and JNK. *Biochem Biophys Res Commun*. 2011 Apr 29;408(1):18-24.

3445 Pang X, Chen Z, Gao X, et al. Potential of a novel polysaccharide preparation (GLPP) from Anhui-grown Ganoderma lucidum in tumor treatment and immunostimulation. *J Food Sci*. 2007 Aug;72(6):S435-42.

3446 Li QZ, Chang YZ, He ZM, et al. Immunomodulatory activity of Ganoderma lucidum immunomodulatory protein via PI3K/Akt and MAPK signaling pathways in RAW264.7 cells. *J Cell Physiol*. 2019 Dec;234(12):23337-23348.

3447 Habijanic J, Berovic M, Boh B, et al. Submerged cultivation of Ganoderma lucidum and the effects of its polysaccharides on the production of human cytokines TNF-α, IL-12, IFN-γ, IL-2, IL-4, IL-10 and IL-17. *N Biotechnol*. 2015 Jan 25;32(1):85-95.

3448 Zhu XL, Lin ZB. Effects of Ganoderma lucidum polysaccharides on proliferation and cytotoxicity of cytokine-induced killer cells. *Acta Pharmacol Sin*. 2005 Sep;26(9):1130-7.

3449 Zhu XL, Chen AF, Lin ZB. Ganoderma lucidum polysaccharides enhance the function of immunological effector cells in immunosuppressed mice. *J Ethnopharmacol*. 2007 May 4;111(2):219-26.

3450 Chan WK, Lam DT, Law HK, et al. Ganoderma lucidum mycelium and spore extracts as natural adjuvants for immunotherapy. *J Altern Complement Med*. 2005 Dec;11(6):1047-57.

3451 Zhang S, Pang G, Chen C, et al. Effective cancer immunotherapy by Ganoderma lucidum polysaccharide-gold nanocomposites through dendritic cell activation and memory T cell response. *Carbohydr Polym*. 2019 Feb 1;205:192-202.

3452 Batbayar S, Kim MJ, Kim HW. Medicinal mushroom Lingzhi or Reishi, Ganoderma lucidum (W.Curt.:Fr.) P. Karst., beta-glucan induces Toll-like receptors and fails to induce inflammatory cytokines in NF-kappaB inhibitor-treated macrophages. *Int J Med Mushrooms*. 2011;13(3):213-25.

3453 Lin YL, Liang YC, Tseng YS, et al. An immunomodulatory protein, Ling Zhi-8, induced activation and maturation of human monocyte-derived dendritic cells by the NF-kappaB and MAPK pathways. *J Leukoc Biol*. 2009 Oct;86(4):877-89.

3454 Su L, Li D, Su J, et al. Polysaccharides of Sporoderm-Broken Spore of Ganoderma lucidum Modulate Adaptive Immune Function via Gut Microbiota Regulation. *Evid Based Complement Alternat Med*. 2021 Mar 23;2021:8842062.

3455 Xu J, Xu D, Hu Q, et al. Immune regulatory functions of biologically active proteins from edible fungi. *Front Immunol*. 2023 Jan 12;13:1034545.

3456 Yue GG, Fung KP, Tse GM, et al. Comparative studies of various ganoderma species and their different parts with regard to their antitumor and immunomodulating activities in vitro. *J Altern Complement Med*. 2006 Oct;12(8):777-89.

3457 Ji Z, Tang Q, Zhang J, et al. Immunomodulation of bone marrow macrophages by GLIS, a proteoglycan fraction from Lingzhi or Reishi medicinal mushroom Ganoderma lucidium (W.Curt.:Fr.) P. Karst. *Int J Med Mushrooms*. 2011;13(5):441-8.

3458 Lin YL, Liang YC, Lee SS, et al. Polysaccharide purified from Ganoderma lucidum induced activation and maturation of human monocyte-derived dendritic cells by the NF-kappaB and p38 mitogen-activated protein kinase pathways. *J Leukoc Biol*. 2005 Aug;78(2):533-43.

3459 Wang PY, Wang SZ, Lin SQ, et al. [Comparison of the immunomodulatory effects of spore polysaccharides and broken spore polysaccharides isolated from Ganoderma lucidum on murine splenic lymphocytes and peritoneal macrophages in vitro]. *Beijing Da Xue Xue Bao Yi Xue Ban*. 2005 Dec 18;37(6):569-74.

3460 Hattori K, Takagi H, Ogata Y, et al. Immunostimulatory effects of a subcritical water extract of Ganoderma. *Biomed Rep*. 2022 Nov 9;18(1):1.

3461 Chen HS, Tsai YF, Lin S, et al. Studies on the immuno-modulating and anti-tumor activities of Ganoderma lucidum (Reishi) polysaccharides. *Bioorg Med Chem*. 2004 Nov 1;12(21):5595-601.

3462 Jeurink PV, Noguera CL, Savelkoul HF, et al. Immunomodulatory capacity of fungal proteins on the cytokine production of human peripheral blood mononuclear cells. *Int Immunopharmacol*. 2008 Aug;8(8):1124-33.

3463 Kino K, Yamashita A, Yamaoka K, et al. Isolation and characterization of a new immunomodulatory protein, ling zhi-8 (LZ-8), from Ganoderma lucidium. *J Biol Chem*. 1989 Jan 5;264(1):472-8.

3464 Chang YH, Yang JS, Yang JL, et al. Ganoderma lucidum extract promotes immune responses in normal BALB/c mice In vivo. *In Vivo*. 2009 Sep-Oct;23(5):755-9.

3465 Wang G, Zhao J, Liu J, et al. Enhancement of IL-2 and IFN-gamma expression and NK cells activity involved in the anti-tumor effect of ganoderic acid Me in vivo. *Int Immunopharmacol*. 2007 Jun;7(6):864-70.

3466 Lin KI, Kao YY, Kuo HK, et al. Reishi polysaccharides induce immunoglobulin production through the TLR4/TLR2-mediated induction of transcription factor Blimp-1. *J Biol Chem*. 2006 Aug 25;281(34):24111-23.

3467 Zhu N, Lv X, Wang Y, et al. Comparison of immunoregulatory effects of polysaccharides from three natural herbs and cellular uptake in dendritic cells. *Int J Biol Macromol*. 2016 Dec;93(Pt A):940-951.

3468 Hsu HY, Hua KF, Wu WC, et al. Reishi immuno-modulation protein induces interleukin-2 expression via protein kinase-dependent signaling pathways within human T cells. *J Cell Physiol*. 2008 Apr;215(1):15-26.

3469 Hsu HY, Hua KF, Lin CC, et al. Extract of Reishi polysaccharides induces cytokine expression via TLR4-modulated protein kinase signaling pathways. *J Immunol*. 2004 Nov 15;173(10):5989-99.

3470 Meng M, Yao J, Zhang Y, et al. Potential Anti-Rheumatoid Arthritis Activities and Mechanisms of Ganoderma lucidum Polysaccharides. *Molecules*. 2023 Mar 8;28(6):2483.

3471 Nizhenkovska IV, Pidchenko VT, Bychkova NG, et al. Influence of Ganoderma lucidum (Curt.: Fr.) P. Karst. on T-cell-mediated immunity in normal and immunosuppressed mice line CBA/Ca. *Ceska Slov Farm*. 2015 Sep;64(4):139-43.

3472 Carrieri R, Manco R, Sapio D, et al. Structural data and immunomodulatory properties of a water-soluble heteroglycan extracted from the mycelium of an Italian isolate of Ganoderma lucidum. *Nat Prod Res*. 2017 Sep;31(18):2119-2125.

3473 Qin C, Wu S, Chen B, et al. Effect of Ganoderma Lucidum Preparation on the Behavior, Biochemistry, and Autoimmune Parameters of Mouse Models of APP/PS1 Double Transgenic Alzheimer's Disease. *Zhongguo Yi Xue Ke Xue Yuan Xue Bao*. 2017 Jun 20;39(3):330-335.

3474 Kino K, Sone T, Watanabe J, et al. Immunomodulator, LZ-8, prevents antibody production in mice. *Int J Immunopharmacol*. 1991;13(8):1109-15.

3475 Jan RH, Lin TY, Hsu YC, et al. Immuno-modulatory activity of Ganoderma lucidum-derived polysacharide on human monocytoid dendritic cells pulsed with Der p 1 allergen. *BMC Immunol*. 2011 May 25;12:31.

3476 Shi Y, Cai D, Wang X, et al. Immunomodulatory effect of ganoderma lucidum polysaccharides (GLP) on long-term heavy-load exercising mice. *Int J Vitam Nutr Res*. 2012 Dec;82(6):383-90.

3477 Lu CC, Hsu YJ, Chang CJ, et al. Immunomodulatory properties of medicinal mushrooms: differential effects of water and ethanol extracts on NK cell-mediated cytotoxicity. *Innate Immun*. 2016 Oct;22(7):522-33.

3478 Spelman K, Aldag R, Hamman A, et al. Traditional herbal remedies that influence cell adhesion molecule activity. *Phytother Res*. 2011 Apr;25(4):473-83.

3479 Miyasaka N, Inoue H, Totsuka T, et al. An immunomodulatory protein, Ling Zhi-8, facilitates cellular interaction through modulation of adhesion molecules. *Biochem Biophys Res Commun*. 1992 Jul 15;186(1):385-90.

3480 Tasaka K, Mio M, Izushi K, et al. Anti-allergic constituents in the culture medium of Ganoderma lucidum. (II). The inhibitory effect of cyclooctasulfur on histamine release. *Agents Actions*. 1988 Apr;23(3-4):157-60.

3481 Mizutani N, Nabe T, Shimazu M, et al. Effect of Ganoderma lucidum on pollen-induced biphasic nasal blockage in a guinea pig model of allergic rhinitis. *Phytother Res*. 2012 Mar;26(3):325-32.

3482 Kohda H, Tokumoto W, Sakamoto K, et al. The biologically active constituents of Ganoderma lucidum (Fr.) Karst. Histamine release-inhibitory triterpenes. *Chem Pharm Bull (Tokyo)*. 1985 Apr;33(4):1367-74.

3483 Tasaka K, Akagi M, Miyoshi K, et al. Anti-allergic constituents in the culture medium of Ganoderma lucidum. (I). Inhibitory effect of oleic acid on histamine release. *Agents Actions*. 1988 Apr;23(3-4):153-6.

3484 Liu YH, Tsai CF, Kao MC, et al. Effectiveness of Dp2 nasal therapy for Dp2- induced airway inflammation in mice: using oral Ganoderma lucidum as an immunomodulator. *J Microbiol Immunol Infect*. 2003 Dec;36(4):236-42.

3485 Zhang Q, Andoh T, Konno M, et al. Inhibitory effect of methanol extract of Ganoderma lucidum on acute itch-associated responses in mice. *Biol Pharm Bull*. 2010;33(5):909-11.

3486 Andoh T, Zhang Q, Yamamoto T, et al. Inhibitory effects of the methanol extract of Ganoderma lucidum on mosquito allergy-induced itch-associated responses in mice. *J Pharmacol Sci*. 2010;114(3):292-7.

3487 Zhang W, Zeng YS, Xiong Y, et al. [Pre-administration of Ganoderma lucidum spore reduces incidence of neural tube defects induced by retinoic acid in pregnant mice]. *Zhong Xi Yi Jie He Xue Bao*. 2006 Jul;4(4):368-73.

3488 Ma HT, Hsieh JF, Chen ST. Anti-diabetic effects of Ganoderma lucidum. *Phytochemistry*. 2015 Jun;114:109-13.

3489 Zhang JJ, Wang DW, Cai D, et al. Meroterpenoids From Ganoderma lucidum Mushrooms and Their Biological Roles in Insulin Resistance and Triple-Negative Breast Cancer. *Front Chem*. 2021 Nov 3;9:772740.

3490 Pan R, Lou J, Wei L. Significant effects of Ganoderma lucidum polysaccharide on lipid metabolism in diabetes may be associated with the activation of the FAM3C-HSF1-CAM signaling pathway. *Exp Ther Med*. 2021 Aug;22(2):820.

3491 Yu F, Teng Y, Yang S, et al. The thermodynamic and kinetic mechanisms of a Ganoderma lucidum proteoglycan inhibiting hIAPP amyloidosis. *Biophys Chem*. 2022 Jan;280:106702.

3492 Bach EE, Hi EMB, Martins AMC, et al. Hypoglicemic and Hypolipedimic Effects of Ganoderma lucidum in Streptozotocin-Induced Diabetic Rats. *Medicines (Basel)*. 2018 Jul 28;5(3):78.

3493 Zhang Y, Pan Y, Li J, et al. Inhibition on α-Glucosidase Activity and Non-Enzymatic Glycation by an Anti-Oxidative Proteoglycan from Ganoderma lucidum. *Molecules*. 2022 Feb 22;27(5):1457.

3494 Sarnthima R, Khammaung S, Sa-Ard P. Culture broth of Ganoderma lucidum exhibited antioxidant, antibacterial and α-amylase inhibitory activities. *J Food Sci Technol*. 2017 Oct;54(11):3724-3730.

3495 Jiang Y, Zhang N, Zhou Y, et al. Manipulations of glucose/lipid metabolism and gut microbiota of resistant starch encapsulated Ganoderma lucidum spores in T2DM rats. *Food Sci Biotechnol*. 2021 Apr 24;30(5):755-764.

3496 Li F, Zhang Y, Zhong Z. Antihyperglycemic effect of ganoderma lucidum polysaccharides on streptozotocin-induced diabetic mice. *Int J Mol Sci*. 2011;12(9):6135-45.

3497 Huang CH, Lin WK, Chang SH, et al. Evaluation of the hypoglycaemic and antioxidant effects of submerged Ganoderma lucidum cultures in type 2 diabetic rats. *Mycology*. 2020 Mar 1;12(2):82-93.

3498 Yang Z, Chen C, Zhao J, et al. Hypoglycemic mechanism of a novel proteoglycan, extracted from Ganoderma lucidum, in hepatocytes. *Eur J Pharmacol*. 2018 Feb 5;820:77-85.

3499 Pan D, Wang L, Chen C, et al. Isolation and characterization of a hyperbranched proteoglycan from Ganoderma lucidum for anti-diabetes. *Carbohydr Polym*. 2015 Mar 6;117:106-114.

3500 Kim SD, Nho HJ. Isolation and characterization of alpha-glucosidase inhibitor from the fungus Ganoderma lucidum. *J Microbiol*. 2004 Sep;42(3):223-7.

3501 Hikino H, Konno C, Mirin Y, et al. Isolation and hypoglycemic activity of ganoderans A and B, glycans of Ganoderma lucidum fruit bodies. *Planta Med*. 1985 Aug;(4):339-40.

3502 Chen B, Tian J, Zhang J, et al. Triterpenes and meroterpenes from Ganoderma lucidum with inhibitory activity against HMGs reductase, aldose reductase and α-glucosidase. *Fitoterapia*. 2017 Jul;120:6-16.

3503 Pan D, Wang L, Hu B, et al. Structural characterization and bioactivity evaluation of an acidic proteoglycan extract from Ganoderma lucidum fruiting bodies for PTP1B inhibition and anti-diabetes. *Biopolymers*. 2014 Jun;101(6):613-23.

3504 Kimura Y, Okuda H, Arichi S. Effects of the extracts of Ganoderma lucidum on blood glucose level in rats. *Planta Med*. 1988 Aug;54(4):290-4.

3505 Fatmawati S, Shimizu K, Kondo R. Ganoderol B: a potent α-glucosidase inhibitor isolated from the fruiting body of Ganoderma lucidum. *Phytomedicine*. 2011 Sep 15;18(12):1053-5.

3506 Abdullah NR, Mohd Nasir MH, Azizan NH, et al. Bioreactor-grown exo- and endo-β-glucan from Malaysian Ganoderma lucidum: An in vitro and in vivo study for potential antidiabetic treatment. *Front Bioeng Biotechnol*. 2022 Aug 25;10:960320.

3507 Yang Z, Zhang Z, Zhao J, et al. Modulation of energy metabolism and mitochondrial biogenesis by a novel proteoglycan from Ganoderma lucidum. *RSC Adv*. 2019 Jan 18;9(5):2591-2598.

3508 Yu F, Teng Y, Li J, et al. Effects of a Ganoderma lucidum Proteoglycan on Type 2 Diabetic Rats and the Recovery of Rat Pancreatic Islets. *ACS Omega*. 2023 May 5;8(19):17304-17316.

3509 Xie F, Wu M, Lai B, et al. Effects of redox interference on the pancreatic mitochondria and the abnormal blood glucose. *Free Radic Res*. 2021 Feb;55(2):119-130.

3510 Hikino H, Mizuno T. Hypoglycemic actions of some heteroglycans of Ganoderma lucidum fruit bodies. *Planta Med*. 1989 Aug;55(4):385.

3511 Zhang HN, He JH, Yuan L, et al. In vitro and in vivo protective effect of Ganoderma lucidum polysaccharides on alloxan-induced pancreatic islets damage. *Life Sci*. 2003 Sep 19;73(18):2307-19.

3512 Lin ZB. Cellular and molecular mechanisms of immuno-modulation by Ganoderma lucidum. *J Pharmacol Sci*. 2005 Oct;99(2):144-53.

3513 Yu F, Wang Y, Teng Y, et al. Interaction and Inhibition of a Ganoderma lucidum Proteoglycan on PTP1B Activity for Anti-diabetes. *ACS Omega*. 2021 Oct 27;6(44):29804-29813.

3514 Ryu DH, Cho JY, Sadiq NB, et al. Optimization of antioxidant, anti-diabetic, and anti-inflammatory activities and ganoderic acid content of differentially dried Ganoderma lucidum using response surface methodology. *Food Chem*. 2021 Jan 15;335:127645.

3515 Shao W, Xiao C, Yong T, et al. A polysaccharide isolated from Ganoderma lucidum ameliorates hyperglycemia through modulating gut microbiota in type 2 diabetic mice. *Int J Biol Macromol*. 2022 Feb 1;197:23-38.

[3516] Shi M, Zhang Z, Yang Y. Antioxidant and immunoregulatory activity of Ganoderma lucidum polysaccharide (GLP). *Carbohydr Polym*. 2013 Jun 5;95(1):200-6.

[3517] Hikino H, Ishiyama M, Suzuki Y, et al. Mechanisms of hypoglycemic activity of ganoderan B: a glycan of Ganoderma lucidum fruit bodies. *Planta Med*. 1989 Oct;55(5):423-8.

[3518] Teng BS, Wang CD, Zhang D, et al. Hypoglycemic effect and mechanism of a proteoglycan from ganoderma lucidum on streptozotocin-induced type 2 diabetic rats. *Eur Rev Med Pharmacol Sci*. 2012 Feb;16(2):166-75.

[3519] Ni T, Hu Y, Sun L, et al. Oral route of mini-proinsulin-expressing Ganoderma lucidum decreases blood glucose level in streptozocin-induced diabetic rats. *Int J Mol Med*. 2007 Jul;20(1):45-51.

[3520] Xiao C, Wu Q, Zhang J, et al. Antidiabetic activity of Ganoderma lucidum polysaccharides F31 down-regulated hepatic glucose regulatory enzymes in diabetic mice. *J Ethnopharmacol*. 2017 Jan 20;196:47-57.

[3521] Zheng J, Yang B, Yu Y, et al. Ganoderma lucidum polysaccharides exert anti-hyperglycemic effect on streptozotocin-induced diabetic rats through affecting β-cells. *Comb Chem High Throughput Screen*. 2012 Aug;15(7):542-50.

[3522] Pan D, Zhang D, Wu J, et al. Antidiabetic, antihyperlipidemic and antioxidant activities of a novel proteoglycan from ganoderma lucidum fruiting bodies on db/db mice and the possible mechanism. *PLoS One*. 2013 Jul 11;8(7):e68332.

[3523] Seto SW, Lam TY, Tam HL, et al. Novel hypoglycemic effects of Ganoderma lucidum water-extract in obese/diabetic (+db/+db) mice. *Phytomedicine*. 2009 May;16(5):426-36.

[3524] Woo CW, Man RY, Siow YL, et al. Ganoderma lucidum inhibits inducible nitric oxide synthase expression in macrophages. *Mol Cell Biochem*. 2005 Jul;275(1-2):165-71.

[3525] Teng BS, Wang CD, Yang HJ, et al. A protein tyrosine phosphatase 1B activity inhibitor from the fruiting bodies of Ganoderma lucidum (Fr.) Karst and its hypoglycemic potency on streptozotocin-induced type 2 diabetic mice. *J Agric Food Chem*. 2011 Jun 22;59(12):6492-500.

[3526] Zhao XR, Huo XK, Dong PP, et al. Inhibitory Effects of Highly Oxygenated Lanostane Derivatives from the Fungus Ganoderma lucidum on P-Glycoprotein and α-Glucosidase. *J Nat Prod*. 2015 Aug 28;78(8):1868-76.

[3527] Khursheed R, Singh SK, Kumar B, et al. Self-nanoemulsifying composition containing curcumin, quercetin, Ganoderma lucidum extract powder and probiotics for effective treatment of type 2 diabetes mellitus in streptozotocin induced rats. *Int J Pharm*. 2022 Jan 25;612:121306.

[3528] Wang CD, Teng BS, He YM, et al. Effect of a novel proteoglycan PTP1B inhibitor from Ganoderma lucidum on the amelioration of hyperglycaemia and dyslipidaemia in db/db mice. *Br J Nutr*. 2012 Dec 14;108(11):2014-25.

[3529] Xiao C, Wu QP, Cai W, et al. Hypoglycemic effects of Ganoderma lucidum polysaccharides in type 2 diabetic mice. *Arch Pharm Res*. 2012 Oct;35(10):1793-801.

[3530] Xiao C, Wu Q, Xie Y, et al. Hypoglycemic mechanisms of Ganoderma lucidum polysaccharides F31 in db/db mice via RNA-seq and iTRAQ. *Food Funct*. 2018 Dec 13;9(12):6495-6507.

[3531] Wu T, Xu B. Antidiabetic and antioxidant activities of eight medicinal mushroom species from China. *Int J Med Mushrooms*. 2015;17(2):129-40.

[3532] Xiao H, Fang Z, He X, et al. Recombinant ling zhi-8 enhances Tregs function to restore glycemic control in streptozocin-induced diabetic rats. *J Pharm Pharmacol*. 2020 Dec;72(12):1946-1955.

[3533] Wang F, Zhou Z, Ren X, et al. Effect of Ganoderma lucidum spores intervention on glucose and lipid metabolism gene expression profiles in type 2 diabetic rats. *Lipids Health Dis*. 2015 May 22;14:49.

[3534] Kino K, Mizumoto K, Sone T, et al. An immunomodulating protein, Ling Zhi-8 (LZ-8) prevents insulitis in non-obese diabetic mice. *Diabetologia*. 1990 Dec;33(12):713-8.

[3535] Jiao J, Yong T, Huang L, et al. A Ganoderma lucidum polysaccharide F31 alleviates hyperglycemia through kidney protection and adipocyte apoptosis. *Int J Biol Macromol*. 2023 Jan 31;226:1178-1191.

[3536] Li L, Xu JX, Cao YJ, et al. Preparation of Ganoderma lucidum polysaccharide-chromium (III) complex and its hypoglycemic and hypolipidemic activities in high-fat and high-fructose diet-induced pre-diabetic mice. *Int J Biol Macromol*. 2019 Nov 1;140:782-793.

[3537] Shafiee-Nick R, Parizadeh SM, Zokaei N, et al. Effect of Ganoderma lucidum hydroalcoholic extract on insulin release in rat-isolated pancreatic islets. *Avicenna J Phytomed*. 2012 Fall;2(4):206-11.

[3538] Zhang JJ, Wang DW, Peng YL, et al. Spiroganodermaines A-G from Ganoderma species and their activities against insulin resistance and renal fibrosis. *Phytochemistry*. 2022 Oct;202:113324.

[3539] Zhang HN, Lin ZB. Hypoglycemic effect of Ganoderma lucidum polysaccharides. *Acta Pharmacol Sin*. 2004 Feb;25(2):191-5.

[3540] Jung KH, Ha E, Kim MJ, et al. Ganoderma lucidum extract stimulates glucose uptake in L6 rat skeletal muscle cells. *Acta Biochim Pol*. 2006;53(3):597-601.

[3541] Thyagarajan-Sahu A, Lane B, Sliva D. ReishiMax, mushroom based dietary supplement, inhibits adipocyte differentiation, stimulates glucose uptake and activates AMPK. *BMC Complement Altern Med*. 2011 Sep 19;11:74.

[3542] Yang Z, Wu F, He Y, Zhang Q et al. A novel PTP1B inhibitor extracted from Ganoderma lucidum ameliorates insulin resistance by regulating IRS1-GLUT4 cascades in the insulin signaling pathway. *Food Funct*. 2018 Jan 24;9(1):397-406.

[3543] Lee HA, Cho JH, Afinanisa Q, et al. Ganoderma lucidum Extract Reduces Insulin Resistance by Enhancing AMPK Activation in High-Fat Diet-Induced Obese Mice. *Nutrients*. 2020 Oct 30;12(11):3338.

[3544] Liang H, Pan Y, Teng Y, et al. A proteoglycan extract from Ganoderma Lucidum protects pancreatic beta-cells against STZ-induced apoptosis. *Biosci Biotechnol Biochem*. 2020 Dec;84(12):2491-2498.

[3545] Zhou S, Zhu H, Xiong P, et al. Spore Oil-Functionalized Selenium Nanoparticles Protect Pancreatic Beta Cells from Palmitic Acid-Induced Apoptosis via Inhibition of Oxidative Stress-Mediated Apoptotic Pathways. *Antioxidants (Basel)*. 2023 Mar 30;12(4):840.

[3546] He YM, Zhang Q, Zheng M, et al. Protective effects of a G. lucidum proteoglycan on INS-1 cells against IAPP-induced apoptosis via attenuating endoplasmic reticulum stress and modulating CHOP/JNK pathways. *Int J Biol Macromol*. 2018 Jan;106:893-900.

[3547] Grienke U, Kaserer T, Pfluger F, et al. Accessing biological actions of Ganoderma secondary metabolites by in silico profiling. *Phytochemistry*. 2015 Jun;114:114-24.

3548 Petryn TS, Nagalievska MR, Wasser SP, et al. Effect of the Lingzi or Reishi Medicinal Mushroom Ganoderma lucidum (Agaricomycetes) on Hyperglycemia and Dyslipidemia with Experimental Metabolic Syndrome. *Int J Med Mushrooms*. 2023;25(5):17-30.

3549 Viroel FJM, Laurino LF, Caetano ÉLA, et al. Ganoderma lucidum Modulates Glucose, Lipid Peroxidation and Hepatic Metabolism in Streptozotocin-Induced Diabetic Pregnant Rats. *Antioxidants (Basel)*. 2022 May 24;11(6):1035.

3550 Xuan M, Okazaki M, Iwata N, et al. Chronic Treatment with a Water-Soluble Extract from the Culture Medium of Ganoderma lucidum Mycelia Prevents Apoptosis and Necroptosis in Hypoxia/Ischemia-Induced Injury of Type 2 Diabetic Mouse Brain. *Evid Based Complement Alternat Med*. 2015;2015:865986.

3551 Li J, Zhang Y, Yu F, et al. Proteoglycan Extracted from Ganoderma lucidum Ameliorated Diabetes-Induced Muscle Atrophy via the AMPK/SIRT1 Pathway In Vivo and In Vitro. *ACS Omega*. 2023 Aug 8;8(33):30359-30373.

3552 Hassan HM, Mahran YF, Ghanim AMH. Ganoderma lucidum ameliorates the diabetic nephropathy via down-regulatory effect on TGFβ-1 and TLR-4/NFκB signalling pathways. *J Pharm Pharmacol*. 2021 Aug 12;73(9):1250-1261.

3553 Zhang JJ, Wang DW, Peng YL, et al. Spiroganodermaines A-G from Ganoderma species and their activities against insulin resistance and renal fibrosis. *Phytochemistry*. 2022 Oct;202:113324.

3554 He CY, Li WD, Guo SX, et al. Effect of polysaccharides from Ganoderma lucidum on streptozotocin-induced diabetic nephropathy in mice. *J Asian Nat Prod Res*. 2006 Dec;8(8):705-11.

3555 Pan Y, Zhang Y, Li J, et al. A proteoglycan isolated from Ganoderma lucidum attenuates diabetic kidney disease by inhibiting oxidative stress-induced renal fibrosis both in vitro and in vivo. *J Ethnopharmacol*. 2023 Jun 28;310:116405.

3556 Pan D, Zhang D, Wu J, et al. A novel proteoglycan from Ganoderma lucidum fruiting bodies protects kidney function and ameliorates diabetic nephropathy via its antioxidant activity in C57BL/6 db/db mice. *Food Chem Toxicol*. 2014 Jan;63:111-8.

3557 Hu Y, Wang SX, Wu FY, et al. Effects and Mechanism of Ganoderma lucidum Polysaccharides in the Treatment of Diabetic Nephropathy in Streptozotocin-Induced Diabetic Rats. *Biomed Res Int*. 2022 Mar 8;2022:4314415.

3558 Tie L, Yang HQ, An Y, et al. Ganoderma lucidum polysaccharide accelerates refractory wound healing by inhibition of mitochondrial oxidative stress in type 1 diabetes. *Cell Physiol Biochem*. 2012;29(3-4):583-94.

3559 Fatmawati S, Kurashiki K, Takeno S, et al. The inhibitory effect on aldose reductase by an extract of Ganoderma lucidum. *Phytother Res*. 2009 Jan;23(1):28-32.

3560 Fatmawati S, Shimizu K, Kondo R. Ganoderic acid Df, a new triterpenoid with aldose reductase inhibitory activity from the fruiting body of Ganoderma lucidum. *Fitoterapia*. 2010 Dec;81(8):1033-6.

3561 Fatmawati S, Shimizu K, Kondo R. Inhibition of aldose reductase in vitro by constituents of Ganoderma lucid. *Planta Med*. 2010 Oct;76(15):1691-3.

3562 Chen B, Tian J, Zhang J, et al. Triterpenes and meroterpenes from Ganoderma lucidum with inhibitory activity against HMGs reductase, aldose reductase and α-glucosidase. *Fitoterapia*. 2017 Jul;120:6-16.

3563 Fatmawati S, Shimizu K, Kondo R. Structure-activity relationships of ganoderma acids from Ganoderma lucidum as aldose reductase inhibitors. *Bioorg Med Chem Lett*. 2011 Dec 15;21(24):7295-7.

3564 Wu T, Xu B. Antidiabetic and antioxidant activities of eight medicinal mushroom species from China. *Int J Med Mushrooms*. 2015;17(2):129-40.

3565 Shaher F, Wang S, Qiu H, et al. Effect and Mechanism of Ganoderma lucidum Spores on Alleviation of Diabetic Cardiomyopathy in a Pilot in vivo Study. *Diabetes Metab Syndr Obes*. 2020 Dec 7;13:4809-4822.

3566 Xue H, Qiao J, Meng G, et al. [Effect of Ganoderma lucidum polysaccharides on hemodynamic and antioxidation in T2DM rats]. *Zhongguo Zhong Yao Za Zhi*. 2010 Feb;35(3):339-43.

3567 Heriansyah T, Nurwidyaningtyas W, Sargowo D, et al. Polysaccharide peptide (PsP) Ganoderma lucidum: a potential inducer for vascular repair in type 2 diabetes mellitus model. *Vasc Health Risk Manag*. 2019 Oct 3;15:419-427.

3568 Huang CH, Lin WK, Chang SH, et al. Ganoderma lucidum culture supplement ameliorates dyslipidemia and reduces visceral fat accumulation in type 2 diabetic rats. *Mycology*. 2020 Mar 23;12(2):94-104.

3569 Pan R, Lou J, Wei L. Significant effects of Ganoderma lucidum polysaccharide on lipid metabolism in diabetes may be associated with the activation of the FAM3C-HSF1-CAM signaling pathway. *Exp Ther Med*. 2021 Aug;22(2):820.

3570 Bach EE, Hi EMB, Martins AMC, et al. Hypoglicemic and Hypolipedimic Effects of Ganoderma lucidum in Streptozotocin-Induced Diabetic Rats. *Medicines (Basel)*. 2018 Jul 28;5(3):78.

3571 Wang BX, Wang SQ, Qin WB, et al. [Effects of ganoderma lucidum spores on cytochrome C and mitochondrial calcium in the testis of NIDDM rats]. *Zhonghua Nan Ke Xue*. 2006 Dec;12(12):1072-5.

3572 Wang SQ, Qin WB, Kang YM, et al. [Intervention effect of ganoderma lucidum spores on the changes of XOD, MPO and SDH in the testis tissue of NIDDM rats]. *Zhonghua Nan Ke Xue*. 2008 Sep;14(9):792-5.

3573 Ma XR, Zhou CF, Wang SQ, et al. [Effects of ganoderma lucidum spores on mitochondrial calcium ion and cytochrome C in epididymal cells of type 2 diabetes rats]. *Zhonghua Nan Ke Xue*. 2007 May;13(5):400-2.

3574 Chen M, Xiao D, Liu W, et al. Intake of Ganoderma lucidum polysaccharides reverses the disturbed gut microbiota and metabolism in type 2 diabetic rats. *Int J Biol Macromol*. 2020 Jul 15;155:890-902.

3575 Yao X, Yuan Y, Jing T, et al. Ganoderma lucidum polysaccharide ameliorated diabetes mellitus-induced erectile dysfunction in rats by regulating fibrosis and the NOS/ERK/JNK pathway. *Transl Androl Urol*. 2022 Jul;11(7):982-995.

3576 Li H, Du Y, Ji H, et al. Adenosine-rich extract of Ganoderma lucidum: A safe and effective lipid-lowering substance. *iScience*. 2022 Sep 26;25(11):105214.

3577 Wu S. Hypolipidaemic and anti-lipidperoxidant activities of Ganoderma lucidum polysaccharide. *Int J Biol Macromol*. 2018 Oct 15;118(Pt B):2001-2005.

3578 Xu Y, Zhang X, Yan XH, et al. Characterization, hypolipidemic and antioxidant activities of degraded polysaccharides from Ganoderma lucidum. *Int J Biol Macromol*. 2019 Aug 15;135:706-716.

3579 Tong A, Wu W, Chen Z, et al. Modulation of gut microbiota and lipid metabolism in rats fed high-fat diets by Ganoderma lucidum triterpenoids. *Curr Res Food Sci*. 2022 Dec 27;6:100427.

[3580] Kim SD. Isolation and structure determination of a cholesterol esterase inhibitor from Ganoderma lucidum. *J Microbiol Biotechnol*. 2010 Nov;20(11):1521-3.

[3581] Chen WQ, Luo SH, Ll HZ, et al. [Effects of ganoderma lucidum polysaccharides on serum lipids and lipoperoxidation in experimental hyperlipidemic rats]. *Zhongguo Zhong Yao Za Zhi*. 2005 Sep;30(17):1358-60.

[3582] Berger A, Rein D, Kratky E, et al. Cholesterol-lowering properties of Ganoderma lucidum in vitro, ex vivo, and in hamsters and minipigs. *Lipids Health Dis*. 2004 Feb 18;3:2.

[3583] Wang W, Zhang Y, Wang Z, et al. Ganoderma lucidum polysaccharides improve lipid metabolism against high-fat diet-induced dyslipidemia. *J Ethnopharmacol*. 2023 Jun 12;309:116321.

[3584] Chen B, Tian J, Zhang J, et al. Triterpenes and meroterpenes from Ganoderma lucidum with inhibitory activity against HMGs reductase, aldose reductase and α-glucosidase. *Fitoterapia*. 2017 Jul;120:6-16.

[3585] Kabir Y, Kimura S, Tamura T. Dietary effect of Ganoderma lucidum mushroom on blood pressure and lipid levels in spontaneously hypertensive rats (SHR). *J Nutr Sci Vitaminol (Tokyo)*. 1988 Aug;34(4):433-8.

[3586] Liang Z, Yuan Z, Li G, et al. Hypolipidemic, Antioxidant, and Antiapoptotic Effects of Polysaccharides Extracted from Reishi Mushroom, Ganoderma lucidum (Leysser: Fr) Karst, in Mice Fed a High-Fat Diet. *J Med Food*. 2018 Dec;21(12):1218-1227.

[3587] Hajjaj H, Macé C, Roberts M, et al. Effect of 26-oxygenosterols from Ganoderma lucidum and their activity as cholesterol synthesis inhibitors. *Appl Environ Microbiol*. 2005 Jul;71(7):3653-8.

[3588] Tong AJ, Hu RK, Wu LX, et al. Ganoderma polysaccharide and chitosan synergistically ameliorate lipid metabolic disorders and modulate gut microbiota composition in high fat diet-fed golden hamsters. *J Food Biochem*. 2020 Jan;44(1):e13109.

[3589] Rahman MA, Abdullah N, Aminudin N. Evaluation of the Antioxidative and Hypo-cholesterolemic Effects of Lingzhi or Reishi Medicinal Mushroom, Ganoderma lucidum (Agaricomycetes), in Ameliorating Cardiovascular Disease. *Int J Med Mushrooms*. 2018;20(10):961-969.

[3590] Romero-Córdoba SL, Salido-Guadarrama I, et al. Mexican Ganoderma Lucidum Extracts Decrease Lipogenesis Modulating Transcriptional Metabolic Networks and Gut Microbiota in C57BL/6 Mice Fed with a High-Cholesterol Diet. *Nutrients*. 2020 Dec 24;13(1):38.

[3591] Komoda Y, Shimizu M, Sonoda Y, et al. Ganoderic acid and its derivatives as cholesterol synthesis inhibitors. *Chem Pharm Bull (Tokyo)*. 1989 Feb;37(2):531-3.

[3592] Guo WL, Pan YY, Li L, et al. Ethanol extract of Ganoderma lucidum ameliorates lipid metabolic disorders and modulates the gut microbiota composition in high-fat diet fed rats. *Food Funct*. 2018 Jun 20;9(6):3419-3431.

[3593] Sobowale MT, Ozolua RI, Uwaya DO, et al. Effects of Concurrently Administered Aqueous Extract of Lingzhi or Reishi Medicinal Mushroom, Ganoderma lucidum (Agaricomycetes), and Lead Acetate in Rats. *Int J Med Mushrooms*. 2019;21(2):143-154.

[3594] Zhang HM, Yao WJ, Tian HK. [Effect of lugu Ganoderma lucidum on low-density lipoprotein oxidation and monocyte adhesion to endothelium]. *Zhongguo Zhong Xi Yi Jie He Za Zhi*. 2002 Jul;22(7):534-7.

[3595] Meneses ME, Martínez-Carrera D, Torres N, et al. Hypocholesterolemic Properties and Prebiotic Effects of Mexican Ganoderma lucidum in C57BL/6 Mice. *PLoS One*. 2016 Jul 20;11(7):e0159631.

[3596] Guo WL, Guo JB, Liu BY, et al. Ganoderic acid A from Ganoderma lucidum ameliorates lipid metabolism and alters gut microbiota composition in hyperlipidemic mice fed a high-fat diet. *Food Funct*. 2020 Aug 1;11(8):6818-6833.

[3597] Ezurike PU, Odunola E, Oke TA, et al. Ganoderma lucidum ethanol extract promotes weight loss and improves depressive-like behaviors in male and female Swiss mice. *Physiol Behav*. 2023 Jun 1;265:114155.

[3598] Sang T, Guo C, Guo D, et al. Suppression of obesity and inflammation by polysaccharide from sporoderm-broken spore of Ganoderma lucidum via gut microbiota regulation. *Carbohydr Polym*. 2021 Mar 15;256:117594.

[3599] Zhong B, Li FL, Zhao JY, et al. Sporoderm-broken spore powder of Ganoderma lucidum ameliorate obesity and inflammation process in high-fat diet-induced obese mice. *Food Nutr Res*. 2022 Oct 12;66.

[3600] Lee I, Seo J, Kim J, et al. Lanostane triterpenes from the fruiting bodies of Ganoderma lucidum and their inhibitory effects on adipocyte differentiation in 3T3-L1 Cells. *J Nat Prod*. 2010 Feb 26;73(2):172-6.

[3601] Lee I, Kim J, Ryoo I, et al. Lanostane triterpenes from Ganoderma lucidum suppress the adipogenesis in 3T3-L1 cells through down-regulation of SREBP-1c. *Bioorg Med Chem Lett*. 2010 Sep 15;20(18):5577-81.

[3602] Lee I, Kim H, Youn U, et al. Effect of lanostane triterpenes from the fruiting bodies of Ganoderma lucidum on adipocyte differentiation in 3T3-L1 cells. *Planta Med*. 2010 Oct;76(14):1558-63.

[3603] Chang CJ, Lin CS, Lu CC, et al. Ganoderma lucidum reduces obesity in mice by modulating the composition of the gut microbiota. *Nat Commun*. 2015 Jun 23;6:7489.

[3604] Jeong YU, Park YJ. Ergosterol Peroxide from the Medicinal Mushroom Ganoderma lucidum Inhibits Differentiation and Lipid Accumulation of 3T3-L1 Adipocytes. *Int J Mol Sci*. 2020 Jan 10;21(2):460.

[3605] Bu S, Zheng H, Yuan C, et al. Lingzhi or Reishi Medicinal Mushroom, Ganoderma lucidum (Agaricomycetes), Polysaccharides Suppressed Adipogenesis and Stimulated Lipolysis in HPA-v and 3T3-L1 Adipocytes. *Int J Med Mushrooms*. 2020;22(9):897-908.

[3606] Krobthong S, Yingchutrakul Y, Visessanguan W, et al. Study of the Lipolysis Effect of Nanoliposome-Encapsulated Ganoderma lucidum Protein Hydrolysates on Adipocyte Cells Using Proteomics Approach. *Foods*. 2021 Sep 12;10(9):2157.

[3607] Milovanovic I, Zengin G, Maksimovic S, et al. Supercritical carbon-oxide extracts from cultivated and wild-grown Ganoderma lucidum mushroom: differences in ergosterol and ganoderic acids content, antioxidative and enzyme inhibitory properties. *Nat Prod Res*. 2023 Feb 6:1-7.

[3608] Wang Y, Yu F, Zheng X, et al. Balancing adipocyte production and lipid metabolism to treat obesity-induced diabetes with a novel proteoglycan from Ganoderma lucidum. *Lipids Health Dis*. 2023 Aug 8;22(1):120.

[3609] Qi G, Hua H, Gao Y, et al. Effects of Ganoderma lucidum spores on sialoadenitis of nonobese diabetic mice. *Chin Med J (Engl)*. 2009 Mar 5;122(5):556-60.

[3610] Lasukova TV, Maslov LN, Arbuzov AG, et al. Cardioprotective Activity of Ganoderma lucidum Extract during Total Ischemia and Reperfusion of Isolated Heart. *Bull Exp Biol Med*. 2015 Apr;158(6):739-41.

[3611] Xie YZ, Yang F, Tan W, et al. The anti-cancer components of Ganoderma lucidum possesses cardiovascular protective effect by regulating circular RNA expression. *Oncoscience*. 2016 Aug 28;3(7-8):203-207.

[3612] Wong KL, Chao HH, Chan P, et al. Antioxidant activity of Ganoderma lucidum in acute ethanol-induced heart toxicity. *Phytother Res*. 2004 Dec;18(12):1024-6.

[3613] Dai C, He L, Ma B, Chen T. Facile Nanolization Strategy for Therapeutic Ganoderma Lucidum Spore Oil to Achieve Enhanced Protection against Radiation-Induced Heart Disease. *Small*. 2019 Sep;15(36):e1902642.

[3614] Lasukova TV, Arbuzov AG, Maslov LN, et al. [Ganoderma lucidum extract in cardiac diastolic dysfunction and irreversible cardiomyocytic damage in ischemia and reperfusion of the isolated heart]. *Patol Fiziol Eksp Ter*. 2008 Jan-Mar;(1):22-5.

[3615] Kirar V, Nehra S, Mishra J, et al. Lingzhi or Reishi Medicinal Mushroom, Ganoderma lucidum (Agaricomycetes), as a Cardioprotectant in an Oxygen-Deficient Environment. *Int J Med Mushrooms*. 2017;19(11):1009-1021.

[3616] Liang CJ, Lee CW, Sung HC, et al. Ganoderma lucidum Polysaccharides Reduce Lipopolysaccharide-Induced Interleukin-1 β Expression in Cultured Smooth Muscle Cells and in Thoracic Aortas in Mice. *Evid Based Complement Alternat Med*. 2014;2014:305149.

[3617] Wang SH, Liang CJ, Weng YW, et al. Ganoderma lucidum polysaccharides prevent platelet-derived growth factor-stimulated smooth cell proliferation in vitro and neointimal hyperplasia in the endothelial-denuded artery in vivo. *J Cell Physiol*. 2012 Aug;227(8):3063-71.

[3618] Zhang X, Xiao C, Liu H. Ganoderic Acid A Protects Rat H9c2 Cardiomyocytes from Hypoxia-Induced Injury via Up-Regulating miR-182-5p. *Cell Physiol Biochem*. 2018;50(6):2086-2096.

[3619] Oh KK, Adnan M, Cho DH. A network pharmacology analysis on drug-like compounds from Ganoderma lucidum for alleviation of atherosclerosis. *J Food Biochem*. 2021 Sep;45(9):e13906.

[3620] Andri Wihastuti T, Sargowo D, Heriansyah T, et al. The reduction of aorta histopathological images through inhibition of reactive oxygen species formation in hypercholesterolemia rattus norvegicus treated with polysaccharide peptide of Ganoderma lucidum. *Iran J Basic Med Sci*. 2015 May;18(5):514-9.

[3621] Wihastuti TA, Amiruddin R, Cesa FY, et al. Decreasing angiogenesis vasa vasorum through Lp-PLA2 and H2O2 inhibition by PSP from Ganoderma lucidum in atherosclerosis: in vivo diabetes mellitus type 2. *J Basic Clin Physiol Pharmacol*. 2020 Feb 7;30(6):/j/jbcpp.2019.30.issue-6/jbcpp-2019-0349/jbcpp-2019-0349.xml.

[3622] Lai P, Cao X, Xu Q, et al. Ganoderma lucidum spore ethanol extract attenuates atherosclerosis by regulating lipid metabolism via upregulation of liver X receptor alpha. *Pharm Biol*. 2020 Dec;58(1):760-770.

[3623] Li Khva Ren, Vasil'ev AV, Orekhov AN, et al. [Anti-atherosclerotic properties of higher mushrooms (a clinico-experimental investigation)]. *Vopr Pitan*. 1989 Jan-Feb;(1):16-9.

[3624] Li Y, Tang J, Gao H, et al. Ganoderma lucidum triterpenoids and polysaccharides attenuate atherosclerotic plaque in high-fat diet rabbits. *Nutr Metab Cardiovasc Dis*. 2021 Jun 7;31(6):1929-1938.

[3625] Wihastuti TA, Heriansyah T. The inhibitory effects of polysaccharide peptides (PsP) of Ganoderma lucidum against atherosclerosis in rats with dyslipidemia. *Heart Int*. 2017 Apr 12;12(1):e1-e7.

[3626] Zheng G, Zhao Y, Li Z, et al. GLSP and GLSP-derived triterpenes attenuate atherosclerosis and aortic calcification by stimulating ABCA1/G1-mediated macrophage cholesterol efflux and inactivating RUNX2-mediated VSMC osteogenesis. *Theranostics*. 2023 Feb 21;13(4):1325-1341.

[3627] Hsu PL, Lin YC, Ni H, et al. Ganoderma Triterpenoids Exert Antiatherogenic Effects in Mice by Alleviating Disturbed Flow-Induced Oxidative Stress and Inflammation. *Oxid Med Cell Longev*. 2018 Apr 11;2018:3491703.

[3628] Sudheesh NP, Ajith TA, Janardhanan KK. Ganoderma lucidum ameliorate mitochondrial damage in isoproterenol-induced myocardial infarction in rats by enhancing the activities of TCA cycle enzymes and respiratory chain complexes. *Int J Cardiol*. 2013 Apr 30;165(1):117-25.

[3629] Xu ZH, Su X, Yang G, et al. Ganoderma lucidum polysaccharides protect against sepsis-induced cardiac dysfunction by activating SIRT1. *J Pharm Pharmacol*. 2022 Jan 5;74(1):124-130.

[3630] Lee SY, Rhee HM. Cardiovascular effects of mycelium extract of Ganoderma lucidum: inhibition of sympathetic outflow as a mechanism of its hypotensive action. *Chem Pharm Bull (Tokyo)*. 1990 May;38(5):1359-64.

[3631] Wu Q, Li Y, Peng K, et al. Isolation and Characterization of Three Antihypertension Peptides from the Mycelia of Ganoderma Lucidum (Agaricomycetes). *J Agric Food Chem*. 2019 Jul 24;67(29):8149-8159.

[3632] Kabir Y, Kimura S, Tamura T. Dietary effect of Ganoderma lucidum mushroom on blood pressure and lipid levels in spontaneously hypertensive rats (SHR). *J Nutr Sci Vitaminol (Tokyo)*. 1988 Aug;34(4):433-8.

[3633] Shevelev OB, Seryapina AA, Zavjalov EL, et al. Hypotensive and neurometabolic effects of intragastric Reishi (Ganoderma lucidum) administration in hypertensive ISIAH rat strain. *Phytomedicine*. 2018 Mar 1;41:1-6.

[3634] Chen Y, Qiao J, Luo J, et al. [Effects of Ganoderma lucidum polysaccharides on advanced glycation end products and receptor of aorta pectoralis in T2DM rats]. *Zhongguo Zhong Yao Za Zhi*. 2011 Mar;36(5):624-7.

[3635] Morigiwa A, Kitabatake K, Fujimoto Y, et al. Angiotensin converting enzyme-inhibitory triterpenes from Ganoderma lucidum. *Chem Pharm Bull (Tokyo)*. 1986 Jul;34(7):3025-8.

[3636] Mohamad Ansor N, Abdullah N, Aminudin N. Anti-angiotensin converting enzyme (ACE) proteins from mycelia of Ganoderma lucidum (Curtis) P. Karst. *BMC Complement Altern Med*. 2013 Oct 4;13:256.

[3637] Kumaran S, Palani P, Nishanthi R, et al. Studies on screening, isolation and purification of a fibrinolytic protease from an isolate (VK12) of Ganoderma lucidum and evaluation of its antithrombotic activity. *Med Mycol J*. 2011;52(2):153-62.

[3638] Yi F, Sun L, Xu LJ, et al. In silico Approach for Anti-Thrombosis Drug Discovery: P2Y1R Structure-Based TCMs Screening. *Front Pharmacol*. 2017 Jan 9;7:531.

[3639] Sharif S, Atta A, Huma T, et al. Anticancer, antithrombotic, antityrosinase, and anti-α-glucosidase activities of selected wild and commercial mushrooms from Pakistan. *Food Sci Nutr*. 2018 Sep 14;6(8):2170-2176.

[3640] Su CY, Shiao MS, Wang CT. Differential effects of ganodermic acid S on the thromboxane A2-signaling pathways in human platelets. *Biochem Pharmacol*. 1999 Aug 15;58(4):587-95.

[3641] Poniedziałek B, Siwulski M, Wiater A, et al. The Effect of Mushroom Extracts on Human Platelet and Blood Coagulation: In vitro Screening of Eight Edible Species. *Nutrients*. 2019 Dec 12;11(12):3040.

3642 Zhen C, Wu X, Zhang J, et al. Ganoderma lucidum polysaccharides attenuates pressure-overload-induced pathological cardiac hypertrophy. *Front Pharmacol*. 2023 Mar 23;14:1127123.

3643 Oluwafemi Adetuyi B, Olamide Okeowo T, et al. Ganoderma Lucidum from Red Mushroom Attenuates Formaldehyde-Induced Liver Damage in Experimental Male Rat Model. *Biology (Basel)*. 2020 Sep 27;9(10):313.

3644 Zhang X, Gao X, Long G, et al. Lanostane-type triterpenoids from the mycelial mat of Ganoderma lucidum and their hepatoprotective activities. *Phytochemistry*. 2022 Jun;198:113131.

3645 Chen S, Guan X, Yong T, et al. Structural characterization and hepatoprotective activity of an acidic polysaccharide from Ganoderma lucidum. *Food Chem X*. 2022 Jan 3;13:100204.

3646 Zhao C, Fan J, Liu Y, et al. Hepatoprotective activity of Ganoderma lucidum triterpenoids in alcohol-induced liver injury in mice, an iTRAQ-based proteomic analysis. *Food Chem*. 2019 Jan 15;271:148-156.

3647 Susilo RJK, Winarni D, Husen SA, et al. Hepatoprotective effect of crude polysaccharides extracted from Ganoderma lucidum against carbon tetrachloride-induced liver injury in mice. *Vet World*. 2019 Dec;12(12):1987-1991.

3648 Shieh YH, Liu CF, Huang YK, et al. Evaluation of the hepatic and renal-protective effects of Ganoderma lucidum in mice. *Am J Chin Med*. 2001;29(3-4):501-7.

3649 Jang SH, Cho SW, Yoon HM, et al. Hepatoprotective Evaluation of Ganoderma lucidum Pharmacopuncture: In vivo Studies of Ethanol-induced Acute Liver Injury. *J Pharmacopuncture*. 2014 Sep;17(3):16-24.

3650 Ha do T, Oh J, Khoi NM, et al. In vitro and in vivo hepatoprotective effect of ganodermanontriol against t-BHP-induced oxidative stress. *J Ethnopharmacol*. 2013 Dec 12;150(3):875-85.

3651 Chen J, He X, Song Y, et al. Sporoderm-broken spores of Ganoderma lucidum alleviates liver injury induced by DBP and BaP co-exposure in rat. *Ecotoxicol Environ Saf*. 2022 Aug;241:113750.

3652 Lakshmi B, Ajith TA, Jose N, et al. Antimutagenic activity of methanolic extract of Ganoderma lucidum and its effect on hepatic damage caused by benzo[a]pyrene. *J Ethnopharmacol*. 2006 Sep 19;107(2):297-303.

3653 Shi Y, Sun J, He H, et al. Hepatoprotective effects of Ganoderma lucidum peptides against D-galactosamine-induced liver injury in mice. *J Ethnopharmacol*. 2008 May 22;117(3):415-9.

3654 Yang XJ, Liu J, Ye LB, et al. In vitro and in vivo protective effects of proteoglycan isolated from mycelia of Ganoderma lucidum on carbon tetrachloride-induced liver injury. *World J Gastroenterol*. 2006 Mar 7;12(9):1379-85.

3655 Leng Y, Wang F, Chen C, et al. Protective Effect of Ganoderma lucidum Spore Powder on Acute Liver Injury in Mice and its Regulation of Gut Microbiota. *Front Biosci (Landmark Ed)*. 2023 Feb 2;28(2):23.

3656 Cao YJ, Huang ZR, You SZ, et al. The Protective Effects of Ganoderic Acids from Ganoderma lucidum Fruiting Body on Alcoholic Liver Injury and Intestinal Microflora Disturbance in Mice with Excessive Alcohol Intake. *Foods*. 2022 Mar 25;11(7):949.

3657 Guo WL, Cao YJ, You SZ, et al. Ganoderic acids-rich ethanol extract from Ganoderma lucidum protects against alcoholic liver injury and modulates intestinal microbiota in mice with excessive alcohol intake. *Curr Res Food Sci*. 2022 Feb 24;5:515-530.

3658 Hu Z, Du R, Xiu L, et al. Protective effect of triterpenes of Ganoderma lucidum on lipopolysaccharide-induced inflammatory responses and acute liver injury. *Cytokine*. 2020 Mar;127:154917.

3659 Chen YS, Chen QZ, Wang ZJ, et al. Anti-Inflammatory and Hepatoprotective Effects of Ganoderma lucidum Polysaccharides against Carbon Tetrachloride-Induced Liver Injury in Kunming Mice. *Pharmacology*. 2019;103(3-4):143-150.

3660 Liu YJ, Du JL, Cao LP, et al. Anti-inflammatory and hepatoprotective effects of Ganoderma lucidum polysaccharides on carbon tetrachloride-induced hepatocyte damage in common carp (Cyprinus carpio L.). *Int Immunopharmacol*. 2015 Mar;25(1):112-20.

3661 Liu Y, Zhang C, Du J, et al. Protective effect of Ganoderma lucidum polysaccharide against carbon tetrachloride-induced hepatic damage in precision-cut carp liver slices. *Fish Physiol Biochem*. 2017 Oct;43(5):1209-1221.

3662 Wu H, Tang S, Huang Z, et al. Hepatoprotective Effects and Mechanisms of Action of Triterpenoids from Lingzhi or Reishi Medicinal Mushroom Ganoderma lucidum (Agaricomycetes) on α-Amanitin-Induced Liver Injury in Mice. *Int J Med Mushrooms*. 2016;18(9):841-850.

3663 Wu X, Zeng J, Hu J, et al. Hepatoprotective effects of aqueous extract from Lingzhi or Reishi medicinal mushroom Ganoderma lucidum (higher basidiomycetes) on α-amanitin-induced liver injury in mice. *Int J Med Mushrooms*. 2013;15(4):383-91.

3664 Wang X, Zhao X, Li D, et al. Effects of Ganoderma lucidum polysaccharide on CYP2E1, CYP1A2 and CYP3A activities in BCG-immune hepatic injury in rats. *Biol Pharm Bull*. 2007 Sep;30(9):1702-6.

3665 Zhang Y, Feng Y, Wang W, et al. Characterization and Hepatoprotections of Ganoderma lucidum Polysaccharides against Multiple Organ Dysfunction Syndrome in Mice. *Oxid Med Cell Longev*. 2021 Feb 3;2021:9703682.

3666 Yuan S, Pan Y, Zhang Z, et al. Amelioration of the Lipogenesis, Oxidative Stress and Apoptosis of Hepatocytes by a Novel Proteoglycan from Ganoderma lucidum. *Biol Pharm Bull*. 2020 Oct 1;43(10):1542-1550.

3667 Aydin S, Aytac E, Uzun H, et al. Effects of Ganoderma lucidum on obstructive jaundice-induced oxidative stress. *Asian J Surg*. 2010 Oct;33(4):173-80.

3668 Chen TQ, Wu JG, Kan YJ, et al. Antioxidant and Hepatoprotective Activities of Crude Polysaccharide Extracts from Lingzhi or Reishi Medicinal Mushroom, Ganoderma lucidum (Agaricomycetes), by Ultrasonic-Circulating Extraction. *Int J Med Mushrooms*. 2018;20(6):581-593.

3669 Jin H, Jin F, Jin JX, et al. Protective effects of Ganoderma lucidum spore on cadmium hepatotoxicity in mice. *Food Chem Toxicol*. 2013 Feb;52:171-5.

3670 Zhang GL, Wang YH, Ni W, et al. Hepatoprotective role of Ganoderma lucidum polysaccharide against BCG-induced immune liver injury in mice. *World J Gastroenterol*. 2002 Aug;8(4):728-33.

3671 Kim DH, Shim SB, Kim NJ, et al. Beta-glucuronidase-inhibitory activity and hepatoprotective effect of Ganoderma lucidum. *Biol Pharm Bull*. 1999 Feb;22(2):162-4.

[3672] Lv XC, Wu Q, Cao YJ, et al. Ganoderic acid A from Ganoderma lucidum protects against alcoholic liver injury through ameliorating the lipid metabolism and modulating the intestinal microbial composition. *Food Funct.* 2022 May 23;13(10):5820-5837.

[3673] Li B, Lee DS, Kang Y, et al. Protective effect of ganodermanondiol isolated from the Lingzhi mushroom against tert-butyl hydroperoxide-induced hepatotoxicity through Nrf2-mediated antioxidant enzymes. *Food Chem Toxicol.* 2013 Mar;53:317-24.

[3674] Lin HJ, Chang YS, Lin LH, et al. An Immunomodulatory Protein (Ling Zhi-8) from a Ganoderma lucidum Induced Acceleration of Wound Healing in Rat Liver Tissues after Monopolar Electrosurgery. *Evid Based Complement Alternat Med.* 2014;2014:916531.

[3675] Jung S, Son H, Hwang CE, et al. Ganoderma lucidum Ameliorates Non-Alcoholic Steatosis by Upregulating Energy Metabolizing Enzymes in the Liver. *J Clin Med.* 2018 Jun 15;7(6):152.

[3676] Zhong D, Xie Z, Huang B, et al. Ganoderma Lucidum Polysaccharide Peptide Alleviates Hepatoteatosis via Modulating Bile Acid Metabolism Dependent on FXR-SHP/FGF. *Cell Physiol Biochem.* 2018;49(3):1163-1179.

[3677] Li HN, Zhao LL, Zhou DY, et al. Ganoderma Lucidum Polysaccharides Ameliorates Hepatic Steatosis and Oxidative Stress in db/db Mice via Targeting Nuclear Factor E2 (Erythroid-Derived 2)-Related Factor-2/Heme Oxygenase-1 (HO-1) Pathway. *Med Sci Monit.* 2020 Apr 4;26:e921905.

[3678] Wang GJ, Huang YJ, Chen DH, et al. Ganoderma lucidum extract attenuates the proliferation of hepatic stellate cells by blocking the PDGF receptor. *Phytother Res.* 2009 Jun;23(6):833-9.

[3679] Kwon SC, Kim YB. Antifibrotic activity a fermentation filtrate of Ganoderma lucidum. *Lab Anim Res.* 2011 Dec;27(4):369-71.

[3680] Wu YW, Fang HL, Lin WC. Post-treatment of Ganoderma lucidum reduced liver fibrosis induced by thioacetamide in mice. *Phytother Res.* 2010 Apr;24(4):494-9. doi: 10.1002/ptr.2949.

[3681] Chen C, Chen J, Wang Y, et al. Ganoderma lucidum polysaccharide inhibits HSC activation and liver fibrosis via targeting inflammation, apoptosis, cell cycle, and ECM-receptor interaction mediated by TGF-β/Smad signaling. *Phytomedicine.* 2023 Feb;110:154626.

[3682] Lin WC, Lin WL. Ameliorative effect of Ganoderma lucidum on carbon tetrachloride-induced liver fibrosis in rats. *World J Gastroenterol.* 2006 Jan 14;12(2):265-70.

[3683] Wang YX, Peng YL, Qiu B, et al. Meroterpenoids with a large conjugated system from Ganoderma lucidum and their inhibitory activities against renal fibrosis. *Fitoterapia.* 2022 Sep;161:105257.

[3684] Shieh YH, Liu CF, Huang YK, et al. Evaluation of the hepatic and renal-protective effects of Ganoderma lucidum in mice. *Am J Chin Med.* 2001;29(3-4):501-7.

[3685] Zhong D, Wang H, Liu M, et al. Ganoderma lucidum polysaccharide peptide prevents renal ischemia reperfusion injury via counteracting oxidative stress. *Sci Rep.* 2015 Nov 25;5:16910.

[3686] Zhang JJ, Qin FY, Meng XH, et al. Renoprotective ganodermaones A and B with rearranged meroterpenoid carbon skelotons from Ganoderma fungi. *Bioorg Chem.* 2020 Jul;100:103930.

[3687] Shao G, He J, Meng J, et al. Ganoderic Acids Prevent Renal Ischemia Reperfusion Injury by Inhibiting Inflammation and Apoptosis. *Int J Mol Sci.* 2021 Sep 23;22(19):10229.

[3688] Peng YL, Wang YX, Cheng YX. Isolation and characterization of dihydropyran-ring containing meroterpenoids from Ganoderma lucidum and their inhibitory activity against renal fibrosis-related protein expression. *Phytochemistry.* 2023 Oct;214:113799.

[3689] Geng XQ, Ma A, He JZ, et al. Ganoderic acid hinders renal fibrosis via suppressing the TGF-β/Smad and MAPK signaling pathways. *Acta Pharmacol Sin.* 2020 May;41(5):670-677.

[3690] Fang H, Li X, Lin D, et al. Inhibition of intrarenal PRR-RAS pathway by Ganoderma lucidum polysaccharide peptides in proteinuric nephropathy. *Int J Biol Macromol.* 2023 Oct 16;253(Pt 7):127336.

[3691] Futrakul N, Panichakul T, Butthep P, et al. Ganoderma lucidum suppresses endothelial cell cytotoxicity and proteinuria in persistent proteinuric focal segmental glomerulosclerosis (FSGS) nephrosis. *Clin Hemorheol Microcirc.* 2004;31(4):267-72.

[3692] Futrakul N, Boongen M, Tosukhowong P, et al. Treatment with vasodilators and crude extract of Ganoderma lucidum suppresses proteinuria in nephrosis with focal segmental glomerulosclerosis. *Nephron.* 2002;92(3):719-20.

[3693] Su L, Liu L, Jia Y, et al. Ganoderma triterpenes retard renal cyst development by downregulating Ras/MAPK signaling and promoting cell differentiation. *Kidney Int.* 2017 Dec;92(6):1404-1418.

[3694] Hossain S, Bhowmick S, Islam S, et al. Oral Administration of Ganoderma lucidum to Lead-Exposed Rats Protects Erythrocytes against Hemolysis: Implicates to Anti-Anemia. *Evid Based Complement Alternat Med.* 2015;2015:463703.

[3695] Seo HW, Hung TM, Na M, et al. Steroids and triterpenes from the fruit bodies of Ganoderma lucidum and their anti-complement activity. *Arch Pharm Res.* 2009 Nov;32(11):1573-9.

[3696] Min BS, Gao JJ, Hattori M, et al. Anticomplement activity of terpenoids from the spores of Ganoderma lucidum. *Planta Med.* 2001 Dec;67(9):811-4.

[3697] Wang Q, Huang Y, Wu B, et al. Inhibitive effect on apoptosis in splenic lymphocytes of mice pretreated with lingzhi (Ganoderma lucidum) spores. *J Tradit Chin Med.* 2014 Apr;34(2):173-7.

[3698] Liang Z, Yuan Z, Guo J, et al. Ganoderma lucidum Polysaccharides Prevent Palmitic Acid-Evoked Apoptosis and Autophagy in Intestinal Porcine Epithelial Cell Line via Restoration of Mitochondrial Function and Regulation of MAPK and AMPK/Akt/mTOR Signaling Pathway. *Int J Mol Sci.* 2019 Jan 23;20(3):478.

[3699] Chen J, Shi Y, He L, et al. Protective roles of polysaccharides from Ganoderma lucidum on bleomycin-induced pulmonary fibrosis in rats. *Int J Biol Macromol.* 2016 Nov;92:278-281.

[3700] Zhan L, Tang J, Lin S, et al. Prophylactic Use of Ganoderma lucidum Extract May Inhibit Mycobacterium tuberculosis Replication in a New Mouse Model of Spontaneous Latent Tuberculosis Infection. *Front Microbiol.* 2016 Jan 8;6:1490.

[3701] Liu H, Qiu F, Wang Y, et al. A recombinant protein rLZ-8, originally extracted from Ganoderma lucidum, ameliorates OVA-induced lung inflammation by regulating Th17/Treg balance. *J Leukoc Biol.* 2020 Aug;108(2):531-545.

3702 Liu C, Yang N, Song Y, et al. Ganoderic acid C1 isolated from the anti-asthma formula, ASHMI™ suppresses TNF-α production by mouse macrophages and peripheral blood mononuclear cells from asthma patients. *Int Immunopharmacol.* 2015 Aug;27(2):224-31.

3703 Zhang X, Wu D, Tian Y, et al. Ganoderma lucidum polysaccharides ameliorate lipopolysaccharide-induced acute pneumonia via inhibiting NRP1-mediated inflammation. *Pharm Biol.* 2022 Dec;60(1):2201-2209.

3704 Liu J, Shiono J, Shimizu K, et al. Ganoderic acids from Ganoderma lucidum: inhibitory activity of osteoclastic differentiation and structural criteria. *Planta Med.* 2010 Feb;76(2):137-9.

3705 Tran PT, Dat NT, Dang NH, et al. Ganomycin I from Ganoderma lucidum attenuates RANKL-mediated osteoclastogenesis by inhibiting MAPKs and NFATc1. *Phytomedicine.* 2019 Mar 1;55:1-8.

3706 Miyamoto I, Liu J, Shimizu K, et al. Regulation of osteoclastogenesis by ganoderic acid DM isolated from Ganoderma lucidum. *Eur J Pharmacol.* 2009 Jan 5;602(1):1-7.

3707 Yang Y, Yang B. Anti-osteoporosis Effect of Ganoderma (Lingzhi) by Inhibition of Osteoclastogenesis. *Adv Exp Med Biol.* 2019;1182:263-269.

3708 Yang Y, Yu T, Tang H, et al. Ganoderma lucidum Immune Modulator Protein rLZ-8 Could Prevent and Reverse Bone Loss in Glucocorticoids-Induced Osteoporosis Rat Model. *Front Pharmacol.* 2020 May 19;11:731.

3709 Wang YQ, Wang NX, Luo Y, et al. Ganoderal A effectively induces osteogenic differentiation of human amniotic mesenchymal stem cells via cross-talk between Wnt/β-catenin and BMP/SMAD signaling pathways. *Biomed Pharmacother.* 2020 Mar;123:109807.

3710 Laçin N, İzol SB, İpek F, et al. Ganoderma lucidum, a promising agent possessing antioxidant and anti-inflammatory effects for treating calvarial defects with graft application in rats. *Acta Cir Bras.* 2019 Nov 25;34(9):e201900904.

3711 Ghajari G, Nabiuni M, Amini E. The association between testicular toxicity induced by Li2Co3 and protective effect of Ganoderma lucidum: Alteration of Bax & c-Kit genes expression. *Tissue Cell.* 2021 Oct;72:101552.

3712 Bin-Jumah MN, Nadeem MS, Gilani SJ, et al. Novelkaraya gum micro-particles loaded Ganoderma lucidum polysaccharide regulate sex hormones, oxidative stress and inflammatory cytokine levels in cadmium induced testicular toxicity in experimental animals. *Int J Biol Macromol.* 2022 Jan 1;194:338-346.

3713 Li Y, Liang W, Han Y, et al. Triterpenoids and Polysaccharides from Ganoderma lucidum Improve the Histomorphology and Function of Testes in Middle-Aged Male Mice by Alleviating Oxidative Stress and Cellular Apoptosis. *Nutrients.* 2022 Nov 9;14(22):4733.

3714 Wu M, Huang B, Hu L, et al. Ganoderma lucidum polysaccharides ameliorates D-galactose-induced aging salivary secretion disorders by upregulating the rhythm and aquaporins. *Exp Gerontol.* 2023 May;175:112147.

3715 Cuong VT, Chen W, Shi J, et al. The anti-oxidation and anti-aging effects of Ganoderma lucidum in Caenorhabditis elegans. *Exp Gerontol.* 2019 Mar;117:99-105.

3716 Weng Y, Lu J, Xiang L, et al. Ganodermasides C and D, two new anti-aging ergosterols from spores of the medicinal mushroom Ganoderma lucidum. *Biosci Biotechnol Biochem.* 2011;75(4):800-3.

3717 Peng HH, Wu CY, Hsiao YC, et al. Ganoderma lucidum stimulates autophagy-dependent longevity pathways in Caenorhabditis elegans and human cells. *Aging (Albany NY).* 2021 May 20;13(10):13474-13495.

3718 Xu Y, Yuan H, Luo Y, et al. Ganoderic Acid D Protects Human Amniotic Mesenchymal Stem Cells against Oxidative Stress-Induced Senescence through the PERK/NRF2 Signaling Pathway. *Oxid Med Cell Longev.* 2020 Jul 27;2020:8291413.

3719 Xie L, Zhong X, Liu D, et al. The effects of freeze-dried Ganoderma lucidum mycelia on a recurrent oral ulceration rat model. *BMC Complement Altern Med.* 2017 Dec 1;17(1):511.

3720 Park JH, Jang KJ, Kim CH, et al. Ganoderma lucidum Pharmacopuncture for the Treatment of Acute Gastric Ulcers in Rats. *J Pharmacopuncture.* 2014 Sep;17(3):40-9.

3721 Tian B, Zhao Q, Xing H, et al. Gastroprotective Effects of Ganoderma lucidum Polysaccharides with Different Molecular Weights on Ethanol-Induced Acute Gastric Injury in Rats. *Nutrients.* 2022 Apr 1;14(7):1476.

3722 Li JP, Chu CL, Chao WR, et al. Ling Zhi-8, a fungal immunomodulatory protein in Ganoderma lucidum, alleviates CPT-11-induced intestinal injury via restoring claudin-1 expression. *Aging (Albany NY).* 2023 May 5;15(9):3621-3634.

3723 Park JH, Jang KJ, Kim CH, et al. Ganoderma lucidum Pharmacopuncture for Teating Ethanol-induced Chronic Gastric Ulcers in Rats. *J Pharmacopuncture.* 2015 Mar;18(1):72-8.

3724 Nagai K, Ueno Y, Tanaka S, et al. Polysaccharides derived from Ganoderma lucidum fungus mycelia ameliorate indomethacin-induced small intestinal injury via induction of GM-CSF from macrophages. *Cell Immunol.* 2017 Oct;320:20-28.

3725 Lin D, Zhang Y, Wang S, et al. Ganoderma lucidum polysaccharide peptides GL-PPSQ2 alleviate intestinal ischemia-reperfusion injury via inhibiting cytotoxic neutrophil extracellular traps. *Int J Biol Macromol.* 2023 Jul 31;244:125370.

3726 Gao Y, Tang W, Gao H, et al. Ganoderma lucidum polysaccharide fractions accelerate healing of acetic acid-induced ulcers in rats. *J Med Food.* 2004 Winter;7(4):417-21.

3727 Gao Y, Zhou S, Wen J, et al. Mechanism of the antiulcerogenic effect of Ganoderma lucidum polysaccharides on indomethacin-induced lesions in the rat. *Life Sci.* 2002 Dec 27;72(6):731-45.

3728 Xie J, Liu Y, Chen B, et al. Ganoderma lucidum polysaccharide improves rat DSS-induced colitis by altering cecal microbiota and gene expression of colonic epithelial cells. *Food Nutr Res.* 2019 Feb 12;63.

3729 Hanaoka R, Ueno Y, Tanaka S, et al. The water-soluble extract from cultured medium of Ganoderma lucidum (Reishi) mycelia (Designated as MAK) ameliorates murine colitis induced by trinitrobenzene sulphonic acid. *Scand J Immunol.* 2011 Nov;74(5):454-62.

3730 Özden H, Şahin Y, Kilitçi A, et al. Comparison of the healing effects of mesazaline and Ganoderma lucidum in acetic acid-induced colitis in rats. *Ann Surg Treat Res.* 2022 Jan;102(1):29-35.

3731 Liu L, Feng J, Jiang S, et al. Anti-inflammatory and intestinal microbiota modulation properties of Ganoderma lucidum β-d-glucans with different molecular weight in an ulcerative colitis model. *Int J Biol Macromol.* 2023 Aug 18;251:126351.

3732 Zhao Y, Zhu L. Oral Lingzhi or Reishi Medicinal Mushroom Ganoderma lucidum (Agaricomycetes) Spore Powder Ameliorates Murine Colitis by Inhibiting Key Kinases Phosphorylation in MAPK Pathway. *Int J Med Mushrooms.* 2023;25(10):39-48.

3733 Li M, Yu L, Zhai Q, et al. Ganoderma lucidum Ethanol Extraction Promotes Dextran Sulphate Sodium Induced Colitis Recovery and Modulation in Microbiota. *Foods*. 2022 Dec 13;11(24):4023.

3734 Chen YH, Shin JY, Wei HM, et al. Prevention of dextran sulfate sodium-induced mouse colitis by the fungal protein Ling Zhi-8 via promoting the barrier function of intestinal epithelial cells. *Food Funct*. 2021 Mar 1;12(4):1639-1650.

3735 Wei B, Zhang R, Zhai J, et al. Suppression of Th17 Cell Response in the Alleviation of Dextran Sulfate Sodium-Induced Colitis by Ganoderma lucidum Polysaccharides. *J Immunol Res*. 2018 May 20;2018:2906494.

3736 Xie J, Liu Y, Chen B, et al. Ganoderma lucidum polysaccharide improves rat DSS-induced colitis by altering cecal microbiota and gene expression of colonic epithelial cells. *Food Nutr Res*. 2019 Feb 12;63.

3737 Hanaoka R, Ueno Y, Tanaka S, et al. The water-soluble extract from cultured medium of Ganoderma lucidum (Reishi) mycelia (Designated as MAK) ameliorates murine colitis induced by trinitrobenzene sulphonic acid. *Scand J Immunol*. 2011 Nov;74(5):454-62.

3738 Talih G, Kantekin ÇÜ, Göçmen Y, et al. Effect of Lingzhi or Reishi Medicinal Mushroom, Ganoderma lucidum (Agaricomycetes), Capsules on Colistin-Induced Nephrotoxicity. *Int J Med Mushrooms*. 2020;22(5):445-453.

3739 Sliva D, Loganathan J, Jiang J, et al. Mushroom Ganoderma lucidum prevents colitis-associated carcinogenesis in mice. *PLoS One*. 2012;7(10):e47873.

3740 Cui XY, Cui SY, Zhang J, et al. Extract of Ganoderma lucidum prolongs sleep time in rats. *J Ethnopharmacol*. 2012 Feb 15;139(3):796-800.

3741 Feng X, Wang Y. Anti-inflammatory, anti-nociceptive and sedative-hypnotic activities of lucidone D extracted from Ganoderma lucidum. *Cell Mol Biol (Noisy-le-grand)*. 2019 Apr 30;65(4):37-42.

3742 Hossen SMM, Yusuf ATM, Emon NU, et al. Biochemical and Pharmacological aspects of Ganoderma lucidum: Exponent from the in vivo and computational investigations. *Biochem Biophys Rep*. 2022 Nov 7;32:101371.

3743 Yao C, Wang Z, Jiang H, et al. Ganoderma lucidum promotes sleep through a gut microbiota-dependent and serotonin-involved pathway in mice. *Sci Rep*. 2021 Jul 1;11(1):13660.

3744 Zhonghui Z, Xiaowei Z, Fang F. Ganoderma lucidum polysaccharides supplementation attenuates exercise-induced oxidative stress in skeletal muscle of mice. *Saudi J Biol Sci*. 2014 Apr;21(2):119-23.

3745 Guo SS, Cui XL, Rausch WD. Ganoderma Lucidum polysaccharides protect against MPP(+) and rotenone-induced apoptosis in primary dopaminergic cell cultures through inhibiting oxidative stress. *Am J Neurodegener Dis*. 2016 Jun 1;5(2):131-44.

3746 Pan Y, Yuan S, Teng Y, et al. Antioxidation of a proteoglycan from Ganoderma lucidum protects pancreatic β-cells against oxidative stress-induced apoptosis in vitro and in vivo. *Int J Biol Macromol*. 2022 Mar 1;200:470-486.

3747 Sudheesh NP, Ajith TA, Mathew J, et al. Ganoderma lucidum protects liver mitochondrial oxidative stress and improves the activity of electron transport chain in carbon tetrachloride intoxicated rats. *Hepatol Res*. 2012 Feb;42(2):181-91.

3748 Lee YH, Kim JH, Song CH, et al. Ethanol Extract of Ganoderma lucidum Augments Cellular Anti-oxidant Defense through Activation of Nrf2/HO-1. *J Pharmacopuncture*. 2016 Mar;19(1):59-69.

3749 Levin RM, Xia L, Wei W, et al. Effects of Ganoderma Lucidum shell-broken spore on oxidative stress of the rabbit urinary bladder using an in vivo model of ischemia/reperfusion. *Mol Cell Biochem*. 2017 Nov;435(1-2):25-35.

3750 Yang Q, Wang S, Xie Y, et al. HPLC analysis of Ganoderma lucidum polysaccharides and its effect on antioxidant enzymes activity and Bax, Bcl-2 expression. *Int J Biol Macromol*. 2010 Mar 1;46(2):167-72.

3751 Xing Z, Zhang C, Zhao C, et al. Targeting oxidative stress using tri-needle electrospray engineered Ganoderma lucidum polysaccharide-loaded porous yolk-shell particles. *Eur J Pharm Sci*. 2018 Dec 1;125:64-73.

3752 Li R, Zhang L, Tang Z, et al. Effects of Fungal Polysaccharide on Oxidative Damage and TLR4 Pathway to the Central Immune Organs in Cadmium Intoxication in Chickens. *Biol Trace Elem Res*. 2019 Oct;191(2):464-473.

3753 You YH, Lin ZB. Protective effects of Ganoderma lucidum polysaccharides peptide on injury of macrophages induced by reactive oxygen species. *Acta Pharmacol Sin*. 2002 Sep;23(9):787-91.

3754 Ding W, Zhang X, Yin X, et al. Ganoderma lucidum aqueous extract inducing PHGPx to inhibit membrane lipid hydroperoxides and regulate oxidative stress based on single-cell animal transcriptome. *Sci Rep*. 2022 Feb 24;12(1):3139.

3755 Chang SS, Zhou D, Meng GL, et al. [Effect of Ganoderma lucidum polysaccharides on oxidative stress of hyperlipidemic fatty liver in rats]. *Zhongguo Zhong Yao Za Zhi*. 2012 Oct;37(20):3102-6.

3756 Johra FT, Hossain S, Jain P, et al. Amelioration of CCl4-induced oxidative stress and hepatotoxicity by Ganoderma lucidum in long evans rats. *Sci Rep*. 2023 Jun 19;13(1):9909.

3757 Hossen SMM, Hossain MS, Yusuf ATM, et al. Profiling of phytochemical and antioxidant activity of wild mushrooms: Evidence from the in vitro study and phytoconstituent's binding affinity to the human erythrocyte catalase and human glutathione reductase. *Food Sci Nutr*. 2021 Nov 2;10(1):88-102.

3758 Tulsawani R, Sharma P, Manimaran M, et al. Effects of Extraction Temperature on Efficacy of Lingzhi or Reishi Medicinal Mushroom, Ganoderma lucidum (Agaricomycetes), Aqueous Extract against Oxidative Stress. *Int J Med Mushrooms*. 2020;22(6):547-558.

3759 Wu JG, Kan YJ, Wu YB, et al. Hepatoprotective effect of ganoderma triterpenoids against oxidative damage induced by tert-butyl hydroperoxide in human hepatic HepG2 cells. *Pharm Biol*. 2016;54(5):919-29.

3760 Tsai IL, Tsai CY, Kuo LL, et al. PLGA nanoparticles containing Lingzhi extracts rescue corneal epithelial cells from oxidative damage. *Exp Eye Res*. 2021 May;206:108539.

3761 Lai KN, Chan LY, Tang SC, et al. Ganoderma extract prevents albumin-induced oxidative damage and chemokines synthesis in cultured human proximal tubular epithelial cells. *Nephrol Dial Transplant*. 2006 May;21(5):1188-97.

3762 Yuan H, Xu Y, Luo Y, et al. Ganoderic acid D prevents oxidative stress-induced senescence by targeting 14-3-3ε to activate CaM/CaMKII/NRF2 signaling pathway in mesenchymal stem cells. *Aging Cell*. 2022 Sep;21(9):e13686.

3763 Çelik B, Özparlak H. Determination of genotoxic and antigenotoxic effects of wild-grown Reishi mushroom (Ganoderma lucidum) using the hen's egg test for analysis of micronucleus induction. *Biotech Histochem*. 2019 Nov;94(8):628-636.

3764 Lee JM, Kwon H, Jeong H, et al. Inhibition of lipid peroxidation and oxidative DNA damage by Ganoderma lucidum. *Phytother Res*. 2001 May;15(3):245-9.

3765 Pillai TG, Maurya DK, Salvi VP, et al. Fungal beta glucan protects radiation induced DNA damage in human lymphocytes. *Ann Transl Med*. 2014 Feb;2(2):13.

3766 Lakshmi B, Ajith TA, Jose N, et al. Antimutagenic activity of methanolic extract of Ganoderma lucidum and its effect on hepatic damage caused by benzo[a]pyrene. *J Ethnopharmacol*. 2006 Sep 19;107(2):297-303.

3767 Wachtel-Galor S, Choi SW, Benzie IF. Effect of Ganoderma lucidum on human DNA is dose dependent and mediated by hydrogen peroxide. *Redox Rep*. 2005;10(3):145-9.

3768 Lakshmi B, Ajith TA, Sheena N, et al. Antiperoxidative, anti-inflammatory, and antimutagenic activities of ethanol extract of the mycelium of Ganoderma lucidum occurring in South India. *Teratog Carcinog Mutagen*. 2003;Suppl 1:85-97.

3769 Cilerdzic J, Stajic M, Zivkovic L, et al. Genoprotective Capacity of Alternatively Cultivated Lingzhi or Reishi Medicinal Mushroom, Ganoderma lucidum (Agaricomycetes), Basidiocarps. *Int J Med Mushrooms*. 2016;18(12):1061-1069.

3770 Hsu HY, Lian SL, Lin CC. Radioprotective effect of Ganoderma lucidum (Leyss. ex. Fr.) Karst after X-ray irradiation in mice. *Am J Chin Med*. 1990;18(1-2):61-9.

3771 Yu C, Fu J, Guo L, et al. UPLC-MS-based serum metabolomics reveals protective effect of Ganoderma lucidum polysaccharide on ionizing radiation injury. *J Ethnopharmacol*. 2020 Aug 10;258:112814.

3772 Pillai TG, Nair CK, Janardhanan KK. Polysaccharides isolated from Ganoderma lucidum occurring in Southern parts of India, protects radiation induced damages both in vitro and in vivo. *Environ Toxicol Pharmacol*. 2008 Jul;26(1):80-5.

3773 Chen WC, Hau DM, Wang CC, et al. Effects of Ganoderma lucidum and krestin on subset T-cell in spleen of gamma-irradiated mice. *Am J Chin Med*. 1995;23(3-4):289-98.

3774 Chen WC, Hau DM, Lee SS. Effects of Ganoderma lucidum and krestin on cellular immunocompetence in gamma-ray-irradiated mice. *Am J Chin Med*. 1995;23(1):71-80.

3775 Smina TP, De S, Devasagayam TP, et al. Ganoderma lucidum total triterpenes prevent radiation-induced DNA damage and apoptosis in splenic lymphocytes in vitro. *Mutat Res*. 2011 Dec 24;726(2):188-94.

3776 Smina TP, Joseph J, Janardhanan KK. Ganoderma lucidum total triterpenes prevent γ-radiation induced oxidative stress in Swiss albino mice in vivo. *Redox Rep*. 2016 Nov;21(6):254-61.

3777 Smina TP, Maurya DK, Devasagayam TP, et al. Protection of radiation induced DNA and membrane damages by total triterpenes isolated from Ganoderma lucidum (Fr.) P. Karst. *Chem Biol Interact*. 2015 May 25;233:1-7.

3778 Cilerdžić J, Vukojević J, Stajić M, et al. Biological activity of Ganoderma lucidum basidiocarps cultivated on alternative and commercial substrate. *J Ethnopharmacol*. 2014 Aug 8;155(1):312-9.

3779 Zhao Y, Li Q, Wang M, et al. Structural characterization of polysaccharides after fermentation from Ganoderma lucidum and its antioxidant activity in HepG2 cells induced by H2O2. *Food Chem X*. 2023 Apr 23;18:100682.

3780 Sarnthima R, Khammaung S, Sa-Ard P. Culture broth of Ganoderma lucidum exhibited antioxidant, antibacterial and α-amylase inhibitory activities. *J Food Sci Technol*. 2017 Oct;54(11):3724-3730.

3781 Lin Z, Deng A. Antioxidative and Free Radical Scavenging Activity of Ganoderma (Lingzhi). *Adv Exp Med Biol*. 2019;1182:271-297.

3782 Fraile-Fabero R, Ozcariz-Fermoselle MV, Oria-de-Rueda-Salgueiro JA, et al. Differences in Antioxidants, Polyphenols, Protein Digestibility and Nutritional Profile between Ganoderma lingzhi from Industrial Crops in Asia and Ganoderma lucidum from Cultivation and Iberian Origin. *Foods*. 2021 Jul 29;10(8):1750.

3783 Veljović S, Veljović M, Nikićević N, et al. Chemical composition, antiproliferative and antioxidant activity of differently processed Ganoderma lucidum ethanol extracts. *J Food Sci Technol*. 2017 Apr;54(5):1312-1320.

3784 Liu SR, Zhang WR. Hyperproduction of exopolysaccharides by submerged mycelial culture of Ganoderma lucidum using a solid seed grown in fine-powder of wheat bran and in vitro evaluation of the antioxidant activity of the exopolysaccharides produced. *Food Sci Biotechnol*. 2018 Feb 28;27(4):1129-1136.

3785 Chen Y, Lan P. Total Syntheses and Biological Evaluation of the Ganoderma lucidum Alkaloids Lucidimines B and C. *ACS Omega*. 2018 Mar 31;3(3):3471-3481.

3786 Zeng X, Li P, Chen X, et al. Effects of deproteinization methods on primary structure and antioxidant activity of Ganoderma lucidum polysaccharides. *Int J Biol Macromol*. 2019 Apr 1;126:867-876.

3787 Zhang J, Meng G, Zhai G, et al. Extraction, characterization and antioxidant activity of polysaccharides of spent mushroom compost of Ganoderma lucidum. *Int J Biol Macromol*. 2016 Jan;82:432-9.

3788 Saltarelli R, Palma F, Gioacchini AM, et al. Phytochemical composition, antioxidant and antiproliferative activities and effects on nuclear DNA of ethanolic extract from an Italian mycelial isolate of Ganoderma lucidum. *J Ethnopharmacol*. 2019 Mar 1;231:464-473.

3789 Deepalakshmi K, Mirunalini S, Krishnaveni M, et al. In vitro and in vivo antioxidant potentials of an ethanolic extract of Ganoderma lucidum in rat mammary carcinogenesis. *Chin J Nat Med*. 2013 Nov;11(6):621-7.

3790 Park M, Kim M. Analysis of Antioxidant and Anti-Inflammatory Activities of Solvent Fractions from Rhynchosia nulubilis Cultivated with Ganoderma lucidum Mycelium. *Prev Nutr Food Sci*. 2017 Dec;22(4):365-371.

3791 Chien YL, Ho CT, Chiang BH, et al. Effect of fermentation time on antioxidative activities of Ganoderma lucidum broth using leguminous plants as part of the liquid fermentation medium. *Food Chem*. 2011 Jun 15;126(4):1586-92.

3792 Tel G, Ozturk M, Duru ME, et al. Antioxidant and anticholinesterase activities of five wild mushroom species with total bioactive contents. *Pharm Biol*. 2015 Jun;53(6):824-30.

3793 Tan X, Sun J, Xu Z, et al. Effect of heat stress on production and in-vitro antioxidant activity of polysaccharides in Ganoderma lucidum. *Bioprocess Biosyst Eng*. 2018 Jan;41(1):135-141.

3794 Vaithanomsat P, Boonlum N, Chaiyana W, et al. Mushroom β-Glucan Recovered from Antler-Type Fruiting Body of Ganoderma lucidum by Enzymatic Process and Its Potential Biological Activities for Cosmeceutical Applications. *Polymers (Basel)*. 2022 Oct 7;14(19):4202.

3795 Kang Q, Chen S, Li S, et al. Comparison on characterization and antioxidant activity of polysaccharides from Ganoderma lucidum by ultrasound and conventional extraction. *Int J Biol Macromol*. 2019 Mar 1;124:1137-1144.

3796 Kan Y, Chen T, Wu Y, et al. Antioxidant activity of polysaccharide extracted from Ganoderma lucidum using response surface methodology. *Int J Biol Macromol*. 2015 Jan;72:151-7.

3797 Wang J, Wang Y, Liu X, et al. Free radical scavenging and immunomodulatory activities of Ganoderma lucidum polysaccharides derivatives. *Carbohydr Polym*. 2013 Jan 2;91(1):33-8.

3798 Zhu M, Chang Q, Wong LK, et al. Triterpene antioxidants from ganoderma lucidum. *Phytother Res*. 1999 Sep;13(6):529-31.

3799 Sudheer S, Alzorqi I, Ali A, et al. Determination of the Biological Efficiency and Antioxidant Potential of Lingzhi or Reishi Medicinal Mushroom, Ganoderma lucidum (Agaricomycetes), Cultivated Using Different Agro-Wastes in Malaysia. *Int J Med Mushrooms*. 2018;20(1):89-100.

3800 Sa-Ard P, Sarnthima R, Khammuang S, et al. Antioxidant, antibacterial and DNA protective activities of protein extracts from Ganoderma lucidum. *J Food Sci Technol*. 2015 May;52(5):2966-73.

3801 Yegenoglu H, Aslim B, Oke F. Comparison of antioxidant capacities of Ganoderma lucidum (Curtis) P. Karst and Funalia trogii (Berk.) Bondartsev & Singer by using different in vitro methods. *J Med Food*. 2011 May;14(5):512-6.

3802 Huang Q, Wang L, Zhang L, et al. Antioxidant Properties of Triterpenoids Isolated from Bagasse-Cultivated Lingzhi or Reishi Medicinal Mushroom, Ganoderma lucidum (Agaricomycetes), at Different Developmental Stages. *Int J Med Mushrooms*. 2022;24(7):41-51.

3803 Zheng S, Zhang W, Liu S. Optimization of ultrasonic-assisted extraction of polysaccharides and triterpenoids from the medicinal mushroom Ganoderma lucidum and evaluation of their in vitro antioxidant capacities. *PLoS One*. 2020 Dec 31;15(12):e0244749.

3804 Mohsin M, Negi P, Ahmed Z. Determination of the antioxidant activity and polyphenol contents of wild Lingzhi or Reishi medicinal mushroom, Ganoderma lucidum (W.Curt. Fr.) P. Karst. (higher Basidiomycetes) from central Himalayan hills of India. *Int J Med Mushrooms*. 2011;13(6):535-44.

3805 Smina TP, Mathew J, Janardhanan KK, et al. Antioxidant activity and toxicity profile of total triterpenes isolated from Ganoderma lucidum (Fr.) P. Karst occurring in South India. *Environ Toxicol Pharmacol*. 2011 Nov;32(3):438-46.

3806 Ryu DH, Cho JY, Sadiq NB, et al. Optimization of antioxidant, anti-diabetic, and anti-inflammatory activities and ganoderic acid content of differentially dried Ganoderma lucidum using response surface methodology. *Food Chem*. 2021 Jan 15;335:127645.

3807 Shi M, Zhang Z, Yang Y. Antioxidant and immunoregulatory activity of Ganoderma lucidum polysaccharide (GLP). *Carbohydr Polym*. 2013 Jun 5;95(1):200-6.

3808 Liang Z, Yi Y, Guo Y, et al. Chemical characterization and antitumor activities of polysaccharide extracted from Ganoderma lucidum. *Int J Mol Sci*. 2014 May 22;15(5):9103-16.

3809 Rani P, Lal MR, Maheshwari U, et al. Antioxidant Potential of Lingzhi or Reishi Medicinal Mushroom, Ganoderma lucidum (Higher Basidiomycetes) Cultivated on Artocarpus heterophyllus Sawdust Substrate in India. *Int J Med Mushrooms*. 2015;17(12):1171-7.

3810 Ren X, Wang J, Huang L, et al. Comparative Studies on Bioactive Compounds, Ganoderic Acid Biosynthesis, and Antioxidant Activity of Pileus and Stipes of Lingzhi or Reishi Medicinal Mushroom, Ganoderma lucidum (Agaricomycetes) Fruiting Body at Different Growth Stages. *Int J Med Mushrooms*. 2020;22(2):133-144.

3811 Zhao W, Jiang X, Deng W, et al. Antioxidant activities of Ganoderma lucidum polysaccharides and their role on DNA damage in mice induced by cobalt-60 gamma-irradiation. *Food Chem Toxicol*. 2012 Feb;50(2):303-9.

3812 Liu W, Wang H, Pang X, et al. Characterization and antioxidant activity of two low-molecular-weight polysaccharides purified from the fruiting bodies of Ganoderma lucidum. *Int J Biol Macromol*. 2010 May 1;46(4):451-7.

3813 Lakshmi B, Ajith TA, Sheena N, et al. Antiperoxidative, anti-inflammatory, and antimutagenic activities of ethanol extract of the mycelium of Ganoderma lucidum occurring in South India. *Teratog Carcinog Mutagen*. 2003;Suppl 1:85-97.

3814 Sun J, He H, Xie BJ. Novel antioxidant peptides from fermented mushroom Ganoderma lucidum. *J Agric Food Chem*. 2004 Oct 20;52(21):6646-52.

3815 Cherian E, Sudheesh NP, Janardhanan KK, et al. Free-radical scavenging and mitochondrial antioxidant activities of Reishi-Ganoderma lucidum (Curt: Fr) P. Karst and Arogyapacha-Trichopus zeylanicus Gaertn extracts. *J Basic Clin Physiol Pharmacol*. 2009;20(4):289-307.

3816 Lou HW, Guo XY, Zhang XC, et al. Optimization of Cultivation Conditions of Lingzhi or Reishi Medicinal Mushroom, Ganoderma lucidum (Agaricomycetes) for the Highest Antioxidant Activity and Antioxidant Content. *Int J Med Mushrooms*. 2019;21(4):353-366.

3817 Xie C, Tang P, Yan S, et al. Comparative Study on Bioactivities from Lingzhi or Reishi Medicinal Mushroom, Ganoderma lucidum (Agaricomycetes), Gives an Insight into the Fermentation Broth Showing Greater Antioxidative Activities. *Int J Med Mushrooms*. 2020;22(7):627-639.

3818 Kebaili FF, Tahar N, Esseddik TM, et al. Antioxidant Activity and Phenolic Content of Extracts of Wild Algerian Lingzhi or Reishi Medicinal Mushroom, Ganoderma lucidum (Agaricomycetes). *Int J Med Mushrooms*. 2021;23(6):79-88.

3819 Wu Y, Wang D. A new class of natural glycopeptides with sugar moiety-dependent antioxidant activities derived from Ganoderma lucidum fruiting bodies. *J Proteome Res*. 2009 Feb;8(2):436-42.

3820 Savin S, Craciunescu O, Oancea A, et al. Antioxidant, Cytotoxic and Antimicrobial Activity of Chitosan Preparations Extracted from Ganoderma Lucidum Mushroom. *Chem Biodivers*. 2020 Jul;17(7):e2000175.

3821 Milovanovic I, Zengin G, Maksimovic S, et al. Supercritical carbon-oxide extracts from cultivated and wild-grown Ganoderma lucidum mushroom: differences in ergosterol and ganoderic acids content, antioxidative and enzyme inhibitory properties. *Nat Prod Res*. 2023 Feb 6:1-7.

3822 Wang ZX, Li N, Xu JW. Effects of Efficient Expression of Vitreoscilla Hemoglobin on Production, Monosaccharide Composition, and Antioxidant Activity of Exopolysaccharides in Ganoderma lucidum. *Microorganisms*. 2021 Jul 21;9(8):1551.

3823 Karaman M, Jovin E, Malbasa R, et al. Medicinal and edible lignicolous fungi as natural sources of antioxidative and antibacterial agents. *Phytother Res*. 2010 Oct;24(10):1473-81.

3824 Kim MY, Seguin P, Ahn JK, et al. Phenolic compound concentration and antioxidant activities of edible and medicinal mushrooms from Korea. *J Agric Food Chem*. 2008 Aug 27;56(16):7265-70.

3825 Mau JL, Lin HC, Chen CC. Antioxidant properties of several medicinal mushrooms. *J Agric Food Chem*. 2002 Oct 9;50(21):6072-7.

3826 Saltarelli R, Ceccaroli P, Buffalini M, et al. Biochemical characterization and antioxidant and antiproliferative activities of different Ganoderma collections. *J Mol Microbiol Biotechnol.* 2015;25(1):16-25.

3827 Aursuwanna T, Noitang S, Sangtanoo P, et al. Investigating the cellular antioxidant and anti-inflammatory effects of the novel peptides in lingzhi mushrooms. *Heliyon.* 2022 Oct 13;8(10):e11067.

3828 Sudheesh NP, Ajith TA, Ramnath V, et al. Therapeutic potential of Ganoderma lucidum (Fr.) P. Karst. against the declined antioxidant status in the mitochondria of post-mitotic tissues of aged mice. *Clin Nutr.* 2010 Jun;29(3):406-12.

3829 Chung WY, Yow CM, Benzie IF. Assessment of membrane protection by traditional Chinese medicines using a flow cytometric technique: preliminary findings. *Redox Rep.* 2003;8(1):31-3.

3830 Sharma P, Tulsawani R, Agrawal U. Pharmacological effects of Ganoderma lucidum extract against high-altitude stressors and its subchronic toxicity assessment. *J Food Biochem.* 2019 Dec;43(12):e13081.

3831 Koganti P, Tulsawani R, Sharma P, et al. Role of Hydroalcoholic Extract of Lingzhi or Reishi Medicinal Mushroom, Ganoderma lucidum (Agaricomycetes), in Facilitating Cellular Acclimatization in a Low-Oxygen Microenvironment. *Int J Med Mushrooms.* 2018;20(5):431-444.

3832 Jatwani A, Tulsawani R. Ganoderma lucidum Induces Myogenesis Markers to Avert Damage to Skeletal Muscles in Rats Exposed to Hypobaric Hypoxia. High Alt Med Biol. 2021 Jun 17. Online ahead of print.

3833 Sudheesh NP, Ajith TA, Janardhanan KK. Ganoderma lucidum (Fr.) P. Karst enhances activities of heart mitochondrial enzymes and respiratory chain complexes in the aged rat. *Biogerontology.* 2009 Oct;10(5):627-36.

3834 Cai M, Xing H, Tian B, et al. Characteristics and antifatigue activity of graded polysaccharides from Ganoderma lucidum separated by cascade membrane technology. *Carbohydr Polym.* 2021 Oct 1;269:118329.

3835 Doğan G, İpek H. The protective effect of Ganoderma lucidum on testicular torsion/detorsion-induced ischemia-reperfusion (I/R) injury. *Acta Cir Bras.* 2020 Mar 20;35(1):e202000103.

3836 Ouyang MZ, Lin LZ, Lv WJ, et al. Effects of the polysaccharides extracted from Ganoderma lucidum on chemotherapy-related fatigue in mice. *Int J Biol Macromol.* 2016 Oct;91:905-10.

3837 Li C, Kim JH, Ji BU, et al. Inhibitory effects of Ganoderma lucidum pharmacopuncture on atopic dermatitis induced by capsaicin in rats. *J Dermatol Sci.* 2015 Dec;80(3):212-4.

3838 Son HU, Lee S, Heo JC, et al. The solid-state fermentation of Artemisia capillaris leaves with Ganoderma lucidum enhances the anti-inflammatory effects in a model of atopic dermatitis. *Int J Mol Med.* 2017 May;39(5):1233-1241.

3839 Shen CY, Xu PH, Shen BD, et al. Nanogel for dermal application of the triterpenoids isolated from Ganoderma lucidum (GLT) for frostbite treatment. *Drug Deliv.* 2016;23(2):610-8.

3840 Shen C, Shen B, Shen G, et al. Therapeutic effects of nanogel containing triterpenoids isolated from Ganoderma lucidum (GLT) using therapeutic ultrasound (TUS) for frostbite in rats. *Drug Deliv.* 2016 Oct;23(8):2643-2650.

3841 Kim KC, Kim IG. Ganoderma lucidum extract protects DNA from strand breakage caused by hydroxyl radical and UV irradiation. *Int J Mol Med.* 1999 Sep;4(3):273-7.

3842 Lee SH, Lee ES, Bae IH, et al. The Protective Effect of Ganoderma lucidum Extract in Ultraviolet B-Induced Human Dermal Fibroblasts and Skin Equivalent Models. *Ann Dermatol.* 2020 Jun;32(3):251-254.

3843 Abate M, Pepe G, Randino R, et al. Ganoderma lucidum Ethanol Extracts Enhance Re-Epithelialization and Prevent Keratinocytes from Free-Radical Injury. *Pharmaceuticals (Basel).* 2020 Aug 29;13(9):224.

3844 Gupta A, Kirar V, Keshri GK, et al. Wound healing activity of an aqueous extract of the Lingzhi or Reishi medicinal mushroom Ganoderma lucidum (higher Basidiomycetes). *Int J Med Mushrooms.* 2014;16(4):345-54.

3845 Cheng PG, Phan CW, Sabaratnam V, et al. Polysaccharides-Rich Extract of Ganoderma lucidum (M.A. Curtis:Fr.) P. Karst Accelerates Wound Healing in Streptozotocin-Induced Diabetic Rats. *Evid Based Complement Alternat Med.* 2013;2013:671252.

3846 Hu F, Yan Y, Wang CW, et al. Article Effect and Mechanism of Ganoderma lucidum Polysaccharides on Human Fibroblasts and Skin Wound Healing in Mice. *Chin J Integr Med.* 2019 Mar;25(3):203-209.

3847 Jiao C, Yun H, Liang H, et al. An active ingredient isolated from Ganoderma lucidum promotes burn wound healing via TRPV1/SMAD signaling. *Aging (Albany NY).* 2022 Jun 13;14(13):5376-5389.

3848 Jiao C, Xie Y, Yun H, et al. The effect of Ganodermalucidum spore oil in early skin wound healing: interactions of skin microbiota and inflammation. *Aging (Albany NY).* 2020 Jul 21;12(14):14125-14140.

3849 Ren H, Meng X, Yin J, et al. Ganoderma lucidum Polysaccharide Peptide Attenuates Skin Flap Ischemia-Reperfusion Injury in a Thioredoxin-Dependent Manner. *Plast Reconstr Surg.* 2018 Jul;142(1):23e-33e.

3850 Jiang L, Huang J, Lu J, et al. Ganoderma lucidum polysaccharide reduces melanogenesis by inhibiting the paracrine effects of keratinocytes and fibroblasts via IL-6/STAT3/FGF2 pathway. *J Cell Physiol.* 2019 Dec;234(12):22799-22808.

3851 Kim JW, Kim HI, Kim JH, et al. Effects of Ganodermanondiol, a New Melanogenesis Inhibitor from the Medicinal Mushroom Ganoderma lucidum. *Int J Mol Sci.* 2016 Oct 27;17(11):1798.

3852 Hu S, Huang J, Pei S, et al. Ganoderma lucidum polysaccharide inhibits UVB-induced melanogenesis by antagonizing cAMP/PKA and ROS/MAPK signaling pathways. *J Cell Physiol.* 2019 May;234(5):7330-7340.

3853 Zeng Q, Zhou F, Lei L, et al. Ganoderma lucidum polysaccharides protect fibroblasts against UVB-induced photoaging. *Mol Med Rep.* 2017 Jan;15(1):111-116.

3854 Shi X, Cheng W, Wang Q, et al. Exploring the Protective and Reparative Mechanisms of G. lucidum Polysaccharides Against H2O2-Induced Oxidative Stress in Human Skin Fibroblasts. *Clin Cosmet Investig Dermatol.* 2021 Oct 14;14:1481-1496.

3855 Vaithanomsat P, Boonlum N, Chaiyana W, et al. Mushroom β-Glucan Recovered from Antler-Type Fruiting Body of Ganoderma lucidum by Enzymatic Process and Its Potential Biological Activities for Cosmeceutical Applications. *Polymers (Basel).* 2022 Oct 7;14(19):4202.

3856 Chien CC, Tsai ML, Chen CC, et al. Effects on tyrosinase activity by the extracts of Ganoderma lucidum and related mushrooms. *Mycopathologia.* 2008 Aug;166(2):117-20.

3857 Sharif S, Atta A, Huma T, et al. Anticancer, antithrombotic, antityrosinase, and anti-α-glucosidase activities of selected wild and commercial mushrooms from Pakistan. *Food Sci Nutr.* 2018 Sep 14;6(8):2170-2176.

3858 Jia D, Tang Y, Qin F, et al. Ganoderma lucidum polysaccharide alleviates Cd toxicity in common carp (Cyprinus carpio): Neuropeptide, growth performance and lipid accumulation. *Comp Biochem Physiol C Toxicol Pharmacol*. 2023 Sep;271:109663.

3859 Dai Z, Li G, Wang X, et al. Mapping the metabolic characteristics of probiotic-fermented Ganoderma lucidum and its protective mechanism against Cd-induced nephrotoxicity. *Food Funct*. 2023 Sep 19;14(18):8615-8630.

3860 Teng X, Zhang W, Song Y, et al. Protective effects of Ganoderma lucidum triterpenoids on oxidative stress and apoptosis in the spleen of chickens induced by cadmium. *Environ Sci Pollut Res Int*. 2019 Aug;26(23):23967-23980.

3861 Zheng DS, Chen LS. Triterpenoids from Ganoderma lucidum inhibit the activation of EBV antigens as telomerase inhibitors. *Exp Ther Med*. 2017 Oct;14(4):3273-3278.

3862 Iwatsuki K, Akihisa T, Tokuda H, et al. Lucidenic acids P and Q, methyl lucidenate P, and other triterpenoids from the fungus Ganoderma lucidum and their inhibitory effects on Epstein-Barr virus activation. *J Nat Prod*. 2003 Dec;66(12):1582-5.

3863 Bharadwaj S, Lee KE, Dwivedi VD, et al. Discovery of Ganoderma lucidum triterpenoids as potential inhibitors against Dengue virus NS2B-NS3 protease. *Sci Rep*. 2019 Dec 13;9(1):19059.

3864 Lim WZ, Cheng PG, Abdulrahman AY, et al. The identification of active compounds in Ganoderma lucidum var. antler extract inhibiting dengue virus serine protease and its computational studies. *J Biomol Struct Dyn*. 2020 Sep;38(14):4273-4288.

3865 Li Y, Yang Y, Fang L, et al. Anti-hepatitis activities in the broth of Ganoderma lucidum supplemented with a Chinese herbal medicine. *Am J Chin Med*. 2006;34(2):341-9.

3866 Li YQ, Zhang KC. [In vitro inhibitory efects on HBsAg and HBeAg secretion of 3 new components produced by Ganoderma lucidum in the medium contained Radix sophorae flavescentis extract]. *Wei Sheng Wu Xue Bao*. 2005 Aug;45(4):643-6.

3867 Li YQ, Wang SF. Anti-hepatitis B activities of ganoderic acid from Ganoderma lucidum. *Biotechnol Lett*. 2006 Jun;28(11):837-41.

3868 Xu J, Yang W, Pan Y, et al. Lucidenic acid A inhibits the binding of hACE2 receptor with spike protein to prevent SARS-CoV-2 invasion. *Food Chem Toxicol*. 2022 Nov;169:113438.

3869 Li Z, Liu J, Zhao Y. Possible mechanism underlying the antiherpetic activity of a proteoglycan isolated from the mycelia of Ganoderma lucidum in vitro. *J Biochem Mol Biol*. 2005 Jan 31;38(1):34-40.

3870 Eo SK, Kim YS, Lee CK, et al. Antiherpetic activities of various protein bound polysaccharides isolated from Ganoderma lucidum. *J Ethnopharmacol*. 1999 Dec 15;68(1-3):175-81.

3871 Eo SK, Kim YS, Lee CK, et al. Antiviral activities of various water and methanol soluble substances isolated from Ganoderma lucidum. *J Ethnopharmacol*. 1999 Dec 15;68(1-3):129-36.

3872 Oh KW, Lee CK, Kim YS, et al. Antiherpetic activities of acidic protein bound polysacchride isolated from Ganoderma lucidum alone and in combinations with acyclovir and vidarabine. *J Ethnopharmacol*. 2000 Sep;72(1-2):221-7.

3873 Liu J, Yang F, Ye LB, et al. Possible mode of action of antiherpetic activities of a proteoglycan isolated from the mycelia of Ganoderma lucidum in vitro. *J Ethnopharmacol*. 2004 Dec;95(2-3):265-72.

3874 Kim YS, Eo SK, Oh KW, et al. Antiherpetic activities of acidic protein bound polysacchride isolated from Ganoderma lucidum alone and in combinations with interferons. *J Ethnopharmacol*. 2000 Oct;72(3):451-8.

3875 Eo SK, Kim YS, Lee CK, et al. Possible mode of antiviral activity of acidic protein bound polysaccharide isolated from Ganoderma lucidum on herpes simplex viruses. *J Ethnopharmacol*. 2000 Oct;72(3):475-81.

3876 Akbar R, Yam WK. Interaction of ganoderic acid on HIV related target: molecular docking studies. *Bioinformation*. 2011;7(8):413-7.

3877 el-Mekkawy S, Meselhy MR, Nakamura N, et al. Anti-HIV-1 and anti-HIV-1-protease substances from Ganoderma lucidum. *Phytochemistry*. 1998 Nov;49(6):1651-7.

3878 Cheng PG, Teoh TC, Rizman-Idid M. Chemical Compounds and Computational Prediction of Their Inhibitory Effects on the HIV-1 gp120 Receptor by Lingzhi or Reishi Medicinal Mushroom, Ganoderma lucidum (Agaricomycetes), with Antler-Like Morphology of Fruiting Bodies. *Int J Med Mushrooms*. 2021;23(7):63-77.

3879 Min BS, Nakamura N, Miyashiro H, et al. Triterpenes from the spores of Ganoderma lucidum and their inhibitory activity against HIV-1 protease. *Chem Pharm Bull (Tokyo)*. 1998 Oct;46(10):1607-12.

3880 Zhang W, Tao J, Yang X, et al. Antiviral effects of two Ganoderma lucidum triterpenoids against enterovirus 71 infection. *Biochem Biophys Res Commun*. 2014 Jul 4;449(3):307-12.

3881 Lin YL, Shih C, Cheng PY, et al. A Polysaccharide Purified From Ganoderma lucidum Acts as a Potent Mucosal Adjuvant That Promotes Protective Immunity Against the Lethal Challenge With Enterovirus A71. *Front Immunol*. 2020 Sep 29;11:561758.

3882 Lu YZ, Wu XX, Chen S, et al. Effectiveness of Ganoderma lucidum preparation in treating simian acquired immune deficiency syndrome. *Zhongguo Yi Xue Ke Xue Yuan Xue Bao*. 2011 Jun;33(3):318-24.

3883 Eo SK, Kim YS, Lee CK, et al. Antiviral activities of various water and methanol soluble substances isolated from Ganoderma lucidum. *J Ethnopharmacol*. 1999 Dec 15;68(1-3):129-36.

3884 Liu Z, Zhu T, He J, et al. Adjuvanticity of Ganoderma lucidum polysaccharide liposomes on porcine circovirus type-II in mice. *Int J Biol Macromol*. 2019 Dec 1;141:1158-1164.

3885 Shamaki BU, Sandabe UK, Ogbe AO, et al. Methanolic soluble fractions of lingzhi or reishi medicinal mushroom, Ganoderma lucidum (higher Basidiomycetes) extract inhibit neuraminidase activity in Newcastle disease virus (LaSota). *Int J Med Mushrooms*. 2014;16(6):579-83.

3886 Grienke U, Kaserer T, Pfluger F, et al. Accessing biological actions of Ganoderma secondary metabolites by in silico profiling. *Phytochemistry*. 2015 Jun;114:114-24.

3887 Constantin M, Răut I, Suica-Bunghez R, et al. Ganoderma lucidum-Mediated Green Synthesis of Silver Nanoparticles with Antimicrobial Activity. *Materials (Basel)*. 2023 Jun 8;16(12):4261.

3888 Cilerdžić J, Vukojević J, Stajić M, et al. Biological activity of Ganoderma lucidum basidiocarps cultivated on alternative and commercial substrate. *J Ethnopharmacol*. 2014 Aug 8;155(1):312-9.

3889 Heleno SA, Ferreira IC, Esteves AP, et al. Antimicrobial and demelanizing activity of Ganoderma lucidum extract, p-hydroxybenzoic and cinnamic acids and their synthetic acetylated glucuronide methyl esters. *Food Chem Toxicol*. 2013 Aug;58:95-100.

[3890] Ergun B. Evaluation of antimicrobial, Cytotoxic and genotoxic activities of Ganoderma lucidum (Reishi mushroom). *Pak J Pharm Sci.* 2017 Sep;30(5(Supplementary)):1991-1995.

[3891] Nayak RN, Dixitraj PT, Nayak A, et al. Evaluation of anti-microbial activity of spore powder of Ganoderma lucidum on clinical isolates of Prevotella intermedia: A pilot study. *Contemp Clin Dent.* 2015 Sep;6(Suppl 1):S248-52.

[3892] Karwa AS, Rai MK. Naturally occurring medicinal mushroom-derived antimicrobials: a case-study using Lingzhi or Reishi Ganoderma lucidum (W. Curt.:Fr.) P. Karst. (higher Basidiomycetes). *Int J Med Mushrooms.* 2012;14(5):481-90.

[3893] Wan-Mohtar WA, Young L, Abbott GM, et al. Antimicrobial Properties and Cytotoxicity of Sulfated (1,3)-β-D-Glucan from the Mycelium of the Mushroom Ganoderma lucidum. *J Microbiol Biotechnol.* 2016 Jun 28;26(6):999-1010.

[3894] Yoon SY, Eo SK, Kim YS, et al. Antimicrobial activity of Ganoderma lucidum extract alone and in combination with some antibiotics. *Arch Pharm Res.* 1994 Dec;17(6):438-42.

[3895] Wang H, Ng TB. Ganodermin, an antifungal protein from fruiting bodies of the medicinal mushroom Ganoderma lucidum. *Peptides.* 2006 Jan;27(1):27-30.

[3896] El Zawawy NA, Ali SS. Anti-proteolytic activity of Ganoderma lucidum methanol extract against Pseudomonas aeruginosa. *J Infect Dev Ctries.* 2016 Sep 30;10(9):1020-1024.

[3897] Zhu H, Liu W, Tian B, et al. Inhibition of quorum sensing in the opportunistic pathogenic bacterium Chromobacterium violaceum by an extract from fruiting bodies of Lingzhi or Reishi medicinal mushroom, Ganoderma lucidum (W.Curt.:Fr.) P. Karst. (higher Basidiomycetes). *Int J Med Mushrooms.* 2011;13(6):559-64.

[3898] Sa-Ard P, Sarnthima R, Khammuang S, et al. Antioxidant, antibacterial and DNA protective activities of protein extracts from Ganoderma lucidum. *J Food Sci Technol.* 2015 May;52(5):2966-73.

[3899] Mishra J, Joshi A, Rajput R, et al. Phenolic Rich Fractions from Mycelium and Fruiting Body of Ganoderma lucidum Inhibit Bacterial Pathogens Mediated by Generation of Reactive Oxygen Species and Protein Leakage and Modulate Hypoxic Stress in HEK 293 Cell Line. *Adv Pharmacol Sci.* 2018 Dec 17;2018:6285615.

[3900] Bhardwaj A, Gupta P, Kumar N, et al. Lingzhi or Reishi Medicinal Mushroom, Ganoderma lucidum (Agaricomycetes), Inhibits Candida Biofilms: A Metabolomic Approach. *Int J Med Mushrooms.* 2017;19(8):685-696.

[3901] Erbiai EH, Amina B, Kaoutar A, et al. Chemical Characterization and Evaluation of Antimicrobial Properties of the Wild Medicinal Mushroom Ganoderma lucidum Growing in Northern Moroccan Forests. *Life (Basel).* 2023 May 19;13(5):1217.

[3902] Vazirian M, Faramarzi MA, Ebrahimi SE, et al. Antimicrobial effect of the Lingzhi or Reishi medicinal mushroom, Ganoderma lucidum (higher Basidiomycetes) and its main compounds. *Int J Med Mushrooms.* 2014;16(1):77-84.

[3903] Lu SY, Shi QQ, Peng XR, et al. Isolation of benzolactones, Ganodumones A-F from Ganoderma lucidum and their antibacterial activities. *Bioorg Chem.* 2020 May;98:103723.

[3904] Savin S, Craciunescu O, Oancea A, et al. Antioxidant, Cytotoxic and Antimicrobial Activity of Chitosan Preparations Extracted from Ganoderma Lucidum Mushroom. *Chem Biodivers.* 2020 Jul;17(7):e2000175.

[3905] Sánchez-Hernández E, Teixeira A, Pereira C, et al. Chemical Constituents and Antimicrobial Activity of a Ganoderma lucidum (Curtis.) P. Karst. Aqueous Ammonia Extract. *Plants (Basel).* 2023 Jun 11;12(12):2271.

[3906] Reid T, Kashangura C, Chidewe C, et al. Characterization of Anti-Salmonella typhi Compounds from Medicinal Mushroom Extracts from Zimbabwe. *Int J Med Mushrooms.* 2019;21(7):713-724.

[3907] Karaman M, Jovin E, Malbasa R, et al. Medicinal and edible lignicolous fungi as natural sources of antioxidative and antibacterial agents. *Phytother Res.* 2010 Oct;24(10):1473-81.

[3908] Kaewjai C, Tonsomboon A, Pawiwongchai J, et al. Antiprotozoal activity of Boesenbergia rotunda (L.) Mansf and Ganoderma lucidum (Fr.) Kart extracts against Blastocystis hominis. *Vet World.* 2023 Jan;16(1):187-193.

[3909] Adams M, Christen M, Plitzko I, et al. Antiplasmodial lanostanes from the Ganoderma lucidum mushroom. *J Nat Prod.* 2010 May 28;73(5):897-900.

[3910] Oluba OM, Olusola AO, Fagbohunka BS, et al. Antimalarial and hepatoprotective effects of crude ethanolic extract of Lingzhi or Reishi medicinal mushroom, Ganoderma lucidum (W.Curt.:Fr.)P.Karst. (higher Basidiomycetes), in Plasmodium berghei-infected mice. *Int J Med Mushrooms.* 2012;14(5):459-66.

[3911] Oluba OM. Ganoderma terpenoid extract exhibited anti-plasmodial activity by a mechanism involving reduction in erythrocyte and hepatic lipids in Plasmodium berghei infected mice. *Lipids Health Dis.* 2019 Jan 12;18(1):12.

[3912] Oluba OM, Olusola AO, Eidangbe GO, et al. Modulation of Lipoprotein Cholesterol Levels in Plasmodium berghei Malarial Infection by Crude Aqueous Extract of Ganoderma lucidum. *Cholesterol.* 2012;2012:536396.

[3913] Oluba OM, Adebisi KE, Eidangbe GO, et al. Modulatory effect of crude aqueous extract of Lingzhi or Reishi Medicinal Mushroom, Ganoderma lucidum (Higher Basidiomycetes), on hematological and antioxidant indices in Plasmodium berghei-infected mice. *Int J Med Mushrooms.* 2014;16(5):499-506.

[3914] Ahmadi M, Salimi M, Saraei M, et al. In vitro anti-Toxoplasma gondii activity of Ganoderma lucidum extracts. *BMC Res Notes.* 2023 May 18;16(1):82.

[3915] Huseein EAM, Samir M, Al-Karmalawy AA, et al. Ganoderma lucidum extract inhibits Schistosoma mansoni survival in silico and in vitro study. *Ann Parasitol.* 2022;68(2):323-330.

[3916] da Silva Coelho J, de Souza CG, de Oliveira AL, et al. Comparative removal of bentazon by Ganoderma lucidum in liquid and solid state cultures. *Curr Microbiol.* 2010 May;60(5):350-5.

[3917] Kaur H, Kapoor S, Kaur G. Application of ligninolytic potentials of a white-rot fungus Ganoderma lucidum for degradation of lindane. *Environ Monit Assess.* 2016 Oct;188(10):588.

[3918] Lin Y, Peng X, Xia B, et al. Investigation of toxicity attenuation mechanism of tetrahydroxy stilbene glucoside in Polygonum multiflorum Thunb. by Ganoderma lucidum. *J Ethnopharmacol.* 2021 Nov 15;280:114421.

[3919] Liao CS, Yuan SY, Hung BH, et al. Removal of organic toxic chemicals using the spent mushroom compost of Ganoderma lucidum. *J Environ Monit.* 2012 Jul;14(7):1983-8.

[3920] Wang H, Deng W, Shen M, et al. A laccase Gl-LAC-4 purified from white-rot fungus Ganoderma lucidum had a strong ability to degrade and detoxify the alkylphenol pollutants 4-n-octylphenol and 2-phenylphenol. *J Hazard Mater.* 2021 Apr 15;408:124775.

3921 Deng W, Zhao W, Yang Y. Degradation and Detoxification of Chlorophenols with Different Structure by LAC-4 Laccase Purified from White-Rot Fungus Ganoderma lucidum. *Int J Environ Res Public Health*. 2022 Jul 2;19(13):8150.

3922 Chen SN, Nan FH, Liu MW, et al. Evaluation of Immune Modulation by β-1,3; 1,6 D-Glucan Derived from Ganoderma lucidum in Healthy Adult Volunteers, A Randomized Controlled Trial. *Foods*. 2023 Feb 3;12(3):659.

3923 Henao SLD, Urrego SA, Cano AM, et al. Randomized Clinical Trial for the Evaluation of Immune Modulation by Yogurt Enriched with β-Glucans from Lingzhi or Reishi Medicinal Mushroom, Ganoderma lucidum (Agaricomycetes), in Children from Medellin, Colombia. *Int J Med Mushrooms*. 2018;20(8):705-716.

3924 Collado Mateo D, Pazzi F, Domínguez Muñoz FJ, et al. Ganoderma lucidum improves physical fitness in women with fibromyalgia. *Nutr Hosp*. 2015 Nov 1;32(5):2126-35.

3925 Pazzi F, Adsuar JC, Domínguez-Muñoz FJ, et al. Ganoderma lucidum Effects on Mood and Health-Related Quality of Life in Women with Fibromyalgia. *Healthcare (Basel)*. 2020 Nov 30;8(4):520.

3926 Donatini B. Control of oral human papillomavirus (HPV) by medicinal mushrooms, Trametes versicolor and Ganoderma lucidum: a preliminary clinical trial. *Int J Med Mushrooms*. 2014;16(5):497-8.

3927 Noguchi M, Kakuma T, Tomiyasu K, et al. Randomized clinical trial of an ethanol extract of Ganoderma lucidum in men with lower urinary tract symptoms. *Asian J Androl*. 2008 Sep;10(5):777-85.

3928 Noguchi M, Kakuma T, Tomiyasu K, et al. Effect of an extract of Ganoderma lucidum in men with lower urinary tract symptoms: a double-blind, placebo-controlled randomized and dose-ranging study. *Asian J Androl*. 2008 Jul;10(4):651-8.

3929 Zhang Y, Lin Z, Hu Y, et al. Effect of Ganoderma lucidum capsules on T lymphocyte subsets in football players on "living high-training low". *Br J Sports Med*. 2008 Oct;42(10):819-22.

3930 Sargowo D, Ovianti N, Susilowati E, et al. The role of polysaccharide peptide of Ganoderma lucidum as a potent antioxidant against atherosclerosis in high risk and stable angina patients. *Indian Heart J*. 2018 Sep-Oct;70(5):608-614.

3931 Susilowati E, Sargowo D, Ovianti N. Oral Presentation Award Winner: Polysaccharide Peptide of Ganoderma lucidum Reduces Endothelial Injury in Stable Angina and High-risk Patients. *Eur Cardiol*. 2021 Dec 14;16:e59.

3932 Chu TT, Benzie IF, Lam CW, et al. Study of potential cardioprotective effects of Ganoderma lucidum (Lingzhi): results of a controlled human intervention trial. *Br J Nutr*. 2012 Apr;107(7):1017-27.

3933 Tao J, Feng KY. Experimental and clinical studies on inhibitory effect of ganoderma lucidum on platelet aggregation. *J Tongji Med Univ*. 1990;10(4):240-3.

3934 Gao Y, Zhou S, Chen G, et al. A Phase I/II Study of a Ganoderma lucidum (Curt.:Fr.) P. Karst. (Ling Zhi, Reishi Mushroom) Extract in Patients with Chronic Hepatitis B. *Int J Med Mushrooms*. 2002;4(4):2321-7.

3935 Gao Y, Zhou S, Jiang W, et al. Effects of ganopoly (a Ganoderma lucidum polysaccharide extract) on the immune functions in advanced-stage cancer patients. *Immunol Invest*. 2003 Aug;32(3):201-15.

3936 Chen X, Hu ZP, Yang XX, et al. Monitoring of immune responses to a herbal immuno-modulator in patients with advanced colorectal cancer. *Int Immunopharmacol*. 2006 Mar;6(3):499-508.

3937 Suprasert P, Apichartpiyakul C, Sakonwasun C, et al. Clinical characteristics of gynecologic cancer patients who respond to salvage treatment with Lingzhi. *Asian Pac J Cancer Prev*. 2014;15(10):4193-6.

3938 Oka S, Tanaka S, Yoshida S, et al. A water-soluble extract from culture medium of Ganoderma lucidum mycelia suppresses the development of colorectal adenomas. *Hiroshima J Med Sci*. 2010 Mar;59(1):1-6.

3939 Zhao H, Zhang Q, Zhao L, et al. Spore Powder of Ganoderma lucidum Improves Cancer-Related Fatigue in Breast Cancer Patients Undergoing Endocrine Therapy: A Pilot Clinical Trial. *Evid Based Complement Alternat Med*. 2012;2012:809614.

3940 Tang W, Gao Y, Chen G, et al. A randomized, double-blind and placebo-controlled study of a Ganoderma lucidum polysaccharide extract in neurasthenia. *J Med Food*. 2005 Spring;8(1):53-8.

3941 Zhang Y, Tang X, Jiang T, et al. The Potential Activity of Lingzhi or Reishi Medicinal Mushroom, Ganoderma lucidum (Agaricomycetes), to Alleviate Liver Injury in Adults with Acute Mushroom Poisoning: A Retrospective Study. *Int J Med Mushrooms*. 2022;24(5):57-72.

3942 Chiu HF, Fu HY, Lu YY, et al. Triterpenoids and polysaccharide peptides-enriched Ganoderma lucidum: a randomized, double-blind placebo-controlled crossover study of its antioxidation and hepatoprotective efficacy in healthy volunteers. *Pharm Biol*. 2017 Dec;55(1):1041-1046.

3943 Wachtel-Galor S, Szeto YT, Tomlinson B, et al. Ganoderma lucidum ('Lingzhi'); acute and short-term biomarker response to supplementation. *Int J Food Sci Nutr*. 2004 Feb;55(1):75-83.

3944 Hijikata Y, Yamada S. Effect of Ganoderma lucidum on postherpetic neuralgia. *Am J Chin Med*. 1998;26(3-4):375-81.

3945 Kuypers KPC. Self-Medication with Ganoderma lucidum ("Reishi") to Combat Parkinson's Disease Symptoms: A Single Case Study. *J Med Food*. 2021 Jul;24(7):766-773.

3946 Fu HD, Wang ZY. The clinical effects of Ganoderma lucidum spore preparations in 10 cases of atrophic myotonia. *J Tradit Chin Med*. 1982 Mar;2(1):63-5.

3947 Din SRU, Zhong M, Nisar MA, et al. Latcripin-7A, derivative of Lentinula edodes C91-3, reduces migration and induces apoptosis, autophagy, and cell cycle arrest at G1 phase in breast cancer cells. *Appl Microbiol Biotechnol*. 2020 Dec;104(23):10165-10179.

3948 Elhusseiny SM, El-Mahdy TS, Awad MF, et al. Proteome Analysis and In Vitro Antiviral, Anticancer and Antioxidant Capacities of the Aqueous Extracts of Lentinula edodes and Pleurotus ostreatus Edible Mushrooms. *Molecules*. 2021 Jul 30;26(15):4623.

3949 Israilides C, Kletsas D, Arapoglou D, et al. In vitro cytostatic and immunomodulatory properties of the medicinal mushroom Lentinula edodes. *Phytomedicine*. 2008 Jun;15(6-7):512-9.

3950 Morales D, Rutckeviski R, Villalva M, et al. Isolation and comparison of α- and β-D-glucans from shiitake mushrooms (Lentinula edodes) with different biological activities. *Carbohydr Polym*. 2020 Feb 1;229:115521.

3951 Elhusseiny SM, El-Mahdy TS, Awad MF, et al. Proteome Analysis and In Vitro Antiviral, Anticancer and Antioxidant Capacities of the Aqueous Extracts of Lentinula edodes and Pleurotus ostreatus Edible Mushrooms. *Molecules*. 2021 Jul 30;26(15):4623.

3952 Finimundy TC, Gambato G, Fontana R, et al. Aqueous extracts of Lentinula edodes and Pleurotus sajor-caju exhibit high antioxidant capability and promising in vitro antitumor activity. *Nutr Res*. 2013 Jan;33(1):76-84.

3953 Elhusseiny SM, El-Mahdy TS, Awad MF, et al. Proteome Analysis and In Vitro Antiviral, Anticancer and Antioxidant Capacities of the Aqueous Extracts of Lentinula edodes and Pleurotus ostreatus Edible Mushrooms. *Molecules*. 2021 Jul 30;26(15):4623.

3954 Yamashita SN, Tanaka Y, Kitagawa T, et al. Down-regulating Effect of a Standardized Extract of Cultured Lentinula edodes mycelia on Cortactin in Prostate Cancer Cells Is Dependent on Malignant Potential. *Anticancer Res*. 2023 Mar;43(3):1159-1166.

3955 Din SRU, Nisar MA, Ramzan MN, et al. Latcripin-7A from Lentinula edodes C91-3 induces apoptosis, autophagy, and cell cycle arrest at G1 phase in human gastric cancer cells via inhibiting PI3K/Akt/mTOR signaling. *Eur J Pharmacol*. 2021 Sep 15;907:174305.

3956 Batool S, Joseph TP, Hussain M, et al. LP1 from Lentinula edodes C91-3 Induces Autophagy, Apoptosis and Reduces Metastasis in Human Gastric Cancer Cell Line SGC-7901. *Int J Mol Sci*. 2018 Sep 30;19(10):2986.

3957 Park HJ, Boo S, Park I, et al. AHCC®, a Standardized Extract of Cultured Lentinula Edodes Mycelia, Promotes the Anti-Tumor Effect of Dual Immune Checkpoint Blockade Effect in Murine Colon Cancer. *Front Immunol*. 2022 Apr 20;13:875872.

3958 Elhusseiny SM, El-Mahdy TS, Awad MF, et al. Proteome Analysis and In Vitro Antiviral, Anticancer and Antioxidant Capacities of the Aqueous Extracts of Lentinula edodes and Pleurotus ostreatus Edible Mushrooms. *Molecules*. 2021 Jul 30;26(15):4623.

3959 Tanaka K, Matsui Y, Ishikawa S, et al. Oral ingestion of Lentinula edodes mycelia extract can restore the antitumor T cell response of mice inoculated with colon-26 cells into the subserosal space of the cecum. *Oncol Rep*. 2012 Feb;27(2):325-32.

3960 Paganelli F, Chiarini F, Palmieri A, et al. The Combination of AHCC and ETAS Decreases Migration of Colorectal Cancer Cells, and Reduces the Expression of LGR5 and Notch1 Genes in Cancer Stem Cells: A Novel Potential Approach for Integrative Medicine. *Pharmaceuticals (Basel)*. 2021 Dec 18;14(12):1325.

3961 Takahashi M, Fujii G, Hamoya T, et al. Activation of NF-E2 p45-related factor-2 transcription and inhibition of intestinal tumor development by AHCC, a standardized extract of cultured Lentinula edodes mycelia. *J Clin Biochem Nutr*. 2019 Nov;65(3):203-208.

3962 Zhao ZZ, Zhang F, Ji BY, et al. Pyrrole alkaloids from the fruiting bodies of edible mushroom Lentinula edodes. *RSC Adv*. 2023 Jun 16;13(27):18223-18228.

3963 Elhusseiny SM, El-Mahdy TS, Awad MF, et al. Proteome Analysis and In Vitro Antiviral, Anticancer and Antioxidant Capacities of the Aqueous Extracts of Lentinula edodes and Pleurotus ostreatus Edible Mushrooms. *Molecules*. 2021 Jul 30;26(15):4623.

3964 Yukawa H, Ishikawa S, Kawanishi T, et al. Direct cytotoxicity of Lentinula edodes mycelia extract on human hepatocellular carcinoma cell line. *Biol Pharm Bull*. 2012;35(7):1014-21.

3965 Finimundy TC, Gambato G, Fontana R, et al. Aqueous extracts of Lentinula edodes and Pleurotus sajor-caju exhibit high antioxidant capability and promising in vitro antitumor activity. *Nutr Res*. 2013 Jan;33(1):76-84.

3966 Islam S, Kitagawa T, Baron B, et al. A standardized extract of cultured Lentinula edodes mycelia downregulates cortactin in gemcitabine-resistant pancreatic cancer cells. *Oncol Lett*. 2021 Sep;22(3):654.

3967 Joseph TP, Zhao Q, Chanda W, et al. Expression and in vitro anticancer activity of Lp16-PSP, a member of the YjgF/YER057c/UK114 protein family from the mushroom Lentinula edodes C91-3. *Arch Microbiol*. 2021 Apr;203(3):1047-1060.

3968 Gao Y, Padhiar AA, Wang J, et al. Recombinant latcripin 11 of Lentinula edodes C91-3 suppresses the proliferation of various cancer cells. *Gene*. 2018 Feb 5;642:212-219.

3969 Ann XH, Lun YZ, Zhang W, et al. Expression and characterization of protein Latcripin-3, an antioxidant and antitumor molecule from Lentinula edodes C91-3. *Asian Pac J Cancer Prev*. 2014;15(12):5055-61.

3970 Tian L, Wang X, Li X, et al. In vitro antitumor activity of Latcripin-15 regulator of chromosome condensation 1 domain protein. *Oncol Lett*. 2016 Nov;12(5):3153-3160.

3971 Wang J, Wan X, Gao Y, et al. Latcripin-13 domain induces apoptosis and cell cycle arrest at the G1 phase in human lung carcinoma A549 cells. *Oncol Rep*. 2016 Jul;36(1):441-7.

3972 Li M, Du X, Yuan Z, et al. Lentinan triggers oxidative stress-mediated anti-inflammatory responses in lung cancer cells. *Mol Cell Biochem*. 2022 Feb;477(2):469-477.

3973 Lo TC, Hsu FM, Chang CA, et al. Branched α-(1,4) glucans from Lentinula edodes (L10) in combination with radiation enhance cytotoxic effect on human lung adenocarcinoma through the Toll-like receptor 4 mediated induction of THP-1 differentiation/activation. *J Agric Food Chem*. 2011 Nov 23;59(22):11997-12005.

3974 Tanaka K, Ishikawa S, Matsui Y, et al. Oral ingestion of Lentinula edodes mycelia extract inhibits B16 melanoma growth via mitigation of regulatory T cell-mediated immunosuppression. *Cancer Sci*. 2011 Mar;102(3):516-21.

3975 Ahn H, Jeon E, Kim JC, et al. Lentinan from shiitake selectively attenuates AIM2 and non-canonical inflammasome activation while inducing pro-inflammatory cytokine production. *Sci Rep*. 2017 May 2;7(1):1314.

3976 Zhao ZZ, Zhang F, Ji BY, et al. Pyrrole alkaloids from the fruiting bodies of edible mushroom Lentinula edodes. *RSC Adv*. 2023 Jun 16;13(27):18223-18228.

3977 Chen Q, Peng H, Dong L, et al. Activation of the NRF2-ARE signalling pathway by the Lentinula edodes polysaccharose LNT alleviates ROS-mediated cisplatin nephrotoxicity. *Int Immunopharmacol*. 2016 Jul;36:1-8.

3978 Gu YH, Belury MA. Selective induction of apoptosis in murine skin carcinoma cells (CH72) by an ethanol extract of Lentinula edodes. *Cancer Lett*. 2005 Mar 18;220(1):21-8.

3979 Ishikawa S, Matsui Y, Wachi S, et al. Age-associated impairment of antitumor immunity in carcinoma-bearing mice and restoration by oral administration of Lentinula edodes mycelia extract. *Cancer Immunol Immunother*. 2016 Aug;65(8):961-72.

3980 Sun B, Wakame K, Sato E, et al. The effect of active hexose correlated compound in modulating cytosine arabinoside-induced hair loss, and 6-mercaptopurine- and methotrexate-induced liver injury in rodents. *Cancer Epidemiol*. 2009 Oct;33(3-4):293-9.

3981 Sun B, Wakame K, Sato E, et al. The effect of active hexose correlated compound in modulating cytosine arabinoside-induced hair loss, and 6-mercaptopurine- and methotrexate-induced liver injury in rodents. *Cancer Epidemiol*. 2009 Oct;33(3-4):293-9.

3982 Liu Q, Dong L, Li H, et al. Lentinan mitigates therarubicin-induced myelosuppression by activating bone marrow-derived macrophages in an MAPK/NF-κB-dependent manner. *Oncol Rep*. 2016 Jul;36(1):315-23.

3983 Kitagawa T, Islam S, Baron B, et al. A Standardized Extract of Cultured Lentinula edodes mycelia Up-regulates COX-2 in Inflammation-related Malignant Progressive Fibrosarcoma Cell Clone QRsP-11. *Anticancer Res*. 2023 Mar;43(3):1239-1244.

3984 Pan W, Jiang P, Zhao J, et al. β-Glucan from Lentinula edodes prevents cognitive impairments in high-fat diet-induced obese mice: involvement of colon-brain axis. *J Transl Med*. 2021 Feb 4;19(1):54.

3985 Xu X, Zhang X. Lentinula edodes-derived polysaccharide alters the spatial structure of gut microbiota in mice. *PLoS One*. 2015 Jan 21;10(1):e0115037.

3986 Yin C, Li C, Ma K, et al. The physicochemical, antioxidant, hypoglycemic and prebiotic properties of γ-irradiated polysaccharides extracted from Lentinula edodes. *Food Sci Biotechnol*. 2023 Jan 25;32(7):987-996.

3987 Xue Z, Ma Q, Chen Y, et al. Structure characterization of soluble dietary fiber fractions from mushroom Lentinula edodes (Berk.) Pegler and the effects on fermentation and human gut microbiota in vitro. *Food Res Int*. 2020 Mar;129:108870.

3988 Chou WT, Sheih IC, Fang TJ. The applications of polysaccharides from various mushroom wastes as prebiotics in different systems. *J Food Sci*. 2013 Jul;78(7):M1041-8.

3989 Matsuhisa K, Watari A, Iwamoto K, et al. Lignosulfonic acid attenuates NF-κB activation and intestinal epithelial barrier dysfunction induced by TNF-α/IFN-γ in Caco-2 cells. *J Nat Med*. 2018 Mar;72(2):448-455.

3990 Doursout MF, Liang Y, Sundaresan A, et al. Active hexose correlated compound modulates LPS-induced hypotension and gut injury in rats. *Int Immunopharmacol*. 2016 Oct;39:280-286.

3991 Li JH, Zhu YY, Gu FT, et al. Efficient isolation of immunostimulatory polysaccharides from Lentinula edodes by autoclaving-ultrasonication extraction and fractional precipitation. *Int J Biol Macromol*. 2023 May 15;237:124216.

3992 Xu X, Yang J, Luo Z, et al. Lentinula edodes-derived polysaccharide enhances systemic and mucosal immunity by spatial modulation of intestinal gene expression in mice. *Food Funct*. 2015 Jun;6(6):2068-80.

3993 Jung BG, Lee JA, Lee BJ. Immunoprophylactic effects of shiitake mushroom (Lentinula edodes) against Bordetella bronchiseptica in mice. *J Microbiol*. 2012 Dec;50(6):1003-8.

3994 Xu X, Yan H, Zhang X. Structure and immuno-stimulating activities of a new heteropolysaccharide from Lentinula edodes. *J Agric Food Chem*. 2012 Nov 21;60(46):11560-6.

3995 Vetvicka V, Vetvickova J. Immune-enhancing effects of Maitake (Grifola frondosa) and Shiitake (Lentinula edodes) extracts. *Ann Transl Med*. 2014 Feb;2(2):14.

3996 Djordjevic B, Skugor S, Jørgensen SM, et al. Modulation of splenic immune responses to bacterial lipopolysaccharide in rainbow trout (Oncorhynchus mykiss) fed lentinan, a beta-glucan from mushroom Lentinula edodes. *Fish Shellfish Immunol*. 2009 Feb;26(2):201-9.

3997 Maji PK, Sen IK, Behera B, et al. Structural characterization and study of immunoenhancing properties of a glucan isolated from a hybrid mushroom of Pleurotus florida and Lentinula edodes. *Carbohydr Res*. 2012 Sep 1;358:110-5.

3998 Zhang J, Tyler HL, Haron MH, et al. Macrophage activation by edible mushrooms is due to the collaborative interaction of toll-like receptor agonists and dectin-1b activating beta glucans derived from colonizing microorganisms. *Food Funct*. 2019 Dec 11;10(12):8208-8217.

3999 Elhusseiny SM, El-Mahdy TS, Elleboudy NS, et al. Immunomodulatory activity of extracts from five edible basidiomycetes mushrooms in Wistar albino rats. *Sci Rep*. 2022 Jul 20;12(1):12423.

4000 Roszczyk A, Turło J, Zagożdżon R, et al. Immunomodulatory Properties of Polysaccharides from Lentinula edodes. *Int J Mol Sci*. 2022 Aug 11;23(16):8980.

4001 Crespo H, Guillén H, de Pablo-Maiso L, et al. Lentinula edodes β-glucan enriched diet induces pro- and anti-inflammatory macrophages in rabbit. *Food Nutr Res*. 2017 Dec 12;61(1):1412791.

4002 Klimaszewska M, Górska S, Łapienis G, et al. Identification of the Primary Structure of Selenium-Containing Polysaccharides Selectively Inhibiting T-Cell Proliferation. *Molecules*. 2021 Sep 6;26(17):5404.

4003 Kajiyama S, Nagatake T, Ishikawa S, et al. Lentinula Edodes Mycelia extract regulates the function of antigen-presenting cells to activate immune cells and prevent tumor-induced deterioration of immune function. *BMC Complement Med Ther*. 2023 Aug 8;23(1):281.

4004 Xu X, Yang J, Ning Z, et al. Lentinula edodes-derived polysaccharide rejuvenates mice in terms of immune responses and gut microbiota. *Food Funct*. 2015 Aug;6(8):2653-63.

4005 López-Cauce B, Urquía A, Menchén L, et al. Lentinula edodes extract increases goblet cell number and Muc2 expression in an intestinal inflammatory model of Trichinella spiralis infection. *Biomed Pharmacother*. 2022 Jun:150:112937.

4006 Pérez-Cantero A, Serrano DR, Navarro-Rodríguez P, et al. Increased Efficacy of Oral Fixed-Dose Combination of Amphotericin B and AHCC® Natural Adjuvant against Aspergillosis. *Pharmaceutics*. 2019 Sep 3;11(9):456.

4007 Yehia RS. Evaluation of the biological activities of β-glucan isolated from Lentinula edodes. *Lett Appl Microbiol*. 2022 Aug;75(2):317-329.

4008 Choi JH, Lee HJ, Park SE, et al. Cytotoxicity, metabolic enzyme inhibitory, and anti-inflammatory effect of Lentinula edodes fermented using probiotic lactobacteria. *J Food Biochem*. 2021 Jul 1:e13838.

4009 Yin C, Li C, Ma K, et al. The physicochemical, antioxidant, hypoglycemic and prebiotic properties of γ-irradiated polysaccharides extracted from Lentinula edodes. *Food Sci Biotechnol*. 2023 Jan 25;32(7):987-996.

4010 Tu J, Adhikari B, Brennan MA, et al. Shiitake polysaccharides acted as a non-competitive inhibitor to α-glucosidase and inhibited glucose transport of digested starch from Caco-2 cells monolayer. *Food Res Int*. 2023 Nov;173(Pt 1):113268.

4011 Alagbaoso CA, Mizuno M. LENTINULA EDODES POLYSACCHARIDES SUPPRESSED PRO-INFLAMMATORY CYTOKINES EXPRESSION AND COLITIS IN MICE. *Arq Gastroenterol*. 2022 Apr-Jun;59(2):288-295.

4012 Xue Z, Li R, Liu J, Zhou J, et al. Preventive and synbiotic effects of the soluble dietary fiber obtained from Lentinula edodes byproducts and Lactobacillus plantarum LP90 against dextran sulfate sodium-induced colitis in mice. *J Sci Food Agric*. 2023 Jan 30;103(2):616-626.

4013 Minato KI, Oura K, Mizuno M. The inhibitory effect of oral administration of lentinan on DSS-induced inflammation is exerted by the migration of T cells activated in the ileum to the colon. *Eur J Pharmacol*. 2023 May 5;946:175631.

[4014] Nishitani Y, Zhang L, Yoshida M, et al. Intestinal anti-inflammatory activity of lentinan: influence on IL-8 and TNFR1 expression in intestinal epithelial cells. *PLoS One*. 2013 Apr 22;8(4):e62441.

[4015] Muszyńska B, Kała K, Włodarczyk A, et al. Lentinula edodes as a Source of Bioelements Released into Artificial Digestive Juices and Potential Anti-inflammatory Material. *Biol Trace Elem Res*. 2020 Apr;194(2):603-613.

[4016] Sun W, Feng Y, Zhang M et al. Protective effects of sulfated polysaccharides from Lentinula edodes on the lung and liver of MODS mice. *Food Funct*. 2021 Jul 21;12(14):6389-6402.

[4017] Zhang Z, Wu D, Li W, et al. Structural elucidation and anti-inflammatory activity of a proteoglycan from spent substrate of Lentinula edodes. *Int J Biol Macromol*. 2023 Jan 1;224:1509-1523.

[4018] Choi JH, Lee HJ, Park SE, et al. Cytotoxicity, metabolic enzyme inhibitory, and anti-inflammatory effect of Lentinula edodes fermented using probiotic lactobacteria. *J Food Biochem*. 2021 Jul 1:e13838.

[4019] Ren Z, Liu W, Song X, et al. Antioxidant and anti-inflammation of enzymatic-hydrolysis residue polysaccharides by Lentinula edodes. *Int J Biol Macromol*. 2018 Dec;120(Pt A):811-822.

[4020] Jafari M, Boskabaday MH, Rezaee SA, et al. Lentinan and β-glucan extract from shiitake mushroom, Lentinula edodes, alleviate acute LPS-induced hematological changes in mice. *Iran J Basic Med Sci*. 2023;26(7):836-842.

[4021] Song X, Ren Z, Wang X, et al. Antioxidant, anti-inflammatory and renoprotective effects of acidic-hydrolytic polysaccharides by spent mushroom compost (Lentinula edodes) on LPS-induced kidney injury. *Int J Biol Macromol*. 2020 May 15;151:1267-1276.

[4022] Morales D, Rutckeviski R, Villalva M, et al. Isolation and comparison of α- and β-D-glucans from shiitake mushrooms (Lentinula edodes) with different biological activities. *Carbohydr Polym*. 2020 Feb 1;229:115521.

[4023] Diallo I, Boudard F, Morel S, et al. Antioxidant and Anti-Inflammatory Potential of Shiitake Culinary-Medicinal Mushroom, Lentinus edodes (Agaricomycetes), Sporophores from Various Culture Conditions. *Int J Med Mushrooms*. 2020;22(6):535-546.

[4024] Paisansak S, Sangtanoo P, Srimongkol P, et al. Angiotensin-I converting enzyme inhibitory peptide derived from the shiitake mushroom (Lentinula edodes). *J Food Sci Technol*. 2021 Jan;58(1):85-97.

[4025] Rahman MA, Abdullah N, Aminudin N. Lentinula edodes (shiitake mushroom): An assessment of in vitro anti-atherosclerotic bio-functionality. *Saudi J Biol Sci*. 2018 Dec;25(8):1515-1523.

[4026] Soroko-Dubrovina M, Górniak W, Zielińska P, et al. Evaluation of Shiitake Mushroom (Lentinula edodes) Supplementation on the Blood Parameters of Young Thoroughbred Racehorses. *Animals (Basel)*. 2022 Nov 19;12(22):3212.

[4027] Spim SRV, de Oliveira BGCC, Leite FG, et al. Effects of Lentinula edodes consumption on biochemical, hematologic and oxidative stress parameters in rats receiving high-fat diet. *Eur J Nutr*. 2017 Oct;56(7):2255-2264.

[4028] Gil-Ramírez A, Caz V, Smiderle FR, et al. Water-Soluble Compounds from Lentinula edodes Influencing the HMG-CoA Reductase Activity and the Expression of Genes Involved in the Cholesterol Metabolism. *J Agric Food Chem*. 2016 Mar 9;64(9):1910-20.

[4029] Morales D, Tejedor-Calvo E, Jurado-Chivato N, et al. In vitro and in vivo testing of the hypocholesterolemic activity of ergosterol- and β-glucan-enriched extracts obtained from shiitake mushrooms (Lentinula edodes). *Food Funct*. 2019 Nov 1;10(11):7325-7332.

[4030] Asada N, Kairiku R, Tobo M, et al. Effects of Shiitake Intake on Serum Lipids in Rats Fed Different High-Oil or High-Fat Diets. *J Diet Suppl*. 2019;16(3):345-356.

[4031] Doursout MF, Liang Y, Sundaresan A, et al. Active hexose correlated compound modulates LPS-induced hypotension and gut injury in rats. *Int Immunopharmacol*. 2016 Oct;39:280-286.

[4032] Tanaka T, Iwamoto K, Wada M, et al. Dietary syringic acid reduces fat mass in an ovariectomy-induced mouse model of obesity. *Menopause*. 2021 Oct 4;28(12):1340-1350.

[4033] Lee H, Lee K, Lee S, et al. Ethyl Acetate Fraction of Aqueous Extract of Lentinula edodes Inhibits Osteoclastogenesis by Suppressing NFATc1 Expression. *Int J Mol Sci*. 2020 Feb 17;21(4):1347.

[4034] Tanaka T, Kawaguchi N, Zaima N, et al. Antiosteoporotic activity of a syringic acid diet in ovariectomized mice. *J Nat Med*. 2017 Oct;71(4):632-641.

[4035] Soroko-Dubrovina M, Górniak W, Zielińska P, et al. Evaluation of Shiitake Mushroom (Lentinula edodes) Supplementation on the Blood Parameters of Young Thoroughbred Racehorses. *Animals (Basel)*. 2022 Nov 19;12(22):3212.

[4036] Spim SRV, de Oliveira BGCC, Leite FG, et al. Effects of Lentinula edodes consumption on biochemical, hematologic and oxidative stress parameters in rats receiving high-fat diet. *Eur J Nutr*. 2017 Oct;56(7):2255-2264.

[4037] Sun W, Feng Y, Zhang M et al. Protective effects of sulfated polysaccharides from Lentinula edodes on the lung and liver of MODS mice. *Food Funct*. 2021 Jul 21;12(14):6389-6402.

[4038] Zhou Z, Ruan B, Hu G. Anti-intoxication and protective effects of a recombinant serine protease inhibitor from Lentinula edodes against acute alcohol-induced liver injury in mice. *Appl Microbiol Biotechnol*. 2020 Jun;104(11):4985-4993.

[4039] Yagi K. [Liver protective effect of Lentinula edodes mycelia(LEM)]. *Gan To Kagaku Ryoho*. 2012 Jul;39(7):1099-102.

[4040] Yoshioka Y, Kojima H, Tamura A, et al. Low-molecular-weight lignin-rich fraction in the extract of cultured Lentinula edodes mycelia attenuates carbon tetrachloride-induced toxicity in primary cultures of rat hepatocytes. *J Nat Med*. 2012 Jan;66(1):185-91.

[4041] Sasidharan S, Aravindran S, Latha LY, et al. In vitro antioxidant activity and hepatoprotective effects of Lentinula edodes against paracetamol-induced hepatotoxicity. *Molecules*. 2010 Jun 23;15(6):4478-89.

[4042] Itoh A, Isoda K, Kondoh M, et al. Hepatoprotective effect of syringic acid and vanillic acid on concanavalin a-induced liver injury. *Biol Pharm Bull*. 2009 Jul;32(7):1215-9.

[4043] Itoh A, Isoda K, Kondoh M, et al. Hepatoprotective effect of syringic acid and vanillic acid on CCl4-induced liver injury. *Biol Pharm Bull*. 2010;33(6):983-7.

[4044] Spim SRV, de Oliveira BGCC, Leite FG, et al. Effects of Lentinula edodes consumption on biochemical, hematologic and oxidative stress parameters in rats receiving high-fat diet. *Eur J Nutr*. 2017 Oct;56(7):2255-2264.

[4045] Song X, Ren Z, Wang X, et al. Antioxidant, anti-inflammatory and renoprotective effects of acidic-hydrolytic polysaccharides by spent mushroom compost (Lentinula edodes) on LPS-induced kidney injury. *Int J Biol Macromol*. 2020 May 15;151:1267-1276.

4046 Sun W, Feng Y, Zhang M et al. Protective effects of sulfated polysaccharides from Lentinula edodes on the lung and liver of MODS mice. *Food Funct.* 2021 Jul 21;12(14):6389-6402.

4047 Zhang Y, Cui Y, Feng Y, et al. Lentinus edodes Polysaccharides Alleviate Acute Lung Injury by Inhibiting Oxidative Stress and Inflammation. *Molecules.* 2022 Oct 28;27(21):7328.

4048 Ren Z, Li J, Song X, et al. The regulation of inflammation and oxidative status against lung injury of residue polysaccharides by Lentinula edodes. *Int J Biol Macromol.* 2018 Jan;106:185-192.

4049 Zhang Y, Cui Y, Feng Y, et al. Lentinus edodes Polysaccharides Alleviate Acute Lung Injury by Inhibiting Oxidative Stress and Inflammation. *Molecules.* 2022 Oct 28;27(21):7328.

4050 Ren Z, Li J, Song X, et al. The regulation of inflammation and oxidative status against lung injury of residue polysaccharides by Lentinula edodes. *Int J Biol Macromol.* 2018 Jan;106:185-192.

4051 Kuppusamy UR, Chong YL, Mahmood AA, et al. Lentinula edodes (Shiitake) mushroom extract protects against hydrogen peroxide induced cytotoxicity in peripheral blood mononuclear cells. *Indian J Biochem Biophys.* 2009 Apr;46(2):161-5.

4052 Takahashi M, Fujii G, Hamoya T, et al. Activation of NF-E2 p45-related factor-2 transcription and inhibition of intestinal tumor development by AHCC, a standardized extract of cultured Lentinula edodes mycelia. *J Clin Biochem Nutr.* 2019 Nov;65(3):203-208.

4053 Muñoz-Castiblanco T, Mejía-Giraldo JC, Puertas-Mejía MÁ. Lentinula edodes, a Novel Source of Polysaccharides with Antioxidant Power. *Antioxidants (Basel).* 2022 Sep 8;11(9):1770.

4054 Dai Y, Wang L, Chen X, et al. Lentinula edodes Sing Polysaccharide: Extraction, Characterization, Bioactivities, and Emulsifying Applications. *Foods.* 2023 Sep 1;12(17):3289.

4055 Yehia RS. Evaluation of the biological activities of β-glucan isolated from Lentinula edodes. *Lett Appl Microbiol.* 2022 Aug;75(2):317-329.

4056 Nam M, Choi JY, Kim MS. Metabolic Profiles, Bioactive Compounds, and Antioxidant Capacity in Lentinula edodes Cultivated on Log versus Sawdust Substrates. *Biomolecules.* 2021 Nov 8;11(11):1654.

4057 Lu X, Wang C, Li Y, et al. Improved production and antioxidant activity of exopolysaccharides by submerged culture of Lentinula edodes by the addition of lignocellulose. *J Biosci Bioeng.* 2022 Aug;134(2):162-166.

4058 Gao Y, Padhiar AA, Wang J, et al. Recombinant latcripin 11 of Lentinula edodes C91-3 suppresses the proliferation of various cancer cells. *Gene.* 2018 Feb 5;642:212-219.

4059 Sun W, Feng Y, Zhang M et al. Protective effects of sulfated polysaccharides from Lentinula edodes on the lung and liver of MODS mice. *Food Funct.* 2021 Jul 21;12(14):6389-6402.

4060 Ren Z, Liu W, Song X, et al. Antioxidant and anti-inflammation of enzymatic-hydrolysis residue polysaccharides by Lentinula edodes. *Int J Biol Macromol.* 2018 Dec;120(Pt A):811-822.

4061 Yin C, Li C, Ma K, et al. The physicochemical, antioxidant, hypoglycemic and prebiotic properties of γ-irradiated polysaccharides extracted from Lentinula edodes. *Food Sci Biotechnol.* 2023 Jan 25;32(7):987-996.

4062 Elhusseiny SM, El-Mahdy TS, Awad MF, et al. Proteome Analysis and In Vitro Antiviral, Anticancer and Antioxidant Capacities of the Aqueous Extracts of Lentinula edodes and Pleurotus ostreatus Edible Mushrooms. *Molecules.* 2021 Jul 30;26(15):4623.

4063 Liu Y, Luo M, Liu F, et al. Effects of freeze drying and hot-air drying on the physicochemical properties and bioactivities of polysaccharides from Lentinula edodes. *Int J Biol Macromol.* 2020 Feb 15;145:476-483.

4064 Finimundy TC, Gambato G, Fontana R, et al. Aqueous extracts of Lentinula edodes and Pleurotus sajor-caju exhibit high antioxidant capability and promising in vitro antitumor activity. *Nutr Res.* 2013 Jan;33(1):76-84.

4065 Song X, Ren Z, Wang X, et al. Antioxidant, anti-inflammatory and renoprotective effects of acidic-hydrolytic polysaccharides by spent mushroom compost (Lentinula edodes) on LPS-induced kidney injury. *Int J Biol Macromol.* 2020 May 15;151:1267-1276.

4066 Ann XH, Lun YZ, Zhang W, et al. Expression and characterization of protein Latcripin-3, an antioxidant and antitumor molecule from Lentinula edodes C91-3. *Asian Pac J Cancer Prev.* 2014;15(12):5055-61.

4067 Morales D, Rutckeviski R, Villalva M, et al. Isolation and comparison of α- and β-D-glucans from shiitake mushrooms (Lentinula edodes) with different biological activities. *Carbohydr Polym.* 2020 Feb 1;229:115521.

4068 Chowdhury M, Kubra K, Ahmed S. Screening of antimicrobial, antioxidant properties and bioactive compounds of some edible mushrooms cultivated in Bangladesh. *Ann Clin Microbiol Antimicrob.* 2015 Feb 7;14:8.

4069 Ao T, Deb CR. Nutritional and antioxidant potential of some wild edible mushrooms of Nagaland, India. *J Food Sci Technol.* 2019 Feb;56(2):1084-1089.

4070 Diallo I, Boudard F, Morel S, et al. Antioxidant and Anti-Inflammatory Potential of Shiitake Culinary-Medicinal Mushroom, Lentinus edodes (Agaricomycetes), Sporophores from Various Culture Conditions. *Int J Med Mushrooms.* 2020;22(6):535-546.

4071 de Lima PL, Sugui MM, Petrício AI, et al. Lentinula edodes (shiitake) modulates chemically induced mutagenesis by enhancing pitting. *J Med Food.* 2013 Aug;16(8):733-9.

4072 Miyaji CK, Poersch A, Ribeiro LR, et al. Shiitake (Lentinula edodes (Berkeley) Pegler) extracts as a modulator of micronuclei induced in HEp-2 cells. *Toxicol In Vitro.* 2006 Dec;20(8):1555-9.

4073 Sugui MM, Alves de Lima PL, Delmanto RD, et al. Antimutagenic effect of Lentinula edodes (BERK.) Pegler mushroom and possible variation among lineages. *Food Chem Toxicol.* 2003 Apr;41(4):555-60.

4074 Soroko-Dubrovina M, Górniak W, Zielińska P, et al. Evaluation of Shiitake Mushroom (Lentinula edodes) Supplementation on the Blood Parameters of Young Thoroughbred Racehorses. *Animals (Basel).* 2022 Nov 19;12(22):3212.

4075 Elhusseiny SM, El-Mahdy TS, Elleboudy NS, et al. In vitro Anti SARS-CoV-2 Activity and Docking Analysis of Pleurotus ostreatus, Lentinula edodes and Agaricus bisporus Edible Mushrooms. *Infect Drug Resist.* 2022 Jul 2;15:3459-3475.

4076 Singh A, Adam A, Rodriguez L, et al. Oral Supplementation with AHCC®, a Standardized Extract of Cultured Lentinula edodes Mycelia, Enhances Host Resistance against SARS-CoV-2 Infection. *Pathogens.* 2023 Apr 3;12(4):554.

4077 Rincão VP, Yamamoto KA, Ricardo NM, et al. Polysaccharide and extracts from Lentinula edodes: structural features and antiviral activity. *Virol J.* 2012 Feb 15;9:37.

[4078] Matsuhisa K, Yamane S, Okamoto T, et al. Anti-HCV effect of Lentinula edodes mycelia solid culture extracts and low-molecular-weight lignin. *Biochem Biophys Res Commun*. 2015 Jun 19;462(1):52-7.

[4079] Elhusseiny SM, El-Mahdy TS, Awad MF, et al. Proteome Analysis and In Vitro Antiviral, Anticancer and Antioxidant Capacities of the Aqueous Extracts of Lentinula edodes and Pleurotus ostreatus Edible Mushrooms. *Molecules*. 2021 Jul 30;26(15):4623.

[4080] Kuroki T, Lee S, Hirohama M, et al. Inhibition of Influenza Virus Infection by Lentinus edodes Mycelia Extract Through Its Direct Action and Immunopotentiating Activity. *Front Microbiol*. 2018 May 29;9:1164.

[4081] Elhusseiny SM, El-Mahdy TS, Awad MF, et al. Proteome Analysis and In Vitro Antiviral, Anticancer and Antioxidant Capacities of the Aqueous Extracts of Lentinula edodes and Pleurotus ostreatus Edible Mushrooms. *Molecules*. 2021 Jul 30;26(15):4623.

[4082] Razumov IA, Kazachinskaia EI, Puchkova LI, et al. [Protective activity of aqueous extracts from higher mushrooms against Herpes simplex virus type-2 on albino mice model]. *Antibiot Khimioter*. 2013;58(9-10):8-12.

[4083] Wang S, Welte T, Fang H, et al. Oral administration of active hexose correlated compound enhances host resistance to West Nile encephalitis in mice. *J Nutr*. 2009 Mar;139(3):598-602.

[4084] Rincao VP, Yamamoto KA, Ricardo NM, et al. Polysaccharide and extracts from Lentinula edodes: Structural features and antiviral activity. *Virol J*. 2012;9:37.

[4085] Tena-Garitaonaindia M, Ceacero-Heras D, Montoro MDMM, et al. A Standardized Extract of Lentinula edodes Cultured Mycelium Inhibits Pseudomonas aeruginosa Infectivity Mechanisms. *Front Microbiol*. 2022 Mar 16;13:814448.

[4086] Yehia RS. Evaluation of the biological activities of β-glucan isolated from Lentinula edodes. *Lett Appl Microbiol*. 2022 Aug;75(2):317-329.

[4087] Erdoğan Eliuz EA. Antibacterial activity and antibacterial mechanism of ethanol extracts of Lentinula edodes (Shiitake) and Agaricus bisporus (button mushroom). *Int J Environ Health Res*. 2022 Aug;32(8):1828-1841.

[4088] Ishihara A, Goto N, Kikkawa M, et al. Identification of antifungal compounds in the spent mushroom substrate of Lentinula edodes. *J Pestic Sci*. 2018 May 20;43(2):108-113.

[4089] Rao JR, Smyth TJ, Millar BC, et al. Antimicrobial properties of shiitake mushrooms (Lentinula edodes). *Int J Antimicrob Agents*. 2009 Jun;33(6):591-2.

[4090] Kwak AM, Lee IK, Lee SY, et al. Oxalic Acid from Lentinula edodes Culture Filtrate: Antimicrobial Activity on Phytopathogenic Bacteria and Qualitative and Quantitative Analyses. *Mycobiology*. 2016 Dec;44(4):338-342.

[4091] Tang L, Shang J, Song C, et al. Untargeted Metabolite Profiling of Antimicrobial Compounds in the Brown Film of Lentinula edodes Mycelium via LC-MS/MS Analysis. *ACS Omega*. 2020 Mar 27;5(13):7567-7575.

[4092] Chowdhury M, Kubra K, Ahmed S. Screening of antimicrobial, antioxidant properties and bioactive compounds of some edible mushrooms cultivated in Bangladesh. *Ann Clin Microbiol Antimicrob*. 2015 Feb 7;14:8.

[4093] Venturini ME, Rivera CS, Gonzalez C, et al. Antimicrobial activity of extracts of edible wild and cultivated mushrooms against foodborne bacterial strains. *J Food Prot*. 2008 Aug;71(8):1701-6.

[4094] Hearst R, Nelson D, McCollum G, et al. An examination of antibacterial and antifungal properties of constituents of Shiitake (Lentinula edodes) and oyster (Pleurotus ostreatus) mushrooms. *Complement Ther Clin Pract*. 2009 Feb;15(1):5-7.

[4095] Yano A, Kikuchi S, Yamashita Y, et al. The inhibitory effects of mushroom extracts on sucrose-dependent oral biofilm formation. *Appl Microbiol Biotechnol*. 2010 Mar;86(2):615-23.

[4096] Yano A, Konno N, Imai S, et al. Inhibitory effects of polysaccharides on the cariogenic activities of Streptococcus mutans. *Biosci Biotechnol Biochem*. 2012;76(12):2313-6.

[4097] Zaura E, Buijs MJ, Hoogenkamp MA, et al. The effects of fractions from shiitake mushroom on composition and cariogenicity of dental plaque microcosms in an in vitro caries model. *J Biomed Biotechnol*. 2011;2011:135034.

[4098] Sharma S, Prakash S. To detect the minimum inhibitory concentration and time-kill curve of shiitake mushroom on periodontal pathogens: An in vitro study. *J Indian Soc Periodontol*. 2019 May-Jun;23(3):216-219.

[4099] Ciric L, Tymon A, Zaura E, et al. In vitro assessment of shiitake mushroom (Lentinula edodes) extract for its antigingivitis activity. *J Biomed Biotechnol*. 2011;2011:507908.

[4100] Choi EJ, Park ZY, Kim EK. Chemical Composition and Inhibitory Effect of Lentinula edodes Ethanolic Extract on Experimentally Induced Atopic Dermatitis in Vitro and in Vivo. *Molecules*. 2016 Jul 29;21(8):993.

[4101] Muszyńska B, Dąbrowska M, Starek M, et al. Lentinula edodes Mycelium as Effective Agent for Piroxicam Mycoremediation. *Front Microbiol*. 2019 Feb 21;10:313.

[4102] Kryczyk-Poprawa A, Piotrowska J, Żmudzki P, et al. Feasibility of the use of Lentinula edodes mycelium in terbinafine remediation. *3 Biotech*. 2020 Apr;10(4):184.

[4103] Muszyńska B, Żmudzki P, Lazur J, et al. Analysis of the biodegradation of synthetic testosterone and 17α-ethynylestradiol using the edible mushroom Lentinula edodes. *3 Biotech*. 2018 Oct;8(10):424.

[4104] Kryczyk-Poprawa A, Żmudzki P, Maślanka A, et al. Mycoremediation of azole antifungal agents using in vitro cultures of Lentinula edodes. *3 Biotech*. 2019 Jun;9(6):207.

[4105] Dong XB, Huang W, Bian YB, et al. Remediation and Mechanisms of Cadmium Biosorption by a Cadmium-Binding Protein from Lentinula edodes. *J Agric Food Chem*. 2019 Oct 16;67(41):11373-11379.

[4106] Tsujiyama S, Muraoka T, Takada N. Biodegradation of 2,4-dichlorophenol by shiitake mushroom (Lentinula edodes) using vanillin as an activator. *Biotechnol Lett*. 2013 Jul;35(7):1079-83.

[4107] Gaitán-Hernández R, Esqueda M, Gutiérrez A, et al. Bioconversion of agrowastes by Lentinula edodes: the high potential of viticulture residues. *Appl Microbiol Biotechnol*. 2006 Jul;71(4):432-9.

[4108] Wang Y, Wang C, Cheng W, et al. Removal of cadmium from contaminated Lentinula edodes by optimized complexation and coagulation. *Food Sci Nutr*. 2016 May 31;5(2):215-222.

[4109] Wong KS, Huang Q, Au CH, et al. Biodegradation of dyes and polyaromatic hydrocarbons by two allelic forms of Lentinula edodes laccase expressed from Pichia pastoris. *Bioresour Technol*. 2012 Jan;104:157-64.

[4110] D'Annibale A, Casa R, Pieruccetti F, et al. Lentinula edodes removes phenols from olive-mill wastewater: impact on durum wheat (Triticum durum Desf.) germinability. *Chemosphere*. 2004 Feb;54(7):887-94.

4111 Barreto-Rodrigues M, Aguiar CM, da Cunha MA. Biotreatment of an effluent from a wood laminate industry using Lentinula edodes UEC 2019. *J Hazard Mater*. 2009 May 30;164(2-3):1556-60.

4112 Pinto AP, Serrano C, Pires T, et al. Degradation of terbuthylazine, difenoconazole and pendimethalin pesticides by selected fungi cultures. *Sci Total Environ*. 2012 Oct 1;435-436:402-10.

4113 Pineda-Alegría JA, Sánchez JE, Ventura-Zapata E, et al. Nematicidal Effect of Shiitake (Lentinula edodes) Extracts Against Haemonchus contortus. *J Med Food*. 2021 Sep;24(9):953-959.

4114 Grotto D, Gerenutti M, Souza VCO, et al. Deficiency of macro- and micronutrients induced by Lentinula edodes. *Toxicol Rep*. 2015 Feb 8;2:401-404.

4115 Smith JA, Gaikwad AA, Mathew L, et al. AHCC® Supplementation to Support Immune Function to Clear Persistent Human Papillomavirus Infections. *Front Oncol*. 2022 Jun 22;12:881902.

4116 Morales D, Shetty SA, López-Plaza B, et al. Modulation of human intestinal microbiota in a clinical trial by consumption of a β-D-glucan-enriched extract obtained from Lentinula edodes. *Eur J Nutr*. 2021 Sep;60(6):3249-3265.

4117 Dai X, Stanilka JM, Rowe CA, et al. Consuming Lentinula edodes (Shiitake) Mushrooms Daily Improves Human Immunity: A Randomized Dietary Intervention in Healthy Young Adults. *J Am Coll Nutr*. 2015;34(6):478-87.

4118 Takanari J, Sato A, Waki H, et al. Effects of AHCC® on Immune and Stress Responses in Healthy Individuals. *J Evid Based Integr Med*. 2018 Jan-Dec;23:2156587218756511.

4119 Zhang M, Zhang Y, Zhang L, et al. Mushroom polysaccharide lentinan for treating different types of cancers: A review of 12 years clinical studies in China. *Prog Mol Biol Transl Sci*. 2019;163:297-328.

4120 Nagashima Y, Yoshino S, Yamamoto S, et al. Lentinula edodes mycelia extract plus adjuvant chemotherapy for breast cancer patients: Results of a randomized study on host quality of life and immune function improvement. *Mol Clin Oncol*. 2017 Sep;7(3):359-366.

4121 Nagashima Y, Maeda N, Yamamoto S, et al. Evaluation of host quality of life and immune function in breast cancer patients treated with combination of adjuvant chemotherapy and oral administration of Lentinula edodes mycelia extract. *Onco Targets Ther*. 2013 Jul 9;6:853-9.

4122 Suzuki N, Takimoto Y, Suzuki R, et al. Efficacy of oral administration of Lentinula eododes mycelia extract for breast cancer patients undergoing postoperative hormone therapy. *Asian Pac J Cancer Prev*. 2013;14(6):3469-72.

4123 Yamaguchi Y, Miyahara E, Hihara J. Efficacy and safety of orally administered Lentinula edodes mycelia extract for patients undergoing cancer chemotherapy: a pilot study. *Am J Chin Med*. 2011;39(3):451-9.

4124 Hashimoto D, Satoi S, Yamamoto T, et al. Nutritional impact of active hexose-correlated compound for patients with resectable or borderline-resectable pancreatic cancer treated with neoadjuvant therapy. *Surg Today*. 2021 Nov;51(11):1872-1876.

4125 Kamiyama T, Orimo T, Wakayama K, et al. Preventing Recurrence of Hepatocellular Carcinoma After Curative Hepatectomy With Active Hexose-correlated Compound Derived From Lentinula edodes Mycelia. *Integr Cancer Ther*. 2022 Jan-Dec;21:15347354211073066.

4126 Tanigawa K, Itoh Y, Kobayashi Y. Improvement of QOL and Immunological Function With Lentinula Edodes Mycelia in Patients Undergoing Cancer Immunotherapy: An Open Pilot Study. *Altern Ther Health Med*. 2016 Jul;22(4):36-42.

4127 Tanigawa K, Ito Y, Sakai M, Kobayashi Y. [Evaluation of quality of life and immune function in cancer patients receiving combined immunotherapy and oral administration of lentinula edodes mycelia extract]. *Gan To Kagaku Ryoho*. 2012 Nov;39(12):1779-81.

4128 Yanagimoto H, Hirooka S, Yamamoto T, et al. Efficacy of Lentinula edodes Mycelia Extract on Chemotherapy-Related Tasted Disorders in Pancreatic Cancer Patients. *Nutr Cancer*. 2023;75(1):236-246.

4129 Hashimoto D, Satoi S, Ishikawa H, et al. Efficacy of active hexose correlated compound on survival of patients with resectable/borderline resectable pancreatic cancer: a study protocol for a double-blind randomized phase II study. *Trials*. 2022 Feb 12;23(1):135.

4130 Okuno K, Uno K. Efficacy of orally administered Lentinula edodes mycelia extract for advanced gastrointestinal cancer patients undergoing cancer chemotherapy: a pilot study. *Asian Pac J Cancer Prev*. 2011;12(7):1671-4.

4131 Aldwinckle J, Kristiansen B. A Quality-of-Life Study in Healthy Adults Supplemented with Lentinex® Beta-Glucan of Shiitake Culinary-Medicinal Mushroom, Lentinus edodes (Agaricomycetes). *Int J Med Mushrooms*. 2020;22(5):407-415.

4132 Ding R, Ning X, Ye M, et al. Antrodia camphorata extract (ACE)-induced apoptosis is associated with BMP4 expression and p53-dependent ROS generation in human colon cancer cells. *J Ethnopharmacol*. 2021 Mar 25;268:113570.

4133 Li B, Lu YY, Lo JY, et al. Chemical constituents from the dish-cultured Antrodia camphorata and their cytotoxic activities. *J Asian Nat Prod Res*. 2021 Jul;23(7):666-674.

4134 Park DK, Lim YH, Park HJ. Antrodia camphorata grown on germinated brown rice inhibits HT-29 human colon carcinoma proliferation through inducing G0/G1 phase arrest and apoptosis by targeting the β-catenin signaling. *J Med Food*. 2013 Aug;16(8):681-91.

4135 Wang G, Wan Y, Zhao J, et al. Ethanol extract of Antrodia camphorata inhibits proliferation of HCT-8 human colorectal cancer cells by arresting cell cycle progression and inducing apoptosis. *Mol Med Rep*. 2017 Oct;16(4):4941-4947.

4136 Yeh CT, Rao YK, Yao CJ, et al. Cytotoxic triterpenes from Antrodia camphorata and their mode of action in HT-29 human colon cancer cells. *Cancer Lett*. 2009 Nov 18;285(1):73-9.

4137 Lien HM, Kuo PT, Huang CL, et al. Study of the Anti-Proliferative Activity of 5-Substituted 4,7-Dimethoxy-1,3-Benzodioxole Derivatives of SY-1 from Antrodia camphorata on Human COLO 205 Colon Cancer Cells. *Evid Based Complement Alternat Med*. 2011;2011:450529.

4138 Tu SH, Wu CH, Chen LC, et al. In vivo antitumor effects of 4,7-dimethoxy-5-methyl-1,3-benzodioxole isolated from the fruiting body of Antrodia camphorata through activation of the p53-mediated p27/Kip1 signaling pathway. *J Agric Food Chem*. 2012 Apr 11;60(14):3612-12.

4139 Chang TC, Yeh CT, Adebayo BO, et al. 4-Acetylantroquinonol B inhibits colorectal cancer tumorigenesis and suppresses cancer stem-like phenotype. *Toxicol Appl Pharmacol*. 2015 Oct 15;288(2):258-68.

[4140] Wei PL, Tu SH, Lien HM, et al. The in vivo antitumor effects on human COLO 205 cancer cells of the 4,7-dimethoxy-5-(2-propen-1-yl)-1,3-benzodioxole (apiole) derivative of 5-substituted 4,7-dimethoxy-5-methyl-1,3-benzodioxole (SY-1) isolated from the fruiting body of Antrodia camphorata. *J Cancer Res Ther*. 2012 Oct-Dec;8(4):532-6.

[4141] Hseu YC, Chao YH, Lin KY, et al. Antrodia camphorata inhibits metastasis and epithelial-to-mesenchymal transition via the modulation of claudin-1 and Wnt/β-catenin signaling pathways in human colon cancer cells. J *Ethnopharmacol*. 2017 Aug 17;208:72-83.

[4142] Lin HC, Lin MH, Liao JH, et al. Antroquinonol, a Ubiquinone Derivative from the Mushroom Antrodia camphorata, Inhibits Colon Cancer Stem Cell-like Properties: Insights into the Molecular Mechanism and Inhibitory Targets. *J Agric Food Chem*. 2017 Jan 11;65(1):51-59.

[4143] Liu FS, Yang PY, Hu DN, et al. Antrodia camphorata induces apoptosis and enhances the cytotoxic effect of paclitaxel in human ovarian cancer cells. *Int J Gynecol Cancer*. 2011 Oct;21(7):1172-9.

[4144] Yang HL, Lin KY, Juan YC, et al. The anti-cancer activity of Antrodia camphorata against human ovarian carcinoma (SKOV-3) cells via modulation of HER-2/neu signaling pathway. *J Ethnopharmacol*. 2013 Jun 21;148(1):254-65.

[4145] Yang PY, Hu DN, Liu FS. Cytotoxic effect and induction of apoptosis in human cervical cancer cells by Antrodia camphorata. *Am J Chin Med*. 2013;41(5):1169-80.

[4146] Hseu YC, Chang GR, Pan JY, et al. Antrodia camphorata inhibits epithelial-to-mesenchymal transition by targeting multiple pathways in triple-negative breast cancers. *J Cell Physiol*. 2019 Apr;234(4):4125-4139.

[4147] Hseu YC, Chen SC, Chen HC, et al. Antrodia camphorata inhibits proliferation of human breast cancer cells in vitro and in vivo. *Food Chem Toxicol*. 2008 Aug;46(8):2680-8.

[4148] Li B, Kuang Y, He JB, et al. Antcamphorols A-K, Cytotoxic and ROS Scavenging Triterpenoids from Antrodia camphorata. *J Nat Prod*. 2020 Jan 24;83(1):45-54.

[4149] Yang HL, Kuo YH, Tsai CT, et al. Anti-metastatic activities of Antrodia camphorata against human breast cancer cells mediated through suppression of the MAPK signaling pathway. *Food Chem Toxicol*. 2011 Jan;49(1):290-8.

[4150] Lin TC, Germagian A, Liu Z. The NF-[Formula: see text]B Signaling and Wnt/[Formula: see text]-catenin Signaling in MCF-7 Breast Cancer Cells in Response to Bioactive Components from Mushroom Antrodia Camphorata. *Am J Chin Med*. 2021;49(1):199-215.

[4151] Wang SC, Lee TH, Hsu CH, et al. Antroquinonol D, isolated from Antrodia camphorata, with DNA demethylation and anticancer potential. *J Agric Food Chem*. 2014 Jun 18;62(24):5625-35.

[4152] Lee WT, Lee TH, Cheng CH, Chen KC, et al. Antroquinonol from Antrodia Camphorata suppresses breast tumor migration/invasion through inhibiting ERK-AP-1- and AKT-NF-κB-dependent MMP-9 and epithelial-mesenchymal transition expressions. *Food Chem Toxicol*. 2015 Apr;78:33-41.

[4153] Hseu YC, Chen SC, Tsai PC, et al. Inhibition of cyclooxygenase-2 and induction of apoptosis in estrogen-nonresponsive breast cancer cells by Antrodia camphorata. *Food Chem Toxicol*. 2007 Jul;45(7):1107-15.

[4154] Yang HL, Lin PY, Vadivalagan C, et al. Coenzyme Q0 defeats NLRP3-mediated inflammation, EMT/metastasis, and Warburg effects by inhibiting HIF-1α expression in human triple-negative breast cancer cells. *Arch Toxicol*. 2023 Apr;97(4):1047-1068.

[4155] Yang HL, Chen CS, Chang WH, et al. Growth inhibition and induction of apoptosis in MCF-7 breast cancer cells by Antrodia camphorata. *Cancer Lett*. 2006 Jan 18;231(2):215-27.

[4156] Rao YK, Wu AT, Geethangili M, et al. Identification of antrocin from Antrodia camphorata as a selective and novel class of small molecule inhibitor of Akt/mTOR signaling in metastatic breast cancer MDA-MB-231 cells. *Chem Res Toxicol*. 2011 Feb 18;24(2):238-45.

[4157] Lee TH, Lee CK, Tsou WL, et al. A new cytotoxic agent from solid-state fermented mycelium of Antrodia camphorata. *Planta Med*. 2007 Oct;73(13):1412-5.

[4158] Lee CC, Yang HL, Way TD, et al. Inhibition of Cell Growth and Induction of Apoptosis by Antrodia camphorata in HER-2/neu-Overexpressing Breast Cancer Cells through the Induction of ROS, Depletion of HER-2/neu, and Disruption of the PI3K/Akt Signaling Pathway. *Evid Based Complement Alternat Med*. 2012;2012:702857.

[4159] Wang HM, Yang HL, Thiyagarajan V, et al. Coenzyme Q0 Enhances Ultraviolet B-Induced Apoptosis in Human Estrogen Receptor-Positive Breast (MCF-7) Cancer Cells. *Integr Cancer Ther*. 2017 Sep;16(3):385-396.

[4160] Li B, Lu YY, Lo JY, et al. Chemical constituents from the dish-cultured Antrodia camphorata and their cytotoxic activities. *J Asian Nat Prod Res*. 2021 Jul;23(7):666-674.

[4161] Chan YY, Chang CS, Chien LH, et al. Apoptotic effects of a high performance liquid chromatography (HPLC) fraction of Antrodia camphorata mycelia are mediated by down-regulation of the expressions of four tumor-related genes in human non-small cell lung carcinoma A549 cell. *J Ethnopharmacol*. 2010 Feb 17;127(3):652-61.

[4162] Chiou JF, Wu AT, Wang WT, et al. A Preclinical Evaluation of Antrodia camphorata Alcohol Extracts in the Treatment of Non-Small Cell Lung Cancer Using Non-Invasive Molecular Imaging. *Evid Based Complement Alternat Med*. 2011;2011:914561.

[4163] Yeh CT, Huang WC, Rao YK, et al. A sesquiterpene lactone antrocin from Antrodia camphorata negatively modulates JAK2/STAT3 signaling via microRNA let-7c and induces apoptosis in lung cancer cells. *Carcinogenesis*. 2013 Dec;34(12):2918-28.

[4164] Wu H, Pan CL, Yao YC, et al. Proteomic analysis of the effect of Antrodia camphorata extract on human lung cancer A549 cell. *Proteomics*. 2006 Feb;6(3):826-35.

[4165] Nakamura N, Hirakawa A, Gao JJ, et al. Five new maleic and succinic acid derivatives from the mycelium of Antrodia camphorata and their cytotoxic effects on LLC tumor cell line. *J Nat Prod*. 2004 Jan;67(1):46-8.

[4166] Wang WJ, Wu YS, Chen S, et al. Mushroom β-Glucan May Immunomodulate the Tumor-Associated Macrophages in the Lewis Lung Carcinoma. *Biomed Res Int*. 2015;2015:604385.

[4167] Kumar VB, Yuan TC, Liou JW, et al. Antroquinonol inhibits NSCLC proliferation by altering PI3K/mTOR proteins and miRNA expression profiles. *Mutat Res*. 2011 Feb 10;707(1-2):42-52.

[4168] Zhu PL, Fu XQ, Li JK, et al. Antrodia camphorata Mycelia Exert Anti-liver Cancer Effects and Inhibit STAT3 Signaling in vitro and in vivo. *Front Pharmacol.* 2018 Dec 17;9:1449.

[4169] Chen YF, Wu HC, Chang JM, et al. Chemical investigations and cytotoxic effects of metabolites from Antrodia camphorata against human hepatocellular carcinoma cells. *Nat Prod Res.* 2023 Feb;37(4):560-570.

[4170] Lee YP, Tsai WC, Ko CJ, et al. Anticancer effects of eleven triterpenoids derived from Antrodia camphorata. *Anticancer Res.* 2012 Jul;32(7):2727-34.

[4171] Chang JS, Kuo HP, Chang KL, et al. Apoptosis of Hepatocellular Carcinoma Cells Induced by Nanoencapsulated Polysaccharides Extracted from Antrodia Camphorata. *PLoS One.* 2015 Sep 1;10(9):e0136782.

[4172] Song TY, Hsu SL, Yeh CT, et al. Mycelia from Antrodia camphorata in Submerged culture induce apoptosis of human hepatoma HepG2 cells possibly through regulation of Fas pathway. *J Agric Food Chem.* 2005 Jul 13;53(14):5559-64.

[4173] Lee TH, Lee CK, Tsou WL, et al. A new cytotoxic agent from solid-state fermented mycelium of Antrodia camphorata. *Planta Med.* 2007 Oct;73(13):1412-5.

[4174] Lin LT, Tai CJ, Su CH, et al. The Ethanolic Extract of Taiwanofungus camphoratus (Antrodia camphorata) Induces Cell Cycle Arrest and Enhances Cytotoxicity of Cisplatin and Doxorubicin on Human Hepatocellular Carcinoma Cells. *Biomed Res Int.* 2015;2015:415269.

[4175] Hsieh YC, Rao YK, Wu CC, et al. Methyl antcinate A from Antrodia camphorata induces apoptosis in human liver cancer cells through oxidant-mediated cofilin- and Bax-triggered mitochondrial pathway. *Chem Res Toxicol.* 2010 Jul 19;23(7):1256-67.

[4176] Hsu YL, Kuo YC, Kuo PL, et al. Apoptotic effects of extract from Antrodia camphorata fruiting bodies in human hepatocellular carcinoma cell lines. *Cancer Lett.* 2005 Apr 18;221(1):77-89.

[4177] Hsieh YC, Rao YK, Whang-Peng J, et al. Antcin B and its ester derivative from Antrodia camphorata induce apoptosis in hepatocellular carcinoma cells involves enhancing oxidative stress coincident with activation of intrinsic and extrinsic apoptotic pathway. *J Agric Food Chem.* 2011 Oct 26;59(20):10943-54.

[4178] Song TY, Hsu SL, Yen GC. Induction of apoptosis in human hepatoma cells by mycelia of Antrodia camphorata in submerged culture. *J Ethnopharmacol.* 2005 Aug 22;100(1-2):158-67.

[4179] Stewart SG, Ho LA, Polomska ME, et al. Rapid evaluation of Antrodia camphorata natural products and derivatives in tumourigenic liver progenitor cells with a novel cell proliferation assay. *ChemMedChem.* 2009 Oct;4(10):1657-67.

[4180] Peng CC, Chen KC, Peng RY, et al. Antrodia camphorata extract induces replicative senescence in superficial TCC, and inhibits the absolute migration capability in invasive bladder carcinoma cells. *J Ethnopharmacol.* 2007 Jan 3;109(1):93-103.

[4181] Peng CC, Chen KC, Peng RY, et al. Human urinary bladder cancer T24 cells are susceptible to the Antrodia camphorata extracts. *Cancer Lett.* 2006 Nov 8;243(1):109-19.

[4182] Lee CI, Wu CC, Hsieh SL, et al. Anticancer effects on human pancreatic cancer cells of triterpenoids, polysaccharides and 1,3-β-D-glucan derived from the fruiting body of Antrodia camphorata. *Food Funct.* 2014 Dec;5(12):3224-32.

[4183] Yu CC, Chiang PC, Lu PH, et al. Antroquinonol, a natural ubiquinone derivative, induces a cross talk between apoptosis, autophagy and senescence in human pancreatic carcinoma cells. *J Nutr Biochem.* 2012 Aug;23(8):900-7.

[4184] Lee YP, Tsai WC, Ko CJ, et al. Anticancer effects of eleven triterpenoids derived from Antrodia camphorata. *Anticancer Res.* 2012 Jul;32(7):2727-34.

[4185] Huang CC, Cheng HH, Wang JL, et al. Effects of Antrodia camphorata extracts on the viability, apoptosis, [Ca2+]i, and MAPKs phosphorylation of OC2 human oral cancer cells. *Chin J Physiol.* 2009 Jun 30;52(3):128-35.

[4186] Tsai WC, Rao YK, Lin SS, et al. Methylantcinate A induces tumor specific growth inhibition in oral cancer cells via Bax-mediated mitochondrial apoptotic pathway. *Bioorg Med Chem Lett.* 2010 Oct 15;20(20):6145-8.

[4187] Lee YP, Tsai WC, Ko CJ, et al. Anticancer effects of eleven triterpenoids derived from Antrodia camphorata. *Anticancer Res.* 2012 Jul;32(7):2727-34.

[4188] Chen KC, Peng CC, Peng RY, et al. Unique formosan mushroom Antrodia camphorata differentially inhibits androgen-responsive LNCaP and -independent PC-3 prostate cancer cells. *Nutr Cancer.* 2007;57(1):111-21.

[4189] Lee TH, Lee CK, Tsou WL, et al. A new cytotoxic agent from solid-state fermented mycelium of Antrodia camphorata. *Planta Med.* 2007 Oct;73(13):1412-5.

[4190] Ho CM, Huang CC, Huang CJ, et al. Effects of antrodia camphorata on viability, apoptosis, and [Ca2+]i in PC3 human prostate cancer cells. *Chin J Physiol.* 2008 Apr 30;51(2):78-84.

[4191] Chen LY, Sheu MT, Liao CK, et al. Taiwanofungus camphoratus (Syn Antrodia camphorata) extract and amphotericin B exert adjuvant effects via mitochondrial apoptotic pathway. *Integr Cancer Ther.* 2013 Mar;12(2):153-64.

[4192] Li B, Lu YY, Lo JY, et al. Chemical constituents from the dish-cultured Antrodia camphorata and their cytotoxic activities. *J Asian Nat Prod Res.* 2021 Jul;23(7):666-674.

[4193] Yang HL, Kumar KJ, Kuo YT, et al. Antrodia camphorata induces G(1) cell-cycle arrest in human premyelocytic leukemia (HL-60) cells and suppresses tumor growth in athymic nude mice. *Food Funct.* 2014 Sep;5(9):2278-88.

[4194] Lee TH, Chen CC, Chen JJ, et al. New and Cytotoxic Components from Antrodia camphorata. *Molecules.* 2014 Dec 19;19(12):21378-85.

[4195] Hseu YC, Chang WC, Hseu YT, et al. Protection of oxidative damage by aqueous extract from Antrodia camphorata mycelia in normal human erythrocytes. *Life Sci.* 2002 Jun 14;71(4):469-82.

[4196] Hseu YC, Yang HL, Lai YC, et al. Induction of apoptosis by Antrodia camphorata in human premyelocytic leukemia HL-60 cells. *Nutr Cancer.* 2004;48(2):189-97.

[4197] Du YC, Chang FR, Wu TY, et al. Antileukemia component, dehydroeburicoic acid from Antrodia camphorata induces DNA damage and apoptosis in vitro and in vivo models. *Phytomedicine.* 2012 Jun 15;19(8-9):788-96.

[4198] Lu MC, Du YC, Chuu JJ, et al. Active extracts of wild fruiting bodies of Antrodia camphorata (EEAC) induce leukemia HL 60 cells apoptosis partially through histone hypoacetylation and synergistically promote anticancer effect of trichostatin A. *Arch Toxicol.* 2009 Feb;83(2):121-9.

[4199] Liu JJ, Huang TS, Hsu ML, et al. Antitumor effects of the partially purified polysaccharides from Antrodia camphorata and the mechanism of its action. *Toxicol Appl Pharmacol.* 2004 Dec 1;201(2):186-93.

[4200] Rao YK, Fang SH, Tzeng YM. Evaluation of the anti-inflammatory and anti-proliferation tumoral cells activities of Antrodia camphorata, Cordyceps sinensis, and Cinnamomum osmophloeum bark extracts. *J Ethnopharmacol*. 2007 Oct 8;114(1):78-85.

[4201] Li B, Lu YY, Lo JY, et al. Chemical constituents from the dish-cultured Antrodia camphorata and their cytotoxic activities. *J Asian Nat Prod Res*. 2021 Jul;23(7):666-674.

[4202] Li B, Kuang Y, He JB, et al. Antcamphorols A-K, Cytotoxic and ROS Scavenging Triterpenoids from Antrodia camphorata. *J Nat Prod*. 2020 Jan 24;83(1):45-54.

[4203] Yang HL, Tsai CH, Shrestha S, et al. Coenzyme Q0, a novel quinone derivative of Antrodia camphorata, induces ROS-mediated cytotoxic autophagy and apoptosis against human glioblastoma cells in vitro and in vivo. *Food Chem Toxicol*. 2021 Sep;155:112384.

[4204] Song M, Park DK, Park HJ. Antrodia camphorata Grown on Germinated Brown Rice Suppresses Melanoma Cell Proliferation by Inducing Apoptosis and Cell Differentiation and Tumor Growth. *Evid Based Complement Alternat Med*. 2013;2013:321096.

[4205] Wang JJ, Wu CC, Lee CL, et al. Antimelanogenic, Antioxidant and Antiproliferative Effects of Antrodia camphorata Fruiting Bodies on B16-F0 Melanoma Cells. *PLoS One*. 2017 Jan 26;12(1):e0170924.

[4206] Hseu YC, Tsou HT, Kumar KJ, et al. The Antitumor Activity of Antrodia camphorata in Melanoma Cells: Modulation of Wnt/β-Catenin Signaling Pathways. *Evid Based Complement Alternat Med*. 2012;2012:197309.

[4207] Chen LY, Sheu MT, Liao CK, et al. Taiwanofungus camphoratus (Syn Antrodia camphorata) extract and amphotericin B exert adjuvant effects via mitochondrial apoptotic pathway. *Integr Cancer Ther*. 2013 Mar;12(2):153-64.

[4208] Yang HL, Chiu LW, Lin YA, et al. In vitro and in vivo anti-tumor activity of Coenzyme Q0 against TWIST1-overexpressing HNSCC cells: ROS-mediated inhibition of EMT/metastasis and autophagy/apoptosis induction. *Toxicol Appl Pharmacol*. 2023 Apr 15;465:116453.

[4209] Ho CL, Wang JL, Lee CC, et al. Antroquinonol blocks Ras and Rho signaling via the inhibition of protein isoprenyltransferase activity in cancer cells. *Biomed Pharmacother*. 2014 Oct;68(8):1007-14.

[4210] Chang CY, Huang ZN, Yu HH, et al. The adjuvant effects of Antrodia Camphorata extracts combined with anti-tumor agents on multidrug resistant human hepatoma cells. *J Ethnopharmacol*. 2008 Aug 13;118(3):387-95.

[4211] Lin LT, Tai CJ, Su CH, et al. The Ethanolic Extract of Taiwanofungus camphoratus (Antrodia camphorata) Induces Cell Cycle Arrest and Enhances Cytotoxicity of Cisplatin and Doxorubicin on Human Hepatocellular Carcinoma Cells. *Biomed Res Int*. 2015;2015:415269.

[4212] Chen LY, Sheu MT, Liu DZ, et al. Pretreatment with an ethanolic extract of Taiwanofungus camphoratus (Antrodia camphorata) enhances the cytotoxic effects of amphotericin B. *J Agric Food Chem*. 2011 Oct 26;59(20):11255-63.

[4213] Lee TH, Chen CC, Chen JJ, et al. New and Cytotoxic Components from Antrodia camphorata. *Molecules*. 2014 Dec 19;19(12):21378-85.

[4214] Liu Y, Ding Y, Ye M, et al. A Novel Heterogalactan from Antrodia camphorata and Anti-Angiogenic Activity of Its Sulfated Derivative. *Polymers (Basel)*. 2017 Jun 16;9(6):228.

[4215] Wang SC, Lee TH, Hsu CH, et al. Antroquinonol D, isolated from Antrodia camphorata, with DNA demethylation and anticancer potential. *J Agric Food Chem*. 2014 Jun 18;62(24):5625-35.

[4216] Mukai M, Hayakawa K, Okamura M, et al. Preferential blockade of dioxin-induced activation of the aryl hydrocarbon receptor by Antrodia camphorata. *Biol Pharm Bull*. 2009 Sep;32(9):1510-5.

[4217] Han C, Shen H, Yang Y, et al. Antrodia camphorata polysaccharide resists 6-OHDA-induced dopaminergic neuronal damage by inhibiting ROS-NLRP3 activation. *Brain Behav*. 2020 Nov;10(11):e01824.

[4218] Yang PS, Lin PY, Chang CC, et al. Antrodia camphorata Potentiates Neuroprotection against Cerebral Ischemia in Rats via Downregulation of iNOS/HO-1/Bax and Activated Caspase-3 and Inhibition of Hydroxyl Radical Formation. *Evid Based Complement Alternat Med*. 2015;2015:232789.

[4219] Kong ZL, Hsu YT, Johnson A, et al. Protective effects of Antrodia camphorata extract against hypoxic cell injury and ischemic stroke brain damage. *Phytother Res*. 2021 Mar;35(3):1609-1620.

[4220] Zou XG, Xu MT, Dong XL, et al. Solid-state-cultured mycelium of Antrodia camphorata exerts potential neuroprotective activities against 6-hydroxydopamine-induced toxicity in PC12 cells. *J Food Biochem*. 2022 Aug;46(8):e14208.

[4221] Huang NK, Cheng JJ, Lai WL, et al. Antrodia camphorata prevents rat pheochromocytoma cells from serum deprivation-induced apoptosis. *FEMS Microbiol Lett*. 2005 Mar 1;244(1):213-9.

[4222] Lee YM, Chang CY, Yen TL, et al. Extract of Antrodia camphorata exerts neuroprotection against embolic stroke in rats without causing the risk of hemorrhagic incidence. *ScientificWorldJournal*. 2014;2014:686109.

[4223] Shi Y, Yang S, Lee DY, et al. Increasing anti-Aβ-induced neurotoxicity ability of Antrodia camphorata-fermented product with deep ocean water supplementary. *J Sci Food Agric*. 2016 Nov;96(14):4690-4701.

[4224] Chen CC, Shiao YJ, Lin RD, et al. Neuroprotective diterpenes from the fruiting body of Antrodia camphorata. *J Nat Prod*. 2006 Apr;69(4):689-91.

[4225] Wang YH, Chern CM, Liou KT, et al. Ergostatrien-7,9(11),22-trien-3β-ol from Antrodia camphorata ameliorates ischemic stroke brain injury via downregulation of p65NF-κ-B and caspase 3, and activation of Akt/GSK3/catenin-associated neurogenesis. *Food Funct*. 2019 Aug 1;10(8):4725-4738.

[4226] Wang LC, Wang SE, Wang JJ, et al. In vitro and in vivo comparisons of the effects of the fruiting body and mycelium of Antrodia camphorata against amyloid β-protein-induced neurotoxicity and memory impairment. *Appl Microbiol Biotechnol*. 2012 Jun;94(6):1505-19.

[4227] Liu HP, Kuo YH, Cheng J, et al. Ergosta-7,9(11),22-trien-3β-ol Rescues AD Deficits by Modulating Microglia Activation but Not Oxidative Stress. *Molecules*. 2021 Sep 2;26(17):5338.

[4228] Chang WH, Chen MC, Cheng IH. Antroquinonol Lowers Brain Amyloid-β Levels and Improves Spatial Learning and Memory in a Transgenic Mouse Model of Alzheimer's Disease. *Sci Rep*. 2015 Oct 15;5:15067.

[4229] Sun P, Li W, Guo J, et al. Ergosterol Isolated from Antrodia camphorata Suppresses LPS-Induced Neuroinflammatory Responses in Microglia Cells and ICR Mice. *Molecules*. 2023 Mar 6;28(5):2406.

[4230] Han C, Guo L, Yang Y, et al. Study on antrodia camphorata polysaccharide in alleviating the neuroethology of PD mice by decreasing the expression of NLRP3 inflammasome. *Phytother Res*. 2019 Sep;33(9):2288-2297.

[4231] Lanza M, Cucinotta L, Casili G, et al. The Transcription Factor Nrf2 Mediates the Effects of Antrodia camphorata Extract on Neuropathological Changes in a Mouse Model of Parkinson's Disease. *Int J Mol Sci*. 2023 May 25;24(11):9250.

[4232] Yang Y, Han C, Sheng Y, et al. Antrodia camphorata polysaccharide improves inflammatory response in liver injury via the ROS/TLR4/NF-κB signal. *J Cell Mol Med*. 2022 May;26(9):2706-2716.

[4233] Ruan S, Yang Y, Li W. Antrodia Camphorata Polysaccharide activates autophagy and regulates NLRP3 degradation to improve liver injury-related inflammatory response. *Aging (Albany NY)*. 2022 Oct 10;14(22):8970-8981.

[4234] Cao C, Zhong H, Chen Z, et al. Triterpene acid from Antrodia camphorata alleviates inflammation in acute liver injury. *Aging (Albany NY)*. 2023 May 26;15(10):4524-4532.

[4235] Hsiao G, Shen MY, Lin KH, et al. Antioxidative and hepatoprotective effects of Antrodia camphorata extract. *J Agric Food Chem*. 2003 May 21;51(11):3302-8.

[4236] Yi Z, Liu X, Liang L, et al. Antrodin A from Antrodia camphorata modulates the gut microbiome and liver metabolome in mice exposed to acute alcohol intake. *Food Funct*. 2021 Apr 7;12(7):2925-2937.

[4237] Yi ZW, Xia YJ, Liu XF, et al. Antrodin A from mycelium of Antrodia camphorata alleviates acute alcoholic liver injury and modulates intestinal flora dysbiosis in mice. *J Ethnopharmacol*. 2020 May 23;254:112681.

[4238] Chen Q, Tang H, Zha Z, et al. β-d-glucan from Antrodia Camphorata ameliorates LPS-induced inflammation and ROS production in human hepatocytes. *Int J Biol Macromol*. 2017 Nov;104(Pt A):768-777.

[4239] Wang HJ, Cui C, Gong XM, et al. Improvement of triterpenoid production in mycelia of Antrodia camphorata through mutagenesis breeding and amelioration of CCl4-induced liver injury in mice. *Heliyon*. 2023 Aug 30;9(9):e19621.

[4240] Li ZW, Kuang Y, Tang SN, et al. Hepatoprotective activities of Antrodia camphorata and its triterpenoid compounds against CCl4-induced liver injury in mice. *J Ethnopharmacol*. 2017 Jul 12;206:31-39.

[4241] Chao TY, Hsieh CC, Hsu SM, et al. Ergostatrien-3β-ol (EK100) from Antrodia camphorata Attenuates Oxidative Stress, Inflammation, and Liver Injury In Vitro and In Vivo. *Prev Nutr Food Sci*. 2021 Mar 31;26(1):58-66.

[4242] Wu Y, Tian WJ, Gao S, et al. Secondary metabolites of petri-dish cultured Antrodia camphorata and their hepatoprotective activities against alcohol-induced liver injury in mice. *Chin J Nat Med*. 2019 Jan;17(1):33-42.

[4243] Wu MT, Tzang BS, Chang YY, et al. Effects of Antrodia camphorata on alcohol clearance and antifibrosis in livers of rats continuously fed alcohol. *J Agric Food Chem*. 2011 Apr 27;59(8):4248-54.

[4244] Chang YY, Liu YC, Kuo YH, et al. Effects of antrosterol from Antrodia camphorata submerged whole broth on lipid homeostasis, antioxidation, alcohol clearance, and anti-inflammation in livers of chronic-alcohol fed mice. *J Ethnopharmacol*. 2017 Apr 18;202:200-207.

[4245] Lu ZM, Tao WY, Zou XL, et al. Protective effects of mycelia of Antrodia camphorata and Armillariella tabescens in submerged culture against ethanol-induced hepatic toxicity in rats. *J Ethnopharmacol*. 2007 Mar 1;110(1):160-4.

[4246] Huang GJ, Deng JS, Huang SS, et al. Hepatoprotective effects of eburicoic acid and dehydroeburicoic acid from Antrodia camphorata in a mouse model of acute hepatic injury. *Food Chem*. 2013 Dec 1;141(3):3020-7.

[4247] Huang CH, Chang YY, Liu CW, et al. Fruiting body of Niuchangchih (Antrodia camphorata) protects livers against chronic alcohol consumption damage. *J Agric Food Chem*. 2010 Mar 24;58(6):3859-66.

[4248] Lu ZM, Tao WY, Xu HY, et al. Further studies on the hepatoprotective effect of Antrodia camphorata in submerged culture on ethanol-induced acute liver injury in rats. *Nat Prod Res*. 2011 Apr;25(7):684-95.

[4249] Song TY, Yen GC. Protective effects of fermented filtrate from Antrodia camphorata in submerged culture against CCl4-induced hepatic toxicity in rats. *J Agric Food Chem*. 2003 Mar 12;51(6):1571-7.

[4250] Xu XY, Geng Y, Xu HX, et al. Antrodia camphorata-Derived Antrodin C Inhibits Liver Fibrosis by Blocking TGF-Beta and PDGF Signaling Pathways. *Front Mol Biosci*. 2022 Feb 15;9:835508.

[4251] Wang LC, Kuo IU, Tsai TY, et al. Antrodia camphorata-fermented product cultured in deep ocean water has more liver protection against thioacetamide-induced fibrosis. *Appl Microbiol Biotechnol*. 2013 Dec;97(23):9955-67.

[4252] Ren Y, Li HX, Zhou L, et al. Protective Effect of Spore Powder of Antrodia camphorata ATCC 200183 on CCl4-Induced Liver Fibrosis in Mice. *Nutrients*. 2020 Sep 11;12(9):2778.

[4253] Geng Y, Wang J, Sun Q, et al. Identification of antrodin B from Antrodia camphorata as a new anti-hepatofibrotic compound using a rapid cell screening method and biological evaluation. *Hepatol Res*. 2016 Mar;46(3):E15-25.

[4254] Lin WC, Kuo SC, Lin WL, et al. Filtrate of fermented mycelia from Antrodia camphorata reduces liver fibrosis induced by carbon tetrachloride in rats. *World J Gastroenterol*. 2006 Apr 21;12(15):2369-74.

[4255] Geng Y, Wang J, Xie M, et al. Screening and isolation for anti-hepatofibrotic components from medicinal mushrooms using TGF-(β1-induced live fibrosis in hepatic stellate cells. *Int J Med Mushrooms*. 2014;16(6):529-39.

[4256] Yang KL, Chang WT, Hong MY, et al. Prevention of TGF-β-induced early liver fibrosis by a maleic acid derivative anti-oxidant through suppression of ROS, inflammation and hepatic stellate cells activation. *PLoS One*. 2017 Apr 6;12(4):e0174008.

[4257] Chang JM, Lee YR, Hung LM, et al. An Extract of Antrodia camphorata Mycelia Attenuates the Progression of Nephritis in Systemic Lupus Erythematosus-Prone NZB/W F1 Mice. *Evid Based Complement Alternat Med*. 2011;2011:465894.

[4258] Tsai PY, Ka SM, Chao TK, et al. Antroquinonol reduces oxidative stress by enhancing the Nrf2 signaling pathway and inhibits inflammation and sclerosis in focal segmental glomerulosclerosis mice. *Free Radic Biol Med*. 2011 Jun 1;50(11):1503-16.

[4259] Yang SM, Ka SM, Hua KF, et al. Antroquinonol mitigates an accelerated and progressive IgA nephropathy model in mice by activating the Nrf2 pathway and inhibiting T cells and NLRP3 inflammasome. *Free Radic Biol Med*. 2013 Aug;61:285-97.

[4260] Tsai PY, Ka SM, Chang JM, et al. Antroquinonol differentially modulates T cell activity and reduces interleukin-18 production, but enhances Nrf2 activation, in murine accelerated severe lupus nephritis. *Arthritis Rheum*. 2012 Jan;64(1):232-42.

[4261] Juan YS, Mannikarottu A, Chuang SM, et al. Protective effect of Antrodia camphorata on bladder ischemia/reperfusion injury. *Int Urol Nephrol*. 2010 Sep;42(3):637-45.

[4262] Huang GJ, Deng JS, Chen CC, et al. Methanol extract of Antrodia camphorata protects against lipopolysaccharide-induced acute lung injury by suppressing NF-κB and MAPK pathways in mice. *J Agric Food Chem*. 2014 Jun 11;62(23):5321-9.

[4263] Yi Z, Liu X, Liang L, et al. Antrodin A from Antrodia camphorata modulates the gut microbiome and liver metabolome in mice exposed to acute alcohol intake. *Food Funct*. 2021 Apr 7;12(7):2925-2937.

[4264] Park DK, Park HJ. Ethanol Extract of Antrodia camphorata Grown on Germinated Brown Rice Suppresses Inflammatory Responses in Mice with Acute DSS-Induced Colitis. *Evid Based Complement Alternat Med*. 2013;2013:914524.

[4265] Liu DZ, Liang YC, Lin SY, et al. Antihypertensive activities of a solid-state culture of Taiwanofungus camphoratus (Changchih) in spontaneously hypertensive rats. *Biosci Biotechnol Biochem*. 2007 Jan;71(1):23-30.

[4266] Wang GJ, Tseng HW, Chou CJ, et al. The vasorelaxation of Antrodia camphorata mycelia: involvement of endothelial Ca(2+)-NO-cGMP pathway. *Life Sci*. 2003 Oct 10;73(21):2769-83.

[4267] Li YH, Chung HC, Liu SL, et al. A novel inhibitory effect of Antrodia camphorata extract on vascular smooth muscle cell migration and neointima formation in mice. *Int Heart J*. 2009 Mar;50(2):207-20.

[4268] Lu CW, Nguyen NTK, Shen SC, et al. Botanical Antcin K Alleviates High-Fat Damage in Palm Acid Oil-Treated Vascular Endothelial Cells and Macrophages. *Plants (Basel)*. 2022 Oct 22;11(21):2812.

[4269] Lu WJ, Lin SC, Lan CC, et al. Effect of Antrodia camphorata on inflammatory arterial thrombosis-mediated platelet activation: the pivotal role of protein kinase C. *ScientificWorldJournal*. 2014;2014:745802.

[4270] Yang HL, Hseu YC, Chen JY, et al. Antrodia camphorata in submerged culture protects low density lipoproteins against oxidative modification. *Am J Chin Med*. 2006;34(2):217-31.

[4271] Kuo YH, Lin CH, Shih CC. Dehydroeburicoic Acid from Antrodia camphorata Prevents the Diabetic and Dyslipidemic State via Modulation of Glucose Transporter 4, Peroxisome Proliferator-Activated Receptor α Expression and AMP-Activated Protein Kinase Phosphorylation in High-Fat-Fed Mice. *Int J Mol Sci*. 2016 Jun 3;17(6):872.

[4272] Lin CH, Kuo YH, Shih CC. Eburicoic Acid, a Triterpenoid Compound from Antrodia camphorata, Displays Antidiabetic and Antihyperlipidemic Effects in Palmitate-Treated C2C12 Myotubes and in High-Fat Diet-Fed Mice. *Int J Mol Sci*. 2017 Nov 2;18(11):2314.

[4273] Kuo YH, Lin CH, Shih CC, et al. Antcin K, a Triterpenoid Compound from Antrodia camphorata, Displays Antidiabetic and Antihyperlipidemic Effects via Glucose Transporter 4 and AMP-Activated Protein Kinase Phosphorylation in Muscles. *Evid Based Complement Alternat Med*. 2016;2016:4867092.

[4274] Lin CH, Hsiao LW, Kuo YH, et al. Antidiabetic and Antihyperlipidemic Effects of Sulphurenic Acid, a Triterpenoid Compound from Antrodia camphorata, in Streptozotocin-Induced Diabetic Mice. *Int J Mol Sci*. 2019 Oct 2;20(19):4897.

[4275] Kuo YH, Lin CH, Shih CC. Antidiabetic and Antihyperlipidemic Properties of a Triterpenoid Compound, Dehydroeburicoic Acid, from Antrodia camphorata in Vitro and in Streptozotocin-Induced Mice. *J Agric Food Chem*. 2015 Nov 25;63(46):10140-51.

[4276] Vong CT, Tseng HH, Kwan YW, et al. Antrodia camphorata Increases Insulin Secretion and Protects from Apoptosis in MIN6 Cells. *Front Pharmacol*. 2016 Mar 21;7:67.

[4277] Kuang Y, Chai Y, Su H, et al. A network pharmacology-based strategy to explore the pharmacological mechanisms of Antrodia camphorata and antcin K for treating type II diabetes mellitus. *Phytomedicine*. 2022 Feb;96:153851.

[4278] Kuo YH, Lin CH, Shih CC. Dehydroeburicoic Acid from Antrodia camphorata Prevents the Diabetic and Dyslipidemic State via Modulation of Glucose Transporter 4, Peroxisome Proliferator-Activated Receptor α Expression and AMP-Activated Protein Kinase Phosphorylation in High-Fat-Fed Mice. *Int J Mol Sci*. 2016 Jun 3;17(6):872.

[4279] Lin CH, Kuo YH, Shih CC. Eburicoic Acid, a Triterpenoid Compound from Antrodia camphorata, Displays Antidiabetic and Antihyperlipidemic Effects in Palmitate-Treated C2C12 Myotubes and in High-Fat Diet-Fed Mice. *Int J Mol Sci*. 2017 Nov 2;18(11):2314.

[4280] Kuo YH, Lin CH, Shih CC. Ergostatrien-3β-ol from Antrodia camphorata inhibits diabetes and hyperlipidemia in high-fat-diet treated mice via regulation of hepatic related genes, glucose transporter 4, and AMP-activated protein kinase phosphorylation. *J Agric Food Chem*. 2015 Mar 11;63(9):2479-89.

[4281] Kuo YH, Lin CH, Shih CC, et al. Antcin K, a Triterpenoid Compound from Antrodia camphorata, Displays Antidiabetic and Antihyperlipidemic Effects via Glucose Transporter 4 and AMP-Activated Protein Kinase Phosphorylation in Muscles. *Evid Based Complement Alternat Med*. 2016;2016:4867092.

[4282] Lin CH, Hsiao LW, Kuo YH, et al. Antidiabetic and Antihyperlipidemic Effects of Sulphurenic Acid, a Triterpenoid Compound from Antrodia camphorata, in Streptozotocin-Induced Diabetic Mice. *Int J Mol Sci*. 2019 Oct 2;20(19):4897.

[4283] Lin CH, Kuo YH, Shih CC. Antidiabetic and hypolipidemic activities of eburicoic acid, a triterpenoid compound from Antrodia camphorata, by regulation of Akt phosphorylation, gluconeogenesis, and PPARα in streptozotocin-induced diabetic mice. *RSC Adv*. 2018 Jun 5;8(37):20462-20476.

[4284] Kuo YH, Lin CH, Shih CC. Antidiabetic and Antihyperlipidemic Properties of a Triterpenoid Compound, Dehydroeburicoic Acid, from Antrodia camphorata in Vitro and in Streptozotocin-Induced Mice. *J Agric Food Chem*. 2015 Nov 25;63(46):10140-51.

[4285] Kuo MC, Chang CY, Cheng TL, et al. Immunomodulatory effect of Antrodia camphorata mycelia and culture filtrate. *J Ethnopharmacol*. 2008 Nov 20;120(2):196-203.

[4286] Lin SY, Sheen LY, Chiang BH, et al. Dietary effect of Antrodia Camphorate extracts on immune responses in WEHI-3 leukemia BALB/c mice. *Nutr Cancer*. 2010;62(5):593-600.

[4287] Chen CJ, Vijaya Krishna R, et al. Structure and functions of gamma-dodecalactone isolated from Antrodia camphorata for NK cell activation. *Bioorg Med Chem*. 2010 Sep 15;18(18):6896-904.

[4288] Song AR, Qin D, Zhao C, et al. Immunomodulatory effect of polysaccharides extracted from the medicinal mushroom Antrodia camphorata (higher Basidiomycetes) in specific pathogen-free chickens. *Int J Med Mushrooms*. 2014;16(1):95-103.

[4289] Sheu F, Chien PJ, Hsieh KY, et al. Purification, cloning, and functional characterization of a novel immunomodulatory protein from Antrodia camphorata (bitter mushroom) that exhibits TLR2-dependent NF-κB activation and M1 polarization within murine macrophages. *J Agric Food Chem*. 2009 May 27;57(10):4130-41.

[4290] Liu KJ, Leu SJ, Su CH, et al. Administration of polysaccharides from Antrodia camphorata modulates dendritic cell function and alleviates allergen-induced T helper type 2 responses in a mouse model of asthma. *Immunology*. 2010 Mar;129(3):351-62.

[4291] Tu PC, Jiang WP, Lin MK, et al. Anti-Inflammatory Constituents of Antrodia camphorata on RAW 264.7 Cells Induced by Polyinosinic-Polycytidylic Acid. *Molecules*. 2022 Aug 20;27(16):5320.

[4292] Hseu YC, Huang HC, Hsiang CY. Antrodia camphorata suppresses lipopolysaccharide-induced nuclear factor-kappaB activation in transgenic mice evaluated by bioluminescence imaging. *Food Chem Toxicol*. 2010 Aug-Sep;48(8-9):2319-25.

[4293] Su HF, Li B, Yi Y, et al. Regio-specific enzymatic glucosylation of triterpenoids from Antrodia camphorata and their biological activities. *Org Biomol Chem*. 2023 Oct 16.

[4294] Chen JJ, Lin WJ, Liao CH, et al. Anti-inflammatory benzenoids from Antrodia camphorata. *J Nat Prod*. 2007 Jun;70(6):989-92.

[4295] Tsai TC, Tung YT, Kuo YH, et al. Anti-inflammatory effects of Antrodia camphorata, a herbal medicine, in a mouse skin ischemia model. *J Ethnopharmacol*. 2015 Jan 15;159:113-21.

[4296] Chen YC, Chiu HL, Chao CY, et al. New Anti-Inflammatory Aromatic Components from Antrodia camphorata. Int *J Mol Sci*. 2013 Feb 26;14(3):4629-39.

[4297] Buccini M, Punch KA, Kaskow B, et al. Ethynylbenzenoid metabolites of Antrodia camphorata: synthesis and inhibition of TNF expression. *Org Biomol Chem*. 2014 Feb 21;12(7):1100-13.

[4298] Liaw CC, Chen YC, Huang GJ, et al. Anti-inflammatory lanostanoids and lactone derivatives from Antrodia camphorata. *J Nat Prod*. 2013 Apr 26;76(4):489-94.

[4299] Hseu YC, Wu FY, Wu JJ, et al. Anti-inflammatory potential of Antrodia Camphorata through inhibition of iNOS, COX-2 and cytokines via the NF-kappaB pathway. *Int Immunopharmacol*. 2005 Dec;5(13-14):1914-25.

[4300] Tang H, Nie W, Xiao J, et al. Structural characterization and anti-inflammatory effect in hepatocytes of a galactoglucan from Antrodia camphorata mycelium. *RSC Adv*. 2019 Mar 8;9(14):7664-7672.

[4301] Lu ZM, Xu ZH. Antcin A contributes to anti-inflammatory effect of Niuchangchih (Antrodia camphorata). *Acta Pharmacol Sin*. 2011 Aug;32(8):981-2.

[4302] Kao ST, Kuo YH, Wang SD, et al. Analogous corticosteroids, 9A and EK100, derived from solid-state-cultured mycelium of Antrodia camphorata inhibit proinflammatory cytokine expression in macrophages. *Cytokine*. 2018 Aug;108:136-144.

[4303] Shie PH, Wang SY, Lay HL, et al. 4,7-Dimethoxy-5-methyl-1,3-benzodioxole from Antrodia camphorata inhibits LPS-induced inflammation via suppression of NF-κB and induction HO-1 in RAW264.7 cells. *Int Immunopharmacol*. 2016 Feb;31:186-94.

[4304] Yang SS, Wang GJ, Wang SY, et al. New constituents with iNOS inhibitory activity from mycelium of Antrodia camphorata. *Planta Med*. 2009 Apr;75(5):512-6.

[4305] Tung YT, Tsai TC, Kuo YH, et al. Comparison of solid-state-cultured and wood-cultured Antrodia camphorata in anti-inflammatory effects using NF-κB/luciferase inducible transgenic mice. *Phytomedicine*. 2014 Oct 15;21(12):1708-16.

[4306] Chen YC, Liu YL, Li FY, et al. Antcin A, a steroid-like compound from Antrodia camphorata, exerts anti-inflammatory effect via mimicking glucocorticoids. *Acta Pharmacol Sin*. 2011 Jul;32(7):904-11.

[4307] Chen CC, Chyau CC, Hseu TH. Production of a COX-2 inhibitor, 2,4,5-trimethoxybenzaldehyde, with submerged cultured Antrodia camphorata. *Lett Appl Microbiol*. 2007 Apr;44(4):387-92.

[4308] Chien SC, Chen ML, Kuo HT, et al. Anti-inflammatory activities of new succinic and maleic derivatives from the fruiting body of Antrodia camphorata. *J Agric Food Chem*. 2008 Aug 27;56(16):7017-22.

[4309] Wu YY, Chen CC, Chyau CC, et al. Modulation of inflammation-related genes of polysaccharides fractionated from mycelia of medicinal basidiomycete Antrodia camphorata. *Acta Pharmacol Sin*. 2007 Feb;28(2):258-67.

[4310] Huang GJ, Huang SS, Lin SS, et al. Analgesic effects and the mechanisms of anti-inflammation of ergostatrien-3beta-ol from Antrodia camphorata submerged whole broth in mice. *J Agric Food Chem*. 2010 Jun 23;58(12):7445-52.

[4311] Shen YC, Wang YH, Chou YC, et al. Evaluation of the anti-inflammatory activity of zhankuic acids isolated from the fruiting bodies of Antrodia camphorata. *Planta Med*. 2004 Apr;70(4):310-4.

[4312] Rao YK, Fang SH, Tzeng YM. Evaluation of the anti-inflammatory and anti-proliferation tumoral cells activities of Antrodia camphorata, Cordyceps sinensis, and Cinnamomum osmophloeum bark extracts. *J Ethnopharmacol*. 2007 Oct 8;114(1):78-85.

[4313] Shen YC, Chou CJ, Wang YH, et al. Anti-inflammatory activity of the extracts from mycelia of Antrodia camphorata cultured with water-soluble fractions from five different Cinnamomum species. *FEMS Microbiol Lett*. 2004 Feb 9;231(1):137-43.

[4314] Chen CC, Liu YW, Ker YB, et al. Chemical characterization and anti-inflammatory effect of polysaccharides fractionated from submerge-cultured Antrodia camphorata mycelia. *J Agric Food Chem*. 2007 Jun 27;55(13):5007-12.

[4315] Chung TY, Li FY, Chang CI, et al. Inhibition of Na(+)/K(+) -ATPase by antcins, unique steroid-like compounds in Antrodia camphorate. *Am J Chin Med*. 2012;40(5):953-65.

[4316] Lee CL, Huang CH, Wang HC, et al. First total synthesis of antrocamphin A and its analogs as anti-inflammatory and anti-platelet aggregation agents. *Org Biomol Chem*. 2011 Jan 7;9(1):70-3.

[4317] Liao YR, Kuo PC, Liang JW, et al. An efficient total synthesis of a potent anti-inflammatory agent, benzocamphorin F, and its anti-inflammatory activity. *Int J Mol Sci*. 2012;13(8):10432-10440.

[4318] Liu DZ, Liang HJ, Chen CH, et al. Comparative anti-inflammatory characterization of wild fruiting body, liquid-state fermentation, and solid-state culture of Taiwanofungus camphoratus in microglia and the mechanism of its action. *J Ethnopharmacol*. 2007 Aug 15;113(1):45-53.

[4319] Meng LM, Pai MH, Liu JJ, et al. Polysaccharides from extracts of Antrodia camphorata mycelia and fruiting bodies modulate inflammatory mediator expression in mice with polymicrobial sepsis. *Nutrition*. 2012 Sep;28(9):942-9.

[4320] Deng JS, Huang SS, Lin TH, et al. Analgesic and anti-inflammatory bioactivities of eburicoic acid and dehydroeburicoic acid isolated from Antrodia camphorata on the inflammatory mediator expression in mice. *J Agric Food Chem*. 2013 May 29;61(21):5064-71.

[4321] Huang GJ, Huang SS, Lin SS, et al. Analgesic effects and the mechanisms of anti-inflammation of ergostatrien-3beta-ol from Antrodia camphorata submerged whole broth in mice. *J Agric Food Chem*. 2010 Jun 23;58(12):7445-52.

[4322] Liu HY, Huang CF, Li CH, et al. Osteoporosis Recovery by Antrodia camphorata Alcohol Extracts through Bone Regeneration in SAMP8 Mice. *Evid Based Complement Alternat Med*. 2016;2016:2617868.

[4323] Yang HL, Korivi M, Chen CH, et al. Antrodia camphorata attenuates cigarette smoke-induced ROS production, DNA damage, apoptosis, and inflammation in vascular smooth muscle cells, and atherosclerosis in ApoE-deficient mice. *Environ Toxicol*. 2017 Aug;32(8):2070-2084.

[4324] Hsieh YL, Wu SP, Fang LW, et al. Effects of Antrodia camphorata extracts on anti-oxidation, anti-mutagenesis and protection of DNA against hydroxyl radical damage. *BMC Complement Altern Med*. 2015 Jul 16;15:237.

[4325] Hsiao G, Shen MY, Lin KH, et al. Antioxidative and hepatoprotective effects of Antrodia camphorata extract. *J Agric Food Chem*. 2003 May 21;51(11):3302-8.

[4326] Hseu YC, Chen SC, Yech YJ, et al. Antioxidant activity of Antrodia camphorata on free radical-induced endothelial cell damage. *J Ethnopharmacol*. 2008 Jul 23;118(2):237-45.

[4327] Zhang F, Cai H, Liu X, et al. Simultaneous determination of 19 fatty acids in Antrodia camphorata by derivatized GC-MS and evaluation of antioxidant activity of Antrodia camphorata crude oil. Arch Pharm Res. 2015 Feb 4. Online ahead of print.

[4328] Wang JJ, Wu CC, Lee CL, et al. Antimelanogenic, Antioxidant and Antiproliferative Effects of Antrodia camphorata Fruiting Bodies on B16-F0 Melanoma Cells. *PLoS One*. 2017 Jan 26;12(1):e0170924.

[4329] Song TY, Yen GC. Antioxidant properties of Antrodia camphorata in submerged culture. *J Agric Food Chem*. 2002 May 22;50(11):3322-7.

[4330] Ken CF, Chen IJ, Lin CT, et al. Monothiol glutaredoxin cDNA from Taiwanofungus camphorata: a novel CGFS-type glutaredoxin possessing glutathione reductase activity. *J Agric Food Chem*. 2011 Apr 27;59(8):3828-35.

[4331] Chen YM, Sung HC, Kuo YH, et al. The Effects of Ergosta-7,9(11),22-trien-3β-ol from Antrodia camphorata on the Biochemical Profile and Exercise Performance of Mice. *Molecules*. 2019 Mar 28;24(7):1225.

[4332] Huang CC, Hsu MC, Huang WC, et al. Triterpenoid-Rich Extract from Antrodia camphorata Improves Physical Fatigue and Exercise Performance in Mice. *Evid Based Complement Alternat Med*. 2012;2012:364741.

[4333] Yang SC, Huang TH, Chiu CH, et al. The atopic dermatitis-like lesion and the associated MRSA infection and barrier dysfunction can be alleviated by 2,4-dimethoxy-6-methylbenzene-1,3-diol from Antrodia camphorata. *J Dermatol Sci*. 2018 Nov;92(2):188-196.

[4334] Amin ZA, Ali HM, Alshawsh MA, et al. Application of Antrodia camphorata Promotes Rat's Wound Healing In Vivo and Facilitates Fibroblast Cell Proliferation In Vitro. *Evid Based Complement Alternat Med*. 2015;2015:317693.

[4335] Kuo YH, Lin TY, You YJ, et al. Antiinflammatory and Antiphotodamaging Effects of Ergostatrien-3β-ol, Isolated from Antrodia camphorata, on Hairless Mouse Skin. *Molecules*. 2016 Sep 10;21(9):1213.

[4336] Lee IH, Huang RL, Chen CT, et al. Antrodia camphorata polysaccharides exhibit anti-hepatitis B virus effects. *FEMS Microbiol Lett*. 2002 Mar 19;209(1):63-7.

[4337] He YC, Lu ZH, Shi P, et al. Anti-herpes simplex virus activities of bioactive extracts from Antrodia camphorata mycelia. *Antivir Ther*. 2016;21(5):377-83.

[4338] Lin CJ, Rao YK, Hung CL, et al. Inhibition of Helicobacter pylori CagA-Induced Pathogenesis by Methylantcinate B from Antrodia camphorata. *Evid Based Complement Alternat Med*. 2013;2013:682418.

[4339] Lien HM, Tseng CJ, Huang CL, et al. Antimicrobial activity of Antrodia camphorata extracts against oral bacteria. *PLoS One*. 2014 Aug 21;9(8):e105286.

[4340] Chen YJ, Cheng PC, Lin CN, et al. Polysaccharides from Antrodia camphorata mycelia extracts possess immunomodulatory activity and inhibits infection of Schistosoma mansoni. *Int Immunopharmacol*. 2008 Mar;8(3):458-67.

[4341] Cheng PC, Hsu CY, Chen CC, et al. In vivo immunomodulatory effects of Antrodia camphorata polysaccharides in a T1/T2 doubly transgenic mouse model for inhibiting infection of Schistosoma mansoni. *Toxicol Appl Pharmacol*. 2008 Mar 1;227(2):291-8.

[4342] Yen YT, Park JH, Kang SH, et al. Clinical Benefits of Golden-Antrodia Camphorata Containing Antroquinonol in Liver Protection and Liver Fat Reduction After Alcoholic Hepatitis. *Front Pharmacol*. 2022 Jun 21;13:757494.

[4343] Janjušević L, Pejin B, Kaišarević S, et al. Trametes versicolor ethanol extract, a promising candidate for health-promoting food supplement. *Nat Prod Res*. 2018 Apr;32(8):963-967.

[4344] Shnyreva AV, Shnyreva AA, Espinoza C, et al. Antiproliferative Activity and Cytotoxicity of Some Medicinal Wood-Destroying Mushrooms from Russia. *Int J Med Mushrooms*. 2018;20(1):1-11.

[4345] Jędrzejewski T, Sobocińska J, Pawlikowska M, et al. Extract from the Coriolus versicolor Fungus as an Anti-Inflammatory Agent with Cytotoxic Properties against Endothelial Cells and Breast Cancer Cells. *Int J Mol Sci*. 2020 Nov 28;21(23):9063.

[4346] Jędrzejewski T, Pawlikowska M, Sobocińska J, et al. Protein-Bound Polysaccharides from Coriolus Versicolor Fungus Disrupt the Crosstalk Between Breast Cancer Cells and Macrophages through Inhibition of Angiogenic Cytokines Production and Shifting Tumour-Associated Macrophages from the M2 to M1 Subtype. *Cell Physiol Biochem*. 2020 Jun 20;54(4):615-628.

[4347] Lu H, Yang Y, Gad E, Inatsuka C, et al. TLR2 agonist PSK activates human NK cells and enhances the antitumor effect of HER2-targeted monoclonal antibody therapy. *Clin Cancer Res*. 2011 Nov 1;17(21):6742-53.

[4348] Pawlikowska M, Jędrzejewski T, Brożyna AA, et al. Protein-Bound Polysaccharides from Coriolus Versicolor Induce RIPK1/RIPK3/MLKL-Mediated Necroptosis in ER-Positive Breast Cancer and Amelanotic Melanoma Cells. *Cell Physiol Biochem*. 2020 Jun 13;54(4):591-604.

[4349] Jędrzejewski T, Pawlikowska M, Sobocińska J, et al. Protein-Bound Polysaccharides from Coriolus Versicolor Fungus Disrupt the Crosstalk Between Breast Cancer Cells and Macrophages through Inhibition of Angiogenic Cytokines Production and Shifting Tumour-Associated Macrophages from the M2 to M1 Subtype. *Cell Physiol Biochem*. 2020 Jun 20;54(4):615-628.

[4350] Kowalczewska M, Piotrowski J, Jędrzejewski T, et al. Polysaccharide peptides from Coriolus versicolor exert differential immunomodulatory effects on blood lymphocytes and breast cancer cell line MCF-7 in vitro. *Immunol Lett*. 2016 Jun;174:37-44.

[4351] Ho CY, Kim CF, Leung KN, et al. Differential anti-tumor activity of coriolus versicolor (Yunzhi) extract through p53- and/or Bcl-2-dependent apoptotic pathway in human breast cancer cells. *Cancer Biol Ther*. 2005 Jun;4(6):638-44.

[4352] Knežević A, Stajić M, Sofrenić I, et al. Antioxidative, antifungal, cytotoxic and antineurodegenerative activity of selected Trametes species from Serbia. *PLoS One*. 2018 Aug 31;13(8):e0203064.

[4353] Shnyreva AV, Shnyreva AA, Espinoza C, et al. Antiproliferative Activity and Cytotoxicity of Some Medicinal Wood-Destroying Mushrooms from Russia. *Int J Med Mushrooms*. 2018;20(1):1-11.

[4354] Jiménez-Medina E, Berruguilla E, Romero I, et al. The immunomodulator PSK induces in vitro cytotoxic activity in tumour cell lines via arrest of cell cycle and induction of apoptosis. *BMC Cancer*. 2008 Mar 24:8:78.

[4355] Hsieh TC, Wu JM. Cell growth and gene modulatory activities of Yunzhi (Windsor Wunxi) from mushroom Trametes versicolor in androgen-dependent and androgen-insensitive human prostate cancer cells. *Int J Oncol*. 2001 Jan;18(1):81-8.

4356 Hsieh TC, Wu JM. Cell growth and gene modulatory activities of Yunzhi (Windsor Wunxi) from mushroom Trametes versicolor in androgen-dependent and androgen-insensitive human prostate cancer cells. *Int J Oncol*. 2001 Jan;18(1):81-8.

4357 Luk SU, Lee TK, Liu J, et al. Chemopreventive effect of PSP through targeting of prostate cancer stem cell-like population. *PLoS One*. 2011;6(5):e19804.

4358 Janjušević L, Pejin B, Kaišarević S, et al. Trametes versicolor ethanol extract, a promising candidate for health-promoting food supplement. *Nat Prod Res*. 2018 Apr;32(8):963-967.

4359 Silva AM, Miranda A, Fernandes E, et al. Endopolysaccharides from Ganoderma resinaceum, Phlebia rufa, and Trametes versicolor affect differently the proliferation rate of HepG2 cells. *Appl Biochem Biotechnol*. 2013 Mar;169(6):1919-26.

4360 Dong Y, Kwan CY, Chen ZN, et al. Antitumor effects of a refined polysaccharide peptide fraction isolated from Coriolus versicolor: in vitro and in vivo studies. *Res Commun Mol Pathol Pharmacol*. 1996 May;92(2):140-8.

4361 Nakajima T, Ichikawa S, Uchida S, et al. Effects of a protein-bound polysaccharide from a basidiomycetes against hepatocarcinogenesis induced by 3'-methyl-4-dimethylaminoazobenzene in rats. *Clin Ther*. 1990 Sep-Oct;12(5):385-92.

4362 He Y, Liu S, Newburg DS. Musarin, a novel protein with tyrosine kinase inhibitory activity from Trametes versicolor, inhibits colorectal cancer stem cell growth. *Biomed Pharmacother*. 2021 Dec;144:112339.

4363 Jian L, Zhicheng H, Shubai L. Polysaccharide Peptide Induced Colorectal Cancer Cells Apoptosis by Down-Regulating EGFR and PD-L1 Expression. *Iran J Pharm Res*. 2022 Jul 2;21(1):e123909.

4364 Roca-Lema D, Martinez-Iglesias O, Fernández de Ana Portela C, et al. In Vitro Anti-proliferative and Anti-invasive Effect of Polysaccharide-rich Extracts from Trametes Versicolor and Grifola Frondosa in Colon Cancer Cells. *Int J Med Sci*. 2019 Jan 1;16(2):231-240.

4365 Shnyreva AV, Shnyreva AA, Espinoza C, et al. Antiproliferative Activity and Cytotoxicity of Some Medicinal Wood-Destroying Mushrooms from Russia. *Int J Med Mushrooms*. 2018;20(1):1-11.

4366 Toth B, Coles M, Lynch J. Effects of VPS extract of Coriolus versicolor on cancer of the large intestine using a serial sacrifice technique. *In Vivo*. 2006 May-Jun;20(3):341-6.

4367 Jiménez-Medina E, Berruguilla E, Romero I, et al. The immunomodulator PSK induces in vitro cytotoxic activity in tumour cell lines via arrest of cell cycle and induction of apoptosis. *BMC Cancer*. 2008 Mar 24:8:78.

4368 Ricciardi MR, Licchetta R, Mirabilii S, et al. Preclinical Antileukemia Activity of Tramesan: A Newly Identified Bioactive Fungal Metabolite. *Oxid Med Cell Longev*. 2017;2017:5061639.

4369 Ho CY, Kim CF, Leung KN, et al. Coriolus versicolor (Yunzhi) extract attenuates growth of human leukemia xenografts and induces apoptosis through the mitochondrial pathway. *Oncol Rep*. 2006 Sep;16(3):609-16.

4370 Wan JM, Sit WH, Yang X, et al. Polysaccharopeptides derived from Coriolus versicolor potentiate the S-phase specific cytotoxicity of Camptothecin (CPT) on human leukemia HL-60 cells. *Chin Med*. 2010 Apr 27;5:16.

4371 Lau CB, Ho CY, Kim CF, et al. Cytotoxic activities of Coriolus versicolor (Yunzhi) extract on human leukemia and lymphoma cells by induction of apoptosis. *Life Sci*. 2004 Jul 2;75(7):797-808.

4372 Yang MM, Chen Z, Kwok JS. The anti-tumor effect of a small polypeptide from Coriolus versicolor (SPCV). *Am J Chin Med*. 1992;20(3-4):221-32.

4373 Zeng F, Hon CC, Sit WH, et al. Molecular characterization of Coriolus versicolor PSP-induced apoptosis in human promyelotic leukemic HL-60 cells using cDNA microarray. *Int J Oncol*. 2005 Aug;27(2):513-23.

4374 Hsieh TC, Kunicki J, Darzynkiewicz Z, et al. Effects of extracts of Coriolus versicolor (I'm-Yunity) on cell-cycle progression and expression of interleukins-1 beta,-6, and -8 in promyelocytic HL-60 leukemic cells and mitogenically stimulated and nonstimulated human lymphocytes. *J Altern Complement Med*. 2002 Oct;8(5):591-602.

4375 Hsieh TC, Wu JM. Regulation of cell cycle transition and induction of apoptosis in HL-60 leukemia cells by the combination of Coriolus versicolor and Ganoderma lucidum. *Int J Mol Med*. 2013 Jul;32(1):251-7.

4376 Dong Y, Yang MM, Kwan CY. In vitro inhibition of proliferation of HL-60 cells by tetrandrine and coriolus versicolor peptide derived from Chinese medicinal herbs. *Life Sci*. 1997;60(8):PL135-40.

4377 Hui KP, Sit WH, Wan JM. Induction of S phase cell arrest and caspase activation by polysaccharide peptide isolated from Coriolus versicolor enhanced the cell cycle dependent activity and apoptotic cell death of doxorubicin and etoposide, but not cytarabine in HL-60 cells. *Oncol Rep*. 2005 Jul;14(1):145-55.

4378 Hirahara N, Fujioka M, Edamatsu T, et al. Protein-bound polysaccharide-K (PSK) induces apoptosis and inhibits proliferation of promyelomonocytic leukemia HL-60 cells. *Anticancer Res*. 2011 Sep;31(9):2733-8.

4379 Hirahara N, Edamatsu T, Fujieda A, et al. Protein-bound polysaccharide-K (PSK) induces apoptosis via p38 mitogen-activated protein kinase pathway in promyelomonocytic leukemia HL-60 cells. *Anticancer Res*. 2012 Jul;32(7):2631-7.

4380 Hirahara N, Edamatsu T, Fujieda A, et al. Protein-bound polysaccharide-K induces apoptosis via mitochondria and p38 mitogen-activated protein kinase-dependent pathways in HL-60 promyelomonocytic leukemia cells. *Oncol Rep*. 2013 Jul;30(1):99-104.

4381 Yang X, Sit WH, Chan DK, et al. The cell death process of the anticancer agent polysaccharide-peptide (PSP) in human promyelotic leukemic HL-60 cells. *Oncol Rep*. 2005 Jun;13(6):1201-10.

4382 Jiménez-Medina E, Berruguilla E, Romero I, et al. The immunomodulator PSK induces in vitro cytotoxic activity in tumour cell lines via arrest of cell cycle and induction of apoptosis. *BMC Cancer*. 2008 Mar 24:8:78.

4383 Hsieh TC, Wu P, Park S, et al. Induction of cell cycle changes and modulation of apoptogenic/anti-apoptotic and extracellular signaling regulatory protein expression by water extracts of I'm-Yunity (PSP). *BMC Complement Altern Med*. 2006 Sep 11;6:30.

4384 Lau CB, Ho CY, Kim CF, et al. Cytotoxic activities of Coriolus versicolor (Yunzhi) extract on human leukemia and lymphoma cells by induction of apoptosis. *Life Sci*. 2004 Jul 2;75(7):797-808.

4385 Shnyreva AV, Shnyreva AA, Espinoza C, et al. Antiproliferative Activity and Cytotoxicity of Some Medicinal Wood-Destroying Mushrooms from Russia. *Int J Med Mushrooms*. 2018;20(1):1-11.

4386 Tsang KW, Lam CL, Yan C, et al. Coriolus versicolor polysaccharide peptide slows progression of advanced non-small cell lung cancer. *Respir Med*. 2003 Jun;97(6):618-24.

4387 Jiménez-Medina E, Berruguilla E, Romero I, et al. The immunomodulator PSK induces in vitro cytotoxic activity in tumour cell lines via arrest of cell cycle and induction of apoptosis. *BMC Cancer*. 2008 Mar 24:8:78.

[4388] Yang CL, Chik SC, Lau AS, et al. Coriolus versicolor and its bioactive molecule are potential immunomodulators against cancer cell metastasis via inactivation of MAPK pathway. *J Ethnopharmacol*. 2023 Jan 30;301:115790.

[4389] Wang DF, Lou N, Li XD. Effect of coriolus versicolor polysaccharide-B on the biological characteristics of human esophageal carcinoma cell line eca109. *Cancer Biol Med*. 2012 Sep;9(3):164-7.

[4390] Jiménez-Medina E, Berruguilla E, Romero I, et al. The immunomodulator PSK induces in vitro cytotoxic activity in tumour cell lines via arrest of cell cycle and induction of apoptosis. *BMC Cancer*. 2008 Mar 24:8:78.

[4391] Jiménez-Medina E, Berruguilla E, Romero I, et al. The immunomodulator PSK induces in vitro cytotoxic activity in tumour cell lines via arrest of cell cycle and induction of apoptosis. *BMC Cancer*. 2008 Mar 24:8:78.

[4392] Lowenthal R, Taylor M, Gidden JA, et al. The mycelium of the Trametes versicolor synn. Coriolus versicolor (Turkey tail mushroom) exhibit anti-melanoma activity in vitro. *Biomed Pharmacother*. 2023 May;161:114424.

[4393] Lowenthal R, Taylor M, Gidden JA, et al. The mycelium of the Trametes versicolor synn. Coriolus versicolor (Turkey tail mushroom) exhibit anti-melanoma activity in vitro. *Biomed Pharmacother*. 2023 May;161:114424.

[4394] Pawlikowska M, Piotrowski J, Jędrzejewski T, et al. Coriolus versicolor-derived protein-bound polysaccharides trigger the caspase-independent cell death pathway in amelanotic but not melanotic melanoma cells. *Phytother Res*. 2020 Jan;34(1):173-183.

[4395] Pawlikowska M, Jędrzejewski T, Brożyna AA, et al. Protein-Bound Polysaccharides from Coriolus Versicolor Induce RIPK1/RIPK3/MLKL-Mediated Necroptosis in ER-Positive Breast Cancer and Amelanotic Melanoma Cells. *Cell Physiol Biochem*. 2020 Jun 13;54(4):591-604.

[4396] Pawlikowska M, Jędrzejewski T, Slominski AT, et al. Pigmentation Levels Affect Melanoma Responses to Coriolus versicolor Extract and Play a Crucial Role in Melanoma-Mononuclear Cell Crosstalk. *Int J Mol Sci*. 2021 May 27;22(11):5735.

[4397] Wenner CA, Martzen MR, Lu H, et al. Polysaccharide-K augments docetaxel-induced tumor suppression and antitumor immune response in an immunocompetent murine model of human prostate cancer. *Int J Oncol*. 2012 Apr;40(4):905-13.

[4398] Kobayashi Y, Kariya K, Saigenji K, et al. Enhancement of anti-cancer activity of cisdiaminedichloroplatinum by the protein-bound polysaccharide of Coriolus versicolor QUEL (PS-K) in vitro. *Cancer Biother*. 1994 Winter;9(4):351-8.

[4399] Wan JM, Sit WH, Louie JC. Polysaccharopeptide enhances the anticancer activity of doxorubicin and etoposide on human breast cancer cells ZR-75-30. *Int J Oncol*. 2008 Mar;32(3):689-99.

[4400] Mao XW, Green LM, Gridley DS. Evaluation of polysaccharopeptide effects against C6 glioma in combination with radiation. *Oncology*. 2001;61(3):243-53.

[4401] Jędrzejewski T, Sobocińska J, Pawlikowska M, et al. Extract from the Coriolus versicolor Fungus as an Anti-Inflammatory Agent with Cytotoxic Properties against Endothelial Cells and Breast Cancer Cells. *Int J Mol Sci*. 2020 Nov 28;21(23):9063.

[4402] Razmovski-Naumovski V, Kimble B, et al. Polysaccharide Peptide Extract From Coriolus versicolor Increased Tmax of Tamoxifen and Maintained Biochemical Serum Parameters, With No Change in the Metabolism of Tamoxifen in the Rat. *Front Pharmacol*. 2022 Apr 1;13:857864.

[4403] Brown DC, Reetz J. Single agent polysaccharopeptide delays metastases and improves survival in naturally occurring hemangiosarcoma. *Evid Based Complement Alternat Med*. 2012;2012:384301.

[4404] Harhaji Lj, Mijatović S, Maksimović-Ivanić D, et al. Anti-tumor effect of Coriolus versicolor methanol extract against mouse B16 melanoma cells: in vitro and in vivo study. *Food Chem Toxicol*. 2008 May;46(5):1825-33.

[4405] Kobayashi Y, Kariya K, Saigenji K, et al. Suppressive effects on cancer cell proliferation of the enhancement of superoxide dismutase (SOD) activity associated with the protein-bound polysaccharide of Coriolus versicolor QUEL. *Cancer Biother*. 1994 Summer;9(2):171-8.

[4406] Luo KW, Yue GG, Ko CH, et al. In vivo and in vitro anti-tumor and anti-metastasis effects of Coriolus versicolor aqueous extract on mouse mammary 4T1 carcinoma. *Phytomedicine*. 2014 Jul-Aug;21(8-9):1078-87.

[4407] Kobayashi Y, Kariya K, Saigenji K, et al. Suppression of cancer cell growth in vitro by the protein-bound polysaccharide of Coriolus versicolor QUEL (PS-K) with SOD mimicking activity. *Cancer Biother*. 1994 Spring;9(1):63-9.

[4408] Fujii T, Saito K, Matsunaga K, et al. Prolongation of the survival period with the biological response modifier PSK in rats bearing N-methyl-N-nitrosourea-induced mammary gland tumors. *In Vivo*. 1995 Jan-Feb;9(1):55-7.

[4409] Awadasseid A, Eugene K, Jamal M, et al. Effect of Coriolus versicolor glucan on the stimulation of cytokine production in sarcoma-180-bearing mice. *Biomed Rep*. 2017 Dec;7(6):567-572.

[4410] Awadasseid A, Hou J, Gamallat Y, et al. Purification, characterization, and antitumor activity of a novel glucan from the fruiting bodies of Coriolus Versicolor. *PLoS One*. 2017 Feb 8;12(2):e0171270.

[4411] Ho JC, Konerding MA, Gaumann A, et al. Fungal polysaccharopeptide inhibits tumor angiogenesis and tumor growth in mice. *Life Sci*. 2004 Jul 30;75(11):1343-56.

[4412] Kanoh T, Matsunaga K, Saito K, et al. Suppression of in vivo tumor-induced angiogenesis by the protein-bound polysaccharide PSK. *In Vivo*. 1994 Mar-Apr;8(2):247-50.

[4413] Yu ZT, Liu B, Mukherjee P, et al. Trametes versicolor extract modifies human fecal microbiota composition in vitro. *Plant Foods Hum Nutr*. 2013 Jun;68(2):107-12.

[4414] Moazzem Hossen SM, Akramul Hoque Tanim M, Shahadat Hossain M, et al. Deciphering the CNS anti-depressant, antioxidant and cytotoxic profiling of methanol and aqueous extracts of Trametes versicolor and molecular interactions of its phenolic compounds. *Saudi J Biol Sci*. 2021 Nov;28(11):6375-6383.

[4415] Janjušević L, Karaman M, Šibul F, et al. The lignicolous fungus Trametes versicolor (L.) Lloyd (1920): a promising natural source of antiradical and AChE inhibitory agents. *J Enzyme Inhib Med Chem*. 2017 Dec;32(1):355-362.

[4416] Knežević A, Stajić M, Sofrenić I, et al. Antioxidative, antifungal, cytotoxic and antineurodegenerative activity of selected Trametes species from Serbia. *PLoS One*. 2018 Aug 31;13(8):e0203064.

[4417] Jin M, Zhou W, Jin C, et al. Anti-inflammatory activities of the chemical constituents isolated from Trametes versicolor. *Nat Prod Res*. 2019 Aug;33(16):2422-2425.

[4418] Bains A, Chawla P. In vitro bioactivity, antimicrobial and anti-inflammatory efficacy of modified solvent evaporation assisted Trametes versicolor extract. *3 Biotech*. 2020 Sep;10(9):404.

[4419] Oyetayo VO, Nieto-Camacho A, Rodriguez BE, et al. Assessment of anti-inflammatory, lipid peroxidation and acute toxicity of extracts obtained from wild higher basidiomycetes mushrooms collected from Akure (southwest Nigeria). *Int J Med Mushrooms*. 2012;14(6):575-80.

[4420] Jędrzejewski T, Pawlikowska M, Piotrowski J, et al. Protein-bound polysaccharides from Coriolus versicolor attenuate LPS-induced synthesis of pro-inflammatory cytokines and stimulate PBMCs proliferation. *Immunol Lett*. 2016 Oct;178:140-7.

[4421] Song LC, Chen HS, Lou N, et al. Effects of Coriolus versicolor polysaccharide B on monocyte chemoattractant protein 1 gene expression in rat. *Acta Pharmacol Sin*. 2002 Jun;23(6):539-43.

[4422] Wang K, Wang Z, Cui R, et al. Polysaccharopeptide from Trametes versicolor blocks inflammatory osteoarthritis pain-morphine tolerance effects via activating cannabinoid type 2 receptor. *Int J Biol Macromol*. 2019 Apr 1;126:805-810.

[4423] Gong S, Zhang HQ, Yin WP, et al. Involvement of interleukin-2 in analgesia produced by Coriolus versicolor polysaccharide peptides. *Zhongguo Yao Li Xue Bao*. 1998 Jan;19(1):67-70.

[4424] Hung PH, Lin CM, Tsai JC, et al. Acetylsalicylic acid-like analgesic effects of Trametes versicolor in Wistar rats. *Biomed Pharmacother*. 2020 Sep;129:110328.

[4425] Ng TB, Chan WY. Polysaccharopeptide from the mushroom Coriolus versicolor possesses analgesic activity but does not produce adverse effects on female reproductive or embryonic development in mice. *Gen Pharmacol*. 1997 Aug;29(2):269-73.

[4426] Chen CH, Kang L, Lo HC, et al. Polysaccharides of Trametes versicolor Improve Bone Properties in Diabetic Rats. *J Agric Food Chem*. 2015 Oct 28;63(42):9232-8.

[4427] Erjavec I, Brkljacic J, Vukicevic S, et al. Mushroom Extracts Decrease Bone Resorption and Improve Bone Formation. *Int J Med Mushrooms*. 2016;18(7):559-69.

[4428] Benson KF, Stamets P, Davis R, et al. The mycelium of the Trametes versicolor (Turkey tail) mushroom and its fermented substrate each show potent and complementary immune activating properties in vitro. *BMC Complement Altern Med*. 2019 Dec 2;19(1):342.

[4429] Li F, Wen H, Zhang Y, et al. Purification and characterization of a novel immunomodulatory protein from the medicinal mushroom Trametes versicolor. *Sci China Life Sci*. 2011 Apr;54(4):379-85.

[4430] Zhang X, Cai Z, Mao H, et al. Isolation and structure elucidation of polysaccharides from fruiting bodies of mushroom Coriolus versicolor and evaluation of their immunomodulatory effects. *Int J Biol Macromol*. 2021 Jan 1;166:1387-1395.

[4431] Yang SF, Zhuang TF, Si YM, et al. Coriolus versicolor mushroom polysaccharides exert immunoregulatory effects on mouse B cells via membrane Ig and TLR-4 to activate the MAPK and NF-κB signaling pathways. *Mol Immunol*. 2015 Mar;64(1):144-51.

[4432] Shi SH, Yang WT, Huang KY, et al. β-glucans from Coriolus versicolor protect mice against S. typhimurium challenge by activation of macrophages. *Int J Biol Macromol*. 2016 May;86:352-61.

[4433] Jędrzejewski T, Sobocińska J, Pawlikowska M, et al. Dual Effect of the Extract from the Fungus Coriolus versicolor on Lipopolysaccharide-Induced Cytokine Production in RAW 264.7 Macrophages Depending on the Lipopolysaccharide Concentration. *J Inflamm Res*. 2022 Jun 20;15:3599-3611.

[4434] Kang SC, Koo HJ, Park S, et al. Effects of β-glucans from Coriolus versicolor on macrophage phagocytosis are related to the Akt and CK2/Ikaros. *Int J Biol Macromol*. 2013 Jun;57:9-16.

[4435] Harikrishnan R, Kim MC, Kim JS, et al. Effect of Coriolus versicolor supplemented diet on innate immune response and disease resistance in kelp grouper Epinephelus bruneus against Listonella anguillarum. *Fish Shellfish Immunol*. 2012 Feb;32(2):339-44.

[4436] Wu ZX, Pang SF, Chen XX, et al. Effect of Coriolus versicolor polysaccharides on the hematological and biochemical parameters and protection against Aeromonas hydrophila in allogynogenetic crucian carp (Carassius auratus gibelio). *Fish Physiol Biochem*. 2013 Apr;39(2):181-90.

[4437] Yu GD, Yin QZ, Hu YM, et al. Effects of Coriolus versicolor polysaccharides peptides on electric activity of mediobasal hypothalamus and on immune function in rats. *Zhongguo Yao Li Xue Bao*. 1996 May;17(3):271-4.

[4438] Li XY, Wang JF, Zhu PP, et al. Immune enhancement of a polysaccharides peptides isolated from Coriolus versicolor. *Zhongguo Yao Li Xue Bao*. 1990 Nov;11(6):542-5.

[4439] Ho CY, Lau CB, Kim CF, et al. Differential effect of Coriolus versicolor (Yunzhi) extract on cytokine production by murine lymphocytes in vitro. *Int Immunopharmacol*. 2004 Nov;4(12):1549-57.

[4440] Liu WK, Ng TB, Sze SF, et al. Activation of peritoneal macrophages by polysaccharopeptide from the mushroom, Coriolus versicolor. *Immunopharmacology*. 1993 Sep-Oct;26(2):139-46.

[4441] Mayer P, Drews J. The effect of a protein-bound polysaccharide from Coriolus versicolor on immunological parameters and experimental infections in mice. *Infection*. 1980;8(1):13-21.

[4442] Jeong SC, Yang BK, Kim GN, et al. Macrophage-stimulating activity of polysaccharides extracted from fruiting bodies of Coriolus versicolor (Turkey Tail Mushroom). *J Med Food*. 2006 Summer;9(2):175-81.

[4443] Wang HX, NG TB, Liu WK, et al. Polysaccharide-peptide complexes from the cultured mycelia of the mushroom Coriolus versicolor and their culture medium activate mouse lymphocytes and macrophages. *Int J Biochem Cell Biol*. 1996 May;28(5):601-7.

[4444] Wang Z, Dong B, Feng Z, et al. A study on immunomodulatory mechanism of Polysaccharopeptide mediated by TLR4 signaling pathway. *BMC Immunol*. 2015 Jun 2;16:34.

[4445] Sekhon BK, Sze DM, Chan WK, et al. PSP activates monocytes in resting human peripheral blood mononuclear cells: immunomodulatory implications for cancer treatment. *Food Chem*. 2013 Jun 15;138(4):2201-9.

[4446] Wang J, Dong B, Tan Y, et al. A study on the immunomodulation of polysaccharopeptide through the TLR4-TIRAP/MAL-MyD88 signaling pathway in PBMCs from breast cancer patients. *Immunopharmacol Immunotoxicol*. 2013 Aug;35(4):497-504.

[4447] Maruyama S, Akasaka T, Yamada K, et al. Protein-bound polysaccharide-K (PSK) directly enhanced IgM production in the human B cell line BALL-1. *Biomed Pharmacother*. 2009 Jul;63(6):409-12.

[4448] Li W, Liu M, Lai S, et al. Immunomodulatory effects of polysaccharopeptide (PSP) in human PBMC through regulation of TRAF6/TLR immunosignal-transduction pathways. *Immunopharmacol Immunotoxicol*. 2010 Dec;32(4):576-84.

4449 Ragupathi G, Yeung KS, Leung PC, et al. Evaluation of widely consumed botanicals as immunological adjuvants. *Vaccine*. 2008 Sep 2;26(37):4860-5.

4450 Kanazawa M, Mori Y, Yoshihara K, et al. Effect of PSK on the maturation of dendritic cells derived from human peripheral blood monocytes. *Immunol Lett*. 2004 Feb 15;91(2-3):229-38.

4451 Asai K, Kato H, Hirose K, et al. PSK and OK-432-induced immunomodulation of inducible nitric oxide (NO) synthase gene expression in mouse peritoneal polymorphonuclear leukocytes and NO-mediated cytotoxicity. *Immunopharmacol Immunotoxicol*. 2000 May;22(2):221-35.

4452 Matsunaga K, Morita I, Iijima H, et al. Effects of biological response modifiers with different modes of action used separately and together on immune responses in mice with syngeneic tumours. *J Int Med Res*. 1992 Sep;20(5):406-21.

4453 Kato H, Yokoe N, Takemura S, et al. Effect of a protein-bound polysaccharide PS-K on the complement system. *Res Exp Med (Berl)*. 1983;182(2):85-94.

4454 Matsunaga K, Morita I, Iijima H, et al. Competitive action of a biological response modifier, PSK, on a humoral immunosuppressive factor produced in tumor-bearing hosts. *J Clin Lab Immunol*. 1990 Mar;31(3):127-36.

4455 Matsunaga K, Morita I, Oguchi Y, et al. Restoration of immune responsiveness by a biological response modifier, PSK, in aged mice bearing syngeneic transplantable tumor. *J Clin Lab Immunol*. 1987 Nov;24(3):143-9.

4456 Matsunaga K, Morita I, Oguchi Y, et al. [Restoration of immunologic responsiveness by PSK in tumor-bearing animals]. *Gan To Kagaku Ryoho*. 1986 Dec;13(12):3468-75.

4457 Matsunaga K, Iijima H, Aota M, et al. Enhancement of effector cell activities in mice bearing syngeneic plasmacytoma X5563 by a biological response modifier, PSK. *J Clin Lab Immunol*. 1992 Jan;37(1):21-37.

4458 Fujii T, Kano T, Saito K, et al. Effect of PSK on prohibited immunity of splenectomized mice. *Anticancer Res*. 1987 Jul-Aug;7(4B):845-8.

4459 Sakagami H, Sugaya K, Utsumi A, et al. Stimulation by PSK of interleukin-1 production by human peripheral blood mononuclear cells. *Anticancer Res*. 1993 May-Jun;13(3):671-5.

4460 Sakagami H, Kim F, Konno K. Stimulation of human peripheral blood polymorphonuclear cell iodination by PSK subfractions. *Anticancer Res*. 1990 May-Jun;10(3):697-702.

4461 Matsunaga K, Morita I, Oguchi Y, et al. [Restoration of depressed immune responses by PSK in C3H/He mice bearing the syngeneic X5563 tumor]. *Gan To Kagaku Ryoho*. 1986 Dec;13(12):3453-60.

4462 Matsunaga K, Morita I, Oguchi Y, et al. [Competitive effect of PSK against the immunosuppressive effect induced in the sera of mice bearing syngeneic tumors]. *Gan To Kagaku Ryoho*. 1986 Dec;13(12):3461-7.

4463 Tsuji K, Takagi M, Kobayashi T, et al. [Effect of a protein-bound polysaccharide, PSK, on human hemopoietic progenitors]. *Nihon Ketsueki Gakkai Zasshi*. 1989 May;52(3):594-600.

4464 Jędrzejewski T, Piotrowski J, Pawlikowska M, et al. Extract from Coriolus versicolor fungus partially prevents endotoxin tolerance development by maintaining febrile response and increasing IL-6 generation. *J Therm Biol*. 2019 Jul;83:69-79.

4465 Pramudya M, Wahyuningsih SPA. Immunomodulatory potential of polysaccharides from Coriolus versicolor against intracellular bacteria Neisseria gonorrhoeae. *Vet World*. 2019 Jun;12(6):735-739.

4466 Qian ZM, Xu MF, Tang PL. Polysaccharide peptide (PSP) restores immunosuppression induced by cyclophosphamide in rats. *Am J Chin Med*. 1997;25(1):27-35.

4467 Williams LM, Berthon BS, Stoodley IL, et al. Medicinal Mushroom Extracts from Hericium coralloides and Trametes versicolor Exert Differential Immunomodulatory Effects on Immune Cells from Older Adults In Vitro. *Nutrients*. 2023 May 8;15(9):2227.

4468 Lee CL, Jiang P, Sit WH, et al. Regulatory properties of polysaccharopeptide derived from Coriolus versicolor and its combined effect with ciclosporin on the homeostasis of human lymphocytes. *J Pharm Pharmacol*. 2010 Aug;62(8):1028-36.

4469 Lee CL, Sit WH, Jiang PP, et al. Polysaccharopeptide mimics ciclosporin-mediated Th1/Th2 cytokine balance for suppression of activated human T cell proliferation by MAPKp38 and STAT5 pathways. *J Pharm Pharmacol*. 2008 Nov;60(11):1491-9.

4470 Sknepnek A, Tomić S, Miletić D, et al. Fermentation characteristics of novel Coriolus versicolor and Lentinus edodes kombucha beverages and immunomodulatory potential of their polysaccharide extracts. *Food Chem*. 2021 Apr 16;342:128344.

4471 Huang Z, Zhang M, Wang Y, et al. Extracellular and Intracellular Polysaccharide Extracts of Trametes versicolor Improve Lipid Profiles Via Serum Regulation of Lipid-Regulating Enzymes in Hyperlipidemic Mice. *Curr Microbiol*. 2020 Nov;77(11):3526-3537.

4472 Kuan YC, Wu YJ, Hung CL, et al. Trametes versicolor protein YZP activates regulatory B lymphocytes - gene identification through de novo assembly and function analysis in a murine acute colitis model. *PLoS One*. 2013 Sep 3;8(9):e72422.

4473 Impellizzeri D, Fusco R, Genovese T, et al. Coriolus Versicolor Downregulates TLR4/NF-κB Signaling Cascade in Dinitrobenzenesulfonic Acid-Treated Mice: A Possible Mechanism for the Anti-Colitis Effect. *Antioxidants (Basel)*. 2022 Feb 17;11(2):406.

4474 Lim BO. Coriolus versicolor suppresses inflammatory bowel disease by Inhibiting the expression of STAT1 and STAT6 associated with IFN-γ and IL-4 expression. *Phytother Res*. 2011 Aug;25(8):1257-61.

4475 Li X, Chen P, Zhang P, et al. Protein-Bound β-glucan from Coriolus Versicolor has Potential for Use Against Obesity. *Mol Nutr Food Res*. 2019 Apr;63(7):e1801231.

4476 Shimokawa K, Mashima I, Asai A, et al. Biological activity, structural features, and synthetic studies of (-)-ternatin, a potent fat-accumulation inhibitor of 3T3-L1 adipocytes. *Chem Asian J*. 2008 Feb 1;3(2):438-46.

4477 Nikolic M, Lazarevic N, Novakovic J, et al. Characterization, In Vitro Biological Activity and In Vivo Cardioprotective Properties of Trametes versicolor (L.:Fr.) Quél. Heteropolysaccharides in a Rat Model of Metabolic Syndrome. *Pharmaceuticals (Basel)*. 2023 May 25;16(6):787.

4478 Teng JF, Lee CH, Hsu TH, et al. Potential activities and mechanisms of extracellular polysaccharopeptides from fermented Trametes versicolor on regulating glucose homeostasis in insulin-resistant HepG2 cells. *PLoS One*. 2018 Jul 19;13(7):e0201131.

4479 Meng F, Lin Y, Hu L, et al. The Therapeutic Effect of Coriolus versicolor Fruiting Body on STZ-Induced ICR Diabetic Mice. *J Healthc Eng*. 2022 Apr 15;2022:7282453.

[4480] Xian HM, Che H, Qin Y, et al. Coriolus versicolor aqueous extract ameliorates insulin resistance with PI3K/Akt and p38 MAPK signaling pathways involved in diabetic skeletal muscle. *Phytother Res*. 2018 Mar;32(3):551-560.

[4481] Hsu WK, Hsu TH, Lin FY, et al. Separation, purification, and α-glucosidase inhibition of polysaccharides from Coriolus versicolor LH1 mycelia. *Carbohydr Polym*. 2013 Jan 30;92(1):297-306.

[4482] Yang JP, Hsu T, Lin F, et al. Potential antidiabetic activity of extracellular polysaccharides in submerged fermentation culture of Coriolus versicolor LH1. *Carbohydr Polym*. 2012 Sep 1;90(1):174-80.

[4483] Su CH, Lai MN, Ng LT. Inhibitory effects of medicinal mushrooms on α-amylase and α-glucosidase - enzymes related to hyperglycemia. *Food Funct*. 2013 Apr 25;4(4):644-9.

[4484] Yang BK, Kim GN, Jeong YT, et al. Hypoglycemic Effects of Exo-biopolymers Produced by Five Different Medicinal Mushrooms in STZ-induced Diabetic Rats. *Mycobiology*. 2008 Mar;36(1):45-9.

[4485] Taguchi T, Haruna M, Okuda J. Effects of 1,5-anhydro-D-fructose on selected glucose-metabolizing enzymes. *Biotechnol Appl Biochem*. 1993 Dec;18(3):275-83.

[4486] Kobayashi M, Kawashima H, Takemori K, et al. Ternatin, a cyclic peptide isolated from mushroom, and its derivative suppress hyperglycemia and hepatic fatty acid synthesis in spontaneously diabetic KK-A(y) mice. *Biochem Biophys Res Commun*. 2012 Oct 19;427(2):299-304.

[4487] Lo HC, Hsu TH, Lee CH. Extracellular Polysaccharopeptides from Fermented Turkey Tail Medicinal Mushroom, Trametes versicolor (Agaricomycetes), Mitigate Oxidative Stress, Hyperglycemia, and Hyperlipidemia in Rats with Type 2 Diabetes Mellitus. *Int J Med Mushrooms*. 2020;22(5):417-429.

[4488] Kobayashi M, Kawashima H, Takemori K, et al. Ternatin, a cyclic peptide isolated from mushroom, and its derivative suppress hyperglycemia and hepatic fatty acid synthesis in spontaneously diabetic KK-A(y) mice. *Biochem Biophys Res Commun*. 2012 Oct 19;427(2):299-304.

[4489] Wang Y, Li H, Li Y, et al. Coriolus versicolor alleviates diabetic cardiomyopathy by inhibiting cardiac fibrosis and NLRP3 inflammasome activation. *Phytother Res*. 2019 Oct;33(10):2737-2748.

[4490] Nikolic M, Lazarevic N, Novakovic J, et al. Characterization, In Vitro Biological Activity and In Vivo Cardioprotective Properties of Trametes versicolor (L.:Fr.) Quél. Heteropolysaccharides in a Rat Model of Metabolic Syndrome. *Pharmaceuticals (Basel)*. 2023 May 25;16(6):787.

[4491] Interdonato L, Impellizzeri D, D'Amico R, et al. Modulation of TLR4/NFκB Pathways in Autoimmune Myocarditis. *Antioxidants (Basel)*. 2023 Jul 27;12(8):1507.

[4492] Yeung JH, Chiu LC, Ooi VE. Effect of polysaccharide peptide (PSP) on glutathione and protection against paracetamol-induced hepatotoxicity in the rat. *Methods Find Exp Clin Pharmacol*. 1994 Dec;16(10):723-9.

[4493] Tang H, Zha Z, Tan Y, et al. Extraction and characterization of polysaccharide from fermented mycelia of Coriolus versicolor and its efficacy for treating nonalcoholic fatty liver disease. *Int J Biol Macromol*. 2023 Sep 1;248:125951.

[4494] Wang KL, Lu ZM, Mao X, et al. Structural characterization and anti-alcoholic liver injury activity of a polysaccharide from Coriolus versicolor mycelia. *Int J Biol Macromol*. 2019 Sep 15;137:1102-1111.

[4495] Ferreiro E, Pita IR, Mota SI, et al. Coriolus versicolor biomass increases dendritic arborization of newly-generated neurons in mouse hippocampal dentate gyrus. *Oncotarget*. 2018 Aug 31;9(68):32929-32942.

[4496] Li L, Li Y, Miao C, Liu Y, et al. Coriolus versicolor polysaccharides (CVP) regulates neuronal apoptosis in cerebral ischemia-reperfusion injury via the p38MAPK signaling pathway. *Ann Transl Med*. 2020 Sep;8(18):1168.

[4497] D'Amico R, Trovato Salinaro A, Fusco R, et al. Hericium erinaceus and Coriolus versicolor Modulate Molecular and Biochemical Changes after Traumatic Brain Injury. *Antioxidants (Basel)*. 2021 Jun 2;10(6):898.

[4498] Kim BC, Kim YS, Lee JW, et al. Protective Effect of Coriolus versicolor Cultivated in Citrus Extract Against Nitric Oxide-Induced Apoptosis in Human Neuroblastoma SK-N-MC Cells. *Exp Neurobiol*. 2011 Jun;20(2):100-9.

[4499] Chen J, Jin X, Zhang L, et al. A study on the antioxidant effect of Coriolus versicolor polysaccharide in rat brain tissues. *Afr J Tradit Complement Altern Med*. 2013 Oct 3;10(6):481-4.

[4500] Cordaro M, Modafferi S, D'Amico R, et al. Natural Compounds Such as Hericium erinaceus and Coriolus versicolor Modulate Neuroinflammation, Oxidative Stress and Lipoxin A4 Expression in Rotenone-Induced Parkinson's Disease in Mice. *Biomedicines*. 2022 Oct 7;10(10):2505.

[4501] D'Amico R, Tomasello M, Impellizzeri D, et al. Mechanism of Action of Natural Compounds in Peripheral Multiorgan Dysfunction and Hippocampal Neuroinflammation Induced by Sepsis. *Antioxidants (Basel)*. 2023 Mar 3;12(3):635.

[4502] Trovato A, Siracusa R, Di Paola R, et al. Redox modulation of cellular stress response and lipoxin A4 expression by Coriolus versicolor in rat brain: Relevance to Alzheimer's disease pathogenesis. *Neurotoxicology*. 2016 Mar;53:350-358.

[4503] Lin IH, Hau DM, Chang YH. Restorative effect of Coriolus versicolor polysaccharides against gamma-irradiation-induced spleen injury in mice. *Zhongguo Yao Li Xue Bao*. 1996 Mar;17(2):102-4.

[4504] Ho CS, Tung YT, Kung WM, et al. Effect of Coriolus versicolor Mycelia Extract on Exercise Performance and Physical Fatigue in Mice. *Int J Med Sci*. 2017 Sep 4;14(11):1110-1117.

[4505] Chong Z, Matsuo H, Kuroda M, et al. Mushroom extract inhibits ultraviolet B-induced cellular senescence in human keratinocytes. *Cytotechnology*. 2018 Jun;70(3):1001-1008.

[4506] Li HY, Wang XM, Tan JQ, et al. [Effects of Coriolus versicolor polysaccharides on productivity and longevity in Drosophila melanogaster]. *Zhongguo Yao Li Xue Bao*. 1993 Nov;14 Suppl:S44-7.

[4507] Kylyc A, Yesilada E. Preliminary results on antigenotoxic effects of dried mycelia of two medicinal mushrooms in Drosophila melanogaster somatic mutation and recombination test. *Int J Med Mushrooms*. 2013;15(4):415-21.

[4508] Knežević A, Živković L, Stajić M, et al. Antigenotoxic Effect of Trametes spp. Extracts against DNA Damage on Human Peripheral White Blood Cells. *ScientificWorldJournal*. 2015;2015:146378.

[4509] Szeto YT, Lau PC, Kalle W, et al. Direct human DNA protection by Coriolus versicolor (Yunzhi) extract. *Pharm Biol*. 2013 Jul;51(7):851-5.

[4510] Janjušević L, Pejin B, Kaišarević S, et al. Trametes versicolor ethanol extract, a promising candidate for health-promoting food supplement. *Nat Prod Res*. 2018 Apr;32(8):963-967.

[4511] Miletić D, Turło J, Podsadni P, et al. Turkey Tail Medicinal Mushroom, Trametes versicolor (Agaricomycetes), Crude Exopolysaccharides with Antioxidative Activity. *Int J Med Mushrooms*. 2020;22(9):885-895.

[4512] Scarpari M, Reverberi M, Parroni A, et al. Tramesan, a novel polysaccharide from Trametes versicolor. Structural characterization and biological effects. *PLoS One*. 2017 Aug 22;12(8):e0171412.

[4513] Janjušević L, Karaman M, Šibul F, et al. The lignicolous fungus Trametes versicolor (L.) Lloyd (1920): a promising natural source of antiradical and AChE inhibitory agents. *J Enzyme Inhib Med Chem*. 2017 Dec;32(1):355-362.

[4514] Michalak K, Winiarczyk S, Adaszek Ł, et al. Antioxidant and antimicrobial properties of an extract rich in proteins obtained from Trametes versicolor. *J Vet Res*. 2023 Jun 16;67(2):209-218.

[4515] Jhan MH, Yeh CH, Tsai CC, et al. Enhancing the Antioxidant Ability of Trametes versicolor Polysaccharopeptides by an Enzymatic Hydrolysis Process. *Molecules*. 2016 Sep 10;21(9):1215.

[4516] Kıvrak I, Kivrak S, Karababa E. Assessment of Bioactive Compounds and Antioxidant Activity of Turkey Tail Medicinal Mushroom Trametes versicolor (Agaricomycetes). *Int J Med Mushrooms*. 2020;22(6):559-571.

[4517] Moazzem Hossen SM, Akramul Hoque Tanim M, Shahadat Hossain M, et al. Deciphering the CNS anti-depressant, antioxidant and cytotoxic profiling of methanol and aqueous extracts of Trametes versicolor and molecular interactions of its phenolic compounds. *Saudi J Biol Sci*. 2021 Nov;28(11):6375-6383.

[4518] Rašeta M, Popović M, Knežević P, et al. Bioactive Phenolic Compounds of Two Medicinal Mushroom Species Trametes versicolor and Stereum subtomentosum as Antioxidant and Antiproliferative Agents. *Chem Biodivers*. 2020 Dec;17(12):e2000683.

[4519] Krsmanović N, Rašeta M, Mišković J, et al. Effects of UV Stress in Promoting Antioxidant Activities in Fungal Species Trametes versicolor (L.) Lloyd and Flammulina velutipes (Curtis) Singer. *Antioxidants (Basel)*. 2023 Jan 28;12(2):302.

[4520] Smith H, Doyle S, Murphy R. Filamentous fungi as a source of natural antioxidants. *Food Chem*. 2015 Oct 15;185:389-97.

[4521] Oyetayo VO, Nieto-Camacho A, Rodriguez BE, et al. Assessment of anti-inflammatory, lipid peroxidation and acute toxicity of extracts obtained from wild higher basidiomycetes mushrooms collected from Akure (southwest Nigeria). *Int J Med Mushrooms*. 2012;14(6):575-80.

[4522] Liu YM, Lai YH, Hsieh FM, et al. Antioxidant Activities of Selected Medicinal Mushroom Submerged Cultivated Mycelia. *Int J Med Mushrooms*. 2020;22(4):367-377.

[4523] Knežević A, Stajić M, Sofrenić I, et al. Antioxidative, antifungal, cytotoxic and antineurodegenerative activity of selected Trametes species from Serbia. *PLoS One*. 2018 Aug 31;13(8):e0203064.

[4524] Sun X, Sun Y, Zhang Q, et al. Screening and comparison of antioxidant activities of polysaccharides from Coriolus versicolor. *Int J Biol Macromol*. 2014 Aug;69:12-9.

[4525] Jun L, Mei Z, Yuan C. Reversal of inhibition of reactive oxygen species on respiratory burst of macrophages by polysaccharide from Coriolus versicolor. *Int J Immunopharmacol*. 1993 Apr;15(3):429-33.

[4526] Mau JL, Lin HC, Chen CC. Antioxidant properties of several medicinal mushrooms. *J Agric Food Chem*. 2002 Oct 9;50(21):6072-7.

[4527] Park KM, Kwon KM, Lee SH. Evaluation of the Antioxidant Activities and Tyrosinase Inhibitory Property from Mycelium Culture Extracts. *Evid Based Complement Alternat Med*. 2015;2015:616298.

[4528] Wei WS, Tan JQ, Guo F, et al. Effects of Coriolus versicolor polysaccharides on superoxide dismutase activities in mice. *Zhongguo Yao Li Xue Bao*. 1996 Mar;17(2):174-8.

[4529] Kobayashi Y, Kariya K, Saigenji K, et al. Suppressive effects on cancer cell proliferation of the enhancement of superoxide dismutase (SOD) activity associated with the protein-bound polysaccharide of Coriolus versicolor QUEL. *Cancer Biother*. 1994 Summer;9(2):171-8.

[4530] Kobayashi Y, Kariya K, Saigenji K, et al. Oxidative stress relief for cancer-bearing hosts by the protein-bound polysaccharide of Coriolus versicolor QUEL with SOD mimicking activity. *Cancer Biother*. 1994 Spring;9(1):55-62.

[4531] Kobayashi Y, Kariya K, Saigenji K, et al. Suppression of cancer cell growth in vitro by the protein-bound polysaccharide of Coriolus versicolor QUEL (PS-K) with SOD mimicking activity. *Cancer Biother*. 1994 Spring;9(1):63-9.

[4532] Kariya K, Nakamura K, Nomoto K, et al. Mimicking of superoxide dismutase activity by protein-bound polysaccharide of Coriolus versicolor QUEL, and oxidative stress relief for cancer patients. *Mol Biother*. 1992 Mar;4(1):40-6.

[4533] Pang ZJ, Chen Y, Zhou M. Polysaccharide Krestin enhances manganese superoxide dismutase activity and mRNA expression in mouse peritoneal macrophages. *Am J Chin Med*. 2000;28(3-4):331-41.

[4534] Nakamura K, Matsunaga K. Susceptibility of natural killer (NK) cells to reactive oxygen species (ROS) and their restoration by the mimics of superoxide dismutase (SOD). *Cancer Biother Radiopharm*. 1998 Aug;13(4):275-90.

[4535] Pang ZJ, Chen Y, Zhou M, et al. Effect of polysaccharide krestin on glutathione peroxidase gene expression in mouse peritoneal macrophages. *Br J Biomed Sci*. 2000;57(2):130-6.

[4536] Yuan C, Mei Z, Liu S, et al. PSK protects macrophages from lipoperoxide accumulation and foam cell formation caused by oxidatively modified low-density lipoprotein. *Atherosclerosis*. 1996 Aug 2;124(2):171-81.

[4537] Shi S, Yin L, Shen X, et al. β-Glucans from Trametes versicolor (L.) Lloyd Is Effective for Prevention of Influenza Virus Infection. *Viruses*. 2022 Jan 25;14(2):237.

[4538] Krupodorova T, Rybalko S, Barshteyn V. Antiviral activity of Basidiomycete mycelia against influenza type A (serotype H1N1) and herpes simplex virus type 2 in cell culture. *Virol Sin*. 2014 Oct;29(5):284-90.

[4539] Collins RA, Ng TB. Polysaccharopeptide from Coriolus versicolor has potential for use against human immunodeficiency virus type 1 infection. *Life Sci*. 1997;60(25):PL383-7.

[4540] Alvarez-Rivera E, Rodríguez-Valentín M, Boukli NM. The Antiviral Compound PSP Inhibits HIV-1 Entry via PKR-Dependent Activation in Monocytic Cells. *Viruses*. 2023 Mar 22;15(3):804.

[4541] Rodríguez-Valentín M, López S, et al. Naturally Derived Anti-HIV Polysaccharide Peptide (PSP) Triggers a Toll-Like Receptor 4-Dependent Antiviral Immune Response. *J Immunol Res*. 2018 Jul 15;2018:8741698.

[4542] Ishimaru H, Umezawa T, Yoshikawa T, et al. Antifungal activity of simply fractionated organosolv lignin against Trametes versicolor. *J Biotechnol*. 2023 Feb 20;364:23-30.

[4543] Michalak K, Winiarczyk S, Adaszek Ł, et al. Antioxidant and antimicrobial properties of an extract rich in proteins obtained from Trametes versicolor. *J Vet Res.* 2023 Jun 16;67(2):209-218.

[4544] Bains A, Chawla P. In vitro bioactivity, antimicrobial and anti-inflammatory efficacy of modified solvent evaporation assisted Trametes versicolor extract. *3 Biotech.* 2020 Sep;10(9):404.

[4545] Orzali L, Valente MT, Scala V, et al. Antibacterial Activity of Essential Oils and Trametes versicolor Extract against Clavibacter michiganensis subsp. michiganensis and Ralstonia solanacearum for Seed Treatment and Development of a Rapid In Vivo Assay. *Antibiotics (Basel).* 2020 Sep 21;9(9):628.

[4546] Hassan F, Ni S, Becker TL, et al. Evaluation of the Antibacterial Activity of 75 Mushrooms Collected in the Vicinity of Oxford, Ohio (USA). *Int J Med Mushrooms.* 2019;21(2):131-141.

[4547] Knežević A, Stajić M, Sofrenić I, et al. Antioxidative, antifungal, cytotoxic and antineurodegenerative activity of selected Trametes species from Serbia. *PLoS One.* 2018 Aug 31;13(8):e0203064.

[4548] Matijašević D, Pantić M, Rašković B, et al. The Antibacterial Activity of Coriolus versicolor Methanol Extract and Its Effect on Ultrastructural Changes of Staphylococcus aureus and Salmonella Enteritidis. *Front Microbiol.* 2016 Aug 4;7:1226.

[4549] Sharma HN, Catrett J, Nwokeocha OD, et al. Anti-Toxoplasma gondii activity of Trametes versicolor (Turkey tail) mushroom extract. *Sci Rep.* 2023 May 29;13(1):8667.

[4550] Leliebre-Lara V, Monzote Fidalgo L, Pferschy-Wenzig EM, et al. In Vitro Antileishmanial Activity of Sterols from Trametes versicolor (Bres. Rivarden). *Molecules.* 2016 Aug 10;21(8):1045.

[4551] Park KM, Kwon KM, Lee SH. Evaluation of the Antioxidant Activities and Tyrosinase Inhibitory Property from Mycelium Culture Extracts. *Evid Based Complement Alternat Med.* 2015;2015:616298.

[4552] Yang P, Xiao W, Lu S, et al. Characterization of a Trametes versicolor aflatoxin B1-degrading enzyme (TV-AFB1D) and its application in the AFB1 degradation of contaminated rice in situ. *Front Microbiol.* 2022 Sep 14;13:960882.

[4553] Zjalic S, Reverberi M, Ricelli A, et al. Trametes versicolor: a possible tool for aflatoxin control. *Int J Food Microbiol.* 2006 Apr 1;107(3):243-9.

[4554] Yang P, Xiao W, Lu S, et al. Recombinant Expression of Trametes versicolor Aflatoxin B1-Degrading Enzyme (TV-AFB1D) in Engineering Pichia pastoris GS115 and Application in AFB1 Degradation in AFB1-Contaminated Peanuts. *Toxins (Basel).* 2021 May 13;13(5):349.

[4555] Suresh G, Cabezudo I, Pulicharla R, et al. Biodegradation of aflatoxin B1 with cell-free extracts of Trametes versicolor and Bacillus subtilis. *Res Vet Sci.* 2020 Dec;133:85-91.

[4556] Dellafiora L, Galaverna G, Reverberi M, et al. Degradation of Aflatoxins by Means of Laccases from Trametes versicolor: An In Silico Insight. *Toxins (Basel).* 2017 Jan 1;9(1):17.

[4557] Loncar J, Bellich B, Cescutti P, et al. The Effect of Mushroom Culture Filtrates on the Inhibition of Mycotoxins Produced by Aspergillus flavus and Aspergillus carbonarius. *Toxins (Basel).* 2023 Feb 25;15(3):177.

[4558] Scarpari M, Bello C, Pietricola C, et al. Aflatoxin control in maize by Trametes versicolor. *Toxins (Basel).* 2014 Dec 17;6(12):3426-37.

[4559] Lou H, Li Y, Yang C, et al. Optimizing the degradation of aflatoxin B1 in corn by Trametes versicolor and improving the nutritional composition of corn. *J Sci Food Agric.* 2023 Aug 31. Online ahead of print.

[4560] Alberts JF, Gelderblom WC, Botha A, et al. Degradation of aflatoxin B(1) by fungal laccase enzymes. *Int J Food Microbiol.* 2009 Sep 30;135(1):47-52.

[4561] Loncar J, Bellich B, Parroni A, et al. Oligosaccharides Derived from Tramesan: Their Structure and Activity on Mycotoxin Inhibition in Aspergillus flavus and Aspergillus carbonarius. *Biomolecules.* 2021 Feb 8;11(2):243.

[4562] Tan Z, Losantos D, Li Y, et al. Biotransformation of chloramphenicol by white-rot-fungi Trametes versicolor under cadmium stress. *Bioresour Technol.* 2023 Feb;369:128508.

[4563] Stenholm Å, Hedeland M, Pettersson CE. Neomycin removal using the white rot fungus Trametes versicolor. *J Environ Sci Health A Tox Hazard Subst Environ Eng.* 2022;57(6):436-447.

[4564] Cruz Del Álamo A, Pariente MI, et al. Trametes versicolor immobilized on rotating biological contactors as alternative biological treatment for the removal of emerging concern micropollutants. *Water Res.* 2020 Mar 1;170:115313.

[4565] Beltrán-Flores E, Sarrà M, et al. Pesticide bioremediation by Trametes versicolor: Application in a fixed-bed reactor, sorption contribution and bioregeneration. *Sci Total Environ.* 2021 Nov 10;794:148386.

[4566] Sun Y, Li Y, Liang H, et al. Distinct laccase expression and activity profiles of Trametes versicolor facilitate degradation of benzo[a]pyrene. *Front Bioeng Biotechnol.* 2023 Sep 21;11:1264135.

[4567] Pezzella C, Macellaro G, Sannia G, et al. Exploitation of Trametes versicolor for bioremediation of endocrine disrupting chemicals in bioreactors. *PLoS One.* 2017 Jun 2;12(6):e0178758.

[4568] Maadani Mallak A, Lakzian A, et al. Effect of Pleurotus ostreatus and Trametes versicolor on triclosan biodegradation and activity of laccase and manganese peroxidase enzymes. *Microb Pathog.* 2020 Dec;149:104473.

[4569] Sun K, Li S, Yu J, et al. Cu2+-assisted laccase from Trametes versicolor enhanced self-polyreaction of triclosan. *Chemosphere.* 2019 Jun;225:745-754.

[4570] Bassanini I, Grosso S, Tognoli C, et al. Studies on the Oxidation of Aromatic Amines Catalyzed by Trametes versicolor Laccase. *Int J Mol Sci.* 2023 Feb 9;24(4):3524.

[4571] Huang Y, Yang J. Kinetics and mechanisms for sulfamethoxazole transformation in the phenolic acid-laccase (Trametes versicolor) system. *Environ Sci Pollut Res Int.* 2022 Sep;29(42):62941-62951.

[4572] Singh J, Kumar P, Saharan V, et al. Simultaneous laccase production and transformation of bisphenol-A and triclosan using Trametes versicolor. *3 Biotech.* 2019 Apr;9(4):129.

[4573] García-Vara M, Hu K, Postigo C, et al. Remediation of bentazone contaminated water by Trametes versicolor: Characterization, identification of transformation products, and implementation in a trickle-bed reactor under non-sterile conditions. *J Hazard Mater.* 2021 May 5;409:124476.

[4574] Hu K, Peris A, Torán J, et al. Exploring the degradation capability of Trametes versicolor on selected hydrophobic pesticides through setting sights simultaneously on culture broth and biological matrix. *Chemosphere.* 2020 Jul;250:126293.

[4575] Li Y, Zhao H, Wang L, et al. New insights in the biodegradation of high-cyclic polycyclic aromatic hydrocarbons with crude enzymes of Trametes versicolor. *Environ Technol*. 2023 Jan 30:1-12.

[4576] Rodríguez-Rodríguez CE, Marco-Urrea E, et al. Naproxen degradation test to monitor Trametes versicolor activity in solid-state bioremediation processes. *J Hazard Mater*. 2010 Jul 15;179(1-3):1152-5.

[4577] Stenholm Å, Hedeland M, Arvidsson T, et al. Removal of nonylphenol polyethoxylates by adsorption on polyurethane foam and biodegradation using immobilized Trametes versicolor. *Sci Total Environ*. 2020 Jul 1;724:138159.

[4578] Trivedi J, Chhaya U. Bioremediation of phenolic pollutant bisphenol A using optimized reverse micelles system of Trametes versicolor laccase in non-aqueous environment. *3 Biotech*. 2021 Jun;11(6):297.

[4579] Hu K, Barbieri MV, López-García E, et al. Fungal degradation of selected medium to highly polar pesticides by Trametes versicolor: kinetics, biodegradation pathways, and ecotoxicity of treated waters. *Anal Bioanal Chem*. 2022 Jan;414(1):439-449.

[4580] Zeng S, Zhao J, Xia L. Simultaneous production of laccase and degradation of bisphenol A with Trametes versicolor cultivated on agricultural wastes. *Bioprocess Biosyst Eng*. 2017 Aug;40(8):1237-1245.

[4581] Hongyan L, Zexiong Z, Shiwei X, et al. Study on transformation and degradation of bisphenol A by Trametes versicolor laccase and simulation of molecular docking. *Chemosphere*. 2019 Jun;224:743-750.

[4582] Trivedi J, Chhaya U. Bioremediation of bisphenol A found in industrial wastewater using Trametes versicolor (TV) laccase nanoemulsion-based bead organogel in packed bed reactor. *Water Environ Res*. 2022 Oct;94(10):e10786.

[4583] Zhang H, Liu X, Liu B, et al. Synergistic degradation of Azure B and sulfanilamide antibiotics by the white-rot fungus Trametes versicolor with an activated ligninolytic enzyme system. *J Hazard Mater*. 2023 Sep 15;458:131939.

[4584] Wang D, Zhu R, Lou J, et al. Plasticizer phthalate esters degradation with a laccase from Trametes versicolor: effects of TEMPO used as a mediator and estrogenic activity removal. *Biodegradation*. 2023 Oct;34(5):431-444.

[4585] Beltrán-Flores E, Torán J, et al. The removal of diuron from agricultural wastewaters by Trametes versicolor immobilized on pinewood in simple channel reactors. *Sci Total Environ*. 2020 Aug 1;728:138414.

[4586] Nowak M, Zawadzka K, Szemraj J, et al. Biodegradation of Chloroxylenol by Cunninghamella elegans IM 1785/21GP and Trametes versicolor IM 373: Insight into Ecotoxicity and Metabolic Pathways. *Int J Mol Sci*. 2021 Apr 22;22(9):4360.

[4587] Pazarlioglu NK, Akkaya A, Akdogan HA, et al. Biodegradation of Direct Blue 15 by free and immobilized Trametes versicolor. *Water Environ Res*. 2010 Jul;82(7):579-85.

[4588] Stenholm Å, Hedeland M, Arvidsson T, et al. Removal of diclofenac from a non-sterile aqueous system using Trametes versicolor with an emphasis on adsorption and biodegradation mechanisms. *Environ Technol*. 2019 Aug;40(19):2460-2472.

[4589] Kolb M, Sieber V, Amann M, et al. Removal of monomer delignification products by laccase from Trametes versicolor. *Bioresour Technol*. 2012 Jan;104:298-304.

[4590] Legerská B, Chmelová D, Ondrejovič M. Decolourization and detoxification of monoazo dyes by laccase from the white-rot fungus Trametes versicolor. *J Biotechnol*. 2018 Nov 10;285:84-90.

[4591] Rodríguez-Rodríguez CE, Jelić A, et al. Bioaugmentation of sewage sludge with Trametes versicolor in solid-phase biopiles produces degradation of pharmaceuticals and affects microbial communities. *Environ Sci Technol*. 2012 Nov 6;46(21):12012-20.

[4592] Ferrando-Climent L, Cruz-Morató C, Marco-Urrea E, et al. Non conventional biological treatment based on Trametes versicolor for the elimination of recalcitrant anticancer drugs in hospital wastewater. *Chemosphere*. 2015 Oct;136:9-19.

[4593] Bernats M, Juhna T. Removal of phenols-like substances in pharmaceutical wastewater with fungal bioreactors by adding Trametes versicolor. *Water Sci Technol*. 2018 Sep;78(3-4):743-750.

[4594] Dalecka B, Strods M, Juhna T, et al. Removal of total phosphorus, ammonia nitrogen and organic carbon from non-sterile municipal wastewater with Trametes versicolor and Aspergillus luchuensis. *Microbiol Res*. 2020 Dec;241:126586.

[4595] Ryan D, Leukes W, Burton S. Improving the bioremediation of phenolic wastewaters by Trametes versicolor. *Bioresour Technol*. 2007 Feb;98(3):579-87.

[4596] Llorens-Blanch G, Badia-Fabregat M, Lucas D, et al. Degradation of pharmaceuticals from membrane biological reactor sludge with Trametes versicolor. *Environ Sci Process Impacts*. 2015 Feb;17(2):429-40.

[4597] Marco-Urrea E, Pérez-Trujillo M, Cruz-Morató C, et al. Degradation of the drug sodium diclofenac by Trametes versicolor pellets and identification of some intermediates by NMR. *J Hazard Mater*. 2010 Apr 15;176(1-3):836-42.

[4598] Blánquez P, Guieysse B. Continuous biodegradation of 17beta-estradiol and 17alpha-ethynylestradiol by Trametes versicolor. *J Hazard Mater*. 2008 Jan 31;150(2):459-62.

[4599] Rodríguez-Rodríguez CE, García-Galán MA, Blánquez P, et al. Continuous degradation of a mixture of sulfonamides by Trametes versicolor and identification of metabolites from sulfapyridine and sulfathiazole. *J Hazard Mater*. 2012 Apr 30;213-214:347-54.

[4600] Cruz-Morató C, Ferrando-Climent L, Rodriguez-Mozaz S, et al. Degradation of pharmaceuticals in non-sterile urban wastewater by Trametes versicolor in a fluidized bed bioreactor. *Water Res*. 2013 Sep 15;47(14):5200-10.

[4601] Aranda E, Marco-Urrea E, Caminal G, et al. Advanced oxidation of benzene, toluene, ethylbenzene and xylene isomers (BTEX) by Trametes versicolor. *J Hazard Mater*. 2010 Sep 15;181(1-3):181-6.

[4602] Rodríguez-Rodríguez CE, Barón E, Gago-Ferrero P, et al. Removal of pharmaceuticals, polybrominated flame retardants and UV-filters from sludge by the fungus Trametes versicolor in bioslurry reactor. *J Hazard Mater*. 2012 Sep 30;233-234:235-43.

[4603] Kurniawati S, Nicell JA. Characterization of Trametes versicolor laccase for the transformation of aqueous phenol. *Bioresour Technol*. 2008 Nov;99(16):7825-34.

[4604] Rodríguez-Rodríguez CE, Marco-Urrea E, et al. Degradation of naproxen and carbamazepine in spiked sludge by slurry and solid-phase Trametes versicolor systems. *Bioresour Technol*. 2010 Apr;101(7):2259-66.

[4605] Badia-Fabregat M, Rodríguez-Rodríguez CE, Gago-Ferrero P, et al. Degradation of UV filters in sewage sludge and 4-MBC in liquid medium by the ligninolytic fungus Trametes versicolor. *J Environ Manage*. 2012 Aug 15;104:114-20.

[4606] Okamoto K, Uchii A, Kanawaku R, et al. Bioconversion of xylose, hexoses and biomass to ethanol by a new isolate of the white rot basidiomycete Trametes versicolor. *Springerplus*. 2014 Mar 3;3:121.

[4607] Han MJ, Choi HT, Song HG. Degradation of phenanthrene by Trametes versicolor and its laccase. *J Microbiol*. 2004 Jun;42(2):94-8.

[4608] Marco-Urrea E, Radjenović J, Caminal G, et al. Oxidation of atenolol, propranolol, carbamazepine and clofibric acid by a biological Fenton-like system mediated by the white-rot fungus Trametes versicolor. *Water Res*. 2010 Jan;44(2):521-32.

[4609] García-Galán MJ, Rodríguez-Rodríguez CE, Vicent T, et al. Biodegradation of sulfamethazine by Trametes versicolor: Removal from sewage sludge and identification of intermediate products by UPLC-QqTOF-MS. *Sci Total Environ*. 2011 Nov 15;409(24):5505-12.

[4610] Bautista LF, Morales G, Sanz R. Biodegradation of polycyclic aromatic hydrocarbons (PAHs) by laccase from Trametes versicolor covalently immobilized on amino-functionalized SBA-15. *Chemosphere*. 2015 Oct;136:273-80.

[4611] Hoff T, Liu SY, Bollag JM. Transformation of Halogen-, Alkyl-, and Alkoxy-Substituted Anilines by a Laccase of Trametes versicolor. *Appl Environ Microbiol*. 1985 May;49(5):1040-5.

[4612] Grey R, Höfer C, Schlosser D. Degradation of 2-chlorophenol and formation of 2-chloro-1,4-benzoquinone by mycelia and cell-free crude culture liquids of Trametes versicolor in relation to extracellular laccase activity. *J Basic Microbiol*. 1998;38(5-6):371-82.

[4613] Uhnáková B, Petríčková A, Biedermann D, et al. Biodegradation of brominated aromatics by cultures and laccase of Trametes versicolor. *Chemosphere*. 2009 Aug;76(6):826-32.

[4614] Demir G. Degradation of toluene and benzene by Trametes versicolor. *J Environ Biol*. 2004 Jan;25(1):19-25.

[4615] Mir-Tutusaus JA, Masís-Mora M, Corcellas C, et al. Degradation of selected agrochemicals by the white rot fungus Trametes versicolor. *Sci Total Environ*. 2014 Dec 1;500-501:235-42.

[4616] Tran NH, Hu J, Urase T. Removal of the insect repellent N,N-diethyl-m-toluamide (DEET) by laccase-mediated systems. *Bioresour Technol*. 2013 Nov;147:667-671.

[4617] Marco-Urrea E, Pérez-Trujillo M, et al. Biodegradation of the analgesic naproxen by Trametes versicolor and identification of intermediates using HPLC-DAD-MS and NMR. *Bioresour Technol*. 2010 Apr;101(7):2159-66.

[4618] Donatini B. Control of oral human papillomavirus (HPV) by medicinal mushrooms, Trametes versicolor and Ganoderma lucidum: a preliminary clinical trial. *Int J Med Mushrooms*. 2014;16(5):497-8.

[4619] Criscuolo AA, Sesti F, Piccione E, et al. Therapeutic Efficacy of a Coriolus versicolor-Based Vaginal Gel in Women with Cervical Uterine High-Risk HPV Infection: A Retrospective Observational Study. *Adv Ther*. 2021 Feb;38(2):1202-1211.

[4620] Serrano L, López AC, González SP, et al. Efficacy of a Coriolus versicolor-Based Vaginal Gel in Women With Human Papillomavirus-Dependent Cervical Lesions: The PALOMA Study. *J Low Genit Tract Dis*. 2021 Apr 1;25(2):130-136.

[4621] Cortés Bordoy J, de Santiago García J, Agenjo González M, et al. Effect of a Multi-Ingredient Coriolus-versicolor-Based Vaginal Gel in Women with HPV-Dependent Cervical Lesions: The Papilobs Real-Life Prospective Study. *Cancers (Basel)*. 2023 Jul 29;15(15):3863.

[4622] Gil-Antuñano SP, Serrano Cogollor L, López Díaz AC, et al. Efficacy of a Coriolusversicolor-Based Vaginal Gel in Human Papillomavirus-Positive Women Older Than 40 Years: A Sub-Analysis of PALOMA Study. *J Pers Med*. 2022 Sep 22;12(10):1559.

[4623] Palacios S, Losa F, Dexeus D, et al. Beneficial effects of a Coriolus versicolor-based vaginal gel on cervical epithelization, vaginal microbiota and vaginal health: a pilot study in asymptomatic women. *BMC Womens Health*. 2017 Mar 16;17(1):21.

[4624] Pallav K, Dowd SE, Villafuerte J, et al. Effects of polysaccharopeptide from Trametes versicolor and amoxicillin on the gut microbiome of healthy volunteers: a randomized clinical trial. *Gut Microbes*. 2014 Jul 1;5(4):458-67.

[4625] Scuto M, Di Mauro P, Ontario ML, et al. Nutritional Mushroom Treatment in Meniere's Disease with Coriolus versicolor: A Rationale for Therapeutic Intervention in Neuroinflammation and Antineurodegeneration. *Int J Mol Sci*. 2019 Dec 31;21(1):284.

[4626] Eliza WL, Fai CK, Chung LP. Efficacy of Yun Zhi (Coriolus versicolor) on survival in cancer patients: systematic review and meta-analysis. *Recent Pat Inflamm Allergy Drug Discov*. 2012 Jan;6(1):78-87.

[4627] Torkelson CJ, Sweet E, Martzen MR, et al. Phase 1 Clinical Trial of Trametes versicolor in Women with Breast Cancer. *ISRN Oncol*. 2012;2012:251632.

[4628] Chay WY, Tham CK, Toh HC, et al. Coriolus versicolor (Yunzhi) Use as Therapy in Advanced Hepatocellular Carcinoma Patients with Poor Liver Function or Who Are Unfit for Standard Therapy. *J Altern Complement Med*. 2017 Aug;23(8):648-652.

[4629] Ito G, Tanaka H, Ohira M, et al. Correlation between efficacy of PSK postoperative adjuvant immunochemotherapy for gastric cancer and expression of MHC class I. *Exp Ther Med*. 2012 Jun;3(6):925-930.

[4630] Stamets P. Trametes versicolor (Turkey Tail Mushrooms) and *the Treatment of Breast Cancer*. *Glob Adv Health Med*. 2012 Nov;1(5):20.

[4631] Han CK, Chiang HC, et al. Comparison of Immunomodulatory and Anticancer Activities in Different Strains of Tremella fuciformis Berk. *Am J Chin Med*. 2015;43(8):1637-55.

[4632] Xie L, Liu G, Huang Z, et al. Tremella fuciformis Polysaccharide Induces Apoptosis of B16 Melanoma Cells via Promoting the M1 Polarization of Macrophages. *Molecules*. 2023 May 11;28(10):4018.

[4633] Ukai S, Hirose K, Kiho T, et al. Antitumor activity on sarcoma 180 of the polysaccharides from Tremella fuciformis Berk. *Chem Pharm Bull (Tokyo)*. 1972 Oct;20(10):2293-4.

[4634] Li X, Su Q, Pan Y. Overcharged lipid metabolism in mechanisms of antitumor by Tremella fuciformis-derived polysaccharide. *Int J Oncol*. 2023 Jan;62(1):11.

[4635] He G, Chen T, Huang L, et al. Tremella fuciformis polysaccharide reduces obesity in high-fat diet-fed mice by modulation of gut microbiota. *Front Microbiol*. 2022 Dec 5;13:1073350.

[4636] Park KJ, Lee SY, Kim HS, et al. The Neuroprotective and Neurotrophic Effects of Tremella fuciformis in PC12h Cells. *Mycobiology*. 2007 Mar;35(1):11-5.

[4637] Jin Y, Hu X, Zhang Y, et al. Studies on the purification of polysaccharides separated from Tremella fuciformis and their neuroprotective effect. *Mol Med Rep*. 2016 May;13(5):3985-92.

[4638] Park KJ, Lee SY, Kim HS, et al. The Neuroprotective and Neurotrophic Effects of Tremella fuciformis in PC12h Cells. *Mycobiology*. 2007 Mar;35(1):11-5.

[4639] Park HJ, Shim HS, Ahn YH, et al. Tremella fuciformis enhances the neurite outgrowth of PC12 cells and restores trimethyltin-induced impairment of memory in rats via activation of CREB transcription and cholinergic systems. *Behav Brain Res*. 2012 Apr 1;229(1):82-90.

4640 Zhang Y, Pei L, Gao L, et al. [A neuritogenic compound from Tremella fuciformis]. *Zhongguo Zhong Yao Za Zhi*. 2011 Sep;36(17):2358-60.

4641 Kim JH, Ha HC, Lee MS, et al. Effect of Tremella fuciformis on the neurite outgrowth of PC12h cells and the improvement of memory in rats. *Biol Pharm Bull*. 2007 Apr;30(4):708-14.

4642 Park HJ, Shim HS, Ahn YH, et al. Tremella fuciformis enhances the neurite outgrowth of PC12 cells and restores trimethyltin-induced impairment of memory in rats via activation of CREB transcription and cholinergic systems. *Behav Brain Res*. 2012 Apr 1;229(1):82-90.

4643 Kim JH, Ha HC, Lee MS, et al. Effect of Tremella fuciformis on the neurite outgrowth of PC12h cells and the improvement of memory in rats. *Biol Pharm Bull*. 2007 Apr;30(4):708-14.

4644 Niu B, Feng S, Xuan S, et al. Moisture and caking resistant Tremella fuciformis polysaccharides microcapsules with hypoglycemic activity. *Food Res Int*. 2021 Aug;146:110420.

4645 Kiho T, Tsujimura Y, Sakushima M, et al. [Polysaccharides in fungi. XXXIII. Hypoglycemic activity of an acidic polysaccharide (AC) from Tremella fuciformis]. *Yakugaku Zasshi*. 1994 May;114(5):308-15.

4646 Wu T, Xu B. Antidiabetic and antioxidant activities of eight medicinal mushroom species from China. *Int J Med Mushrooms*. 2015;17(2):129-40.

4647 Lee J, Ha SJ, Lee HJ, et al. Protective effect of Tremella fuciformis Berk extract on LPS-induced acute inflammation via inhibition of the NF-κB and MAPK pathways. *Food Funct*. 2016 Jul 13;7(7):3263-72.

4648 Li H, Lee HS, Kim SH, et al. Antioxidant and anti-inflammatory activities of methanol extracts of Tremella fuciformis and its major phenolic acids. *J Food Sci*. 2014 Apr;79(4):C460-8.

4649 Ukai S, Kiho T, Hara C, et al. Polysaccharides in fungi. XIV. Anti-inflammatory effect of the polysaccharides from the fruit bodies of several fungi. *J Pharmacobiodyn*. 1983 Dec;6(12):983-90.

4650 Huang TY, Yang FL, Chiu HW, et al. An Immunological Polysaccharide from Tremella fuciformis: Essential Role of Acetylation in Immunomodulation. *Int J Mol Sci*. 2022 Sep 8;23(18):10392.

4651 Gao Y, Yang X, Zheng W, et al. Preparation, characterization, and cytokine-stimulating activity of oligosaccharides from Tremella fuciformis Berk. *J Food Biochem*. 2020 Jul;44(7):e13212.

4652 Gao QP, Jiang RZ, Chen HQ, et al. Characterization and cytokine stimulating activities of heteroglycans from Tremella fuciformis. *Planta Med*. 1996 Aug;62(4):297-302.

4653 Hung CL, Chang AJ, Kuo XK, et al. Molecular cloning and function characterization of a new macrophage-activating protein from Tremella fuciformis. *J Agric Food Chem*. 2014 Feb 19;62(7):1526-35.

4654 Gao Q, Killie MK, Chen H, et al. Characterization and cytokine-stimulating activities of acidic heteroglycans from Tremella fuciformis. *Planta Med*. 1997 Oct;63(5):457-60.

4655 Gao Q, Seljelid R, Chen H, et al. Characterisation of acidic heteroglycans from Tremella fuciformis Berk with cytokine stimulating activity. *Carbohydr Res*. 1996 Jul 19;288:135-42.

4656 Gao Q, Berntzen G, Jiang R, et al. Conjugates of Tremella polysaccharides with microbeads and their TNF-stimulating activity. *Planta Med*. 1998 Aug;64(6):551-4.

4657 Han CK, Chiang HC, et al. Comparison of Immunomodulatory and Anticancer Activities in Different Strains of Tremella fuciformis Berk. *Am J Chin Med*. 2015;43(8):1637-55.

4658 Ma L, Lin ZB. [Effect of Tremella polysaccharide on IL-2 production by mouse splenocytes]. *Yao Xue Xue Bao*. 1992;27(1):1-4.

4659 Xiao H, Li H, Wen Y, et al. Tremella fuciformis polysaccharides ameliorated ulcerative colitis via inhibiting inflammation and enhancing intestinal epithelial barrier function. *Int J Biol Macromol*. 2021 Jun 1;180:633-642.

4660 Xu Y, Xie L, Zhang Z, et al. Tremella fuciformis Polysaccharides Inhibited Colonic Inflammation in Dextran Sulfate Sodium-Treated Mice via Foxp3+ T Cells, Gut Microbiota, and Bacterial Metabolites. *Front Immunol*. 2021 Apr 1;12:648162.

4661 He G, Chen T, Huang L, et al. Tremella fuciformis polysaccharide reduces obesity in high-fat diet-fed mice by modulation of gut microbiota. *Front Microbiol*. 2022 Dec 5;13:1073350.

4662 Chiu CH, Chiu KC, Yang LC. Amelioration of Obesity in Mice Fed a High-Fat Diet with Uronic Acid-Rich Polysaccharides Derived from Tremella fuciformis. *Polymers (Basel)*. 2022 Apr 8;14(8):1514.

4663 Cheng HH, Hou WC, Lu ML. Interactions of lipid metabolism and intestinal physiology with Tremella fuciformis Berk edible mushroom in rats fed a high-cholesterol diet with or without Nebacitin. *J Agric Food Chem*. 2002 Dec 4;50(25):7438-43.

4664 Khan TJ, Xu X, Xie X, et al. Tremella fuciformis Crude Polysaccharides Attenuates Steatosis and Suppresses Inflammation in Diet-Induced NAFLD Mice. *Curr Issues Mol Biol*. 2022 Mar 3;44(3):1224-1234.

4665 Cui JY, Lin ZB. [Effects of Tremella polysaccharide on cytoplasmic free calcium concentration in murine splenocytes]. *Yao Xue Xue Bao*. 1997 Aug;32(8):561-4.

4666 Ruan Y, Li H, Pu L, et al. Tremella fuciformis Polysaccharides Attenuate Oxidative Stress and Inflammation in Macrophages through miR-155. *Anal Cell Pathol (Amst)*. 2018 May 2;2018:5762371.

4667 Ge X, Huang W, Xu X, et al. Production, structure, and bioactivity of polysaccharide isolated from Tremella fuciformis XY. *Int J Biol Macromol*. 2020 Apr 1;148:173-181.

4668 Li M, Ma F, Li R, et al. Degradation of Tremella fuciformis polysaccharide by a combined ultrasound and hydrogen peroxide treatment: Process parameters, structural characteristics, and antioxidant activities. *Int J Biol Macromol*. 2020 Oct 1;160:979-990.

4669 Lee Q, Han X, Zheng M, et al. Preparation of low molecular weight polysaccharides from Tremella fuciformis by ultrasonic-assisted H2O2-Vc method: Structural characteristics, in vivo antioxidant activity and stress resistance. *Ultrason Sonochem*. 2023 Oct;99:106555.

4670 Ji YW, Rao GW, Xie GF. Ultrasound-assisted aqueous two-phase extraction of total flavonoids from Tremella fuciformis and antioxidant activity of extracted flavonoids. *Prep Biochem Biotechnol*. 2022;52(9):1060-1068.

4671 Wang X, Zhang Z, Zhao M. Carboxymethylation of polysaccharides from Tremella fuciformis for antioxidant and moisture-preserving activities. *Int J Biol Macromol*. 2015 Jan;72:526-30.

[4672] Chen X, Tian Y, Zhang J, et al. Study on effects of preparation method on the structure and antioxidant activity of protein-Tremella fuciformis polysaccharide complexes by asymmetrical flow field-flow fractionation. *Food Chem*. 2022 Aug 1;384:132619.

[4673] Liu J, Meng CG, Yan YH, et al. Structure, physical property and antioxidant activity of catechin grafted Tremella fuciformis polysaccharide. *Int J Biol Macromol*. 2016 Jan;82:719-24.

[4674] Zhang Z, Wang X, Zhao M, et al. Free-radical degradation by Fe2+/Vc/H2O2 and antioxidant activity of polysaccharide from Tremella fuciformis. *Carbohydr Polym*. 2014 Nov 4;112:578-82.

[4675] Zheng Q, He BL, Wang JY, et al. Structural Analysis and Antioxidant Activity of Extracellular Polysaccharides Extracted from Culinary-Medicinal White Jelly Mushroom Tremella fuciformis (Tremellomycetes) Conidium Cells. *Int J Med Mushrooms*. 2020;22(5):489-500.

[4676] Li H, Lee HS, Kim SH, et al. Antioxidant and anti-inflammatory activities of methanol extracts of Tremella fuciformis and its major phenolic acids. *J Food Sci*. 2014 Apr;79(4):C460-8.

[4677] Zou Y, Hou X. Extraction Optimization, Composition Analysis, and Antioxidation Evaluation of Polysaccharides from White Jelly Mushroom, Tremella fuciformis (Tremellomycetes). *Int J Med Mushrooms*. 2017;19(12):1113-1121.

[4678] Gusman JK, Lin CY, Shih YC. The optimum submerged culture condition of the culinary-medicinal white jelly mushroom (Tremellomycetes) and its antioxidant properties. *Int J Med Mushrooms*. 2014;16(3):293-302.

[4679] Xu W, Shen X, Yang F, et al. Protective effect of polysaccharides isolated from Tremella fuciformis against radiation-induced damage in mice. *J Radiat Res*. 2012;53(3):353-60.

[4680] Xie L, Yang K, Liang Y, et al. Tremella fuciformis polysaccharides alleviate induced atopic dermatitis in mice by regulating immune response and gut microbiota. *Front Pharmacol*. 2022 Aug 25;13:944801.

[4681] Fu H, You S, Zhao D, et al. Tremella fuciformis polysaccharides inhibit UVA-induced photodamage of human dermal fibroblast cells by activating up-regulating Nrf2/Keap1 pathways. *J Cosmet Dermatol*. 2021 Dec;20(12):4052-4059.

[4682] Lin M, Bao C, Chen L, et al. Tremella fuciformis polysaccharides alleviates UV-provoked skin cell damage via regulation of thioredoxin interacting protein and thioredoxin reductase 2. *Photochem Photobiol Sci*. 2023 Oct;22(10):2285-2296.

[4683] Shen T, Duan C, Chen B, et al. Tremella fuciformis polysaccharide suppresses hydrogen peroxide-triggered injury of human skin fibroblasts via upregulation of SIRT1. *Mol Med Rep*. 2017 Aug;16(2):1340-1346.

[4684] Chiang JH, Tsai FJ, Lin TH, et al. Tremella fuciformis Inhibits Melanogenesis in B16F10 Cells and Promotes Migration of Human Fibroblasts and Keratinocytes. *In Vivo*. 2022 Mar-Apr;36(2):713-722.

[4685] Chiang JH, Tsai FJ, Lin TH, et al. Tremella fuciformis Inhibits Melanogenesis in B16F10 Cells and Promotes Migration of Human Fibroblasts and Keratinocytes. *In Vivo*. 2022 Mar-Apr;36(2):713-722.

[4686] Shin DI, Song KS, Park HS. Oral vaccination of mice with Tremella fuciformis yeast-like conidium cells expressing HBsAg. *Biotechnol Lett*. 2015 Mar;37(3):539-44.

[4687] Chen A, Pan F, Zhang T, et al. Characterization of chitin-glucan complex from Tremella fuciformis fermentation residue and evaluation of its antibacterial performance. *Int J Biol Macromol*. 2021 Sep 1;186:649-655.

[4688] Zhu H, Sun SJ. Inhibition of bacterial quorum sensing-regulated behaviors by Tremella fuciformis extract. *Curr Microbiol*. 2008 Nov;57(5):418-22.

[4689] Ban S, Lee SL, Jeong HS, et al. Efficacy and Safety of Tremella fuciformis in Individuals with Subjective Cognitive Impairment: A Randomized Controlled Trial. *J Med Food*. 2018 Apr;21(4):400-407.

[4690] Wu F, Yuan Y, Malysheva VF, et al. Species clarification of the most important and cultivated Auricularia mushroom "Heimuer": evidence from morphological and molecular data. *Phytotaxa*. 2014;186(5):241–253.

[4691] Wu F, Yuan Y, He S, et al. Global diversity and taxonomy of the Auricularia auricula-judae complex (Auriculariales, Basidiomycota). *Mycological Progress*. 2015;14(10).

[4692] Wu F, Tohtirjap A, Fan L, et al. Global diversity and updated phylogeny of Auricularia (Auriculariales, Basidiomycota). *J Fungi*. 2021;7(11):933.

[4693] Ping Z, Xu H, Liu T, et al. Anti-hepatoma activity of the stiff branched β-d-glucan and effects of molecular weight. *J Mater Chem B*. 2016 Jul 14;4(26):4565-4573.

[4694] Reza MA, Jo WS, Park SC. Comparative antitumor activity of wood ear culinary-medicinal mushroom, Auricularia auricula-judae (Bull.) J. Schrot. (higher basidiomycetes) extracts against tumor cells in vitro. *Int J Med Mushrooms*. 2012;14(4):403-9.

[4695] Reza MA, Hossain MA, Lee SJ, et al. Dichlormethane extract of the wood ear mushroom Auricularia auricula-judae (higher Basidiomycetes) inhibits tumor cell growth in vitro. *Int J Med Mushrooms*. 2014;16(1):37-47.

[4696] Reza MA, Jo WS, Park SC. Comparative antitumor activity of wood ear culinary-medicinal mushroom, Auricularia auricula-judae (Bull.) J. Schrot. (higher basidiomycetes) extracts against tumor cells in vitro. *Int J Med Mushrooms*. 2012;14(4):403-9.

[4697] Reza MA, Hossain MA, Lee SJ, et al. Dichlormethane extract of the wood ear mushroom Auricularia auricula-judae (higher Basidiomycetes) inhibits tumor cell growth in vitro. *Int J Med Mushrooms*. 2014;16(1):37-47.

[4698] Panthong S, Boonsathorn N, Chuchawankul S. Antioxidant activity, anti-proliferative activity, and amino acid profiles of ethanolic extracts of edible mushrooms. *Genet Mol Res*. 2016 Oct 17;15(4).

[4699] Shahar O, Pereman I, Khamisie H, et al. Compounds originating from the edible mushroom Auricularia auricula-judae inhibit tropomyosin receptor kinase B activity. *Heliyon*. 2023 Feb 16;9(3):e13756.

[4700] Reza MA, Jo WS, Park SC. Comparative antitumor activity of wood ear culinary-medicinal mushroom, Auricularia auricula-judae (Bull.) J. Schrot. (higher basidiomycetes) extracts against tumor cells in vitro. *Int J Med Mushrooms*. 2012;14(4):403-9.

[4701] Reza A, Choi MJ, Damte D, et al. Comparative Antitumor Activity of Different Solvent Fractions from an Auricularia auricula-judae Ethanol Extract in P388D1 and Sarcoma 180 Cells. *Toxicol Res*. 2011 Jun;27(2):77-83.

[4702] Misaki A, Kakuta M, Sasaki T, et al. Studies on interrelation of structure and antitumor effects of polysaccharides: antitumor action of periodate-modified, branched (1 goes to 3)-beta-D-glucan of Auricularia auricula-judae, and other polysaccharides containing (1 goes to 3)-glycosidic linkages. *Carbohydr Res*. 1981 May 18;92(1):115-29.

[4703] Reza A, Choi MJ, Damte D, et al. Comparative Antitumor Activity of Different Solvent Fractions from an Auricularia auricula-judae Ethanol Extract in P388D1 and Sarcoma 180 Cells. *Toxicol Res*. 2011 Jun;27(2):77-83.

4704 Zhou Y, Jia Y, Xu N, et al. Auricularia auricula-judae (Bull.) polysaccharides improve obesity in mice by regulating gut microbiota and TLR4/JNK signaling pathway. *Int J Biol Macromol*. 2023 Oct 1;250:126172

4705 Liu N, Chen M, Song J, et al. Effects of Auricularia auricula Polysaccharides on Gut Microbiota Composition in Type 2 Diabetic Mice. *Molecules*. 2022 Sep 16;27(18):6061.

4706 Zhou Y, Jia Y, Xu N, et al. Auricularia auricula-judae (Bull.) polysaccharides improve obesity in mice by regulating gut microbiota and TLR4/JNK signaling pathway. *Int J Biol Macromol*. 2023 Oct 1;250:126172

4707 Ohiri RC, Odey OP. Human Hemoglobin S Erythrocyte-Stabilizing and Antisickling Potential of Extract of Wood Ear Mushroom, Auricularia auricula (Agaricomycetes). *Int J Med Mushrooms*. 2022;24(3):25-34

4708 Zhou Y, Jia Y, Xu N, et al. Auricularia auricula-judae (Bull.) polysaccharides improve obesity in mice by regulating gut microbiota and TLR4/JNK signaling pathway. *Int J Biol Macromol*. 2023 Oct 1;250:126172

4709 Liu Q, Ma R, Li S, et al. Dietary Supplementation of Auricularia auricula-judae Polysaccharides Alleviate Nutritional Obesity in Mice via Regulating Inflammatory Response and Lipid Metabolism. *Foods*. 2022 Mar 24;11(7):942.

4710 Zong X, Zhang H, Zhu L, et al. Auricularia auricula polysaccharides attenuate obesity in mice through gut commensal Papillibacter cinnamivorans. *J Adv Res*. 2023 Oct;52:203-218.

4711 Takeujchi H, He P, Mooi LY. Reductive effect of hot-water extracts from woody ear (Auricularia auricula-judae Quel.) on food intake and blood glucose concentration in genetically diabetic KK-Ay mice. *J Nutr Sci Vitaminol (Tokyo)*. 2004 Aug;50(4):300-4.

4712 Xu N, Zhou Y, Lu X, et al. Auricularia auricula-judae (Bull.) polysaccharides improve type 2 diabetes in HFD/STZ-induced mice by regulating the AKT/AMPK signaling pathways and the gut microbiota. *J Food Sci*. 2021 Dec;86(12):5479-5494.

4713 Shen M, Fang Z, Chen Y, et al. Hypoglycemic Effect of the Degraded Polysaccharides from the Wood Ear Medicinal Mushroom Auricularia auricula-judae (Agaricomycetes). *Int J Med Mushrooms*. 2019;21(10):1033-1042.

4714 Yuan Z, He P, Cui J, et al. Hypoglycemic effect of water-soluble polysaccharide from Auricularia auricula-judae Quel. on genetically diabetic KK-Ay mice. *Biosci Biotechnol Biochem*. 1998 Oct;62(10):1898-903.

4715 Yuan Z, He P, Takeuchi H. Ameliorating effects of water-soluble polysaccharides from woody ear (Auricularia auricula-judae Quel.) in genetically diabetic KK-Ay mice. *J Nutr Sci Vitaminol (Tokyo)*. 1998 Dec;44(6):829-40.

4716 Liu N, Chen M, Song J, et al. Effects of Auricularia auricula Polysaccharides on Gut Microbiota Composition in Type 2 Diabetic Mice. *Molecules*. 2022 Sep 16;27(18):6061.

4717 Liu N, Chen X, Song J, et al. Hypoglycemic effects of Auricularia auricula polysaccharides on high fat diet and streptozotocin-induced diabetic mice using metabolomics analysis. *Food Funct*. 2021 Oct 19;12(20):9994-10007.

4718 Takeujchi H, He P, Mooi LY. Reductive effect of hot-water extracts from woody ear (Auricularia auricula-judae Quel.) on food intake and blood glucose concentration in genetically diabetic KK-Ay mice. *J Nutr Sci Vitaminol (Tokyo)*. 2004 Aug;50(4):300-4.

4719 Jeong H, Yang BK, Jeong YT, et al. Hypolipidemic Effects of Biopolymers Extracted from Culture Broth, Mycelia, and Fruiting Bodies of Auricularia auricula-judae in Dietary-induced Hyperlipidemic Rats. *Mycobiology*. 2007 Mar;35(1):16-20.

4720 Reza MA, Hossain MA, Damte D, et al. Hypolipidemic and Hepatic Steatosis Preventing Activities of the Wood Ear Medicinal Mushroom Auricularia auricula-judae (Higher Basidiomycetes) Ethanol Extract In Vivo and In Vitro. *Int J Med Mushrooms*. 2015;17(8):723-34.

4721 Xiao B, Chen S, Huang Q, et al. The lipid lowering and antioxidative stress potential of polysaccharide from Auricularia auricula prepared by enzymatic method. *Int J Biol Macromol*. 2021 Sep 30;187:651-663.

4722 Zhang Y, Li X, Yang Q, et al. Antioxidation, anti-hyperlipidaemia and hepatoprotection of polysaccharides from Auricularia auricular residue. *Chem Biol Interact*. 2021 Jan 5;333:109323.

4723 Zhang Y, Li X, Yang Q, et al. Antioxidation, anti-hyperlipidaemia and hepatoprotection of polysaccharides from Auricularia auricular residue. *Chem Biol Interact*. 2021 Jan 5;333:109323.

4724 Reza MA, Hossain MA, Damte D, et al. Hypolipidemic and Hepatic Steatosis Preventing Activities of the Wood Ear Medicinal Mushroom Auricularia auricula-judae (Higher Basidiomycetes) Ethanol Extract In Vivo and In Vitro. *Int J Med Mushrooms*. 2015;17(8):723-34.

4725 Shu Y, Huang Y, Dong W, et al. The polysaccharides from Auricularia auricula alleviate non-alcoholic fatty liver disease via modulating gut microbiota and bile acids metabolism. *Int J Biol Macromol*. 2023 Aug 15;246:125662.

4726 Yu X, Wang R, Lai B, et al. Effect of Auricularia auricula fermentation broth on the liver and stomach of mice with acute alcoholism. *Food Funct*. 2021 Jan 7;12(1):191-202.

4727 Chen Y, Xu M, Wang X, et al. Preparation of Wood Ear Medicinal Mushroom, Auricularia auricula-judae (Agaricomycetes), Melanin and Its Antioxidant Properties: Evaluation In Vitro and In Vivo. *Int J Med Mushrooms*. 2021;23(6):89-100.

4728 Han Q, Li H, Zhao F, et al. Auricularia auricula Peptides Nutritional Supplementation Delays H2O2-Induced Senescence of HepG2 Cells by Modulation of MAPK/NF-κB Signaling Pathways. *Nutrients*. 2023 Aug 25;15(17):3731.

4729 Zhang Y, Shi Q, Jiang W, et al. Comparison of the chemical composition and antioxidant stress ability of polysaccharides from Auricularia auricula under different drying methods. *Food Funct*. 2022 Mar 7;13(5):2938-2951.

4730 Damte D, Reza MA, Lee SJ, et al. Anti-inflammatory Activity of Dichloromethane Extract of Auricularia auricula-judae in RAW264.7 Cells. *Toxicol Res*. 2011 Mar;27(1):11-4.

4731 Ukai S, Kiho T, Hara C, et al. Polysaccharides in fungi. XIV. Anti-inflammatory effect of the polysaccharides from the fruit bodies of several fungi. *J Pharmacobiodyn*. 1983 Dec;6(12):983-90.

4732 Zhang Y, Zeng Y, Men Y, et al. Structural characterization and immunomodulatory activity of exopolysaccharides from submerged culture of Auricularia auricula-judae. *Int J Biol Macromol*. 2018 Aug;115:978-984.

4733 Perera N, Yang FL, Chiu HW, et al. Phagocytosis enhancement, endotoxin tolerance, and signal mechanisms of immunologically active glucuronoxylomannan from Auricularia auricula-judae. *Int J Biol Macromol*. 2020 Dec 15;165(Pt A):495-505.

4734 Ibe V, Ihim SA, Ikegbunam M, et al. Influence of Nigerian Wood Ear Culinary-Medicinal Mushroom, Auricularia auricula-judae (Agaricomycetes), on Humoral and Cellular Immunity. *Int J Med Mushrooms*. 2020;22(5):467-478.

[4735] Perera N, Yang FL, Chern J, et al. Carboxylic and O-acetyl moieties are essential for the immunostimulatory activity of glucuronoxylomannan: a novel TLR4 specific immunostimulator from Auricularia auricula-judae. *Chem Commun (Camb)*. 2018 Jun 21;54(51):6995-6998.

[4736] Jeong SC, Cho SP, Yang BK, et al. Production of an anti-complement exo-polymer produced by Auricularia auricula-judae in submerged culture. *Biotechnol Lett*. 2004 Jun;26(11):923-7.

[4737] Bian C, Wang Z, Shi J. Extraction Optimization, Structural Characterization, and Anticoagulant Activity of Acidic Polysaccharides from Auricularia auricula-judae. *Molecules*. 2020 Feb 6;25(3):710.

[4738] Chen Y, Xu M, Wang X, et al. Preparation of Wood Ear Medicinal Mushroom, Auricularia auricula-judae (Agaricomycetes), Melanin and Its Antioxidant Properties: Evaluation In Vitro and In Vivo. *Int J Med Mushrooms*. 2021;23(6):89-100.

[4739] Xiao B, Chen S, Huang Q, et al. Preparation of Wood Ear Mushroom, Auricularia auricula-judae (Agaricomycetes), Polysaccharides by Neutral Protease and Their Antioxidant Stress Capacity. *Int J Med Mushrooms*. 2021;23(5):41-53.

[4740] Dai Y, Ma Y, Liu X, et al. Formation Optimization, Characterization and Antioxidant Activity of Auricularia auricula-judae Polysaccharide Nanoparticles Obtained via Antisolvent Precipitation. *Molecules*. 2022 Oct 18;27(20):7037.

[4741] Kho YS, Vikineswary S, Abdullah N, et al. Antioxidant capacity of fresh and processed fruit bodies and mycelium of Auricularia auricula-judae (Fr.) Quél. *J Med Food*. 2009 Feb;12(1):167-74.

[4742] Ma YP, Bao YH, Kong XH, et al. Optimization of Melanin Extraction from the Wood Ear Medicinal Mushroom, Auricularia auricula-judae (Agaricomycetes), by Response Surface Methodology and Its Antioxidant Activities In Vitro. *Int J Med Mushrooms*. 2018;20(11):1087-1095.

[4743] Choi YJ, Park IS, Kim MH, et al. The medicinal mushroom Auricularia auricula-judae (Bull.) extract has antioxidant activity and promotes procollagen biosynthesis in HaCaT cells. *Nat Prod Res*. 2019 Nov;33(22):3283-3286.

[4744] Cai M, Lin Y, Luo YL, et al. Extraction, Antimicrobial, and Antioxidant Activities of Crude Polysaccharides from the Wood Ear Medicinal Mushroom Auricularia auricula-judae (Higher Basidiomycetes). *Int J Med Mushrooms*. 2015;17(6):591-600.

[4745] Shi Q, Yang Z, Fan R, et al. Isolation, Characterization, and Antioxidant Activity of Melanin from Auricularia auricula (Agaricomycetes). *Int J Med Mushrooms*. 2023;25(6):55-73.

[4746] Xiao B, Huang Q, Chen S, et al. Comparison on chemical features and antioxidant activity of polysaccharides from Auricularia auricula by three different enzymes. *J Food Biochem*. 2022 May;46(5):e14051.

[4747] Zhang Y, Shi Q, Jiang W, et al. Comparison of the chemical composition and antioxidant stress ability of polysaccharides from Auricularia auricula under different drying methods. *Food Funct*. 2022 Mar 7;13(5):2938-2951.

[4748] Yin CM, Yao F, Wu W, et al. Physicochemical Properties and Antioxidant Activity of Natural Melanin Extracted from the Wild Wood Ear Mushroom, Auricularia auricula (Agaricomycetes). *Int J Med Mushrooms*. 2022;24(1):67-82.

[4749] Huang Q, Xiao B, Chen S, et al. Effect of Enzyme-Assisted Extraction on the Chemical Properties and Antioxidant Activities of Polysaccharides Obtained from the Wood Ear Mushroom, Auricularia auricula (Agaricomycetes). *Int J Med Mushrooms*. 2022;24(2):49-62.

[4750] Yao J, Zeng JY, Tang YX, et al. Effects of the Extraction Solvents on Dissolution Rate and Antioxidant Capacity of Auricularia auricula (Agaricomycetes) Polysaccharides In Vitro and In Vivo. *Int J Med Mushrooms*. 2023;25(5):61-74.

[4751] Panthong S, Boonsathorn N, Chuchawankul S. Antioxidant activity, anti-proliferative activity, and amino acid profiles of ethanolic extracts of edible mushrooms. *Genet Mol Res*. 2016 Oct 17;15(4).

[4752] Zhang Y, Li X, Yang Q, et al. Antioxidation, anti-hyperlipidaemia and hepatoprotection of polysaccharides from Auricularia auricular residue. *Chem Biol Interact*. 2021 Jan 5;333:109323.

[4753] Mapoung S, Umsumarng S, Semmarath W, et al. Skin Wound-Healing Potential of Polysaccharides from Medicinal Mushroom Auricularia auricula-judae (Bull.). *J Fungi (Basel)*. 2021 Mar 25;7(4):247.

[4754] Choi YJ, Park IS, Kim MH, et al. The medicinal mushroom Auricularia auricula-judae (Bull.) extract has antioxidant activity and promotes procollagen biosynthesis in HaCaT cells. *Nat Prod Res*. 2019 Nov;33(22):3283-3286.

[4755] Oli AN, Edeh PA, Al-Mosawi RM, et al. Evaluation of the phytoconstituents of Auricularia auricula-judae mushroom and antimicrobial activity of its protein extract. *Eur J Integr Med*. 2020 Sep;38:101176.

[4756] Cai M, Lin Y, Luo YL, et al. Extraction, Antimicrobial, and Antioxidant Activities of Crude Polysaccharides from the Wood Ear Medicinal Mushroom Auricularia auricula-judae (Higher Basidiomycetes). *Int J Med Mushrooms*. 2015;17(6):591-600.

INDEX

A

Agaricus blazei
   see almond mushroom
Agaricus brasiliensis
   see almond mushroom
Agaricus fiardii
   see almond mushroom
Agaricus rufotegulis
   see almond mushroom
Agaricus subrufescens, 21
agarikon mushroom, 17-19, 188
almond mushroom, 21-29, 189
Amanita bisporigera, 187, 188
Amanita muscaria, 11, 187, 188
Amanita phalloides, 187, 188
Antrodia camphorata, 141
Antrodia cinnamonea
   see Antrodia camphorata
Armillaria mellea, 13, 55
Auricularia auricula-judae, 159

B

Brazilian mushroom
   see almond mushroom

C

chaga mushroom, 31-35, 189
Chlorophyllum molybdites, 187, 188
cordyceps mushroom, 37-48, 189
Cordyceps militaris, 37
Cordyceps sinensis, 37
Coriolus versicolor
   see Trametes versicolor

D

death caps, 187, 188
destroying angel, 187, 188

E

enoki mushroom, 49-53, 189

F

false parasol, 187, 188
Flammulina velutipes, 49
fly agaric, 11, 187, 188
Fomitopsis officinalis
   see Laricifomes officinalis
French horn mushroom
   see king oyster mushroom

G

Ganoderma lucidum, 119

H

hen of the woods mushroom
   see maitake mushroom
Hericium erinaceus, 65
honey mushroom/fungus, 55-58, 189

I

Inonotus obliquus, 31

K

king oyster mushroom, 59-63, 190
king trumpet mushroom
   see king oyster mushroom

L

Laricifomes officinalis, 17
Lentinula edodes, 133
lion's mane mushroom, 65-70, 190

M

magic mushroom
   see psilocybe mushroom
maitake mushroom, 71-76, 190
mesima mushroom, 77-82, 190
militaris mushroom
   see Cordyceps militaris
military cordyceps
   see Cordyceps militaris
monkey head mushroom
   see lion's mane mushroom
mushroom of the sun
   see almond mushroom

N

Niu-Chang-Chih
see stout camphor mushroom

O

Orphiocordyceps sinensis
see Cordyceps sinensis
oyster mushroom, 83-89, 190

P

Pachyma cocos
see poria mushroom
Phellinus linteus, 77
pink oyster mushroom, 91-93, 190
Pleurotus djamor, 91
Pleurotus eryngii, 59
Pleurotus ostreatus, 83
Polyporous versicolor
see Trametes versicolor
pom pom blanc
see lion's mane mushroom
poria mushroom, 95-101, 191
Psilocybe azurescens
see psilocybe mushroom
Psilocybe bohemica
see psilocybe mushroom
Psilocybe cubensis
see psilocybe mushroom
Psilocybe cyanescens
see psilocybe mushroom
Psilocybe haeocystitis
see psilocybe mushroom
Psilocybe hoogshagenii
see psilocybe mushroom
psilocybe mushroom,103-118, 191
Psilocybe semilanceata
see psilocybe mushroom
Psilocybe serbica
see psilocybe mushroom
Psilocybe spp.
see psilocybe mushroom
Psilocybe tampanensis
see psilocybe mushroom

Psilocybe weilii
see psilocybe mushroom
psilocybin, 103-118
psilocin, 103-118

R

reishi mushroom, 119-131, 191
royal sun mushroom
see almond mushroom

S

shiitake mushroom, 133-139, 191
stout camphor mushroom, 141-145, 191

T

Taiwanofungus camphoratus
see Antrodia camphorata
Trametes versicolor, 147
Tremella fuciformis, 155
turkey tail mushroom, 147-153, 191

W

white jelly mushroom, 155-158, 192
wood ear mushroom, 159-162, 192
Wolfiporia extensa, 95
Wolfporia cocous
see poria mushroom

Y

yamabushitake mushroom
see lion's mane mushroom

www.ingramcontent.com/pod-product-compliance
Lightning Source LLC
Chambersburg PA
CBHW080227270326
41926CB00020B/4172